MW00749411

Atlas of INFECTIOUS DISEASES

Volume III

CENTRAL NERVOUS SYSTEM AND EYE INFECTIONS

Atlas of INFECTIOUS DISEASES

Volume III

Central Nervous System and Eye Infections

Editor-in-Chief

Gerald L. Mandell, MD

Professor of Medicine
Owen R. Cheatham Professor of the Sciences
Chief, Division of Infectious Diseases
University of Virginia Health Sciences Center
Charlottesville, Virginia, USA

Editor

Thomas P. Bleck, MD

Associate Professor of Neurology and Neurological Surgery
The John T. and Louise Nerancy Chairholder in Neurology
Division of Critical Care, Department of Neurology
University of Virginia Health Sciences Center
Charlottesville, Virginia, USA

Churchill Livingstone

Developed by Current Medicine, Inc.
Philadelphia

CURRENT MEDICINE
400 MARKET STREET, SUITE 700
PHILADELPHIA, PA 19106

Library of Congress Cataloging-in-Publication Data

Central nervous system and eye infections/editor-in-chief, Gerald L. Mandell;
editor, Thomas P. Bleck.
p. cm.–(Atlas of infectious diseases; v. 3)
Includes bibliographical references and index.
ISBN 0-443-07700-2 (hardcover)
1. Central nervous system–Infections–Atlases. 2. Eye–Infections–Atlases.
I. Mandell, Gerald L. II. Bleck, Thomas P., 1951- . III. Series
[DNLM: 1. Central Nervous System Diseases–diagnosis–atlases
2. Central Nervous System Diseases–microbiology–atlases. 3. Eye
Infections–diagnosis–atlases. WL 17 C397 1995]
RC359.5.C46 1995
616.8–dc20
DNLM/DLC
for Library of Congress 94-41262
CIP

Managing Editor: ....**Lori J. Bainbridge**
Development Editor: ....**Elizabeth Howard**
Editorial Assistant: ....**Jabin White**
Art Director: ....**Paul Fennessy**
Design and Layout: ....**Patrick Whelan and Jerilyn Bockorick**
Illustration Director: ....**Ann Saydlowski**
Illustrators: ....**Liz Carrozza, Wiesia Langenfeld, Ann Saydlowski, Rick Ward, and Gary Welch**
Production: ....**David Myers and Wendy Feinstein**
Typesetting Director: ....**Colleen Ward**

Printed in Hong Kong by Paramount Printing Group Limited.

10 9 8 7 6 5 4 3 2 1

Preface

The diagnosis and management of patients with infectious diseases are based in large part on visual clues. Skin and mucous membrane lesions, eye findings, imaging studies, Gram stains, culture plates, insect vectors, preparations of blood, urine, pus, cerebrospinal fluid, and biopsy specimens are studied to establish the proper diagnosis and to choose the most effective therapy. The Atlas of Infectious Diseases is a modern, complete collection of these images. Current Medicine, with its capability of superb color reproduction and its state-of-the-art computer imaging facilities, is the ideal publisher for the atlas. Infectious diseases physicians, scientists, microbiologists, and pathologists frequently teach other healthcare professionals, and this comprehensive atlas with available slides is an effective teaching tool.

Dr. Thomas Bleck, the volume editor, is uniquely suited to cover this subject. He is an expert in both neurology and infectious diseases. He and his contributors have assembled a remarkable collection of images to aid in our understanding and management of central nervous system and eye infections.

Gerald L. Mandell, MD
Professor of Medicine
Owen R. Cheatham Professor of the Sciences
Chief, Division of Infectious Diseases
University of Virginia Health Sciences Center
Charlottesville, Virginia

CONTRIBUTORS

Sebastian R. Alston, MD
Assistant Professor of Pathology (Neuropathology)
Department of Pathology
University of Virginia Health Sciences Center
Charlottesville, Virginia, USA

Joseph R. Berger, MD, FACP
Professor and Chairman
Department of Neurology
University of Kentucky
Lexington, Kentucky, USA

Thomas P. Bleck, MD
Associate Professor of Neurology and Neurological Surgery
The John T. and Louise Nerancy Chairholder in Neurology
Division of Critical Care, Department of Neurology
University of Virginia Health Sciences Center
Charlottesville, Virginia, USA

Jose M. Bonnin, MD
Neuropathologist
Methodist Hospital of Indiana
Indianapolis, Indiana, USA

David G. Brock, MD
Instructor in Neurology
Department of Neurology
University of Virginia Health Sciences Center
Charlottesville, Virginia, USA

Sidney E. Croul, MD
Assistant Professor of Pathology
Medical College of Pennsylvania and Hahnemann University School of Medicine
Philadelphia, Pennsylvania, USA

Thomas A. Deutsch, MD
Program Director of Ophthalmology
Professor, Rush Medical College
Chicago, Illinois, USA

Jonathan D. Glass, MD
Assistant Professor of Neurology
Department of Neurology
Johns Hopkins University School of Medicine
Baltimore, Maryland, USA

Daniel F. Hanley, MD
Director of Neurosciences Critical Care Unit
Professor, Departments of Neurology, Neurosurgery and Anesthesiology/Critical Care Medicine
Johns Hopkins University School of Medicine
Baltimore, Maryland, USA

Richard T. Johnson, MD
Chairman, Department of Neurology
Johns Hopkins University School of Medicine
Baltimore, Maryland, USA

Justin C. McArthur, MBBS
Assistant Professor of Neurology
Department of Neurology
Johns Hopkins University School of Medicine
Baltimore, Maryland, USA

Hans-Walter Pfister, MD
Department of Neurology
Klinikum Grosshadern
Ludwig-Maximilians-University of Munich
Munich, Germany

David A. Ramsay, MB, ChB, DPhil, FRCPC
Assistant Professor
Departments of Pathology and Clinical Neurological Sciences
University of Western Ontario
London, Ontario, Canada

Karen L. Roos, MD
Associate Professor of Neurology
Indiana University School of Medicine
Indianapolis, Indiana, USA

Oren Sagher, MD
Assistant Professor of Neurosurgery
University of Michigan
Chief of Neurosurgery
Ann Arbor Veterans Administration Hospital
Ann Arbor, Michigan, USA

Allan R. Tunkel, MD, PhD
Associate Professor of Medicine
Medical College of Pennsylvania and Hahnemann University School of Medicine
Philadelphia, Pennsylvania, USA

Eberhard Wilmes, MD
Department of ENT and Head and Neck Surgery
Klinikum Grosshadern
Ludwig-Maximilians-University of Munich
Munich, Germany

Brian Wispelwey, MD
Associate Professor of Medicine
Director, Infectious Diseases Clinic
University of Virginia Health Sciences Center
Charlottesville, Virginia, USA

G. Bryan Young, MD, FRCPC
Associate Professor
Department of Clinical Neurological Sciences
University of Western Ontario
London, Ontario, Canada

CONTENTS

CHAPTER 1

Acute Bacterial Meningitides

Karen L. Roos
Jose M. Bonnin

Etiology and Epidemiology

Common meningeal pathogens by age group	
Neonates	Group B streptococci
	Escherichia coli
Children	*Haemophilus influenzae* type b
	Neisseria meningitidis
	Streptococcus pneumoniae
Adults	*S. pneumoniae*
	Neisseria meningitidis
Older adults (> 50 yrs)	*S. pneumoniae*
	Enteric gram-negative bacilli
	Haemophilus influenzae
	Listeria monocytogenes

Figure 1-1 Common meningeal pathogens by age group. The choice of empiric antimicrobial therapy for bacterial meningitis should be based on the most likely meningeal pathogen, which depends on the patient's age and associated conditions increasing the risk for bacterial infections.

Epidemiologic features of *Haemophilus influenzae* meningitis
Causes 40%–50% of cases in US
Capsular type b involved in > 90% of serious infections
Concurrent pharyngitis or otitis media in > 50% of cases
Suspected nasopharyngeal acquisition of bacteria
Usually occurs in children < 6 years of age
Disease in persons > 6 years of age is associated with:
Chronic parameningeal infection (sinusitis or mastoiditis)
Pneumonia
Sickle cell disease
Splenectomy
Diabetes mellitus
Immune deficiency (hypogammaglobulinemia)
Head trauma with CSF leak
Alcoholism

Figure 1-2 Epidemiologic features of *Haemophilus influenzae* meningitis. *H. influenzae* type b is the most common etiologic agent of bacterial meningitis in childhood. Most cases occur between 4 months and 2 years of age. Its incidence has declined since the availability of the first Hib conjugate vaccine in 1987 for routine use in children. *H. influenzae* is an important etiologic organism of bacterial meningitis also in the elderly and in individuals with immunoglobulin or complement deficiencies, alcoholism, sickle cell anemia, splenectomy, chronic pulmonary infections, diabetes mellitus, chronic sinusitis or mastoiditis, and cerebrospinal fluid (CSF) fistulas.

A. Epidemiologic features of meningococcal meningitis
Affects mostly children and young adults
Epidemics usually due to serogroups A and C
Nasopharyngeal acquisition of infection
Congenital late complement component (C5–C8, and perhaps C9) deficiency predisposes to meningococcemia

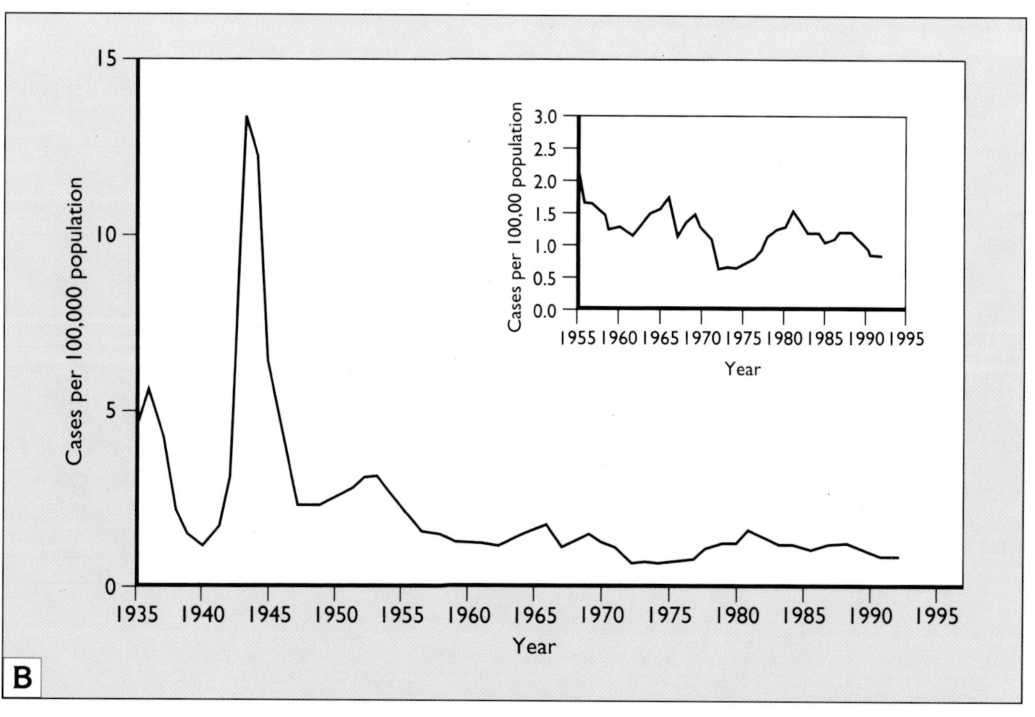

Figure 1-3 Epidemiologic features of meningococcal meningitis. **A**, Meningococcal meningitis, caused by *Neisseria meningitidis*, is primarily a disease of children and young adults. Invasive disease follows nasopharyngeal colonization by the organism. As with colonization, the age-specific incidence of meningococcal meningitis is inversely proportional to the concentration of serum anticapsular antibodies. Congenital deficiency of the terminal complement components (C5, C6, C7, C8, and perhaps C9) predisposes to meningococcemia. Large-scale epidemics of meningococcal meningitis in the "meningitis belt" of sub-Saharan Africa are associated with a "shift to the right," toward an older age group of infected individuals. **B**, Incidence of meningococcal infection, by year, United States, 1935–1992. Meningococcal meningitis tends to occur in epidemics. (*Panel B from* CDC: Summary of notifiable diseases, United States, 1992, *MMWR* 1992, 41(55):41.)

Epidemiologic features of pneumococcal meningitis
Most common etiologic organism of meningitis in adults in US
Mortality of 19%–30%
Associated with other suppurative foci of infection:
Pneumonia (25%)
Otitis media or mastoiditis (30%)
Sinusitis (10%–15%)
Endocarditis (< 5%)
Head trauma (10%)

FIGURE 1-4 Epidemiologic features of pneumococcal meningitis. *Streptococcus pneumoniae* is the most common cause of bacterial meningitis in adults. Like *Haemophilus influenzae* and *Neisseria meningitidis* meningitis, pneumococcal meningitis follows nasopharyngeal colonization by the organism. Of the factors that predispose an individual to pneumococcal meningitis, pneumonia and acute otitis media are the most important. Pneumococci are the most common cause of recurrent meningitis in the setting of head trauma with a chronic CSF fistula.

Epidemiologic features of group B streptococcal meningitis
Important etiologic organism in neonates
(approx 1–3 cases/1000 births/y in US)
Two presentations in the neonate
1. Early-onset septicemia—associated with:
Prematurity
Premature rupture of membranes
Low birth weight < 2.5 kg
2. Late-onset meningitis (> 7 days after birth)

FIGURE 1-5 Epidemiologic features of group B streptococcal meningitis. Neonatal group B streptococcal meningitis is divided into two types: early-onset disease associated with premature birth, prolonged rupture of membranes, or low birth weight (< 2.5 kg); and late onset disease (> 7 days after birth). In early-onset meningitis, the organism is acquired from the maternal genital tract during delivery, and in late-onset disease the organism is most likely acquired by nosocomial transmission from other colonized infants or nursery personnel.

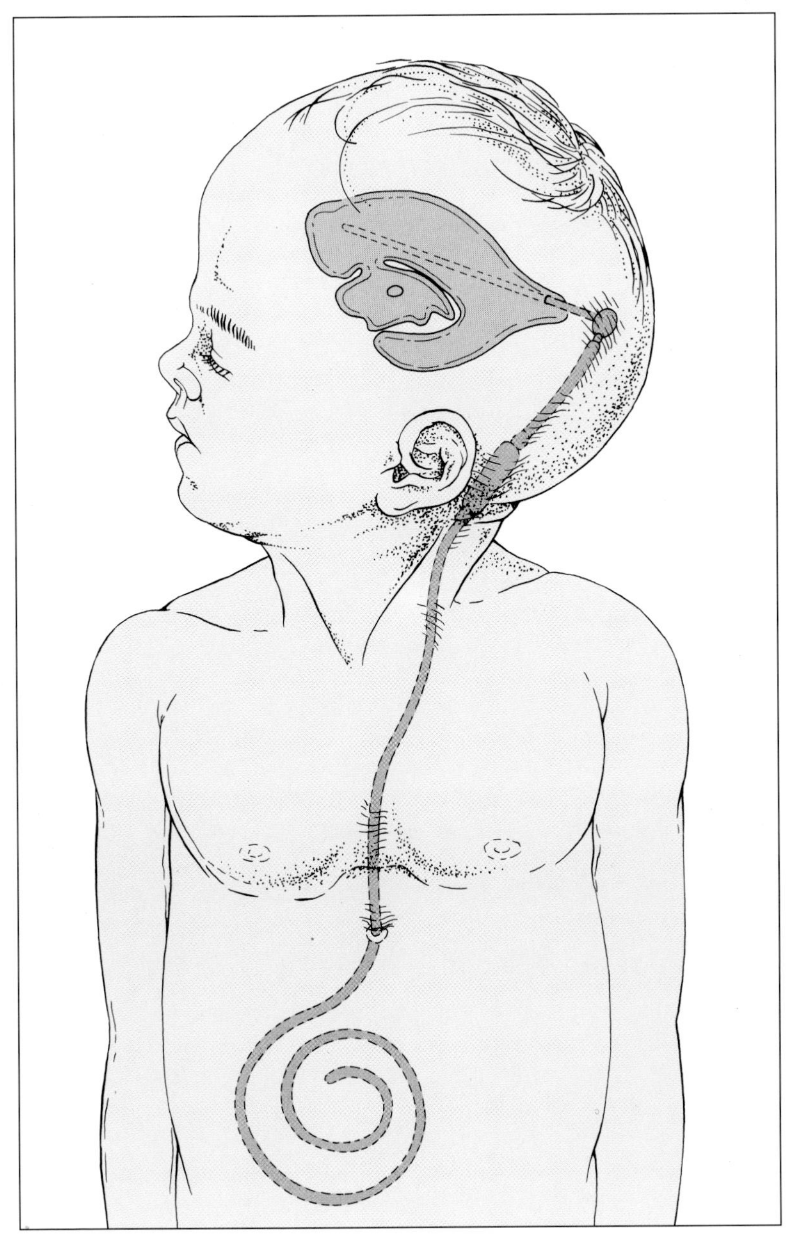

FIGURE 1-6 A ventriculoperitoneal shunt is inserted into a lateral ventricle and drains CSF into the abdominal cavity. The most common organisms infecting these shunts are coagulase-negative staphylococci and *Staphylococcus aureus*. In general, the most common etiologic organisms of bacterial meningitis complicating neurosurgical procedures are gram-negative bacilli, *S. aureus*, and *Pseudomonas aeruginosa*.

Pathogenesis

Pathogenesis of meningitis
1. Nasopharyngeal acquisition and mucosal colonization 2. Bloodstream invasion and survival 3. Bacterial entry into CSF 4. Multiplication within the CSF 5. Subarachnoid space inflammation 6. Increased blood-brain barrier permeability and vasogenic, cytotoxic, and interstitial edema 7. Increased intracranial pressure

Figure 1-7 Pathogenesis of meningitis. The neurologic manifestations and complications of bacterial meningitis develop following a series of steps that is initiated by nasopharyngeal colonization by the meningeal pathogen. The eventual development of increased intracranial pressure and the associated neurologic complications is the result of bacterial replication and lysis in the subarachnoid space, the recruitment of inflammatory cells with the production of a purulent exudate, and an increase in the permeability of the blood-brain barrier. Interstitial edema develops as a result of obstruction of flow of CSF by the purulent exudate in the subarachnoid space. Vasogenic cerebral edema is primarily a result of the increased blood-brain barrier permeability. The factors contributing to the development of cytotoxic cerebral edema are less well understood, but cytotoxic edema is most likely the result of release of toxic oxygen metabolites from neutrophils with subsequent swelling of the cellular elements of the brain.

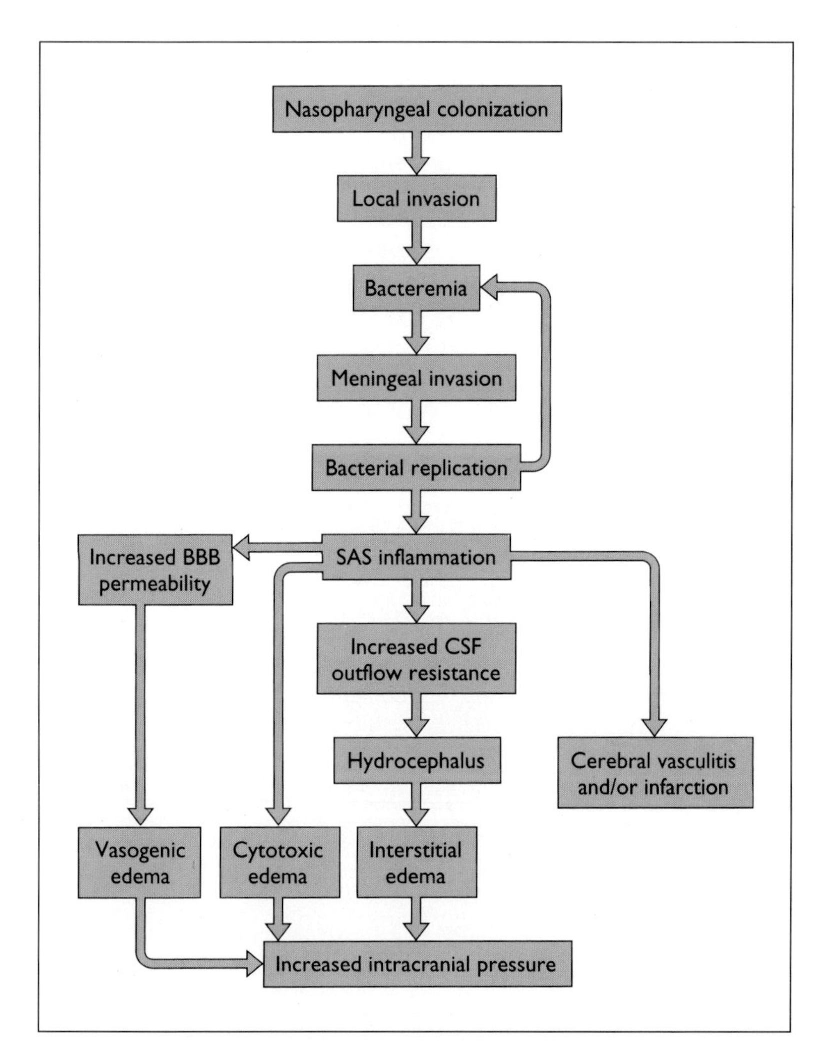

Figure 1-8 Scheme of pathogenic and pathophysiologic mechanisms in bacterial meningitis. BBB—blood–brain barrier; SAS—subarachnoid space. (*From* Roos KL, Tunkel AR, Scheld WM: Acute bacterial meningitis in children and adults. In Scheld WM, Whitley RJ, Durack DT (eds.): *Infections of the Central Nervous System.* New York: Raven Press; 1991:335–410; with permission.)

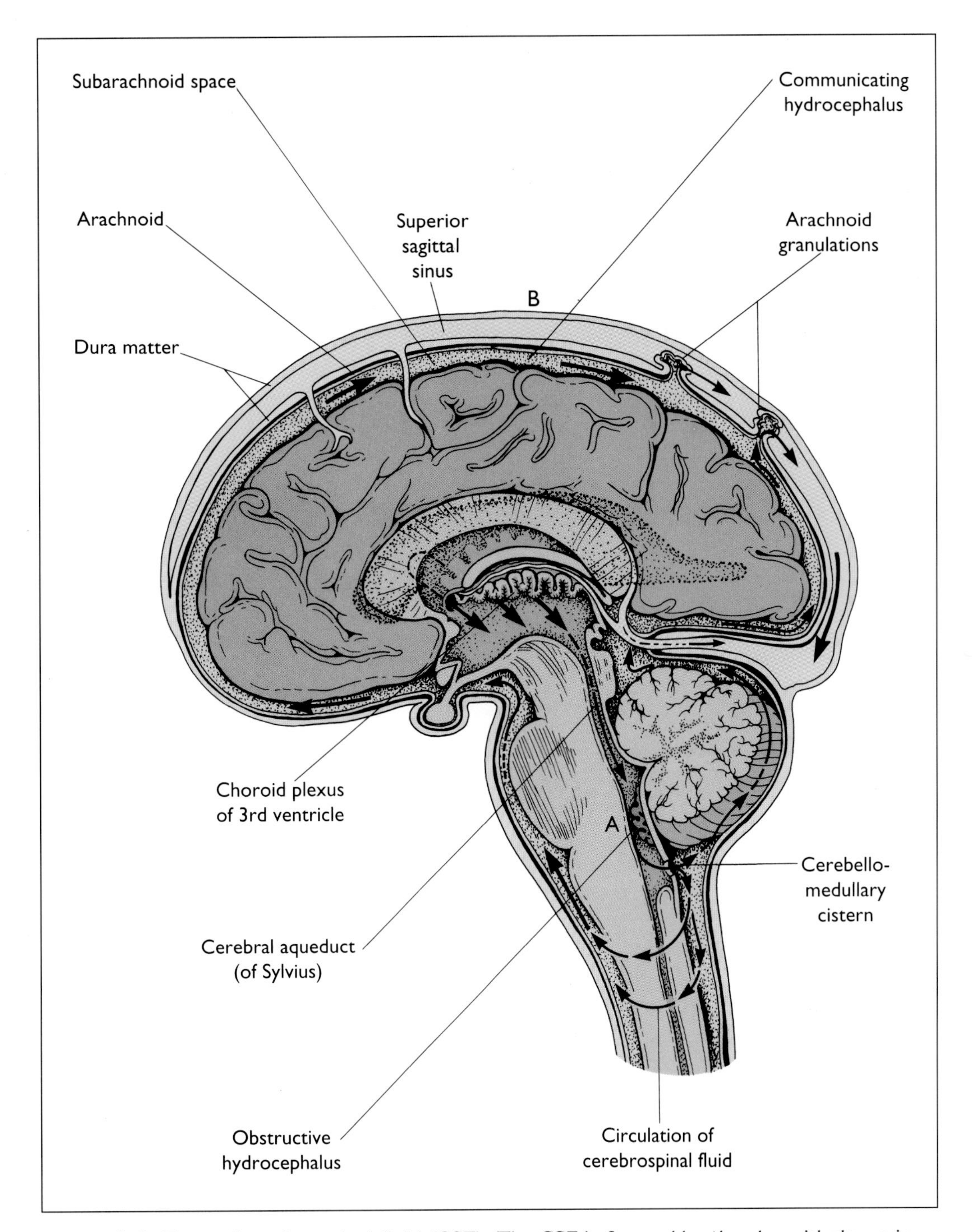

FIGURE 1-9 Flow of cerebrospinal fluid (CSF). The CSF is formed by the choroid plexus in the lateral and third ventricles and flows through the cerebral aqueduct into the fourth ventricle. The CSF leaves the fourth ventricle through the foramina of Luschka and Magendie and flows into the subarachnoid space at the base of the brain. From there, CSF flows up over the convexity of the hemispheres to be resorbed by the arachnoid villi in the venous sinuses. The accumulation of a purulent exudate in the subarachnoid space at the base of the brain (*A*) blocks the outflow of CSF through the foramina of Luschka and Magendie, resulting in obstructive hydrocephalus. The accumulation of purulent exudate in other areas of the subarachnoid space (*B*) obstructs the resorption of CSF by the arachnoid villi, resulting in a communicating hydrocephalus. The end result of obstruction to the flow and resorption of CSF through the normal pathways is interstitial edema.

CLINICAL MANIFESTATIONS

Frequency of symptoms and signs in bacterial meningitis

Findings	Relative frequency, %
Headache	≥ 90
Fever	≥ 90
Meningismus	≥ 85
Brudzinski's sign	≥ 50
Kernig's sign	≥ 50
Altered sensorium	> 80
Vomiting	~ 35
Seizures	~ 30
Petechiae	~ 50
Focal findings	10–20
Cranial nerves	~ 10
Hemiparesis	< 5
Papilledema	< 1
Myalgia	30–60
Other suppurative foci (pneumonia, otitis, sinusitis, etc.)	0–30

FIGURE 1-10 Frequency of symptoms and signs in bacterial meningitis. The classic presentation of bacterial meningitis in an adult is headache, fever, an altered level of consciousness, and a meningeal sign (meningismus, Brudzinski's sign, or Kernig's sign). (*From* Tunkel AR, Scheld WM: Acute meningitis. *In* Stein JH (ed.): *Internal Medicine*, 4th ed. St. Louis: Mosby; 1994:1890; with permission.)

Clinical signs of acute bacterial meningitis

Infants (≤ 2 years)	Children and adults
Fever	Fever
Lethargy, irritability	Headache
Apnea	Nuchal rigidity
Poor feeding	Lethargy, stupor, coma
Seizures	Nausea and vomiting
Bulging fontanel	Photophobia
	Ataxia (in children)
	Seizures

FIGURE 1-11 Clinical signs and symptoms of acute bacterial meningitis. The clinical presentation of bacterial meningitis in infants is nonspecific and typical of sepsis. The clinical presentation of bacterial meningitis in children and adults consists of the classic triad of fever, headache, and nuchal rigidity. The illness can progress rapidly, within minutes to hours, and demands rapid diagnosis and therapeutic intervention.

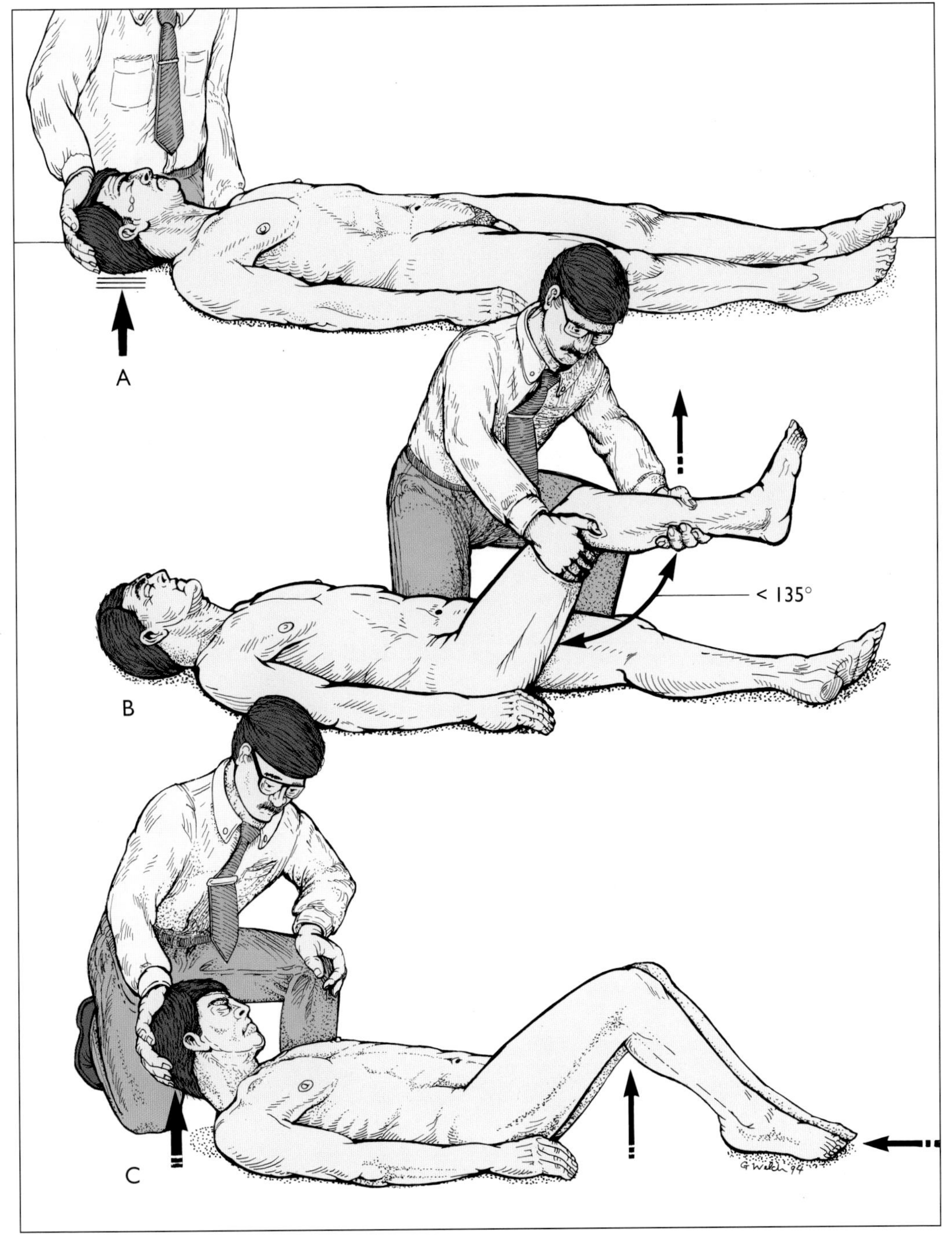

Figure 1-12 Classic signs of meningeal irritation. The classic signs of meningeal irritation are nuchal rigidity, Kernig's sign, and Brudzinski's sign. **A**, Nuchal rigidity is present as resistance to passive flexion of the neck. **B**, Kernig's sign is elicited by flexing the thigh and knee while the patient is in the supine position; in the presence of meningeal inflammation, there is resistance to passive extension of the leg at the knee. **C**, Brudzinski's sign is positive when passive flexion of the neck causes flexion of the hips and knees.

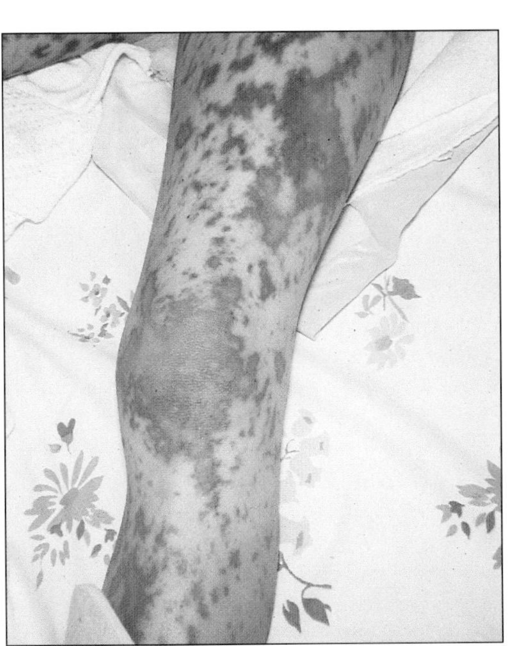

Figure 1-13 Meningococcemial rash. The initial rash of meningococcemia is often characterized by discrete, round, erythematous macules. Petechiae can be found in the skin, mucous membranes, and conjunctivae, but the nailbeds are spared. As the rash evolves, petechial and/or purpuric lesions are most pronounced on the trunk and lower extremities. (Feigin RD, McCracken GH, Klein JO: Diagnosis and management of meningitis. *Pediatr Infect Dis J* 1992, 11:785–814.)

NEUROLOGIC FINDINGS

Seizures

Pathogenesis of seizures in bacterial meningitis
Fever
Focal ischemia
Hyponatremia
Intracranial mass lesion (abscess, subdural effusion, empyema)
Antimicrobial agents

FIGURE 1-14 Pathogenesis of seizures. Seizures occur in 29% to 40% of children and adults with bacterial meningitis, usually within the first few days of illness. Generalized seizures may be due to fever or to a metabolic (hyponatremia) or toxic encephalopathy (due to antimicrobial therapy). Focal seizures may develop as a complication of arterial thrombosis or ischemia, cortical venous thrombosis with hemorrhage, or a focal intracranial mass lesion.

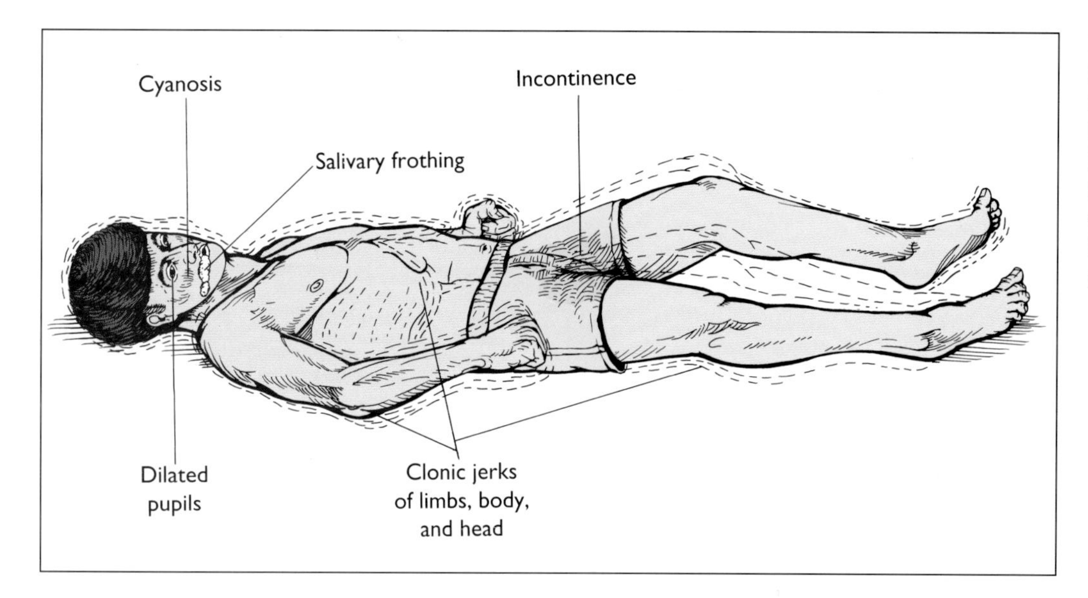

FIGURE 1-15 Generalized tonic clonic seizures. The clinical characteristics of a generalized tonic clonic seizure are as follows: dilated pupils; clonic jerking of arms, legs, and head alternating with tonic extension of the limbs and extension of the head and neck; cyanosis; tongue biting; urinary incontinence; and postictal unresponsiveness or confusion.

Cranial Nerve Dysfunction

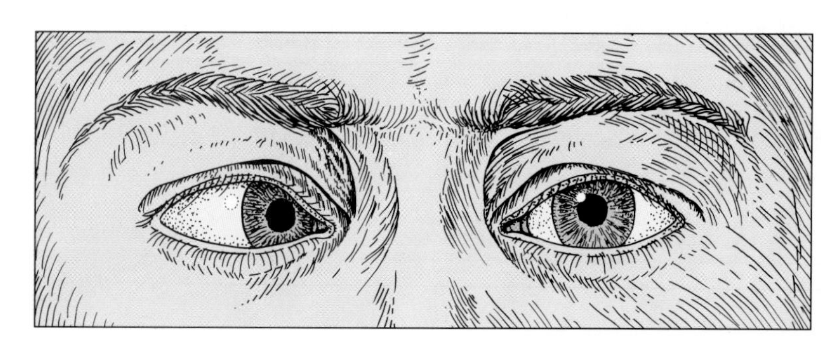

FIGURE 1-16 Cranial nerve palsies. Cranial nerve palsies may develop during the course of bacterial meningitis due to the purulent exudate within the arachnoidal sheath enveloping the nerve or due to raised intracranial pressure. Typically, cranial nerves III, VI, VII, and VIII are involved. This drawing demonstrates a right cranial nerve VI palsy.

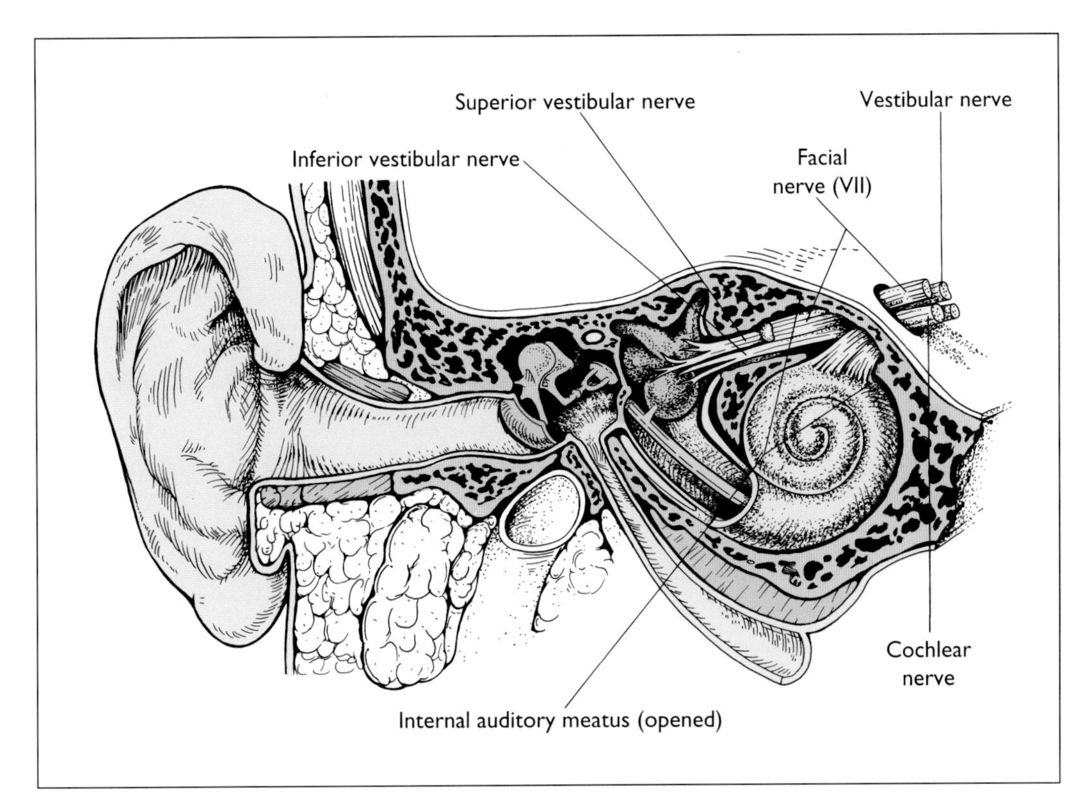

FIGURE 1-17 Sensorineural hearing loss. Sensorineural hearing loss and facial palsy result from purulent exudate in the arachnoidal sheaths of cranial nerves VII and VIII as they course through the bony canal.

Pathogenesis of sensorineural hearing loss
Cochlear dysfunction due to a direct invasion of bacteria into the cochlea via the cochlear aqueduct
Cochlear nerve inflammation
Vascular occlusion
Cochlear or nerve toxicity due to antimicrobial agents

FIGURE 1-18 Pathogenesis of sensorineural hearing loss. A moderate-to-severe unilateral or bilateral sensorineural hearing loss occurs as a complication of bacterial meningitis in 10% to 30% of infants and children and is the leading cause of acquired deafness in infants and children. (Dodge PR, Davis H, Feigin RD, *et al.*: Prospective evaluation of hearing impairment as a sequela of acute bacterial meningitis. *N Engl J Med* 1984, 311:869–874.)

Cerebral Edema and Increased Intracranial Pressure

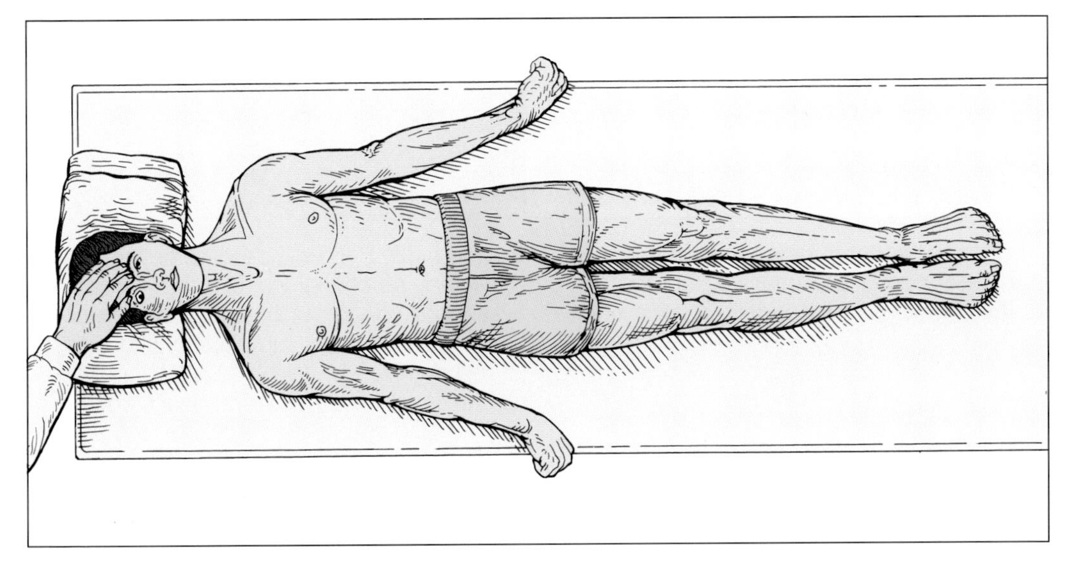

FIGURE 1-19 Decorticate or decerebrate posturing. Patients with increasing intracranial pressure may demonstrate spontaneous decorticate or decerebrate posturing or posture to noxious stimuli. In a decerebrate posture, the arms and legs are held in rigid extension. In a decorticate posture, the arms are held in flexion and the legs in extension.

Focal Cerebral Signs

Focal cerebral signs
Hemiparesis
Ataxia
Seizures
Cranial nerve palsies
Gaze preference

Figure 1-20 Focal cerebral signs. Focal neurologic signs may occur early or late in the course of bacterial meningitis. Hemiparesis is either due to vasculitis with cerebral ischemia and/or infarction or is a sign of a large subdural effusion causing a mass effect. Ataxia is a common presenting sign of *Haemophilus influenzae* meningitis in a child. Ataxia is typically a transient symptom, but because auditory and vestibular cranial nerve involvement tends to occur together and because ataxia is a sign of vestibular dysfunction, ataxia is associated with postmeningitic hearing loss. Seizures occur in 30% to 40% of children with acute bacterial meningitis and typically occur within the first 3 days of illness. Cranial nerve palsies develop as the nerve becomes enveloped by exudate in the arachnoidal sheath surrounding the nerve, or alternatively, cranial nerve palsies are a sign of increased intracranial pressure. In a recent review of acute bacterial meningitis in adults, the most common focal neurologic deficit was a gaze preference. A gaze preference is due to either a hemispheral lesion or a lesion in the horizontal gaze center in the pons. (Durand ML, Calderwood SB, Weber DJ, *et al.*: Acute bacterial meningitis in adults: A review of 493 episodes. *N Engl J Med* 1993, 328:21–28.)

Pathologic Findings

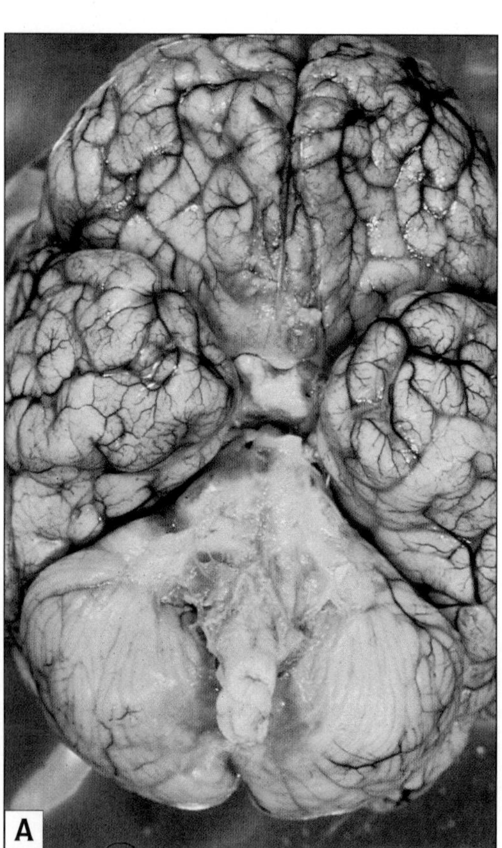

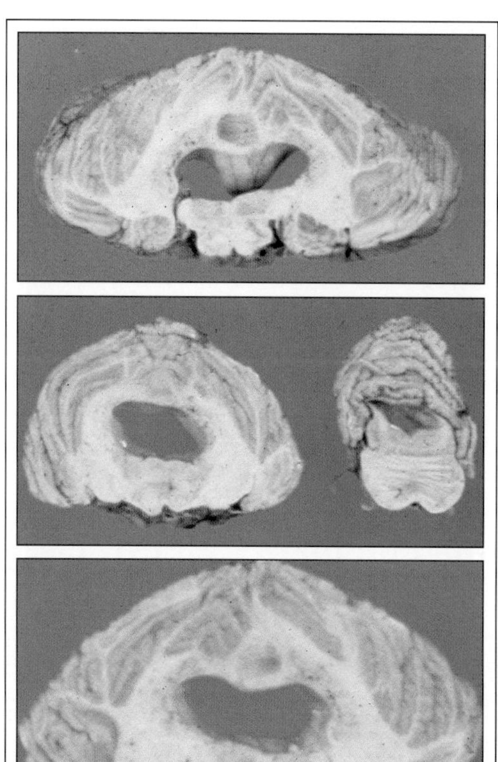

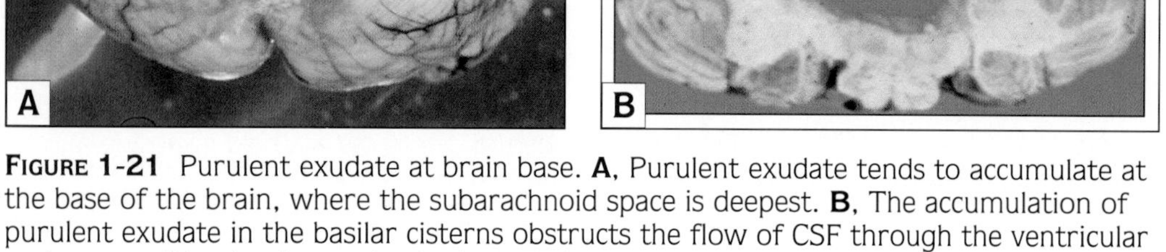

Figure 1-21 Purulent exudate at brain base. **A**, Purulent exudate tends to accumulate at the base of the brain, where the subarachnoid space is deepest. **B**, The accumulation of purulent exudate in the basilar cisterns obstructs the flow of CSF through the ventricular system, resulting in obstructive hydrocephalus.

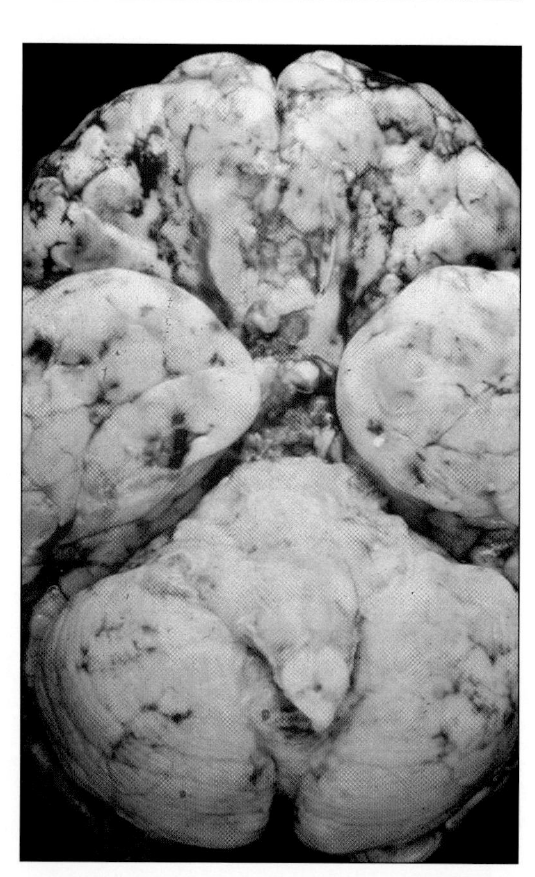

Figure 1-22 Purulent exudate of bacterial meningitis surrounding the temporal cortices, optic chiasm, brainstem, and cerebellum. The neurologic complications of bacterial meningitis, which include raised intracranial pressure, seizures, focal neurologic deficits, and cranial nerve palsies, are all a result of the accumulation of this purulent exudate around the base of the brain.

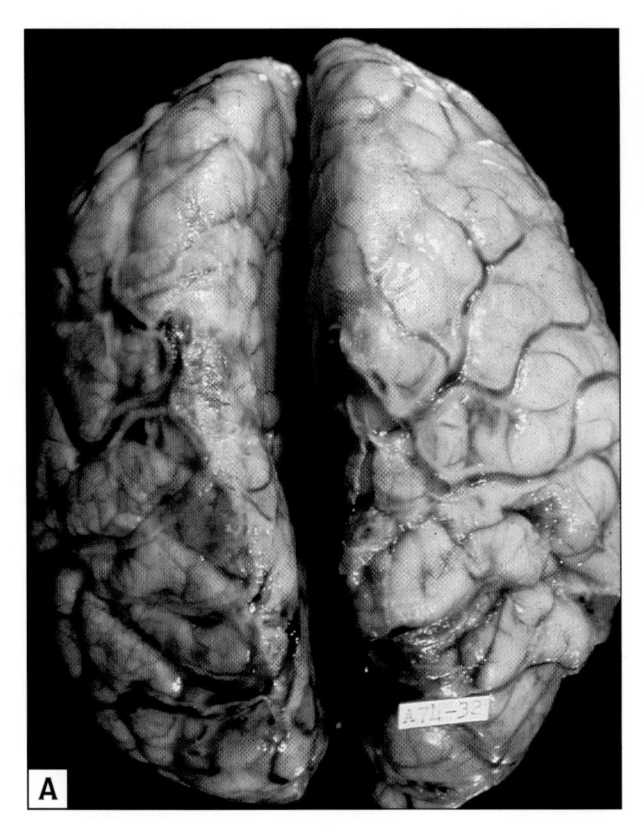

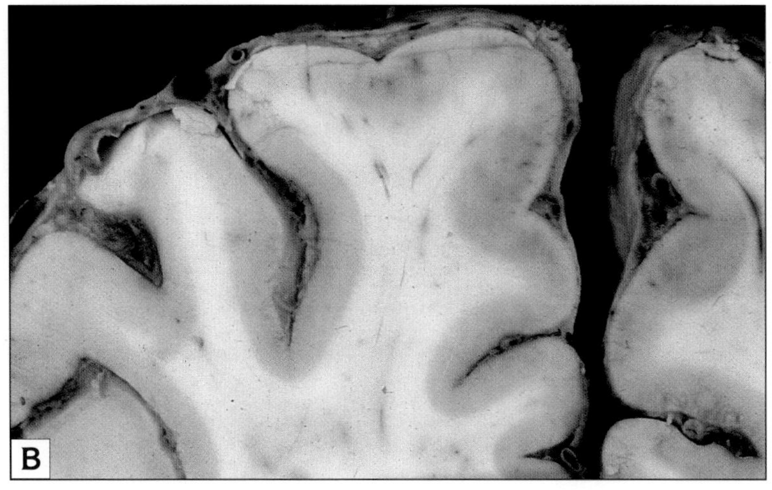

FIGURE 1-23 Purulent exudate in the convexities of the cerebral cortex. **A**, On gross examination of the brain, the purulent exudate in the convexities of the cerebral cortex has a gray-yellow appearance . The superficial cerebral veins are prominent due to venous outflow obstruction. The small hemorrhages are the result of cortical venous infarction. **B**, Cross-section of the brain demonstrates purulent exudate in the cerebral sulci. (*From* Roos KL, Tunkel AR, Scheld WM: Acute bacterial meningitis in children and adults. In Scheld WM, Whitley RJ, Durack DT (eds.): *Infections of the Central Nervous System*. New York: Raven Press; 1991:335–409; with permission.)

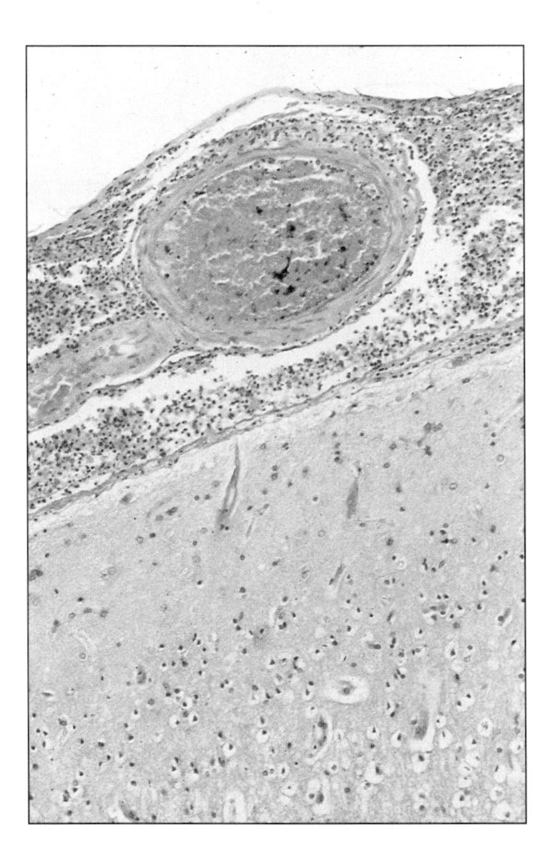

FIGURE 1-24 The subarachnoid space is expanded by inflammatory exudate with extension of the exudate into the perivascular space and into the wall of the artery. There is edema of the underlying cerebral cortex.

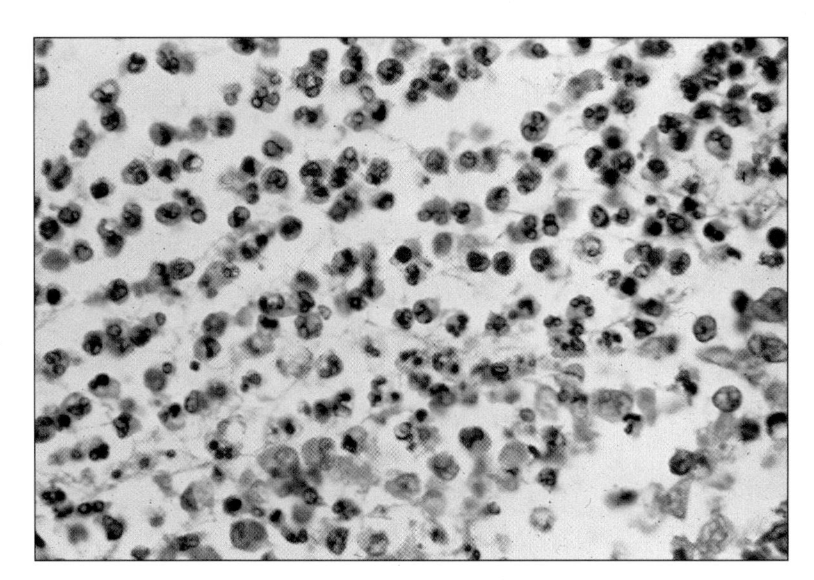

FIGURE 1-25 Microscopic examination of the inflammatory exudate demonstrates large numbers of polymorphonuclear leukocytes.

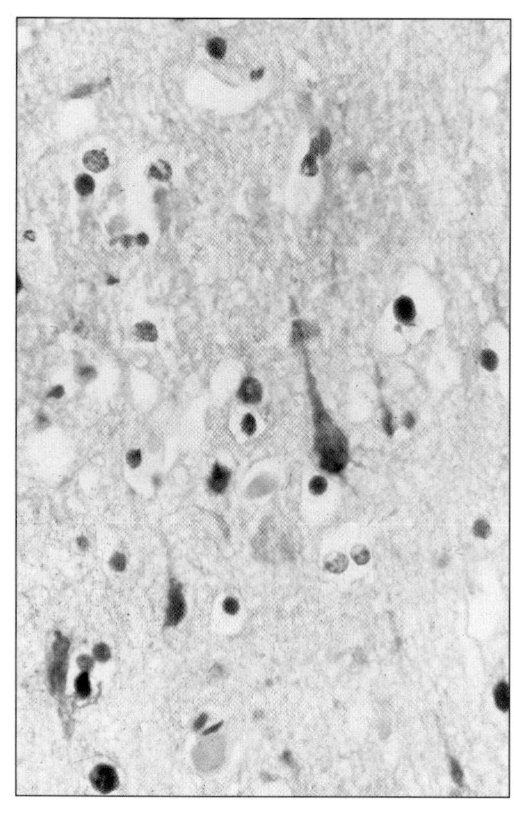

FIGURE 1-26 Microscopic examination of the brain parenchyma reveals shrunken and darkly staining "red" neurons, the result of ischemic and hypoxic cortical injury.

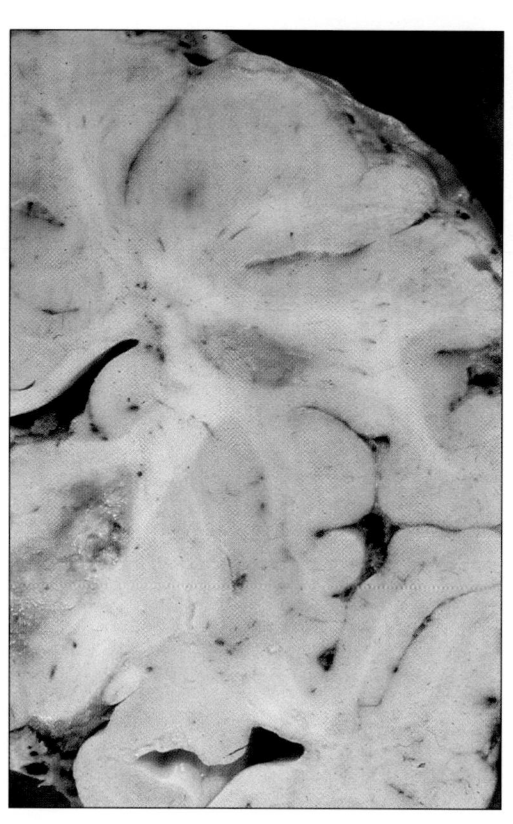

FIGURE 1-27 Loss of distinction between gray and white matter due to cerebral edema.

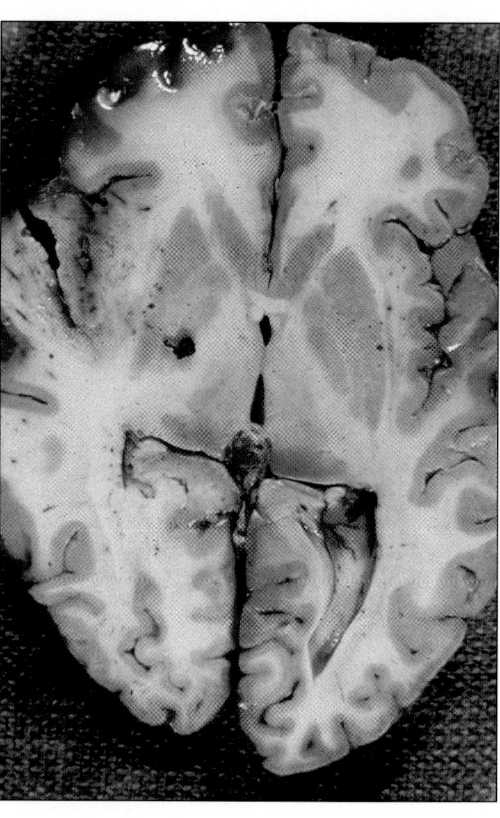

FIGURE 1-28 Cerebral edema of subcortical white matter.

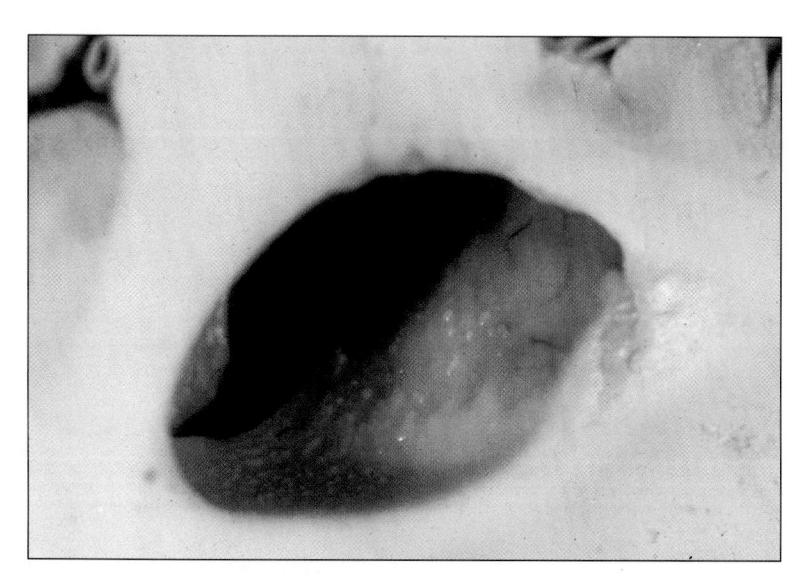

FIGURE 1-29 Purulent exudate in the ventricular fluid and attached to the ventricular walls (ventriculitis) complicating meningitis.

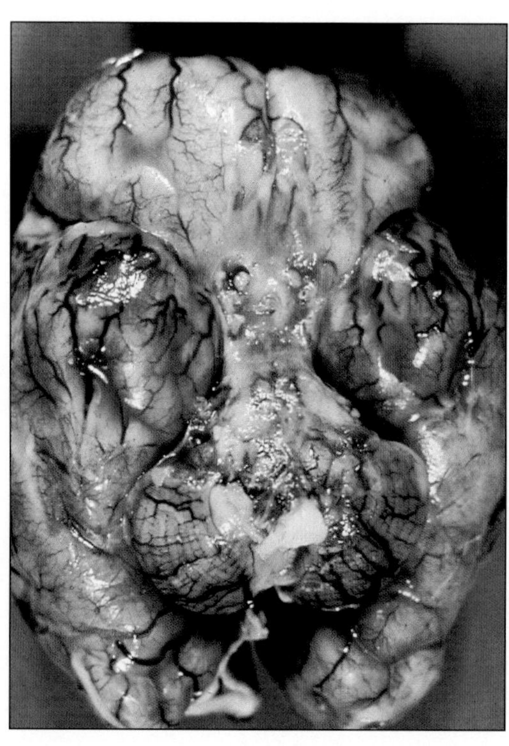

FIGURE 1-30 Brain of a premature infant with bacterial meningitis. There is marked swelling of the cerebral hemispheres and purulent exudate in the Sylvian fissures and interpeduncular cistern.

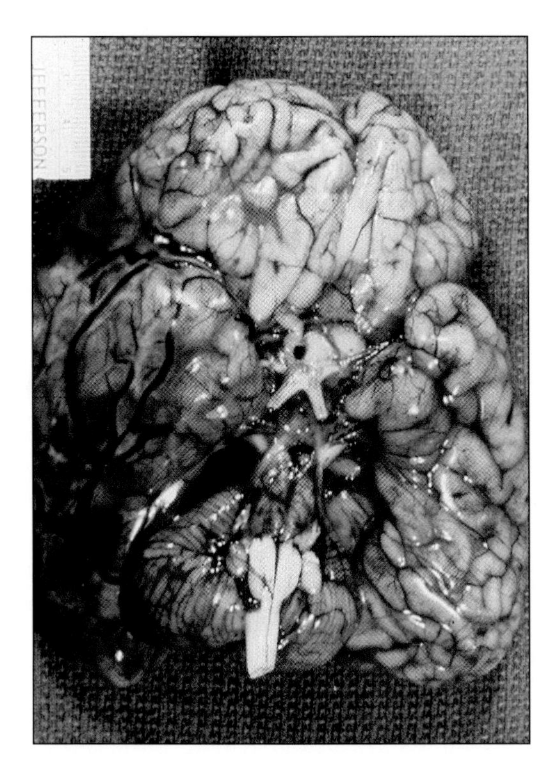

FIGURE 1-31 Brain of a full-term infant with bacterial meningitis. There is marked overall softening of the brain secondary to cerebral edema with prominent dilatation of superficial cerebral veins.

DIAGNOSTIC EVALUATIONS

Diagnostic studies in acute bacterial meningitis
1. Neuroimaging (CT or MRI)
2. CSF examination
Opening pressure
Chemistries
Cell count
Gram stain
Culture
3. Blood cultures

FIGURE 1-32 Diagnostic studies in acute bacterial meningitis. A neuroimaging procedure, either computed tomography (CT) or magnetic resonance imaging (MRI), is recommended prior to lumbar puncture in patients with coma, focal neurologic deficit, dilated nonreactive pupil, papilledema, or AIDS. In patients with AIDS, the occurrence of CNS toxoplasmosis may not be heralded by a focal neurologic deficit but will be detected with neuroimaging. Measurement of the opening pressure should be routine practice in the CSF analysis so that increased intracranial pressure can be diagnosed and managed aggressively. The Gram stain is positive in identifying the meningeal pathogen in 60% to 90% of cases of bacterial meningitis. If the CSF is cloudy, smears should be obtained from fresh, uncentrifuged fluid for Gram stain. If the CSF is clear, the smear should be obtained from the centrifuged sediment. Culture of CSF is positive in approximately 80% of cases of bacterial meningitis. Blood cultures should be part of the routine evaluation of patients with suspected meningitis. In the presence of raised intracranial pressure or a focal neurologic deficit, blood cultures may reveal the organism, and thus the lumbar puncture may be avoided or delayed.

Lumbar Puncture

Clinical signs of increased intracranial pressure
Altered level of consciousness
Cushing reflex (bradycardia and elevated blood pressure)
Dilated, nonreactive pupil
Bilateral cranial nerve VI palsies
Papilledema
Decorticate or decerebrate posturing

FIGURE 1-33 Clinical signs of increased intracranial pressure. Increased intracranial pressure is a common complication of bacterial meningitis and a major cause of neurologic morbidity.

Indications for neuroimaging prior to lumbar puncture
Coma
Focal neurologic deficit
Dilated nonreactive pupil
Papilledema
Signs of a posterior fossa lesion (cranial-nerve abnormalities, vomiting, gait disturbance, cerebellar deficit on exam)
AIDS

FIGURE 1-34 Indications for neuroimaging studies prior to lumbar puncture. Brain herniation is a rare complication of lumbar puncture but may occur when CSF is removed in the presence of cerebral edema or an intracranial mass lesion. A neuroimaging study, either by CT or MRI, should be performed prior to lumbar puncture when the neurologic examination reveals focal neurologic deficit, papilledema, or signs of a mass lesion in the posterior fossa.

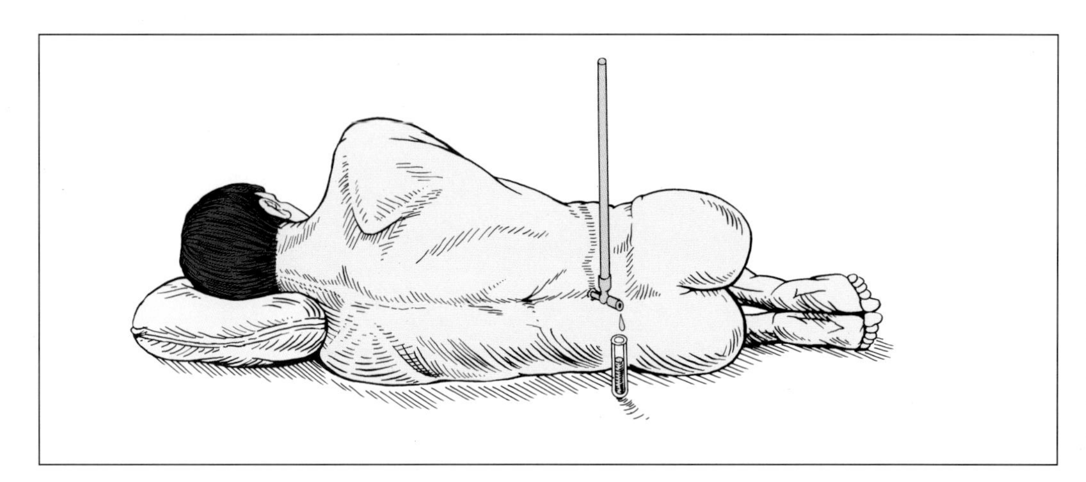

FIGURE 1-35 The technique of lumbar puncture. The patient is placed in the lateral recumbent position with the knees and neck flexed. A 22- or 20-gauge needle is inserted below the conus medullaris (L2) between the L4 and L5 or the L3 and L4 vertebrae into the subarachnoid space. Four tubes of CSF are collected for analysis. (Fishman RA: Examination of the cerebrospinal fluid: Techniques and complications. *In* Fishman RA (ed.): *Cerebrospinal Fluid in Diseases of the Central Nervous System*, 2nd ed. Philadelphia: W.B. Saunders; 1992:157–182.)

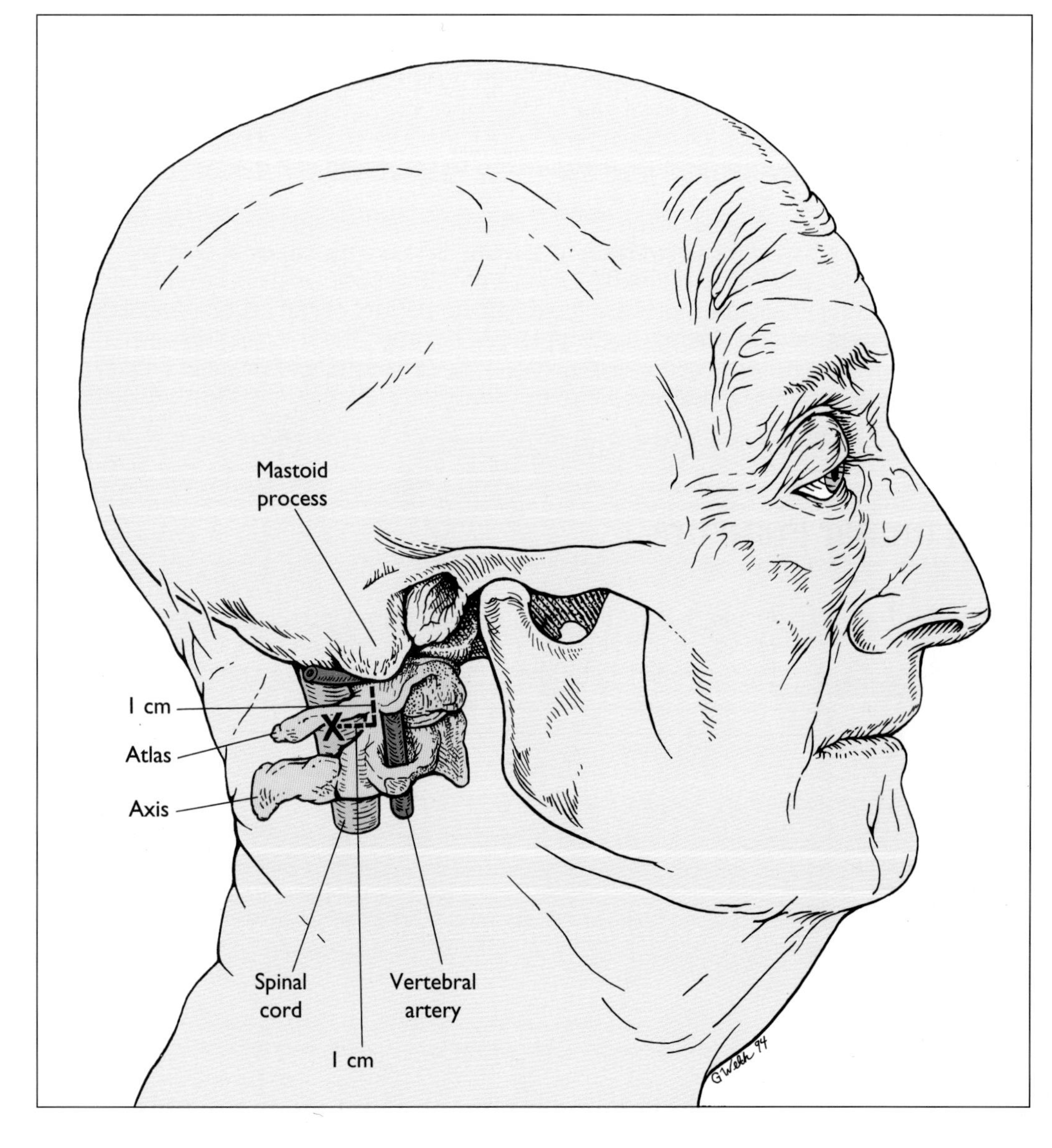

FIGURE 1-36 Lateral cervical puncture. This procedure can also be used to obtain CSF. It is performed with the patient in the supine position, and a 20-gauge spinal needle is inserted parallel to the plane of the bed in a site 1 cm caudal to and 1 cm dorsal to the tip of the mastoid process. The complications of lateral cervical puncture include injury to the spinal cord and puncture of the vertebral artery. (Silverberg GD: Intracranial pressure monitoring. *In* Wilkins RH, Rengachary SS (eds.): *Neurosurgery*. New York: McGraw-Hill Book Company; 1985:156–174.)

Range of normal values for opening pressure in lumbar puncture

Age group	Opening pressure
Neonates	10–100 mm H_2O
Children (< age 6)	10 –100 mm H_2O
Children (> age 6)	60–200 mm H_2O
Adults	60–200 mm H_2O
Obese adults	<250 mm H_2O

FIGURE 1-37 Opening pressure in lumbar puncture. A critical step in performing a lumbar puncture is the measurement of the opening pressure. The normal range for opening pressure in an adult in the lateral recumbent position is 60 to 200 mm H_2O, except in the markedly obese adult, who may have a normal opening pressure as high as 250 mm H_2O. The normal opening pressure in infants and children ranges from 10 to 100 mm H_2O. Children reach the adult range of opening pressure at about 6 to 8 years of age. (Fishman RA: Examination of the cerebrospinal fluid: Techniques and complications. *In* Fishman RA (ed.): *Cerebrospinal Fluid in Diseases of the Nervous System*, 2nd ed. Philadelphia: W.B. Saunders; 1992:157–182. Corbett JJ, Mehta MP: Cerebrospinal fluid pressure in normal obese subjects and patients with pseudotumor cerebri. *Neurology* 1983, 33:1386–1388.)

Lumbar puncture in increased intracranial pressure

Mannitol, in bolus dose of 1 g/kg iv, 20 min before procedure
Intubate and hyperventilate to $PaCO_2$ of 25–30 mm Hg, plus iv mannitol
Use smaller 22-gauge needle

FIGURE 1-38 Lumbar puncture in the setting of increased intracranial pressure. A lumbar puncture can be performed safely for the diagnosis of bacterial meningitis even though cerebral edema and increased intracranial pressure are present. When the clinical examination reveals signs of increased intracranial pressure, one technique is to infuse mannitol intravenously (iv) in a bolus dose of 1 g/kg of body weight 20 minutes before lumbar puncture, or in addition to administering mannitol, to intubate and hyperventilate the patient to achieve an arterial PCO_2 of 25 to 30 mm Hg. Lumbar puncture should be performed with a 22-gauge needle to avoid creating a large rent in the dura through which CSF will continue to leak.

CSF Examination and Bacteriologic Culture

Cerebrospinal fluid abnormalities in bacterial meningitis

Increased opening pressure (200–500 mm H_2O)
Decreased glucose (< 40 mg/dL)
Decreased CSF/serum glucose ratio (< 0.31)
Increased protein (> 50 mg/dL)
Increased leukocyte count (PMNL predominance)

FIGURE 1-39 CSF abnormalities in bacterial meningitis. CSF abnormalities characteristic of bacterial meningitis are an elevated opening pressure, low glucose concentration and CSF/serum glucose ratio, increased CSF protein, and elevated leukocyte count with a predominance of polymorphonuclear leukocytes (PMNL).

Rapid diagnostic studies on cerebrospinal fluid

Latex agglutination (LA)
Coagglutination (CoA)
Limulus amoebocyte assay (indicates gram-negative meningitis)
Counterimmunoelectrophoresis (CIE)

FIGURE 1-40 Rapid diagnostic studies on CSF. Several techniques are available to detect bacterial antigens in CSF including the Phadebact coagglutination (CoA) test, the Directigen latex agglutination (LA) test, counterimmunoelectrophoresis (CIE), and the *Limulus* amoebocyte lysate (LAL) test. These tests are particularly useful in patients who have been pretreated with antibiotics. In cases in which the Gram stain is negative, the *Limulus* amoebocyte lysate test is reported to have a sensitivity of 77% to 99.5% and a specificity of 86% to 99.8% for the detection of gram-negative endotoxin in CSF. Both the latex agglutination and coagglutination tests are highly sensitive and specific for the detection of *Haemophilus influenzae* in CSF, moderately sensitive but highly specific for the detection of *Streptococcus pneumoniae* in CSF, but only about 50% sensitive for the detection of *Neisseria meningitidis* in CSF. The latex agglutination and coagglutination tests have replaced the counterimmunoelectrophoresis test because they are easier and quicker to do.

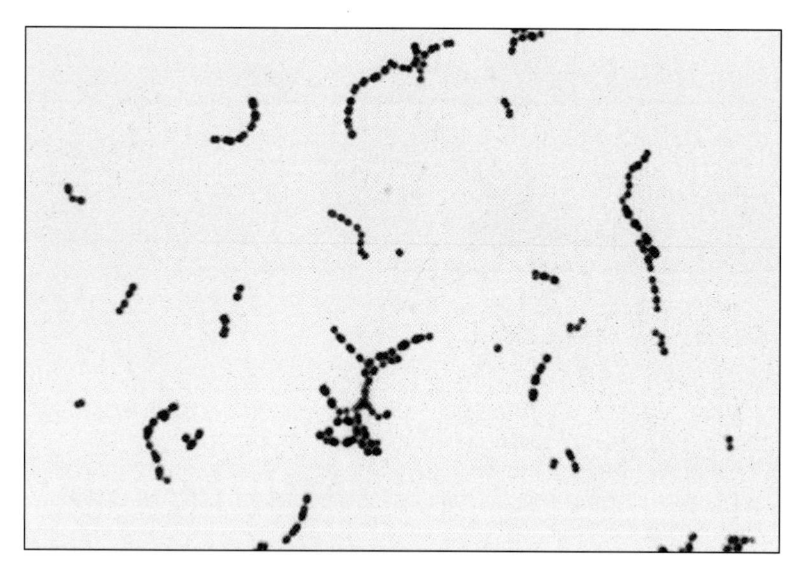

FIGURE 1-41 Group B streptococci. Gram stain demonstrating gram-positive organisms in culture which are group B streptococci. This organism, in addition to *Escherichia coli* and *Listeria monocytogenes*, is the most common etiologic organism of bacterial meningitis in the neonatal age group.

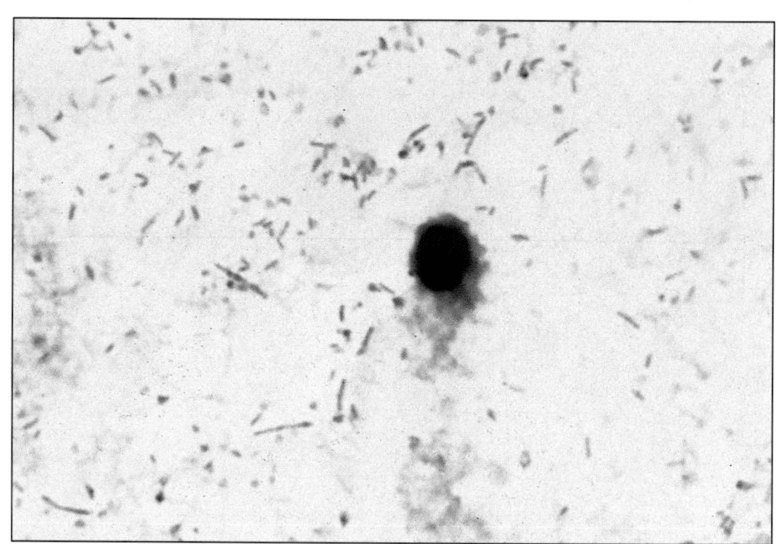

FIGURE 1-42 *Haemophilus influenzae* type b. Gram stain of CSF demonstrating *H. influenzae* type b, small gram-negative coccobacilli. This organism, in addition to *Neisseria meningitidis* and *Streptococcus pneumoniae*, is the most common etiologic organism of bacterial meningitis in children.

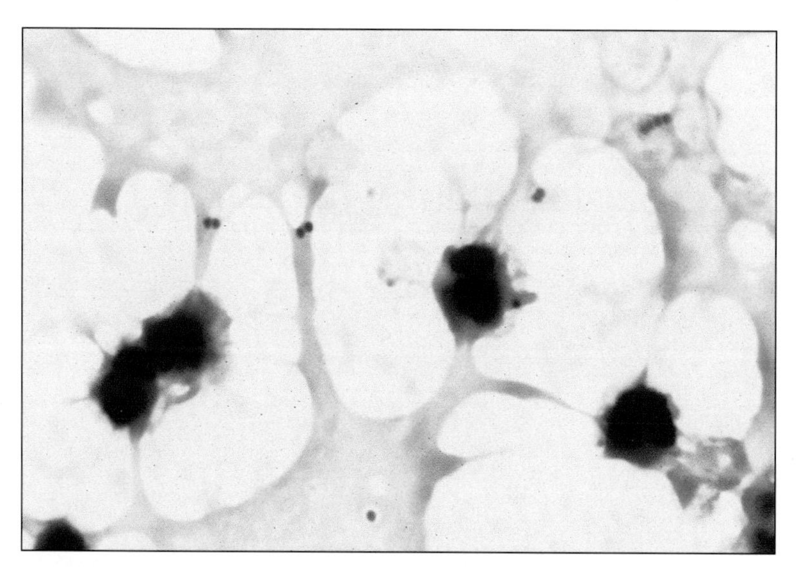

FIGURE 1-43 *Neisseria meningitidis.* Gram stain of CSF demonstrating gram-negative diplococci which are *N. meningitidis*. This organism, in addition to *Streptococcus pneumoniae*, is the most common causative organism of bacterial meningitis in adults.

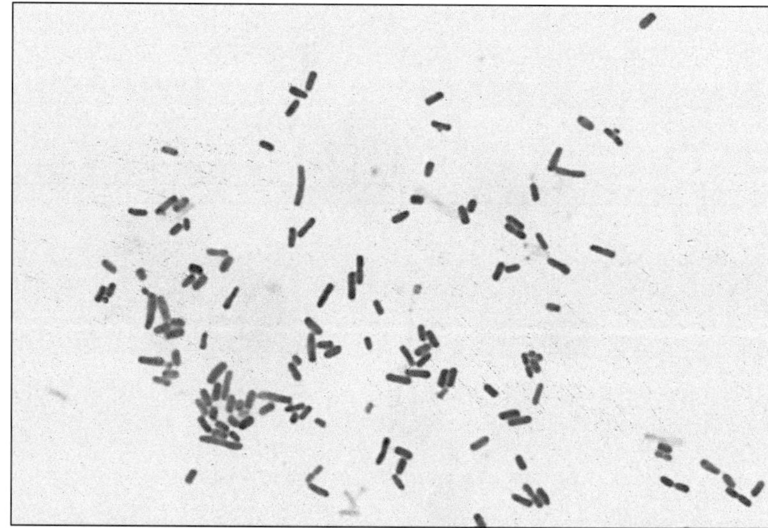

FIGURE 1-44 Gram-negative bacilli. Gram stain demonstrating gram-negative rods. Meningitis due to gram-negative organisms occurs in four clinical settings: neonates, the elderly, in association with head trauma, and following neurosurgical procedures.

Radiologic Findings

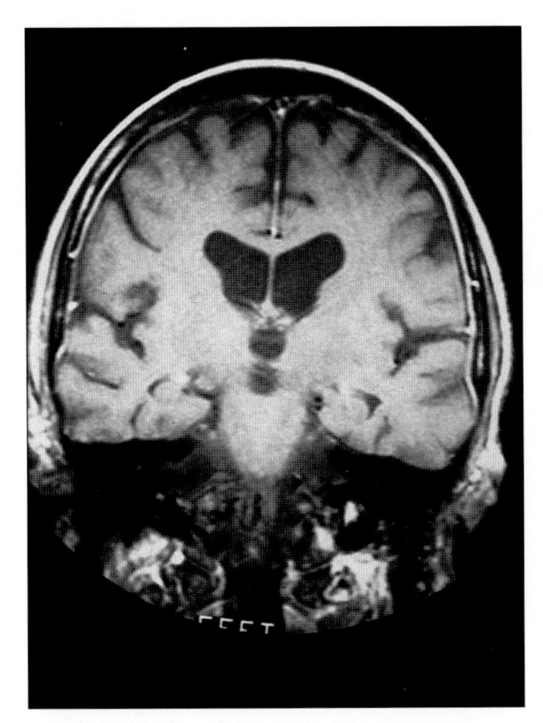

FIGURE 1-45 Meningeal inflammation. T1-weighted MR scan following administration of gadolinium-DTPA (Gd-DTPA) demonstrates diffuse enhancement of the meninges due to purulent meningitis. Gd-DTPA is an intravenous MR contrast agent that enhances areas of blood-brain barrier breakdown. MR with Gd-DTPA is a very sensitive method for demonstrating meningeal inflammation.

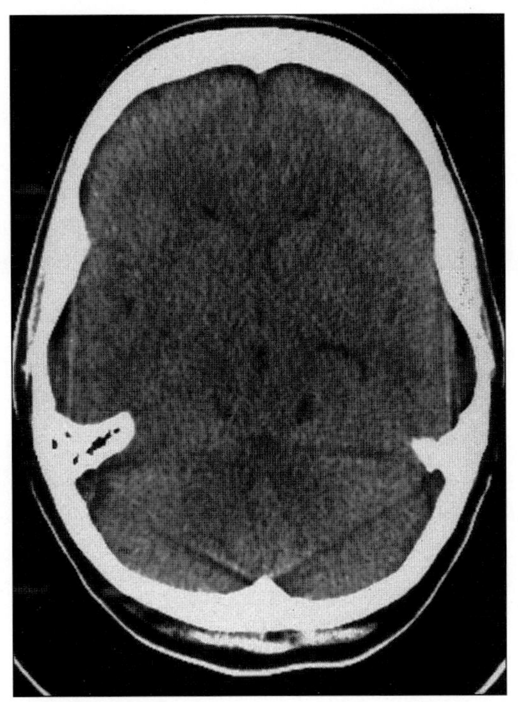

FIGURE 1-46 Diffuse cerebral edema. CT scan demonstrates diffuse cerebral edema. In bacterial meningitis, cerebral edema is due to a combination of vasogenic, interstitial, and cytotoxic edema. Vasogenic edema is due to the altered blood-brain barrier permeability. Interstitial edema results from obstruction to CSF resorption due to inflammatory changes in the arachnoid granulations. Cytotoxic edema is due to the intracellular accumulation of water and sodium. Bacterial cell wall components and the degranulation of leukocytes contribute to the development of cytotoxic edema. Increasing intracranial pressure develops as cerebral edema increases and adversely affects cerebral perfusion pressure.

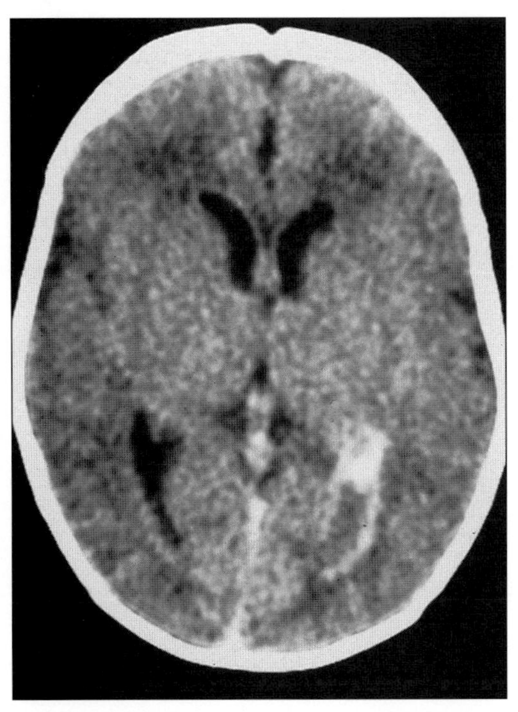

FIGURE 1-47 Ventriculitis and choroid plexitis. CT scan following contrast administration demonstrates enlargement of the left ventricular atrium and abnormal enhancement of the left ventricular wall and choroid plexus. Ventriculitis and choroid plexitis may develop as complications of the inflammation in the leptomeninges and may contribute to the development of hydrocephalus due to obstruction to the flow of CSF through the foramen of Monroe, cerebral aqueduct, and foramina of Magendie and Luschka.

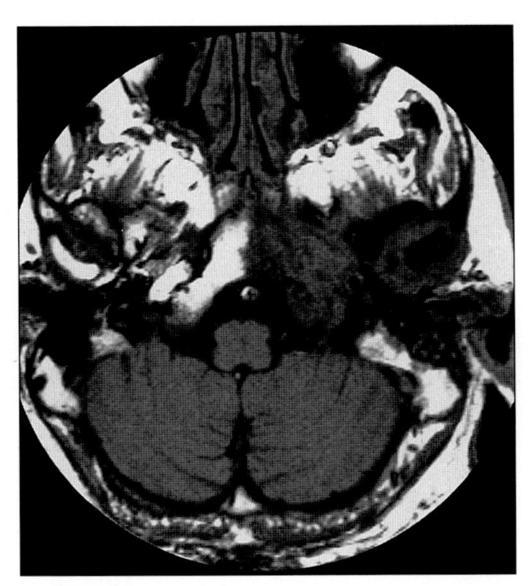

FIGURE 1-48 Pneumococcal meningitis. T1-weighted MR image in an adult with pneumococcal meningitis due to acute otitis media shows spread of infection to the clivus. The most common predisposing conditions for pneumococcal meningitis are pneumonia, acute and chronic otitis media, and congenital or traumatic dural sinus fistula. *Streptococcus pneumoniae* is the most common causative organism in meningitis due to head trauma with basilar skull fracture; in these cases, the fracture creates a fistula between the paranasal sinuses, nasopharynx, or middle ear and the subarachnoid space.

Differential Diagnosis

Differential diagnoses in acute bacterial meningitis

	Diagnostic test/finding
Viral meningitis	CSF
Meningoencephalitis (HSV-1)	CSF, EEG, brain biopsy
Rocky Mountain spotted fever	Skin biopsy, IFA
Subarachnoid hemorrhage	CSF
Tuberculous meningitis	CSF
Fungal meningitis	CSF
Brain abscess	CT, MRI
Subdural empyema	CT, MRI
Staphylococcal endocarditis	Cardiac murmur
Neuroleptic malignant syndrome	↑ serum CK

Figure 1-49 Differential diagnoses in acute bacterial meningitis. *Viral meningitis* is typically the leading alternative diagnostic consideration in patients with suspected acute bacterial meningitis. The distinction between viral and bacterial meningitis is classically made by examination of the CSF, but several clinical features also may help to distinguish these: patients with viral meningitis typically complain of a grippe-like headache but are otherwise awake and alert; the fever is usually higher in bacterial than in viral meningitis; viral meningitis has a more insidious onset than does bacterial meningitis; and stupor, obtundation, and coma are rare in viral meningitis. *Herpes simplex virus* (HSV) encephalitis cannot typically be distinguished from acute bacterial meningitis by clinical presentation. HSV has a predilection for the temporal and orbitofrontal areas, causing a change in behavior, confusion, focal neurologic deficits, and new-onset seizure activity. The electroencephalogram (EEG) and CSF examination are helpful in diagnosis. *Rocky Mountain spotted fever* is characterized by headache, fever, rash, and altered mental status. Diagnosis may be made by biopsy of the skin lesions and staining with immunofluorescent antibodies (IFA) to *Rickettsia rickettsii*. *Subarachnoid hemorrhage* is usually heralded by the sudden onset of a severe, excruciating headache or a sudden transient loss of consciousness followed by an explosive headache. This diagnosis is made by evidence of xanthochromia on CSF examination. *Tuberculous* and *fungal meningitis* also can be distinguished by examination of the CSF. The most common symptom of *brain abscess* or *subdural empyema* is hemicranial headache. A brain abscess presents as an expanding intracranial mass lesion with headache and a focal neurologic deficit or new-onset focal or generalized seizure activity. A subdural empyema is manifested by a headache localized to the side of the subdural infection, and as the subdural empyema creates a mass effect, a focal neurologic deficit develops with focal or generalized seizure activity and an altered level of consciousness. *Staphylococcal endocarditis* can be distinguished by the characteristic findings of a new cardiac murmur and petechial lesions in the nailbeds, mucous membranes, and extremities. The symptoms of *neuroleptic malignant syndrome* are fever, generalized lead-pipe rigidity, fluctuating consciousness, and autonomic instability. The most specific laboratory abnormality in this disorder is marked elevation in the serum creatine kinase (CK) concentration.

Differential diagnosis of erythematous or petechial rash in acute bacterial meningitis

- Meningococcal meningitis
- Enteroviral meningitis
- ECHO virus type 9
- *Haemophilus influenzae* meningitis
- *Streptococcus pneumoniae* meningitis
- Rocky Mountain spotted fever
- *Staphylococcus aureus* endocarditis

Figure 1-50 Differential diagnosis of an erythematous or petechial rash in acute bacterial meningitis. The rash of meningococcemia may initially be diffuse, erythematous, and maculopapular (*see* Figure 1-13). It typically then becomes a petechial or purpuric rash that is present on the trunk and lower extremities. Petechiae are found in the skin, mucous membranes, or conjunctivae, but never in the nailbeds of patients with meningococcemia. Biopsy of the purpuric lesions may reveal the organism on Gram smear. The characteristic rash of Rocky Mountain spotted fever is petechial rash which, in contrast, is evident first on the wrists and ankles prior to spreading centrally to the chest, face, and abdomen. The rash of Rocky Mountain spotted fever usually does not involve the mucous membranes. Diagnosis may be made by biopsy of the skin lesions and staining of the specimen with immunofluorescent antibodies to *Rickettsia rickettsii*. The petechial lesions in staphylococcal endocarditis involve the nailbeds, as well as the mucous membranes and extremities.

Cerebrospinal fluid abnormalities in bacterial versus viral meningitis

	Bacterial	Viral
Opening pressure	200–500 mm H_2O	≤ 250 mm H_2O
White blood cells	10–10,000 mm^3 (predominance of PMNLs)	50–2000 mm^3 (predominance of lymphocytes)
Glucose concentration	< 40 mg/dL	> 45 mg/dL
CSF/serum glucose ratio	< 0.31	> 0.6
Protein concentration	> 50 mg/dL	< 200 mg/dL

Figure 1-51 CSF abnormalities in bacterial versus viral meningitis. A variety of CSF abnormalities help to distinguish bacterial from viral meningitis. The opening pressure, the degree and type of CSF pleocytosis, and the glucose concentration are particularly useful in making the distinction between these two types of meningitis. PMNLs–polymorphonuclear leukocytes.

Complications

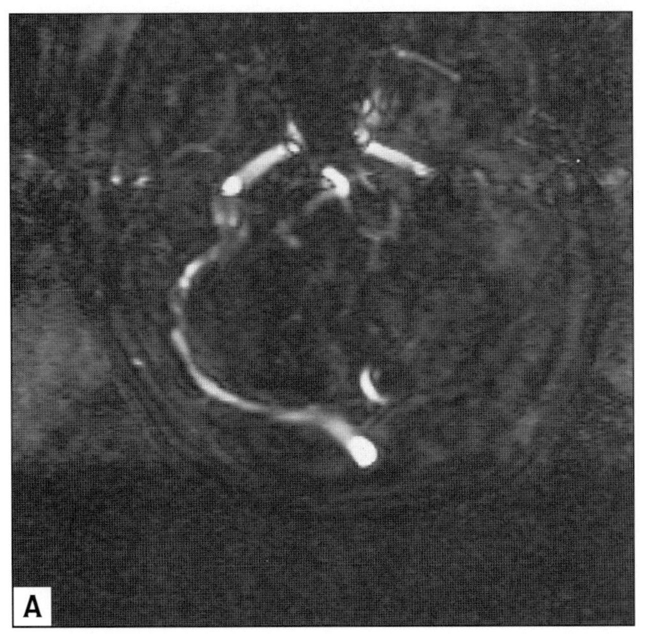

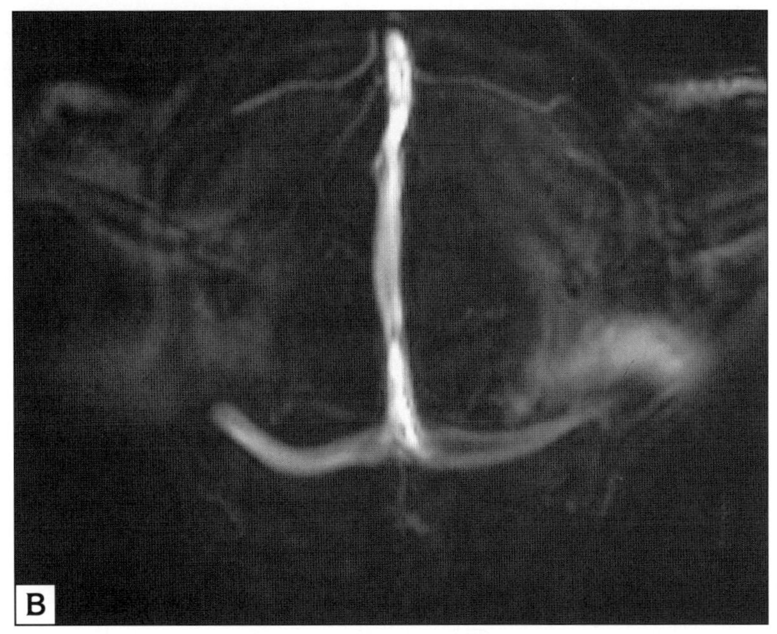

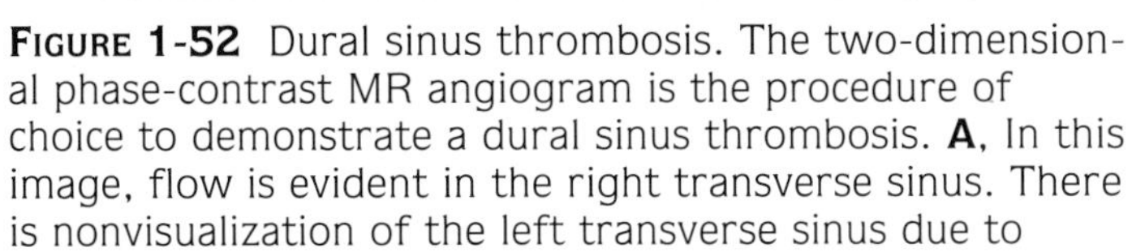

Figure 1-52 Dural sinus thrombosis. The two-dimensional phase-contrast MR angiogram is the procedure of choice to demonstrate a dural sinus thrombosis. **A**, In this image, flow is evident in the right transverse sinus. There is nonvisualization of the left transverse sinus due to occlusion of the left transverse sinus by thrombosis. **B**, Two-dimensional contrast MR angiogram demonstrating normal visualization of the superior sagittal sinus and the right and left transverse sinuses.

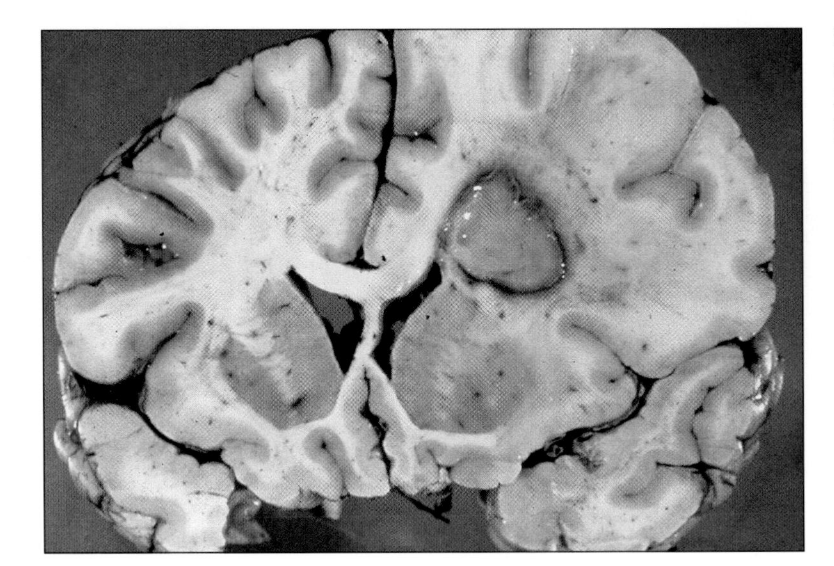

Figure 1-53 Brain abscess. Brain abscess is a rare complication of meningitis, but it may develop in an area of brain that has become necrotic due to infarction from arteritis or altered cerebral perfusion pressure.

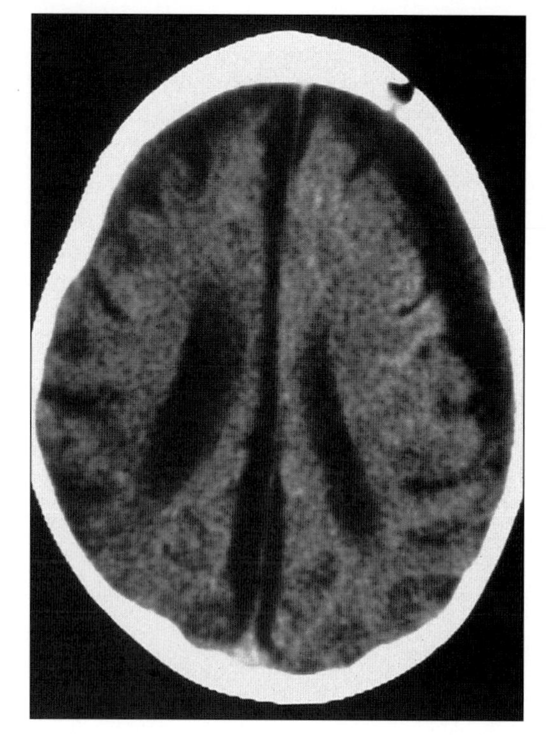

Figure 1-54 Subdural effusion in meningitis. CT scan demonstrates bilateral subdural effusions in *Haemophilus influenzae* meningitis. Subdural effusions develop during the course of bacterial meningitis in children due to an increase in the permeability of the thin-walled capillaries and veins in the inner layer of the dura, with subsequent leakage of albumin-rich fluid into the subdural space. These effusions are not usually symptomatic unless they become very large and produce a mass effect on the underlying hemisphere or unless they become infected. The fluid in the subdural space is usually resorbed when the infection in the subarachnoid space resolves. Subdural effusion is a rare complication of meningitis, but it may develop in an area of brain that has become necrotic due to infarction from arteritis or altered cerebral perfusion pressure.

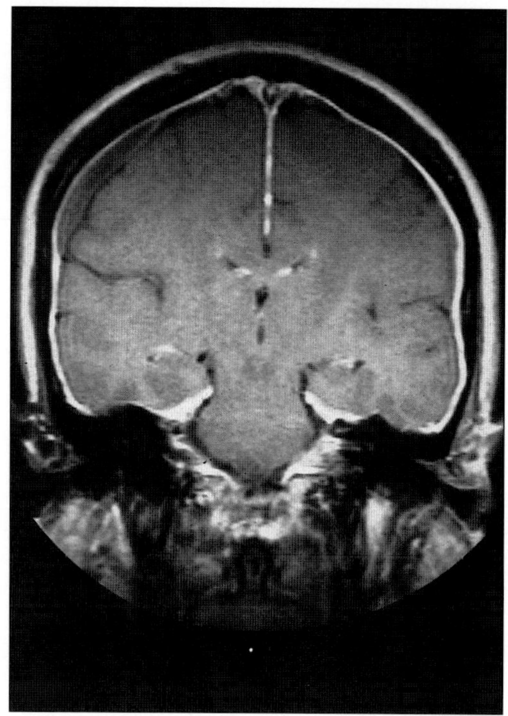

Figure 1-55 Subdural empyema. T1-weighted MR coronal image after Gd-DTPA administration demonstrates subdural empyema on the right side. This is a rare complication of meningitis but should be considered in a patient with prolonged fever. A subdural effusion is isointense with CSF on the T1-weighted image and appears continuous with the subarachnoid space. A subdural empyema is isointense or slightly hypointense to brain parenchyma on a T1-weighted image, and a medial enhancing rim is often present, as evident on this slide. Unlike a subdural effusion, a subdural empyema will not be resorbed as the meningitis resolves and requires neurosurgical intervention.

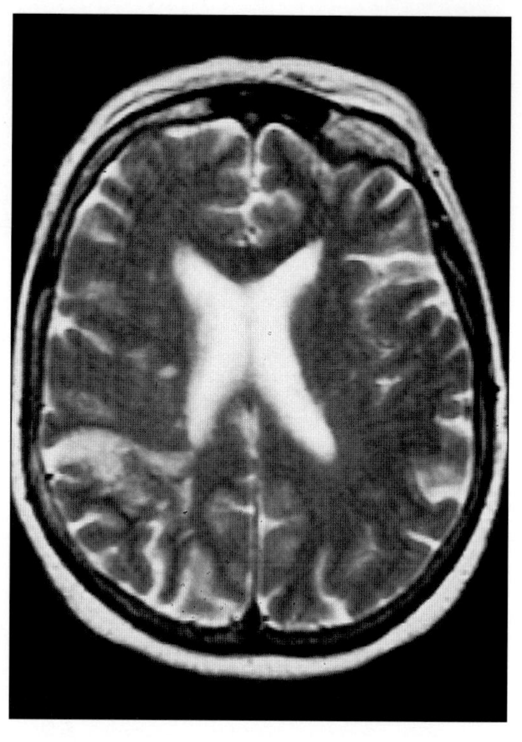

Figure 1-56 A T2-weighted MR scan demonstrates a cortical infarction due to occlusion of one of the posterior branches of the middle cerebral artery.

Cerebrovascular complications of bacterial meningitis
Narrowing of large arteries at the base of brain
Narrowing of medium-sized arteries and occlusion of distal branches of middle cerebral artery, resulting in cerebral ischemia and infarction
Septic dural sinus thrombosis and thrombophlebitis of cortical veins

Figure 1-57 Cerebrovascular complications of bacterial meningitis. Cerebrovascular complications of bacterial meningitis are the result of the accumulation of a purulent exudate in the basilar cisterns compressing the large arteries at the base of the brain and the result of arteritis and thrombophlebitis. Additionally, cerebral blood flow is affected by a loss of autoregulation and the decreased cerebral perfusion pressure that develops as a result of increased intracranial pressure.

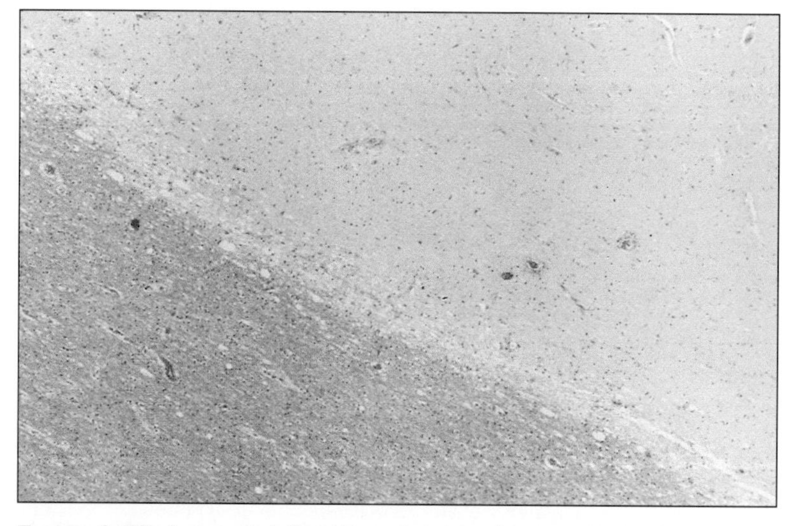

Figure 1-58 Ischemic infarction of cerebral cortex and subcortical white matter. This cerebrovascular complication of bacterial meningitis is typically manifest clinically by a focal neurologic deficit.

Predisposing factors to recurrent bacterial meningitis

Head injury with CSF fistula
Chronic otitis media or mastoiditis
Neurosurgical complication
Splenectomy
Hypogammaglobulinemia
Complement deficiencies
Neutropenia
Immunosuppressant therapy

FIGURE 1-59 Predisposing factors to recurrent bacterial meningitis. A state of immunosuppression, a parameningeal suppurative focus, and a dural sinus fistula predispose an individual to recurrent bacterial meningitis.

THERAPY

Initial approach to the patient

1. Dexamethasone, 0.15 mg/kg, at 15–20 min before the first dose of antibiotic
2. Empiric antimicrobial therapy
3. Neuroimaging procedure (CT or MRI)
4. CSF analysis

FIGURE 1-60 Initial approach to the patient with bacterial meningitis. Therapy for bacterial meningitis should be initiated in the patient with suspected bacterial meningitis, and then a diagnostic evaluation performed.

Antimicrobial Therapy

Empiric antimicrobial therapy for bacterial meningitis

	Antimicrobial agent
Neonates	Ampicillin plus cefotaxime
Infants and children	Cefotaxime or ceftriaxone
Adults (15–50 yrs)	Third-generation cephalosporin or penicillin G
Older adults	Third-generation cephalosporin (ceftriaxone or ceftazidime) plus ampicillin
Neurosurgical procedure	Third-generation cephalosporin (ceftazidime) plus aminoglycoside plus vancomycin
Immunocompromised state	Ampicillin plus third-generation cephalosporin
Neutropenic state	Ceftazidime plus ampicillin

FIGURE 1-61 Empiric antimicrobial therapy for bacterial meningitis. The choice of an empiric agent for the treatment of bacterial meningitis should be based on the patient's age and any associated conditions (recent neurosurgical procedure, immunocompromised state, and so forth).

Recommended antibiotics for the treatment of bacterial meningitis by organism

Organism	Antibiotic
Haemophilus influenzae type b	Third-generation cephalosporin or ampicillin plus chloramphenicol
Neisseria meningitidis	Penicillin G or ampicillin
Streptococcus pneumoniae	Penicillin G or ampicillin
Pseudomonas aeruginosa	Ceftazidime (plus aminoglycoside)
Staphylococcus aureus (methicillin-sensitive)	Nafcillin or oxacillin
Staphylococcus aureus (methicillin-resistant)	Vancomycin
Coagulase-negative staphylococci	Vancomycin
Listeria monocytogenes	Ampicillin (plus aminoglycoside)
Enterobacteriaceae	Third-generation cephalosporin
Streptococcus agalactiae	Penicillin G or ampicillin (plus aminoglycoside)

FIGURE 1-62 Recommended antibiotics for treatment of bacterial meningitis by organism. Effective third-generation cephalosporins include cefotaxime or ceftriaxone. For meningitis due to coagulase-negative staphylococci, rifampin is added to vancomycin when there is no improvement after 48 hours of therapy. For that due to the Enterobacteriaceae, ceftazidime is used if *Pseudomonas aeruginosa* is suspected or proven. (*From* Roos KL, Tunkel AR, Scheld WM: Acute bacterial meningitis in children and adults. *In* Scheld WM, Whitley RJ, Durack DT (eds.): *Infections of the Central Nervous System*. New York: Raven Press; 1991:335–410; with permission.)

A. Recommended doses of antibiotics for bacterial meningitis in children

Antibiotic	Daily dose, *mg/kg/d*	Dosing interval, *hr*
Penicillin G	250,000–400,000 U	4–6
Ampicillin	150–200	4–6
Chloramphenicol	100	6
Ceftriaxone	80–100	12–24
Cefotaxime	200	6
Cefuroxime	240	8
Ceftazidime	125–150	8
Nafcillin	100–150	4
Vancomycin	40–60	6
Rifampin	20	
Gentamicin	5	8
Amikacin	20	8
TMP-SMX	10 (based on TMP)	12

B. Recommended doses of antibiotics for bacterial meningitis in adults

Antibiotic	Total daily dose	Dosing interval, *hr*
Penicillin G	20–24 mL U	4
Ampicillin	12 g	4
Ceftriaxone	4–6 g	12
Cefotaxime	8–12 g	4
Ceftazidime	6 g	8
Vancomycin	2 g	12
Nafcillin, oxacillin	9–12 g	4
Chloramphenicol	4 g	6
Gentamicin, tobramycin	5 mg/kg	8
Amikacin	15 mg/kg	8
TMP/SMX	10 mg/kg (based on TMP)	12

FIGURE 1-63 Recommended doses of antibiotics for bacterial meningitis. **A**, Dosages in children. If a once-daily regimen of cefotaxime is used, an 80-mg/kg dose should be given on the first day at diagnosis, at 12 and 24 hours, and then every 24 hours thereafter. **B**, Dosages in adults (≥ 15 yrs). For nafcillin and oxacillin, higher dosages are used if leukopenia is present. With chloramphenicol, the dosage is increased to 6 g/d for pneumococcal meningitis. TMP-SMX—trimethoprim-sulfamethoxazole. (*From* Roos KL, Tunkel AR, Scheld WM: Acute bacterial meningitis in children and adults. *In* Scheld WM, Whitley RJ, Durack DT (eds): *Infections of the Central Nervous System*. New York: Raven Press; 1991:335–410; with permission.)

Management of Complications

Complications of bacterial meningitis

Neurologic	Systemic
Cerebral edema	Pneumonia
Increased ICP	ARDS
Seizures	Deep vein thrombosis
Cerebral infarction	Disseminated intravascular coagulation
Hydrocephalus	Pulmonary embolism
Subdural effusion	Electrolyte abnormalities
Hyponatremia	
Sensorineural hearing loss	

FIGURE 1-64 Neurologic and systemic complications of bacterial meningitis. The successful treatment of bacterial meningitis requires not only antimicrobial agents but also the successful management of the neurologic complications, including raised intracranial pressure (ICP) due to cerebral edema, seizures, stroke, and sensorineural hearing loss. These complications are due to a cascade of events that are initiated by the lysis of bacteria in the subarachnoid space. ARDS—acute respiratory distress syndrome.

Initial management of increased intracranial pressure

Elevate the head of the bed 30 degrees
Hyperventilation to lower $PaCO_2$ to 25 mm Hg
Mannitol 1.0 g/kg bolus injection
Dexamethasone 0.15 mg/kg every 6 hours
Barbiturate coma (therapeutic pentobarbital level, 25 to 40 mg/L)

FIGURE 1-65 Initial management of increased intracranial pressure. Increased intracranial pressure is present when an opening pressure of > 250 mm H_2O is measured from the L3 to L4 interspace or a pressure of > 15 mm Hg is recorded from an intracranial pressure monitoring device. The barbiturate coma is induced with a pentobarbital loading dose of 5 to 10 mg/kg, with a maintenance infusion rate of 1 to 3 mg/kg/hr to achieve a burst-suppression pattern on the electroencephalogram

Management of stroke during meningitis

Recommended	Of unclear benefit
CT scan to rule out hemorrhage	Hypervolemic hemodilution therapy
If ICP is increased, hyperventilation and iv hyperosmolar therapy (mannitol, 1.0 g/kg)	Intravenous heparin
Subcutaneous heparin to prevent deep venous thrombosis	

FIGURE 1-66 Management of stroke during the course of meningitis. When a focal neurologic deficit suggestive of a stroke develops, a CT scan should be obtained to rule out the presence of hemorrhage, abscess, subdural effusion, or empyema. Careful attention must be given to cerebral perfusion pressure, which is defined as the difference between systemic mean arterial pressure and intracranial pressure. Systemic mean arterial pressure should be conservatively managed, and rapid lowering of blood pressure avoided. Only systolic pressures > 210 mm Hg and diastolic pressures > 110 mm Hg should be treated. Intracranial pressure should be aggressively controlled with hyperventilation and hyperosmolar therapy. Therapies of unclear benefit include hypervolemic hemodilution therapy, which lowers blood viscosity and thus increases cerebral blood flow poststroke; this therapy has been investigated in the general management of acute stroke, but its role in stroke complicating bacterial meningitis has not been established. Intravenous heparin therapy, likewise, may have a role in the management of septic dural sinus thrombosis, but no firm recommendations can be made at this time.

Management of seizures

1. Lorazepam, 2 mg iv, may be repeated once
2. Phenytoin, 20 mg/kg iv, at a rate of 50 mg/min (or 25 mg/min for elderly patient)
   Monitor heart rate and blood pressure
3. Endotracheal intubation, then phenobarbital, 20 mg/kg, at a rate of 100 mg/min

FIGURE 1-67 Management of generalized and focal seizure activity. Failure to control status epilepticus is often due to an inadequate loading dose of phenytoin or too slow of an infusion rate of phenobarbital. An additional 500 mg of phenytoin may be administered intravenously if the loading dose does not stop seizure activity. If seizure activity is controlled with phenytoin, step 3—intubation and phenobarbital—is not necessary.

Adjunctive Treatment

Adjunctive therapy in bacterial meningitis
Dexamethasone, 0.15 mg/kg, every 6 hours for the first 4 days of therapy
Initial dose of dexamethasone should be given before or with the initial dose of antimicrobial therapy
Concomitant use of an intravenous H_2 antagonist is recommended

FIGURE 1-68 Adjunctive therapy in bacterial meningitis. In experimental studies, dexamethasone has inhibited the production of the inflammatory cytokines, tumor necrosis factor–alpha and interleukin-1; decreased cerebral edema and intracranial pressure; and decreased the leakage of serum proteins into the CSF by minimizing the damage to the blood-brain barrier. In clinical trials, dexamethasone has reduced the frequency of bilateral sensorineural hearing loss in patients with bacterial meningitis and reduced the inflammation in the subarachnoid space. The American Academy of Pediatrics recommends the consideration of dexamethasone therapy in infants and children 2 months of age and older with proven or suspected bacterial meningitis. Although the clinical trials to determine the efficacy of dexamethasone in adults with bacterial meningitis have not been completed, dexamethasone is most likely beneficial in adults as well, as the pathophysiology of bacterial meningitis in children and adults is the same.

Clinical trials of dexamethasone in bacterial meningitis

Author, year	Study population	Findings associated with dexamethasone use
Lebel, 1988	200 infants and children with Hib meningitis	Reduced bilateral sensorineural hearing loss vs antimicrobial therapy alone
Odio, 1991	101 infants and children with bacterial meningitis	Improved opening CSF lumbar pressure, cerebral perfusion pressure, and CSF abnormalities within 12 hrs of administration; had significantly better clinical condition at 24 hrs
Girgis, 1989	106 adults and children with pneumococcal meningitis	Significant decrease in mortality
Schaad, 1993	115 children with acute bacterial meningitis	Significant decrease in neurologic and audiologic sequelae

FIGURE 1-69 Dexamethasone as adjunctive therapy in bacterial meningitis. All clinical trials to date demonstrate the efficacy of adjunctive therapy with dexamethasone. Lebel *et al.* conducted two consecutive prospective, double-blind, placebo-controlled trials in 200 infants and children with bacterial meningitis. In these clinical trials, the children with *Haemophilus influenzae* type b (Hib) meningitis who received dexamethasone in addition to antimicrobial therapy had a significantly reduced frequency of bilateral sensorineural hearing loss as compared to the placebo group who received antimicrobial therapy only. (Lebel MH, *et al.*: Dexamethasone therapy for bacterial meningitis: Results of two double-blind, placebo-controlled trials. *N Engl J Med* 1988, 319:964–971.) Odio *et al.* conducted a placebo-controlled, double-blind trial of dexamethasone therapy in 101 infants and children with bacterial meningitis. The initial dose of dexamethasone was administered before the initial dose of antibiotic. In the dexamethasone group, there was a significant improvement in the opening lumbar CSF pressure, the estimated cerebral perfusion pressure, and the CSF lactate, leukocyte, glucose, and protein concentrations within 12 hours compared to the children who received antimicrobial therapy only. The rapid improvement in these indices of inflammation correlated with a significantly better clinical condition in the dexamethasone-treated patients after a 24-hour treatment period. (Odio CM, *et al.*: The beneficial effects of early dexamethasone administration in infants and children with bacterial meningitis. *N Engl J Med* 1991, 324:1525–1531.) In the study by Girgis *et al.*, the use of dexamethasone therapy was associated with a significant decrease in mortality in patients with pneumococcal meningitis. (Girgis NI, *et al.*: Dexamethasone treatment for bacterial meningitis in children and adults. *Pediatr Infect Dis J* 1989, 8:848–851.) Schaad *et al.* conducted a prospective study of dexamethasone in 115 children with acute bacterial meningitis and demonstrated a significant decrease in neurologic and audiologic sequelae. At follow-up examinations 3, 9, and 15 months after hospital discharge, nine (16%) of 55 placebo recipients and three (5%) of 60 dexamethasone recipients had one or more neurologic or audiologic sequelae ($P = 0.066$). (Schaad UB, *et al.*: Dexamethasone therapy for bacterial meningitis in children. *Lancet* 1993, 342:457–461.)

Experimental adjunctive therapies
Leukocyte monoclonal antibodies
Anticytokine antibodies
Pentoxifylline
Nonsteroidal antiinflammatory agents

FIGURE 1-70 Experimental adjunctive therapies. Other adjunctive agents may have a role in the treatment of bacterial meningitis. Leukocyte monoclonal antibodies prevent circulating leukocytes from getting into the CSF, where in the subarachnoid space they contribute to the purulent exudate and obstruct the flow of CSF while doing little to eradicate the infection. The permeability of cerebral capillary endothelial cells is also increased by the adherence of leukocytes, thus allowing for the leakage of plasma proteins into the CSF. Antibodies to the many inflammatory cytokines that contribute to meningeal inflammation may have a role in limiting the degree of inflammation in the subarachnoid space. Pentoxifylline, likewise, may help reduce the meningeal inflammatory response. Nonsteroidal antiinflammatory agents inhibit prostaglandin synthesis, counteracting the production-stimulating effects of the inflammatory cytokines tumor necrosis factor and interleukin-1. Prostaglandins are potent mediators of inflammation.

Prognosis

Mortality with treatment

Organism	Percent
Haemophilus influenzae	3–6
Neisseria meningitis	5–10
Streptococcus pneumoniae	20–35
Escherichia coli	30
Listeria monocytogenes	15–40
Group B streptococci	10–30

FIGURE 1-71 Mortality of bacterial meningitis with treatment. The mortality from *Streptococcus pneumoniae*, *Escherichia coli*, and *Listeria monocytogenes* meningitis is high despite adequate antimicrobial treatment. The mortality is due to the underlying conditions that predispose to infection with these organisms and to the systemic and neurologic complications associated with bacterial meningitis.

PREVENTION

Chemoprophylaxis for meningococcal meningitis

Recommended for close contacts:
- Household
- Day care centers
- Medical personnel

Rifampin dosages:
- Adults 600 mg orally q12h × 2 d
- Children 10 mg/kg orally q12h × 2 d
- Neonates < 1 mo 5 mg/kg orally q12h × 2 d

FIGURE 1-72 Chemoprophylaxis for meningococcal meningitis. Chemoprophylaxis for eradication of bacteria from the nasopharynx with rifampin is recommended for all close contacts of any individuals with meningococcal meningitis. A single oral dose of ciprofloxacin (750 mg) has also been demonstrated to be efficacious in the eradication of the carrier state in meningococcal infection.

Chemoprophylaxis for *Haemophilus influenzae* type b meningitis

Recommended for close contacts and patient:
- Household
- Day care centers
- Medical personnel
- Patient

Rifampin dosages:
- Adults 600 mg/d orally × 4 d
- Children 20 mg/kg orally (max. 600 mg/d) × 4 d
- Neonates < 1 mo 10 mg/kg/d orally × 4 d

FIGURE 1-73 Chemoprophylaxis for *Haemophilus influenzae* type b meningitis. Chemoprophylaxis with rifampin for meningitis due to *H. influenzae* is recommended not only for close contacts of patients with Hib meningitis, but also for the patient, as the meningeal pathogen is usually not eradicated from the nasopharynx by systemic antimicrobial therapy. Rifampin is not recommended for pregnant women.

Recommendations for use of the Hib conjugate vaccine
1. Vaccinate all infants at age 2, 4, and 6 mo Unvaccinated infants 7–11 mo of age should receive two doses 2 mo apart Unvaccinated children 12–14 mo of age should receive one dose plus a booster dose after 15 mo of age
2. Unvaccinated children 15–60 mo of age should receive a single dose and do not require a booster
3. Children > 60 mo should be vaccinated based on disease risk (asplenia, sickle-cell disease, immunosuppressive malignancy)
4. Use of Hib vaccine does not preclude rifampin prophylaxis of Hib contacts or timing of other vaccines
5. Children with a history of invasive Hib disease or vaccinated at ≥ age 24 mo with PRP vaccine do not need revaccination

FIGURE 1-74 Recommendations for use of the Hib conjugate vaccine. The routine use of the *Haemophilus influenzae* type b (Hib) conjugate vaccine in children has significantly decreased the incidence of meningitis due to this pathogen. PRP—*H. influenzae* b polysaccharide. (CDC: Standards for pediatric immunization practices. *MMWR* 1993, 42(RR-5):1. *Adapted from* Roos KL, Tunkel AR, Scheld WM: Acute bacterial meningitis in children and adults. *In* Scheld WM, Whitley RJ, Durack DT (eds.): *Infections of the Central Nervous System*. New York: Raven Press; 1991:335–410; with permission.)

SELECTED BIBLIOGRAPHY

Roos KL, Tunkel AR, Scheld WM: Acute bacterial meningitis in children and adults. *In* Scheld WM, Whitley RJ, Durack DT, eds.: *Infections of the Central Nervous System*. New York: Raven Press; 1991:335–410.

Fishman RA: *Cerebrospinal Fluid in Diseases of the Nervous System*, 2nd ed. Philadelphia: W.B. Saunders Company; 1992.

Roos KL: New treatment strategies for bacterial meningitis. *Clin Neuropharmacol* 1993, 16:373–386.

Pfister W, Roos KL: The neurocritical care of bacterial meningitis. *In* Hacke W, Hanley DF, Einhaupl KM, *et al.*, eds.: *Neurocritical Care*. Berlin: Springer-Verlag; 1994: 377–397.

CHAPTER 2

Subacute and Chronic Meningitides

Allan R. Tunkel
Sidney E. Croul

Etiology and Diagnosis

Diseases sometimes resembling chronic meningitis
Infectious etiologies
Aseptic meningitis
Viral and nonviral encephalitis
Partially treated bacterial meningitis
Parameningeal infections
Infective endocarditis
Noninfectious etiologies
Metabolic and other encephalopathies
Brain tumor
Subarachnoid hemorrhage
Subdural hematoma
Multiple sclerosis
Systemic lupus erythematosus
Postinfectious encephalitis
Giant cell arteritis
Thrombotic thrombocytopenic purpura

Figure 2-1 Diseases resembling chronic meningitis. A number of infectious conditions may cause syndromes resembling chronic meningitis superficially, but these are usually distinguishable from it on clinical grounds at presentation or during evaluation and observation of the patient. (*From* Gripshover BM, Ellner JJ: Chronic meningitis. *In* Mandell GL, Bennett JE, Dolin R (eds.): *Principles and Practice of Infectious Diseases*, 4th ed. New York: Churchill-Livingstone; 1994:868; with permission.)

Common causes of chronic meningitis

Infectious	Noninfectious
Mycobacterium tuberculosis	Carcinoma
Cryptococcus neoformans	Sarcoid
Treponema pallidum	Granulomatous angiitis
Coccidioides immitis	Systemic lupus erythematosus
Histoplasma capsulatum	Behçet's disease
Borrelia burgdorferi	Vogt-Koyanagi-Harada syndrome

Figure 2-2 Common causes of chronic meningitis. (*From* Tucker T, Ellner JJ: Chronic meningitis. *In* Scheld WM, Whitley RJ, Durack DT (eds.): *Infections of the Central Nervous System*. New York: Raven Press; 1991:704; with permission.)

Infectious causes of chronic meningitis

Tuberculosis	Actinomycosis
Cryptococcosis	Phaeohyphomycosis (chromomycosis)
Coccidioidomycosis	Cysticercosis
Histoplasmosis	Rarer etiologies
Candidiasis	*Pseudallescheria boydii*
Blastomycosis	*Sporothrix schenckii*
Syphilis	Agents of mucormycosis
Brucellosis	*Coenurus cerebralis*
Toxoplasmosis	*Leptospira icterohaemorrhagiae*
Nocardiosis	*Angiostrongylus cantonensis*
Lyme disease	

Figure 2-3 Infectious causes of chronic meningitis. Blastomycosis, toxoplasmosis, nocardiosis, actinomycosis, phaeohypomycosis, and cysticercosis more commonly occur as brain abscesses or focal lesions. (*From* Katzman M, Ellner JJ: Chronic meningitis. *In* Mandell GL, Douglas RG, Bennett JE (eds.): *Principles and Practice of Infectious Diseases*, 3rd ed. New York: Churchill-Livingstone; 1990:758; with permission.)

Noninfectious causes of chronic meningitis
Neoplasm
Sarcoidosis
Granulomatous angiitis
Uveomeningoencephalitis
Behçet's disease
Chronic benign lymphocytic meningitis
Chronic meningitis of unknown etiology

Figure 2-4 Noninfectious causes of chronic meningitis. The noninfectious diseases causing chronic meningitis may be difficult to diagnose and distinguish from occult infections. (*From* Gripshover BM, Ellner JJ: Chronic meningitis. *In* Mandell GL, Bennett JE, Dolin R (eds.): *Principles and Practice of Infectious Diseases*, 4th ed. New York: Churchill-Livingstone; 1994:865; with permission.)

A. Differential diagnosis of chronic meningitis by predominant type of CSF inflammatory response: viral and bacterial causes

	Lymphocytic	Neutrophilic	Eosinophilic
Viral			
Lymphocytic choriomeningitis	x		
Mumps	x		
Herpes simplex	x	x	
Herpes zoster	x		
Arbovirus	x		
Flavivirus	x		
Echovirus	x		
Bacterial			
Tuberculosis	x	x	x
Brucellosis	x	x	
Tularemia	x		
Syphilis	x		x
Lyme disease	x		
Leptospirosis	x		
Recurrent fever	x		
Nocardiosis	x	x	
Actinomycosis	x	x	
Listeriosis	x	x	
Subacute bacterial endocarditis	x		
Meningococcus in complement deficiency		x	

B. Differential diagnosis of chronic meningitis by predominant type of CSF inflammatory response: fungal and parasitic causes

	Lymphocytic	Neutrophilic	Eosinophilic
Fungal			
Cryptococcosis	x		
Coccidioidomycosis	x	x	x
Candidiasis	x	x	
Histoplasmosis	x	x	
Blastomycosis	x	x	
Aspergillosis	x	x	
Dermatomycosis	x	x	
Zygomycosis	x	x	
Pseudallescheria boydii	x	x	
Parasitic			
Cysticercosis	x		x
Paragonimiasis	x		x
Schistosomiasis	x		x
Fascioliasis	x		x
Echinococcosis	x		x
Trichinosis	x		x
Visceral larva migrans	x		x
Angiostrongylus cantonensis			x
Gnathostoma spinigerum			x

FIGURE 2-5 Differential diagnosis of chronic meningitis by predominant type of cerebrospinal fluid (CSF) inflammatory response. Knowledge of the inflammatory cell type in the CSF in patients with chronic meningitis is useful for formulating the appropriate differential diagnosis and is the basis for categorizing the specific disease entities. **A**, Viral and bacterial causes. **B**, Fungal and parasitic causes. (*continued*)

C. Differential diagnosis of chronic meningitis by predominant type of CSF inflammatory response: noninfectious and other causes

	Lymphocytic	Neutrophilic	Eosinophilic
Noninfectious disease			
Solid neoplasm	x	x	
Lymphoma	x		x
Leukemia	x		
Sarcoidosis	x	x	x
Vasculitis	x		
Collagen vascular disease	x		
Behçet's disease	x		
Vogt-Koyanagi-Harada syndrome	x		
Foreign body in CNS		x	x
Drug or chemical toxicity		x	
Other			
Parameningeal focus	x	x	
Benign chronic lymphocytic meningitis	x		

Figure 2-5 (*continued*) **C**, Noninfectious and other causes. (*Adapted from* Hirsch DJ, Harris AA, Levin S: Chronic meningitis. *In* Gorbach SL, Bartlett JG, Blacklow NR (eds.): *Infectious Diseases.* Philadelphia: W.B. Saunders; 1992:1182; with permission.)

Causes of chronic meningitis resulting in low CSF glucose concentrations

Mycobacterial meningitis
Fungal meningitis
Carcinomatous meningitis
Meningeal cysticercosis/trichinosis
Drug-induced meningitis (NSAIDs)
Acute syphilitic meningitis
Chemical meningitis (direct intrathecal injections)
Viral meningitis (occasionally; *ie*, mumps)
Rheumatoid meningitis
Lupus myelopathy
Amebic meningitis

Figure 2-6 Causes of chronic meningitis resulting in low CSF glucose concentrations. Hypoglycorrhachia in a patient with meningitis suggests an infectious cause, but noninfectious processes also can produce low CSF glucose concentrations. NSAIDs—nonsteroidal antiinflammatory drugs. (*Adapted from* Perfect JR: Diagnosis and treatment of fungal meningitis. *In* Scheld WM, Whitley RJ, Durack DT (eds.): *Infections of the Central Nervous System.* New York: Raven Press; 1991:730; with permission.)

A. Diagnostic evaluation of chronic meningitis for all patients

Complete blood count
Chemistry panel
Blood, urine, and sputum cultures
Chest radiography
Head CT with contrast enhancement
ANA, RF, ESR
Serologic tests for histoplasmosis, coccidioidomycosis, syphilis, Lyme disease
Skin test with 5 TU PPD (second-strength PPD and anergy profile if intermediate test is negative)
CSF examination:

Glucose	Protein
Cell count	India ink stain
Culture for bacteria, fungus, AFB	CSF VDRL
Cryptococcal antigen and antibody	Cytology

Figure 2-7 Diagnostic evaluation of chronic meningitis. **A**, Suggested diagnostic evaluation for all patients with chronic meningitis. History and physical examination are the major tools for the diagnosis. Laboratory confirmation of the suspected diagnosis is often difficult. CSF cultures should optimally propagate the pathogen, or serologic studies should suggest local antibody production. The CSF formula (*ie*, cell count and differential, glucose, and protein) is rarely diagnostic but assists in guiding therapy. (*continued*)

B. Diagnostic evaluation of chronic meningitis: additional studies

CSF serologic examination:

Histoplasmosis	Coccidioidomycosis
Borreliosis	Aspergillosis
Sporotrichosis tuberculous	Brucellosis

CSF for tuberculous antigens or antibodies, IgG-albumin ratio
Serum or CSF cultures for *Brucella*
MRI of head or spine for parameningeal and parenchymal lesions
EEG
Biopsy of enlarged lymph node
Bone marrow and liver biopsy for pathology and culture
Skin and muscle biopsy for vasculitis or sarcoid
Cerebral angiography

Figure 2-7 (*continued*) **B**, Additional studies, if indicated. AFB—acid-fast bacilli; ANA—antinuclear antibody; CT—computed tomography; EEG—electroencephalography; ESR—erythrocyte sedimentation rate; MRI—magnetic resonance imaging; PPD—purified protein derivative; RF—rheumatoid factor; TU—tuberculin units. (*Adapted from* Hirsch DJ, Harris AA, Levin S: Chronic meningitis. *In* Gorbach SL, Bartlett JG, Blacklow NR (eds.): *Infectious Diseases*. Philadelphia: W.B. Saunders; 1992:1181; with permission.)

Spirochetal Meningitis

Neurosyphilis

Classification of neurosyphilis

Asymptomatic	Parenchymal
Meningovascular	General paresis
Syphilitic meningitis	Tabes dorsalis
Cerebrovascular	Taboparesis
Gumma	Ocular
Spinal	Otic
	Congenital syphilis

Figure 2-8 Classification of neurosyphilis. Dissemination of *Treponema pallidum* is associated with vague symptoms, including headache or stiff neck, photophobia, and nonspecific flu-like symptoms. If these patients are not treated, almost 10% eventually develop late (tertiary stage) disease involving the central nervous system (CNS). Individual patients often have combinations of these syndromes. (*From* Coyle PK, Dattwyler R: Spirochetal infection of the central nervous system. *Infect Dis Clin North Am* 1990, 4:732; with permission.)

Relative frequencies of major types of neurosyphilis

	Frequency, %	
Type	1932–1942	1970–1980
Asymptomatic	27	20
Acute syphilitic meningitis	4	2
Meningovascular	15	34
General paresis	17	28
Tabes dorsalis	37	16

Figure 2-9 Relative frequencies of major types of neurosyphilis. There is a decreased frequency of tabes dorsalis since the introduction of antibiotics. (*From* Davis LE: Spirochetal disease. *In* Asbury AK, McKhann GM, McDonald WI (eds.): *Diseases of the Nervous System: Clinical Neurobiology*, 2nd ed. Philadelphia: W.B. Saunders; 1992:1361; with permission.)

Time course of CNS involvement in syphilis

Stage	Peak incidence, *yrs*
Asymptomatic neurosyphilis	Any time
Syphilitic meningitis	1–2
Meningovascular syphilis	6–8
Parenchymatous neurosyphilis	
General paresis	8–10
Tabes dorsalis	15–20
Gummatous neurosyphilis	Any time

Figure 2-10 Time course of CNS involvement in syphilis. Clinical neurosyphilis syndromes can be divided into several distinct clinical syndromes which tend to occur at somewhat different points in the natural history of untreated syphilis. (Hook EW III: Central nervous system syphilis. *In* Scheld WM, Whitley RJ, Durack DT (eds.): *Infections of the Central Nervous System*. New York: Raven Press; 1991:644.)

Clinical manifestations of neurosyphilis

- Meningovascular
  - Hemiplegia or hemiparesis
  - Seizures
    - Generalized
    - Focal
  - Aphasia
- General paresis
  - Changes in personality, affect, sensorium, intellect, insight, judgment
  - Hyperactive reflexes
  - Speech disturbances (slurring)
  - Pupillary disturbances (Argyll Robertson pupils)
  - Optic atrophy tremors (face, tongue, hands, legs)
- Tabes dorsalis
  - Shooting or lightning pains
  - Ataxia
  - Pupillary disturbances (Argyll Robertson pupils)
  - Impotence
  - Bladder disturbances
  - Fecal incontinence
  - Peripheral neuropathy
  - Romberg's sign
  - Cranial nerve involvement (II–VII)

Figure 2-11 Clinical manifestation of neurosyphilis. (*From* Tramont EC: *Treponema pallidum* (syphilis). *In* Mandell GL, Bennett JE, Dolin R (eds.): *Principles and Practice of Infectious Diseases*, 4th ed. New York: Churchill-Livingstone; 1994:2124; with permission.)

Clinical features of meningovascular syphilis

- Peak incidence 5–7 yrs after infection
- Abrupt onset of stroke syndromes following prodrome
  - Hemiparesis (80%)
  - Aphasia (30%)
  - Seizures (14%)
- Focal neurologic deficits result from vasculitis of small- to medium-sized arterial blood vessels
- Cerebral infarctions evident on CT or MRI

Figure 2-12 Clinical features of meningovascular syphilis. Meningovascular syphilis is found in 10% to 12% of individuals with CNS involvement, occurring months to years following the initial acquisition of syphilis (peak incidence ~ 7 years), and is characterized by an obliterative endarteritis affecting the small blood vessels of the meninges, brain, and spinal cord. The clinical symptoms and signs of progressive syphilitic vasculitis may result from the accompanying local inflammation, transient vascular insufficiency related to spasm of involved vessels, lasting tissue hypoxia related to irreversible vascular involvement, or the fibrosis and scarring following hypoxic damage. Most patients experience weeks to months of episodic prodromal symptoms and signs including headache or vertiginous episodes, personality changes (*eg*, apathy or inattention), behavioral changes (*eg*, irritability or memory impairment), insomnia, or occasional seizures. Focal deficits reflecting episodes of ischemia to regions of the brain by involved vessels may also occur.

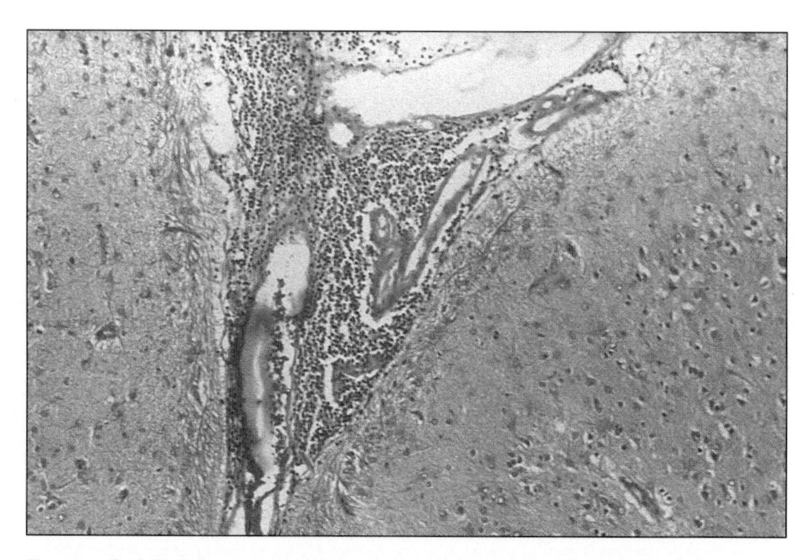

Figure 2-13 Meningovascular involvement in neurosyphilis demonstrating lymphoplasmacytic meningeal infiltrate in sulcus. There is neuronal loss and marked gliosis in the underlying cortex. (Hematoxylin-eosin stain.) (From *Infectious Diseases: Text and Color Atlas*, 2nd ed. by WE Farrar, MJ Wood, JA Innes, H Tubbs. Gower Medical Publishing; an imprint of Times Mirror International Publishers Ltd., London, UK, 1992; with permission. *Courtesy of* Dr. P. Garen.)

Signs and symptoms of general paresis

Personality	Irritability, emotional lability (agitation, euphoria, depression), paranoia
Affect	Carelessness of appearance, apathy, expressionless facies, inappropriate behavior
Reflex	Abnormal reflexes (usually hyperactive), tremors of tongue, hands, face
Eye	Pupillary abnormalities, Argyll Robertson pupils
Sensorium	Illusions, hallucinations, delusions of grandeur
Intellect	Memory loss, impaired learning, lack of insight, confusion, disorientation
Speech	Slurred speech

FIGURE 2-14 Signs and symptoms of general paresis. General paresis is relatively rare today and does not become apparent until 10 to 20 years following acquisition of infection. There is probable invasion of the brain substance by spirochetes with destruction of nerve cells, principally in the cerebral cortex. Clinical manifestations include changes in personality, intellect, affect, and judgment; abnormalities correspond to the mnemonic "paresis." (*From* Tramont EC: Syphilis of the central nervous system. *In* Lambert HP (ed.): *Infections of the Central Nervous System.* Philadelphia: B.C. Decker; 1991:212; with permission.)

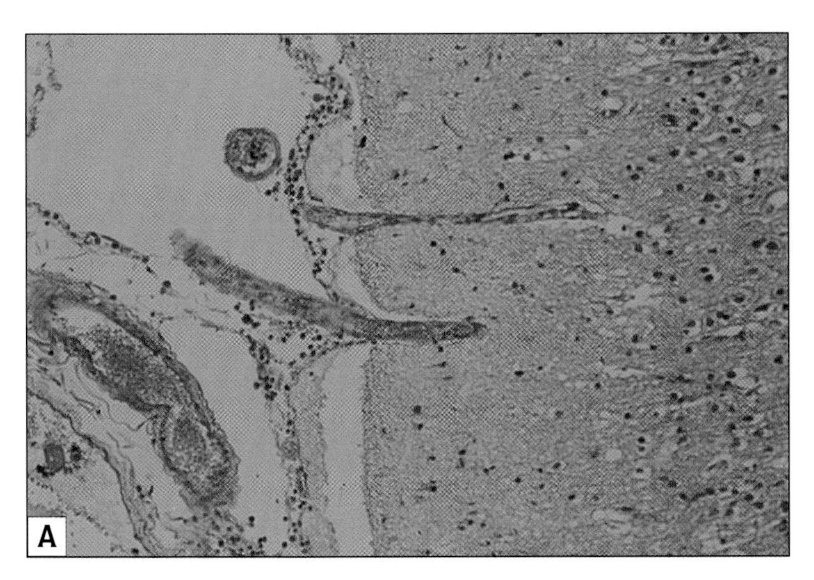

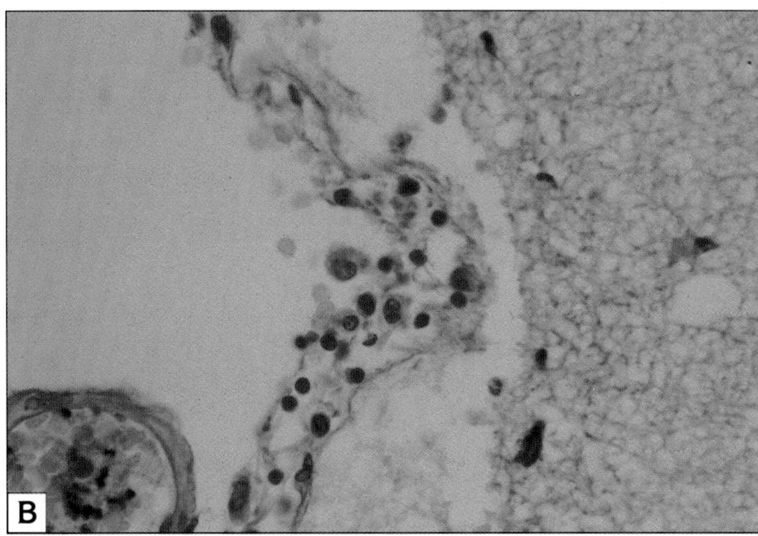

FIGURE 2-15 Brain invasion in general paresis. **A**, Compared with Figure 2-13, the cellular infiltrate is much less marked. In the superficial layers, there is marked loss of neurons. **B**, A higher power view reveals the predominance of plasma cells.

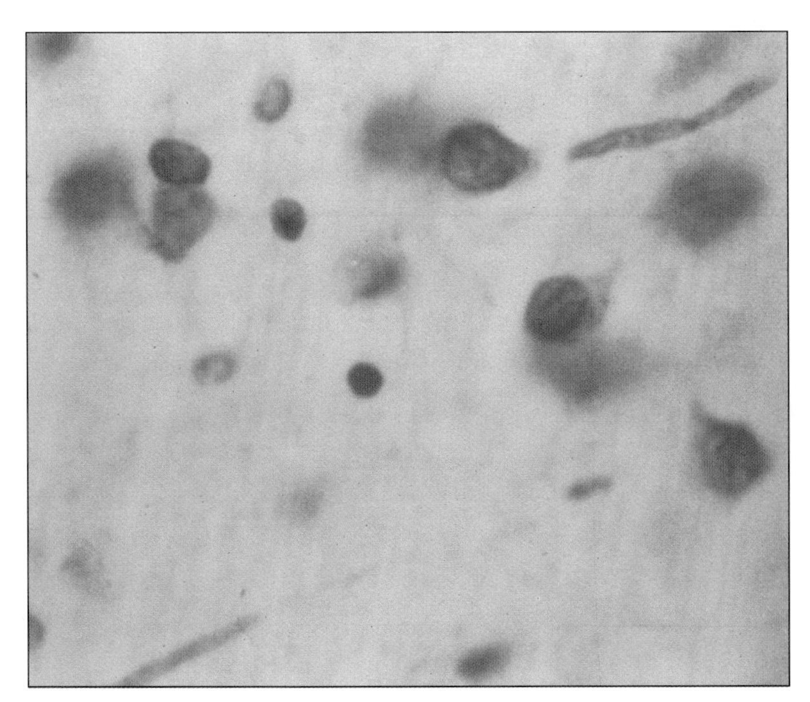

FIGURE 2-16 Microglial rod cells in general paresis. Histologic section of the frontal cortex reveals elongate nuclei of microglial rod cells. The finding of rod cells is a hallmark of general paresis and connotes activation of resident microglial cells in response to the primary disease process (Nissl stain). (From *Infectious Diseases: Text and Color Atlas*, 2nd ed. by WE Farrar, MJ Wood, JA Innes, H Tubbs. Gower Medical Publishing; an imprint of Times Mirror International Publishers Ltd., London, UK, 1992; with permission.)

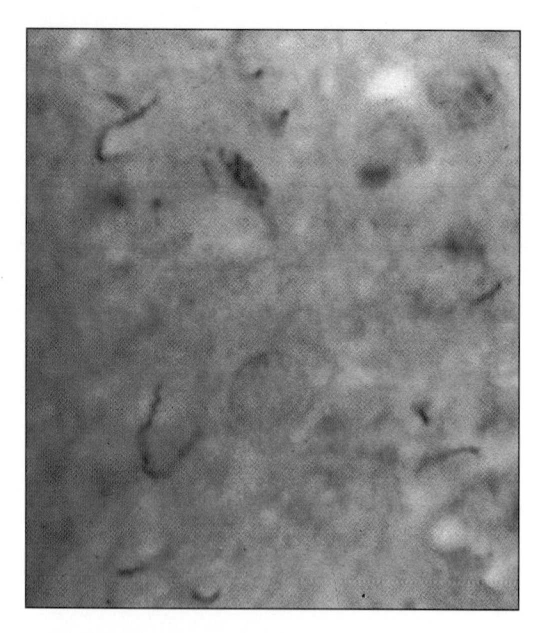

FIGURE 2-17 Histologic section of the frontal cortex showing the corkscrew appearance of spirochetes in general paresis. (Levaditi silver stain.) (From *Infectious Diseases: Text and Color Atlas*, 2nd ed. by WE Farrar, MJ Wood, JA Innes, H Tubbs. Gower Medical Publishing; an imprint of Times Mirror International Publishers Ltd., London, UK, 1992; with permission.)

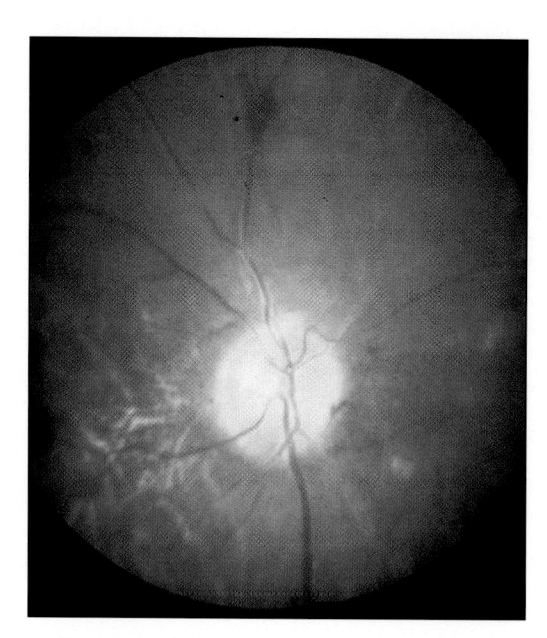

FIGURE 2-18 Optic atrophy in general paresis. Ocular manifestations of neurosyphilis include the Argyll Robertson pupil and optic atrophy. (From *Infectious Diseases: Text and Color Atlas*, 2nd ed. by WE Farrar, MJ Wood, JA Innes, H Tubbs. Gower Medical Publishing; an imprint of Times Mirror International Publishers Ltd., London, UK, 1992; with permission.)

Signs and symptoms of tabes dorsalis

Signs and symptoms	Range, %
Pupillary abnormalities (Argyll Robertson pupils)	94–97
Absent reflexes, lower extremities	78–94
Lightening pains	70–75
Romberg's sign	51–55
Impaired position sense	44–45
Ataxia	42–46
Bladder disturbances	28–33
Visual loss	16–43
Impaired vibratory sense	17–52
Visceral crisis	15–18
Impaired pain sense	13–18
Cranial nerve palsy	9–10
Paresthesias	7–24
Charcot joints	6–7
Anal sphincter atony	3–14
Perforating ulcers (mal perforans)	5–6

FIGURE 2-19 Signs and symptoms of tabes dorsalis. Clinically, tabes dorsalis is characterized by concurrent development of a broad-based ataxic gait, foot slap, paresthesias, lightening pains, positive Romberg's sign, hyporeflexia, degenerative joint disease (Charcot joint), impotence, disturbance of bowel and bladder function, and sensory losses. (*From* Tramont EC: Syphilis of the central nervous system. *In* Lambert HP (ed.): *Infections of the Central Nervous System*. Philadelphia: B.C. Decker; 1991:213; with permission.)

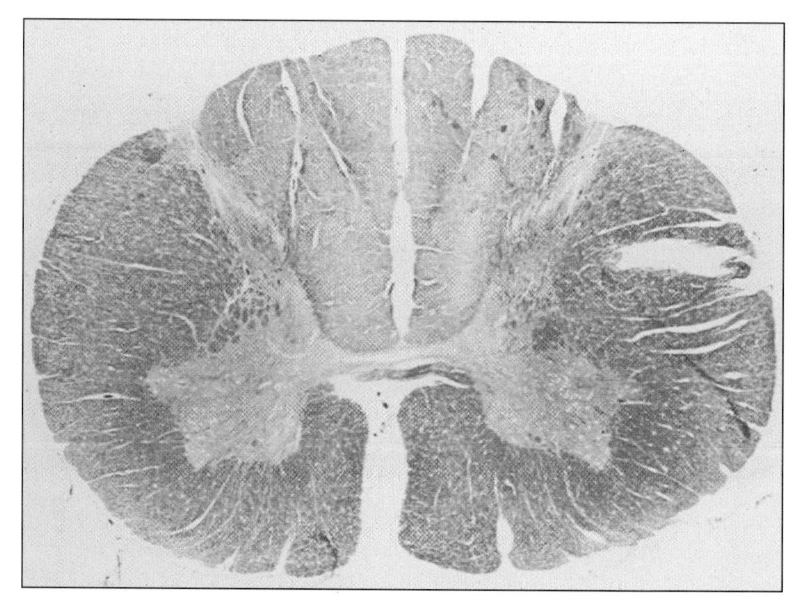

FIGURE 2-20 Degeneration of the posterior columns of spinal cord in tabes dorsalis. Tabes dorsalis is characterized by degeneration of the posterior columns of the spinal cord, dorsal root ganglia, and dorsal roots. (Myelin stain.) (From *Infectious Diseases: Text and Color Atlas*, 2nd ed. by WE Farrar, MJ Wood, JA Innes, H Tubbs. Gower Medical Publishing; an imprint of Times Mirror International Publishers Ltd., London, UK, 1992; with permission. *Courtesy of* Dr. H. Whitwell.)

CSF findings in neurosyphilis	
Measure	**Value**
Elevated opening pressure (> 200 mm H_2O)	10%
Total white blood cells	10–500/mm^3
% mononuclear	50%–99%
Total red blood cells	0–5/mm^3
Glucose level	35–75 mg/dL
Total protein level	30–250 mg/dL
Elevated gamma globulin level (> 11% of total protein)	>70%
Oligoclonal bands	>50%
Reactive with CSF VDRL test	50%–85%
Reactive with CSF FTA-ABS test	75%–95%

FIGURE 2-21 Cerebrospinal fluid findings in neurosyphilis. These changes in CSF parameters are seen in virtually all stages of neurosyphilis. For diagnosis of CNS involvement, no single routine laboratory test is definitive. Although the specificity of the CSF VDRL for the diagnosis of neurosyphilis is high, the specificity is low (reactive tests in only 50% to 85% of patients). The CSF fluorescent treponemal antibody absorption (FTA-ABS) test has also been examined as a possible diagnostic test for neurosyphilis; a nonreactive test effectively rules out the likelihood of neurosyphilis, but the specificity of the test is much less than that of the CSF VDRL because of the possibility of leakage of small amounts of antibody from the serum into CSF. From these data, the diagnosis of neurosyphilis is based upon elevated CSF concentrations of white blood cells and/or protein in the appropriate clinical and serologic setting. (*From* Davis LE: Spirochetal disease. *In* Asbury AK, McKhann GM, McDonald WI (eds.): *Diseases of the Nervous System: Clinical Neurobiology*, 2nd ed. Philadelphia: W.B. Saunders; 1992:1360; with permission.)

Recommended regimens for therapy of CNS syphilis	
Preferred regimen	
Aqueous crystalline penicillin G	12–24 MU/d iv q4h x 10–14 d
Alternate regimen	
Procaine penicillin	2.4 MU/d im x 10–14 d
plus	
Probenecid	500 mg po qid x 10–14 d

FIGURE 2-22 Recommended regimens for therapy of CNS syphilis. At present, the Centers for Disease Control and Prevention recommend high-dose parenteral penicillin as the drug of choice for therapy of syphilis in patients with CNS involvement. Alternative agents, such as the third-generation cephalosporins, chloramphenicol, and the tetracyclines, have not been adequately studied in patients to determine their efficacy in therapy for neurosyphilis. (*Adapted from* Hook EW III: Central nervous system syphilis. *In* Scheld WM, Whitley RJ, Durack DT (eds.): *Infections of the Central Nervous System*. New York: Raven Press; 1991:653; with permission.)

Lyme Disease

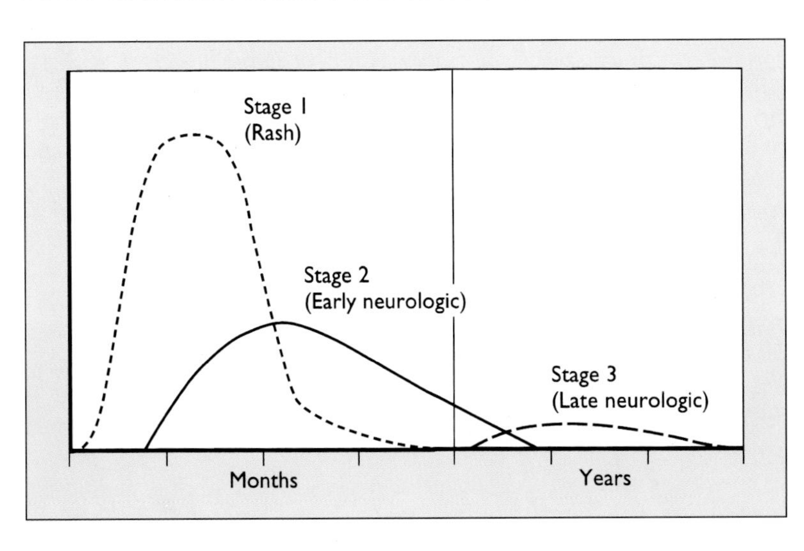

FIGURE 2-23 Stages of Lyme disease. The nervous system eventually is involved clinically in at least 10% to 15% of patients with Lyme disease, either early while erythema chronicum migrans is still present or 1 to 6 months later. (*From* Davis LE: Spirochetal disease. *In* Asbury AK, McKhann GM, McDonald WI (eds.): *Diseases of the Nervous System: Clinical Neurobiology*, 2nd ed. Philadelphia: W.B. Saunders; 1992:1365; with permission.)

Neurologic abnormalities in Lyme disease

Stage	CNS	PNS
I	Headache Neck stiffness without pleocytosis	
II	Lymphocytic meningitis Encephalitis Myelitis	Cranial neuritis Radiculitis Plexitis Mononeuritis Guillain-Barré syndrome
III	Progressive encephalomyelitis Late mental changes with MRI abnormalities Latent CNS borreliosis ? Amyotrophic lateral sclerosis ? Others	Distal axonopathy Neuropathy of ACA

Figure 2-24 Neurologic abnormalities in Lyme disease. ACA—acrodermatitis chronica atrophicans; PNS—peripheral nervous system. (*From* Reik L Jr: Lyme disease. *In* Scheld WM, Whitley RJ, Durack DT (eds.): *Infections of the Central Nervous System*. New York: Raven Press; 1991:668; with permission.)

Neurologic conditions in which Lyme disease should be considered

Acute aseptic meningitis	Cranial neuritis (Bell's palsy)
Chronic lymphocytic meningitis	Mononeuritis simplex or multiplex
Acute meningoencephalitis	Radiculoneuritis
Acute focal encephalitis	Plexitis
Brainstem encephalitis	Distal axonal neuropathy
Progressive encephalomyelitis	Demyelinating neuropathy
Cerebral demyelination	Carpal tunnel syndrome
Cerebral vasculitis	Focal myositis
Dementia	
Transverse myelitis	

Figure 2-25 Neurologic conditions in which Lyme disease should be considered. Lyme disease should be suspected in any patient with chronic lymphocytic meningitis or mild meningoencephalitis with superimposed cranial neuritis or radiculitis, although patients with other neurologic abnormalities may have the same illness. (*From* Reik L Jr: Lyme disease. *In* Scheld WM, Whitley RJ, Durack DT (eds.): *Infections of the Central Nervous System*. New York: Raven Press; 1991:678; with permission.)

Minimal diagnostic criteria for Lyme neuroborreliosis

Definite neuroborreliosis
- Compatible neurologic abnormality without other cause and with one of the following:
  - History of well-documented ECM
  - Presence of ACA
  - Serum *and* CSF immunoreactivity, or CSF reactivity alone, against *B. burgdorferi* by ELISA or Western blot
  - Both other organ system involvement typical of Lyme disease (*eg*, Lyme arthritis) and serum immunoreactivity to *B. burgdorferi*
  - Seroconversion or 4-fold rise in titer of *B. burgdorferi* antibody between acute and convalescent sera

Probable neuroborreliosis
- Compatible neurologic abnormality without other cause and with serum immunoreactivity to *B. burgdorferi*

Possible neuroborreliosis
- Compatible neurologic abnormality without other cause and with tick bite or travel or residence in endemic area

Figure 2-26 Minimal diagnostic criteria for Lyme neuroborreliosis. The best laboratory test for diagnosing Lyme disease is the demonstration of specific antibody to *Borrelia burgdorferi*; a positive test in a patient with a compatible neurologic abnormality is strong evidence of the diagnosis. However, even though laboratory tests are widely used, they are not standardized, and there is a great deal of interlaboratory variability. Specific antibody also appears in the CSF, and calculation of a specific antibody/IgG index for serum and CSF often indicates intrathecal synthesis of anti–*B. burgdorferi* antibody. ACA—acrodermatitis chronica atrophicans; ECM—erythema chronicum migrans; ELISA—enzyme-linked immunosorbent assay. (*From* Reik L Jr: Lyme disease. *In* Scheld WM, Whitley RJ, Durack DT (eds.): *Infections of the Central Nervous System*. New York: Raven Press; 1991:678; with permission.)

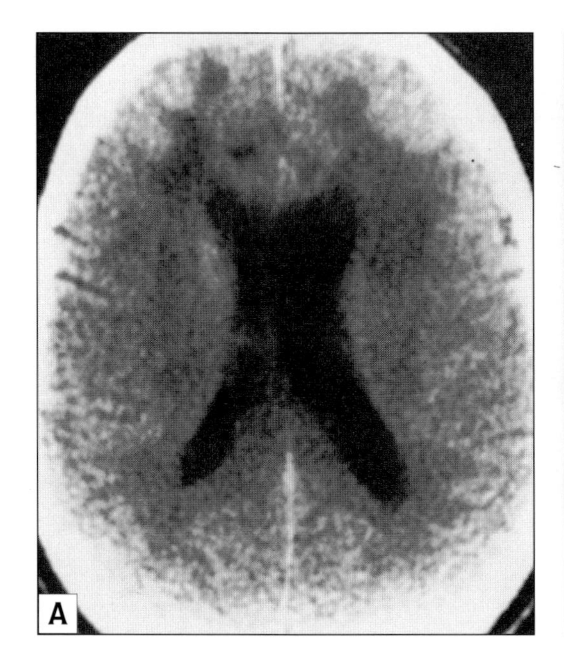

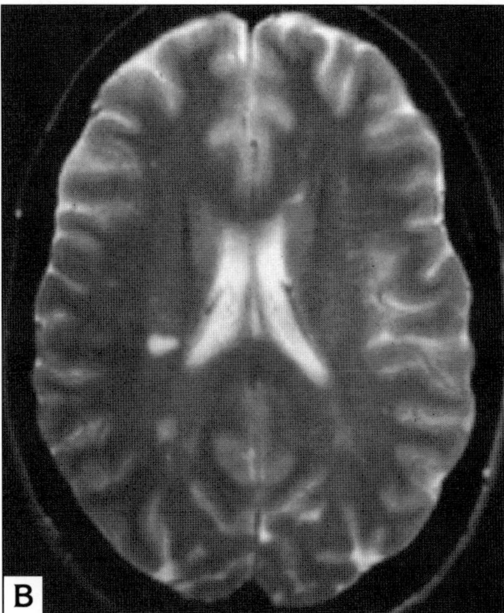

FIGURE 2-27 Radiologic findings in Lyme disease. Radiologic studies may be useful in patients with CNS manifestations of Lyme disease. CT has shown both enhancing and nonenhancing low-density lesions, mass effect, and cerebral demyelination. MRI may reveal punctate hyperresonant areas, without mass effect, within cerebral white matter. **A**, Postcontrast cranial CT scan demonstrates extensive areas of low density in the white matter of the frontal lobes and centrum semiovale in a patient with stage II Lyme disease and encephalitis. (*From* Reik L Jr: Lyme disease. *In* Scheld WM, Whitley RJ, Durack DT (eds.): *Infections of the Central Nervous System*. New York: Raven Press; 1991:672; with permission.) **B**, MRI scan (T2-weighted) in a patient with Lyme disease reveals areas of increased signal intensity in the cerebral white matter. (*From* Tunkel AR, Scheld WM: Acute meningitis. *In* Mandell GL, Bennett JE, Dolin CR (eds.): *Principles and Practice of Infectious Diseases*, 4th ed. New York: Churchill-Livingstone; 1994:847; with permission.)

Antibiotic therapy for neurologic abnormalities of Lyme disease

Facial palsy alone
Adults
- Amoxicillin, 500 mg orally qid x 2–4 wks (± probenecid, 500 mg orally qid)
- Doxycycline, 100 mg orally bid x 2–4 wks

Children
- Amoxicillin, 20–40 mg/kg/d orally qid x 2–4 wks
- Erythromycin, 30 mg/kg/d orally qid x 2–4 wks

All other neurologic abnormalities
Adults
- Ceftriaxone, 2 g/d iv x 2–4 wks
- Penicillin G, 20–24 MU/d iv for 10–14 d
- Doxycycline, 100 mg orally bid x 10–30 d *or* 200 mg iv x 2 d, then 100 mg/d iv x 8 d

Children
- Ceftriaxone, 50–80 mg/kg/d iv x 2–4 wks
- Penicillin G, 250,000 U/kg/d iv in divided doses

FIGURE 2-28 Antibiotic therapy for neurologic abnormalities of Lyme disease. The current recommendation is to treat most patients having Lyme meningitis with intravenous ceftriaxone at a dosage of 2 g/d for 2 to 4 weeks; the literature contains no agreement on the duration of therapy or on the minimal adequate dosage of antimicrobial. There is no evidence to support treatment durations longer than 4 weeks. No regimen has proven to be universally effective. (*Adapted from* Reik L Jr: Lyme disease. *In* Scheld WM, Whitley RS, Durack DT (eds.): *Infections of the Central Nervous System*. New York: Raven Press; 1991:681; with permission.)

Tuberculous Meningitis

Clinical staging of tuberculous meningitis

Stage	Features
Stage I (early)	Nonspecific symptoms and signs No clouding of consciousness No neurologic deficits
Stage II (intermediate)	Lethargy or alteration in behavior Meningeal irritation Minor neurologic deficits (cranial nerve palsies)
Stage III (advanced)	Abnormal movements Convulsions Stupor or coma Severe neurologic deficits (paresis)

Figure 2-29 Clinical staging of tuberculous meningitis. The clinical picture of tuberculous meningitis is quite variable, with substantial differences seen among patients of different ages. Therefore, a staging system was introduced to systematize the spectrum of clinical findings in tuberculous meningitis. Patients in stage I have only nonspecific manifestations of infection without neurologic signs or symptoms. In stage II, patients have symptoms and signs of meningeal irritation with cranial nerve palsies but no other neurologic deficits and no clouding of consciousness. In stage III, patients are severely ill with gross neurologic deficits, stupor, or coma. (*From* Zuger A, Lowy FD: Tuberculosis of the central nervous system. *In* Scheld WM, Whitley RJ, Durack DT (eds.): *Infections of the Central Nervous System*. New York: Raven Press; 1991:430; with permission.)

Clinical presentations of patients with tuberculous meningitis

	Children, %	Adults, %
Symptoms		
Headache	20–50	50–60
Nausea/vomiting	50–75	8–40
Apathy/behavioral changes	30–70	30–70
Seizures	10–20	0–13
Prior history of TB	55	8–12
Signs		
Fever	50–100	60–100
Meningismus	70–100	60–70
Cranial nerve palsy	15–30	15–40
Coma	30–45	20–30
PPD-positive	85–90	40–65

Figure 2-30 Clinical presentations of patients with tuberculous meningitis. Symptoms among adult patients are frequently, although not invariably, more specifically neurologic than they are among children. (*Adapted from* Zuger A, Lowy FD: Tuberculosis of the central nervous system. *In* Scheld WM, Whitley RJ, Durack DT (eds.): *Infections of the Central Nervous System*. New York: Raven Press; 1991:430–431; with permission.)

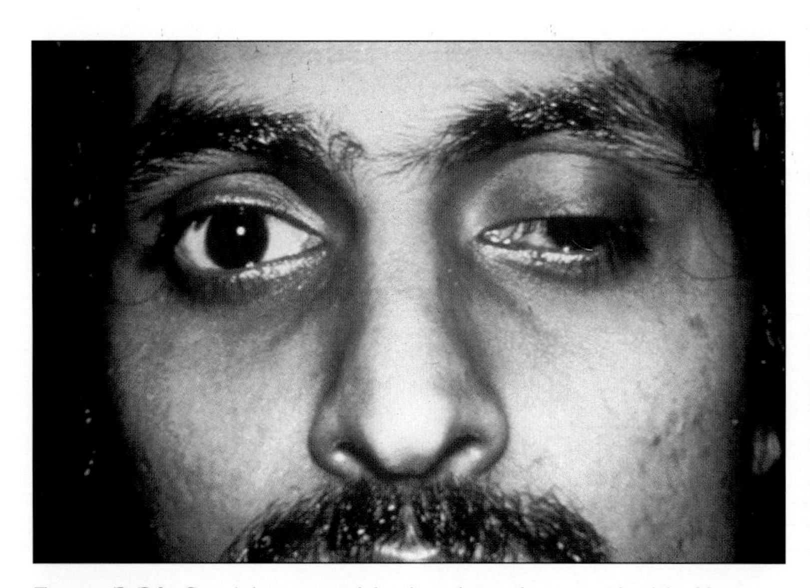

Figure 2-31 Cranial nerve palsies in tuberculous meningitis. Up to 30% of patients with tuberculous meningitis have focal neurologic signs on presentation, most frequently consisting of unilateral or, less commonly, bilateral cranial nerve palsies. The most frequently affected is cranial nerve VI, followed by cranial nerves III, IV, and VIII. During antituberculous therapy, this patient developed left cranial nerve III paralysis, shown here by ptosis and lateral deviation of the eye caused by unopposed action of the lateral rectus muscle. (From *Infectious Diseases: Text and Color Atlas*, 2nd ed. by WE Farrar, MJ Wood, JA Innes, H Tubbs. Gower Medical Publishing; an imprint of Times Mirror International Publishers Ltd., London, UK, 1992; with permission.)

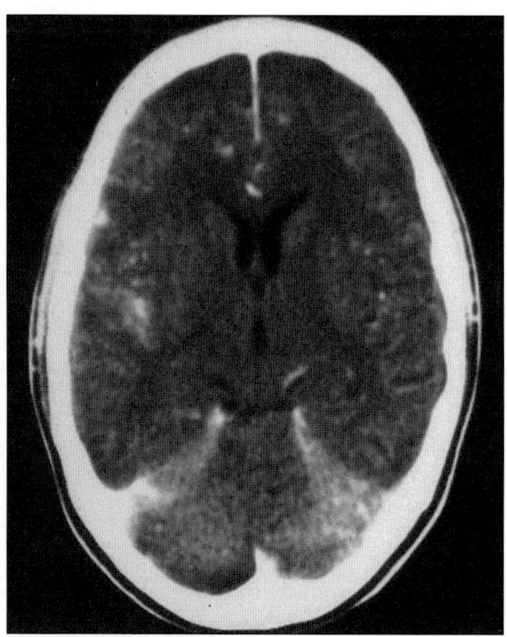

Figure 2-32 Cranial CT scan in a patient with tuberculous meningitis revealing basilar enhancement and periventricular lesions. There are no radiologic changes pathognomonic for a diagnosis of tuberculous meningitis. Enhancement of the basal cisterns, following the intravenous administration of contrast material, with widening and blurring of the basilar artery structures may be seen. Periventricular lucencies, reflecting the presence of tuberculous exudate and tubercle formation adjacent to the choroid and ependyma, may also be evident.

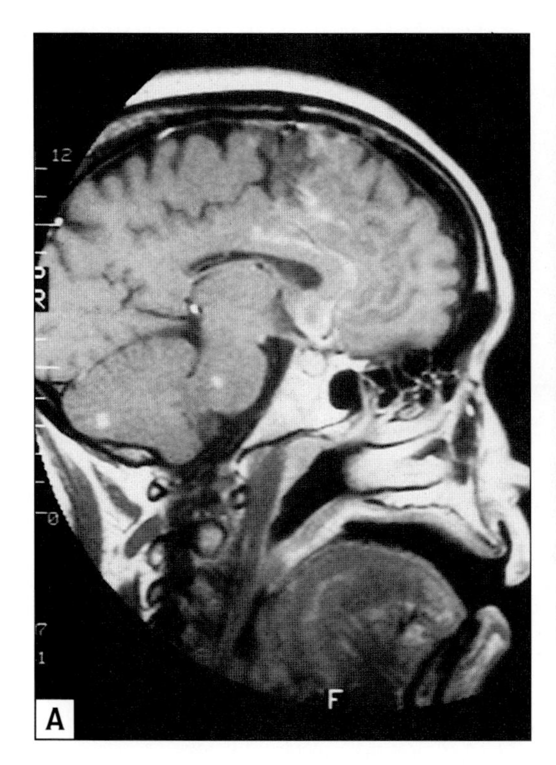

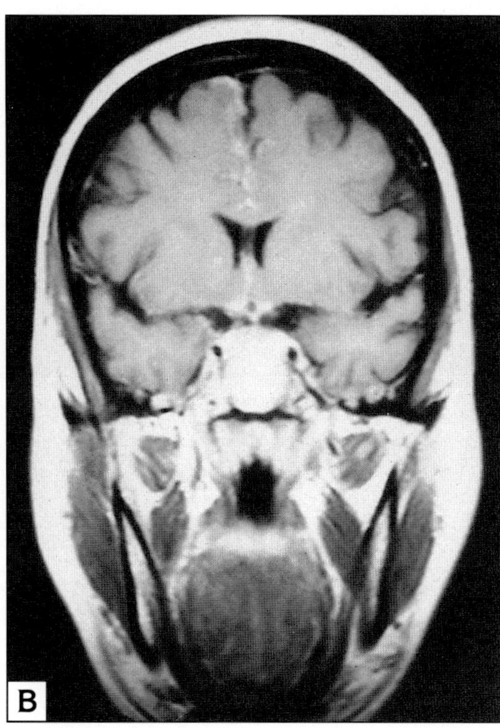

Figure 2-33 Cranial MRI in a patient with tuberculous meningitis revealing extensive leptomeningeal contrast enhancement. On this T1-weighted image with gadolinium, enhancement is particularly evident within the interhemispheric fissure; additional lesions are present in the pons and cerebellum. **A**, Sagittal view; **B**, Coronal view. MRI may be superior to CT scanning in the identification of basilar meningeal inflammation and small tuberculoma formation.

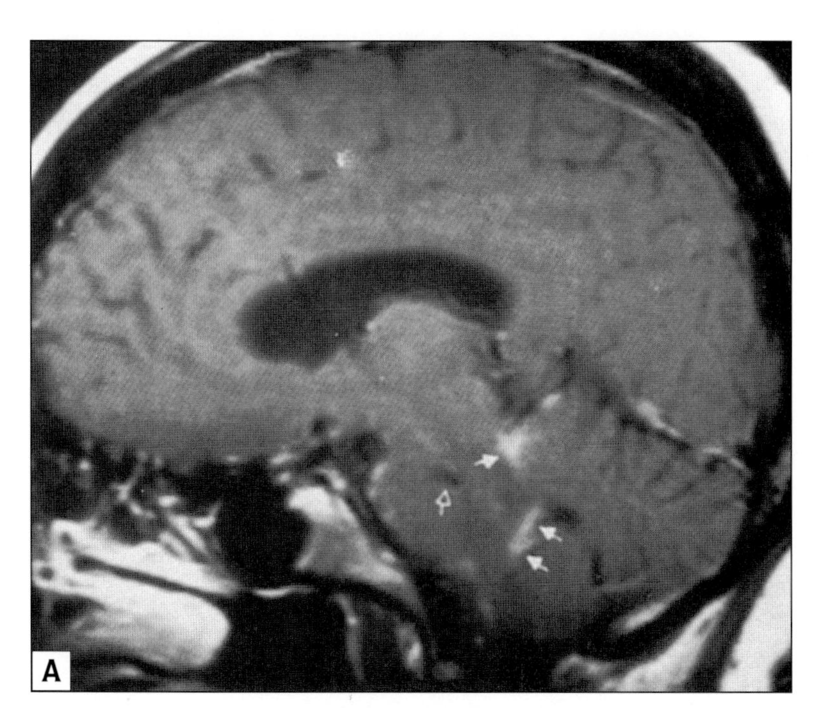

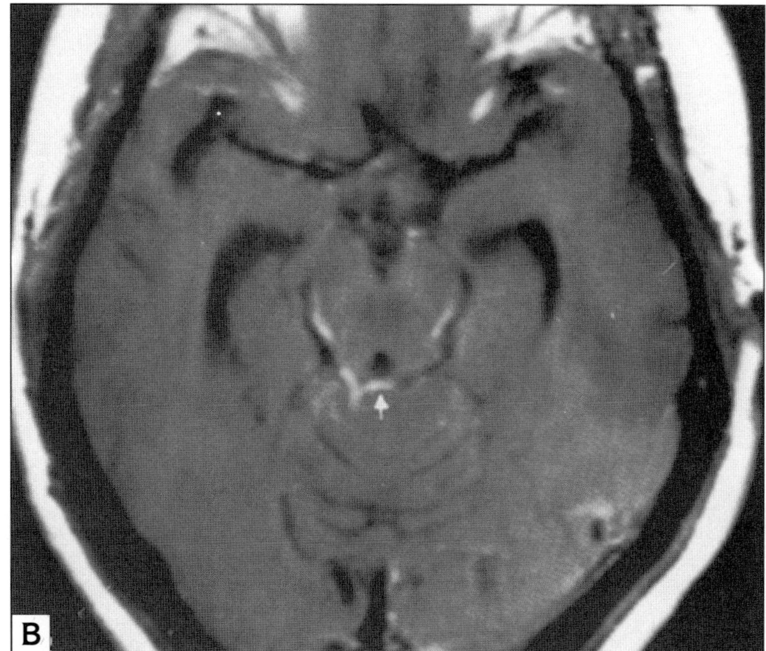

Figure 2-34 Chronic tuberculous meningitis with communicating hydrocephalus. An MRI scan of the head (T1-weighted with gadolinium enhancement) shows abnormal enhancement of the meninges anterior to the pons and medulla (*solid arrows*), within the perimesencephalic and quadrigeminal cisterns, and at the outlet of the fourth ventricle. A well-circumscribed focal hypointensity, without enhancement or mass effect, is seen in the pons (*open arrow*) and represents an old infarct. **A**, Left parasagittal view; **B**, axial view. Hydrocephalus is a characteristic feature of tuberculous meningitis, resulting from profound disturbances in the circulation of CSF; this finding is more often seen in children than adults. An obstructive hydrocephalus may be induced by exudate or local cerebral edema blocking the spinal aqueduct or the foramina of Luschka. More often, however, there is communicating hydrocephalus with exudate blocking the basal cisterns and impeding the resorption of CSF. (*From* Bowen BC, Donovan Post MJ: Intracranial infection. *In* Atlas SE (ed.): *Magnetic Resonance Imaging of the Brain and Spine*. New York: Raven Press; 1991:501–538; with permission.)

Typical CSF findings in tuberculous meningitis

Opening pressure	180–300 mm H_2O
CSF WBC	50–300 cells/mm^3, usually lymphocytic
CSF glucose	< 45 mg/dL
CSF protein	50–200 mg/dL
Positive CSF smear	8%–29%
Positive CSF culture	25%–70%

FIGURE 2-35 Typical CSF findings in tuberculous meningitis. Because of the small population of tuberculous organisms in CSF, identification by specific stains is difficult; in many series, < 25% of specimens are smear-positive. One study found a rate of positive smears of 86% using multiple testing. False-negative CSF cultures are also common in patients with tuberculous meningitis, and even with as many as four CSF specimens, almost 20% of patients have persistently negative CSF cultures. WBC—white blood cell. (Zuger A, Lowy FD: Tuberculosis of the central nervous system. *In* Scheld WM, Whitley RJ, Durack DT (eds.): *Infections of the Central Nervous System*. New York: Raven Press; 1991:424–455.)

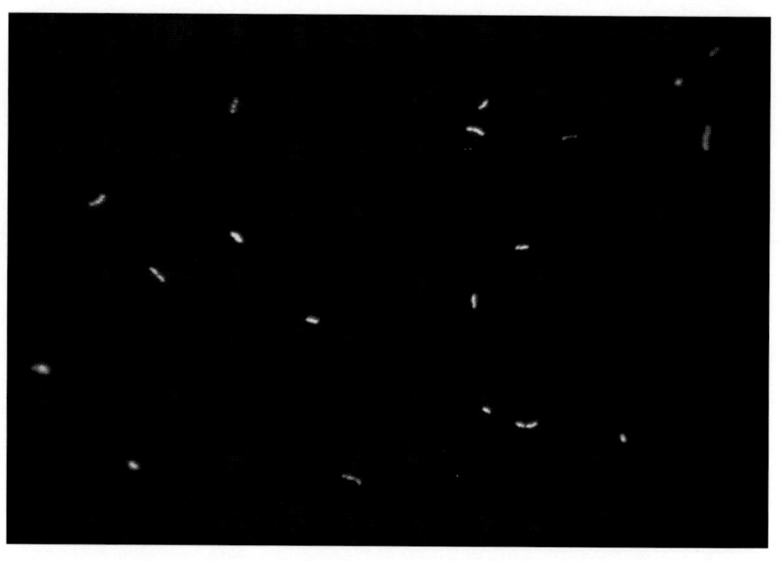

FIGURE 2-36 Auramine smear of CSF. An auramine smear in a patient with tuberculous meningitis reveals fluorescent bacteria; culture subsequently revealed *Mycobacterium tuberculosis*. Because of the small numbers of tuberculous organisms in CSF, identification by specific stains (*ie*, Kinyoun stain) is difficult. Auramine-conjugated material specifically binds to mycolic acids and lipid layers of mycobacteria, causing the organisms to fluoresce. (*From* Kaplan MH: *Meningitis and CNS Infection: Part II. Chronic Forms and Focal Lesions*. Medcom, Inc; 1985; with permission.)

Newer diagnostic tests for tuberculous meningitis

Test	Sensitivity, %	Specificity, %	Time required, *h*
Radiolabeled bromide partition ratio	90–94	88–96	48
CSF adenosine deaminase level	73–100	71–99	< 24
CSF tuberculostearic acid level	95	99	< 24
CSF mycobacterial antigen	79–94	95–100	< 24
CSF mycobacterial antibody	27–100	94–100	< 24
CSF polymerase chain reaction	83	100	< 24

FIGURE 2-37 Newer diagnostic tests for tuberculous meningitis. The deficiencies of most ordinary tests for the diagnosis of tuberculous meningitis have kindled great interest in the development of clinically useful alternatives. Over the past 40 years, a variety of alternatives have been proposed to fit the qualifications of a rapid, sensitive, and highly specific test; all have been promising in some respects and disappointing in others. The usefulness of these tests in the diagnosis of tuberculous meningitis requires large-scale confirmatory studies. (*From* Zuger A, Lowy FD: Tuberculosis of the central nervous system. *In* Scheld WM, Whitley RJ, Durack DT (eds.): *Infections of the Central Nervous System*. New York: Raven Press; 1991:435; with permission.)

Differential diagnosis of tuberculous meningitis

Fungal meningitis
Neurobrucellosis
Neurosyphilis
Neuroborreliosis
Focal parameningeal infection (sphenoid sinusitis, endocarditis)
Pyogenic brain abscess
CNS toxoplasmosis
Partially treated bacterial meningitis
Neoplastic meningitis (lymphoma, carcinoma)
Cerebrovascular accident
CNS sarcoidosis

FIGURE 2-38 Differential diagnosis of tuberculous meningitis. (*From* Leonard JM, Des Prez RM: Tuberculous meningitis. *Infect Dis Clin North Am* 1990, 4:769–788; with permission.)

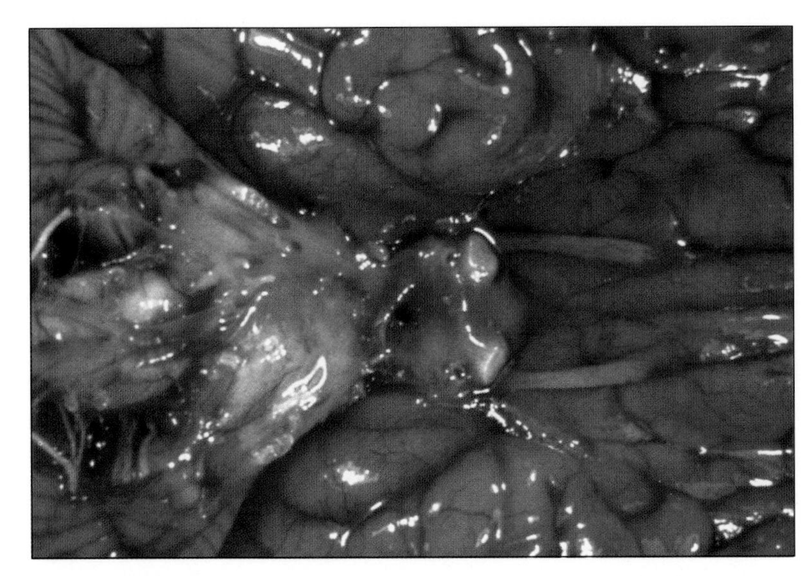

Figure 2-39 Autopsy specimen of the brain in a patient with tuberculous meningitis showing thickened gelatinous basal meninges. The thickening is especially prominent in the region of the optic chiasm and over the pons. The primary pathologic event in patients with tuberculous meningitis is formation of a thick exudate within the subarachnoid space; the exudate is usually diffuse and particularly prominent at the base of the brain, but it may be localized to the immediate vicinity of a tubercle rupture. (From *Infectious Diseases: Text and Color Atlas*, 2nd ed. by WE Farrar, MJ Wood, JA Innes, H Tubbs. Gower Medical Publishing; an imprint of Times Mirror International Publishers Ltd., London, UK, 1992; with permission.)

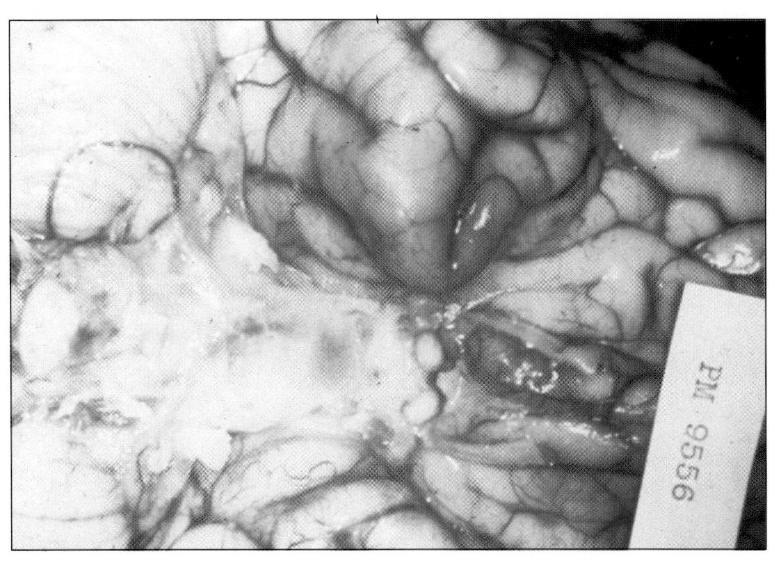

Figure 2-40 Autopsy specimen of the brain of a child with tuberculous meningitis showing a sheet of white exudate which encompasses and obscures the basal cranial nerves. (From *Infectious Diseases: Text and Color Atlas*, 2nd ed. by WE Farrar, MJ Wood, JA Innes, H Tubbs. Gower Medical Publishing; an imprint of Times Mirror International Publishers Ltd., London, UK, 1992; with permission.)

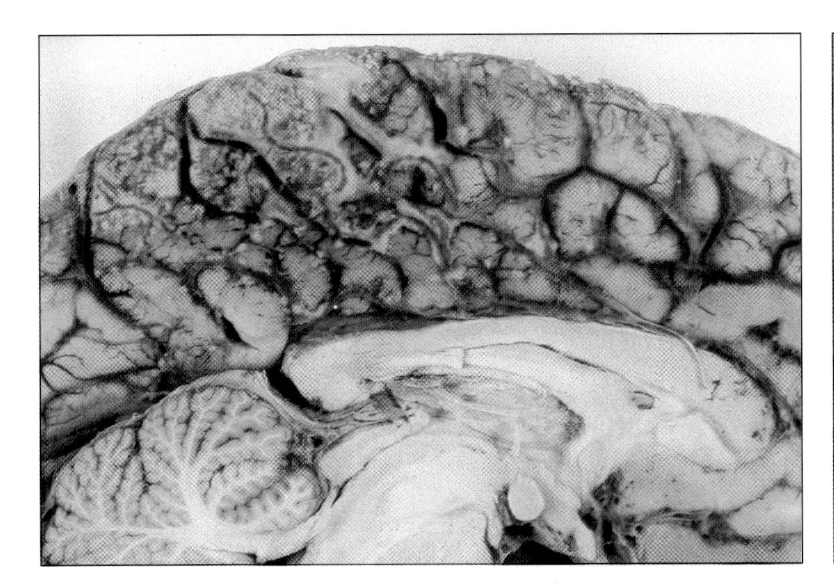

Figure 2-41 Sagittal section of the brain in a patient with tuberculous meningitis showing a thick, grayish-white inflammatory exudate, especially prominent over the vertex and spreading over medially to the subarachnoid space. Note that the exudate is most marked along the course of adjacent blood vessels. (*From* Turk JL (ed.): *Royal College of Surgeons of England Slide Atlas of Pathology.* London: Gower Medical Publishing; 1985; with permission.)

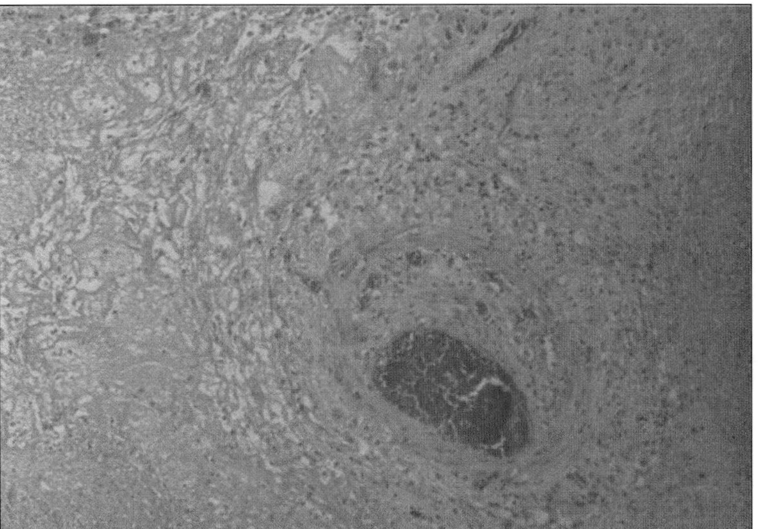

Figure 2-42 Tuberculous meningitis with granulomatous inflammation. A section through a meningeal vessel demonstrates partial occlusion and organization; adjacent acute necrosis is apparent. Along with exudate, an inflammatory response affecting primarily small and medium-sized arteries traversing the exudate is observed in tuberculous meningitis; capillaries and veins may also be affected. There may be ischemic cerebral infarction resulting from vascular occlusion in patients with tuberculous arteritis, most often in the distribution of the middle cerebral artery and the lateral striate arteries as they penetrate the base of the brain. Thrombosed vessels frequently result in zones of hemorrhage and infarction in adjacent brain tissue. (Hematoxylin-eosin stain.) (From *Infectious Diseases: Text and Color Atlas*, 2nd ed. by WE Farrar, MJ Wood, JA Innes, H Tubbs. Gower Medical Publishing; an imprint of Times Mirror International Publishers Ltd., London, UK, 1992; with permission. *Courtesy of* Dr. P. Garen.)

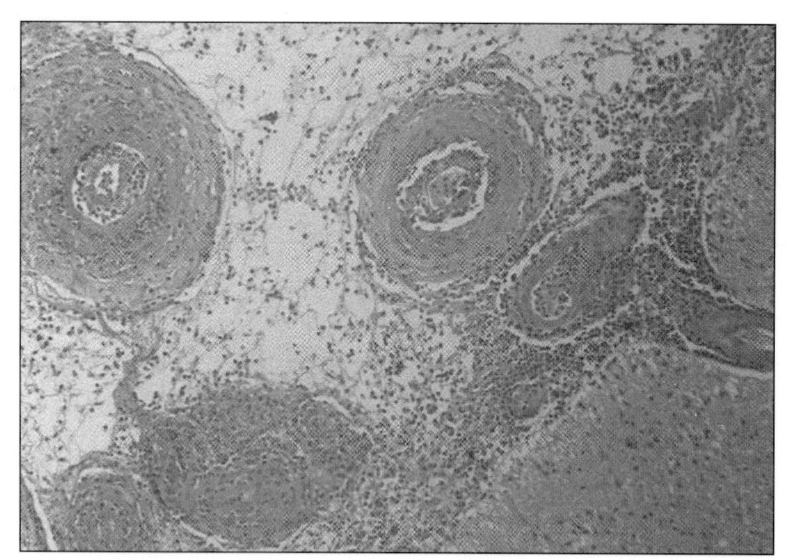

FIGURE 2-43 Acute tuberculous meningitis with marked involvement of the vessel walls and occlusion of smaller vessels. The vascular involvement can result in infarction. (Hematoxylin-eosin stain.) (From *Infectious Diseases: Text and Color Atlas*, 2nd ed. by WE Farrar, MJ Wood, JA Innes, H Tubbs. Gower Medical Publishing; an imprint of Times Mirror International Publishers Ltd., London, UK, 1992; with permission. *Courtesy of* Dr. P. Garen.)

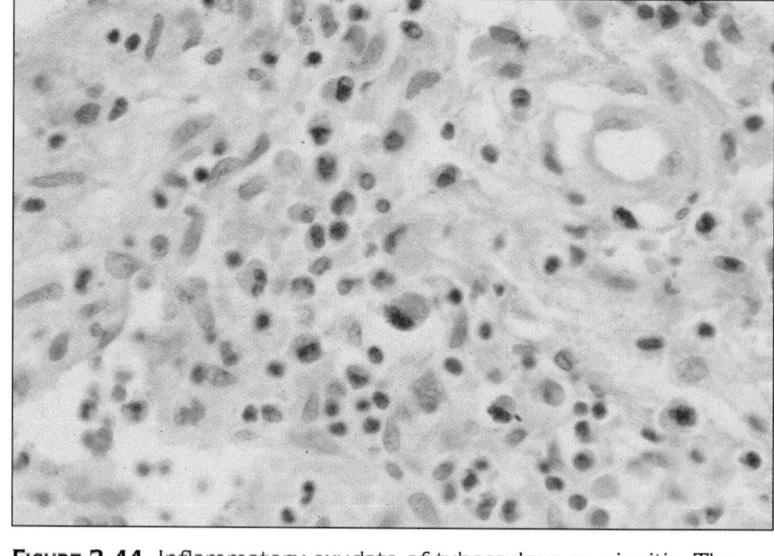

FIGURE 2-44 Inflammatory exudate of tuberculous meningitis. The exudate typically consists of neutrophils, red blood cells, macrophages, and lymphocytes within a fibrin network. Lymphocytes predominate as the disease progresses, and typical tubercles may subsequently develop within the exudate. In brain parenchyma adjacent to zones of exudate, the brain tissue softens, and astrocytic, microglial, and diffuse inflammatory reactions can be seen.

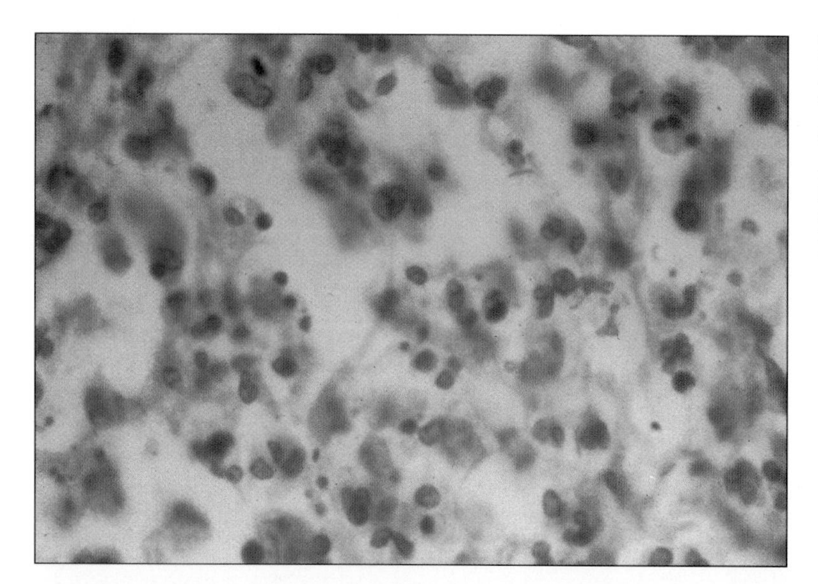

FIGURE 2-45 Inflammatory exudate containing multiple acid-fast bacilli. There are usually a variable number of mycobacteria within the exudate of tuberculous meningitis, ranging from none to enormous numbers. (Kinyoun carbolfuchsin stain.) (From *Infectious Diseases: Text and Color Atlas*, 2nd ed. by WE Farrar, MJ Wood, JA Innes, H Tubbs. Gower Medical Publishing; an imprint of Times Mirror International Publishers Ltd., London, UK, 1992; with permission. *Courtesy of* Dr. P. Garen.)

Penetration of antimycobacterial agents into the CSF

Agent	Usual daily dose, *mg/kg/d*	Range of mean peak concentrations (μg/mL)		
		Serum	CSF, normal meninges	CSF, inflamed meninges
Isoniazid	5–10	3.0–5.0	0.6–1.6	2.0
Rifampin	10–20	0.4–12.0	0	0.4–1.0
Ethambutol	15–25	1.0–7.7	0	0.5–2.5
Pyrazinamide	20–35	45–50	—	50
Streptomycin	15–40	25–50	Trace	9

FIGURE 2-46 Penetration of antimycobacterial agents into CSF. Antimycobacterial agents must penetrate the blood-brain barrier in concentrations sufficient to eliminate small numbers of both intracellular and extracellular *Mycobacterium tuberculosis*. For pyrazinamide, the value of 50 μg/mL in CSF with inflamed meninges resulted after a 50 mg/kg dose. (*From* Zuger A, Lowy FD: Tuberculosis of the central nervous system. *In* Scheld WM, Whitley RJ, Durack DT (eds.): *Infections of the Central Nervous System*. New York: Raven Press; 1991:443; with permission.)

Signs and symptoms of fungal meningitis

	Fever (> 101°F)	Headache	Stiff neck	Change in mentation	Focal signs	Visual disturbance
Blastomyces	+	+++	+++	+	++	+
Candida	+++	+++	++	+	+	+
Coccidioides	+	+++	+	++	++	++
Cryptococcus	+	+++	+++	+	+	+++
Histoplasma	++	+	++	+	+	+
Sporothrix	+	++	++	++	+	?

FIGURE 2-53 Signs and symptoms of fungal meningitis. The frequency of presentations is noted as usually (+++), occasionally to moderately frequently (++), or rare (+). (*From* Tucker T, Ellner JJ: Chronic meningitis. *In* Scheld WM, Whitley RJ, Durack DT (eds.): *Infections of the Central Nervous System*. New York: Raven Press; 1991:714; with permission.)

General clinical parameters for diagnosis of fungal meningitis

History
Physical examination
Serum chemistries
Cultures and smears
Biopsy, histopathology
Serodiagnostic tests

FIGURE 2-54 General clinical parameters for the diagnosis of fungal meningitis. The clinical findings in fungal meningitis depend upon interactions between the specific etiologic agents and predominant host factors in the involved patient. In general, fungal meningitis occurring in the absence of apparent immunocompromise tends to be subacute or chronic, whereas in immunosuppressed patients, the course tends to be more rapid or even acute. (*Adapted from* Diamond RD: Fungal meningitis. *In* Lambert HP (ed.): *Infections of the Central Nervous System*. Philadelphia: B.C. Decker; 1991:236; with permission.)

CSF parameters for diagnosis of fungal meningitis

General	Opening pressure
	Cell count and differential
	Glucose
	Protein
Culture	Use ≥ 10–15 mL of fluid
	Culture on multiple occasions
Direct smears	India ink for *Cryptococcus neoformans*
Serologies	Cryptococcal antigen
	Coccidioides immitis antibody by complement fixation

FIGURE 2-55 CSF parameters for the diagnosis of fungal meningitis. It is seldom possible to presume that fungal meningitis is present without definitive evidence of infection; therefore, careful examination of the CSF is critical. (*Adapted from* Diamond RD: Fungal meningitis. *In* Lambert HP (ed.): *Infections of the Central Nervous System*. Philadelphia: B.C. Decker; 1991:236; with permission.)

A. Diagnostic characteristics of fungi causing CNS infection

	CSF culture positive	CSF serologies
Aspergillus spp.	Rare	Ab/An
Blastomyces dermatitidis	Rare	Ab
Candida spp.	50%	Ab/An
Coccidioides immitis	25%–45%	Ab
Cryptococcus neoformans	75%–80%	An
Dematiaceous fungi	Rare	None
Histoplasma capsulatum	50%	Ab
Paracoccidioides brasiliensis	Rare	Ab
Pseudallescheria boydii	Rare	None
Sporothrix schenckii	Rare	Ab
Zygomycetes spp.	Rare	Ab

B. Primary antifungal therapy for fungal meningitides

Aspergillus spp.	Amphotericin B
Blastomyces dermatitidis	Amphotericin B
Candida spp.	Amphotericin B, fluconazole
Coccidioides immitis	Amphotericin B (intrathecal), fluconazole
Cryptococcus neoformans	Amphotericin B, fluconazole
Dematiaceous fungi	Surgery
Histoplasma capsulatum	Amphotericin B
Paracoccidioides brasiliensis	Ketoconazole
Pseudallescheria boydii	Miconazole, fluconazole
Sporothrix schenckii	Amphotericin B
Zygomycetes spp.	Amphotericin B

FIGURE 2-56 Diagnostic and therapeutic characteristics of fungi causing CNS infection. **A**, Diagnostic characteristics. Conclusive proof for a fungal infection is provided by identification of the fungus in brain tissue or in CSF. Unfortunately, CSF cultures are not always positive in patients with fungal meningitis; to improve the yield, large volumes (10–30 mL) of CSF should be withdrawn and sent for culture. **B**, Primary antifungal therapy for fungal meningitides. Ab—antibody test; An—antigen test. (*Adapted from* Perfect JR: Diagnosis and treatment of fungal meningitis. *In* Scheld WM, Whitley RJ, Durack DT (eds.): *Infections of the Central Nervous System*. New York: Raven Press; 1991:731; with permission.)

Cryptococcal Meningitis

Clinical presentation of cryptococcal meningitis in non-AIDS and AIDS patients

	Non-AIDS, %	AIDS, %
Headache	87	81
Fever	60	88
Nausea, vomiting, malaise	53	38
Mental status changes	52	19
Meningeal signs	50	31
Visual changes, photophobia	33	19
Seizures	15	8
No symptoms or signs	10	12

Figure 2-57 Clinical presentation of cryptococcal meningitis. In non-AIDS patients, cryptococcal meningitis typically manifests as a subacute process after days to weeks of symptoms. In AIDS patients, the presentation of cryptococcal meningitis can be very subtle, with minimal, if any, symptoms. AIDS patients may present only with fever and headache. (*From* Tunkel AR, Scheld WM: Central nervous system infections in the compromised host. *In* Rubin RH, Young LS (eds.): *Clinical Approach to Infection in the Compromised Host*, 3rd ed. New York: Plenum; 1994:187; with permission.)

Laboratory findings in cryptococcal meningitis

	Non-AIDS, %	AIDS, %
Positive blood culture	—	30–63
Positive serum cryptococcal antigen	66	99
CSF opening pressure > 200 mm H_2O	72	62
CSF glucose < 2.2 mmol/L (40 mg/dL)	73	33
CSF protein > 0.45 g/L (45 mg/dL)	89	58
CSF leukocytes > 20 X 10^6/L	70	23
Positive CSF India ink	60	74
Positive CSF culture	96	95
Positive CSF cryptococcal antigen	86	91–100

Figure 2-58 Laboratory findings in cryptococcal meningitis. AIDS patients with cryptococcal meningitis may have very low or even normal CSF leukocyte counts during active infection; 65% of patients have < 5 cells/mm^3. (*From* Tunkel AR, Scheld WM: Central nervous system infections in the compromised host. *In* Rubin RH, Young LS (eds.): *Clinical Approach to Infection in the Compromised Host*, 3rd ed. New York: Plenum; 1994:187; with permission.)

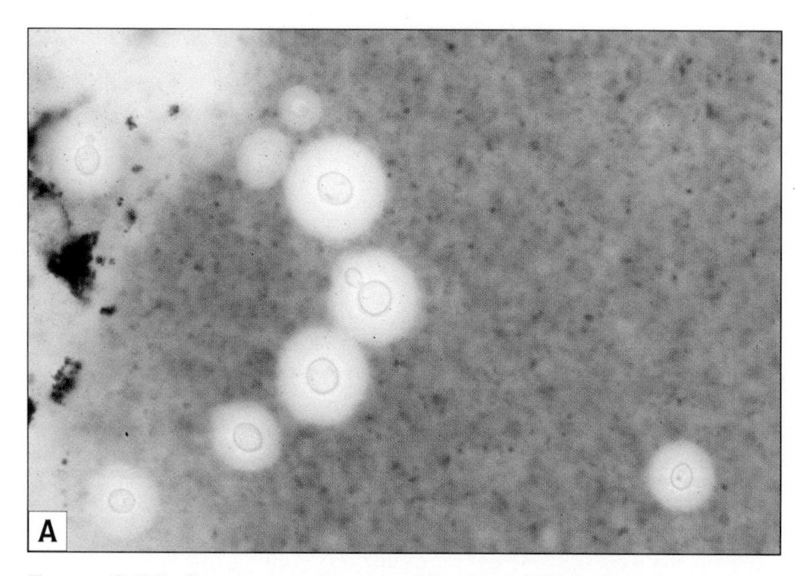

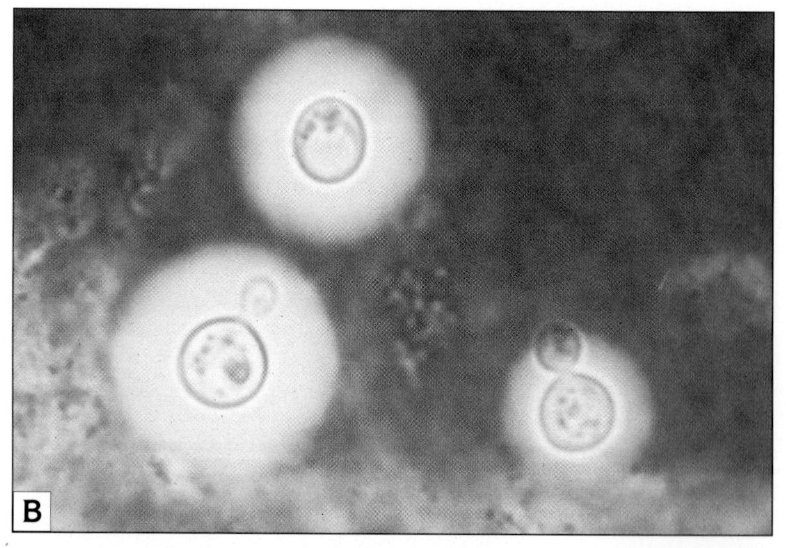

Figure 2-59 Cryptococcal meningitis. **A** and **B**, India ink preparation of CSF sediment demonstrates the prominent capsule of *Cryptococcus neoformans*. Note the highly refractile cell wall and internal structure of the yeast. The India ink test is positive in 50% to 75% of patients with cryptococcal meningitis; this yield increases up to 88% in patients with AIDS. (From *Infectious Diseases: Text and Color Atlas*, 2nd ed. by WE Farrar, MJ Wood, JA Innes, H Tubbs. Gower Medical Publishing; an imprint of Times Mirror International Publishers Ltd., London, UK, 1992; with permission. *Courtesy of* AE Prevost.)

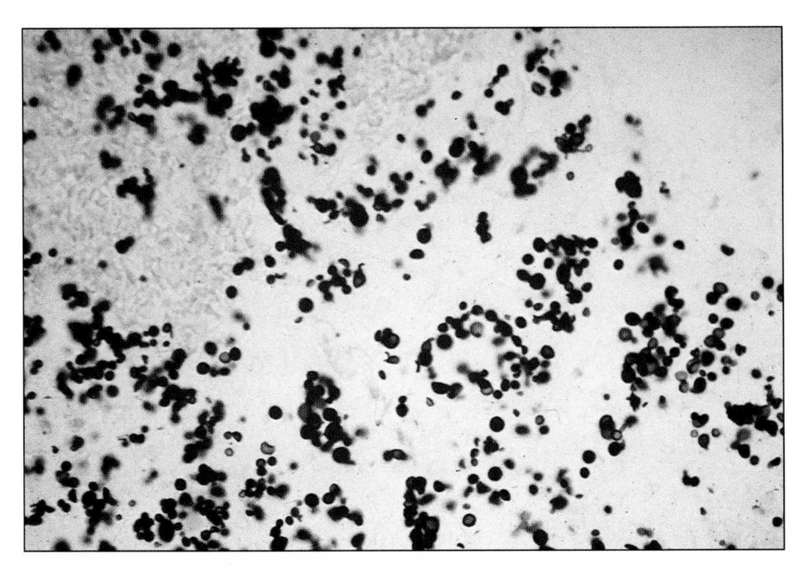

FIGURE 2-60 *Cryptococcus neoformans* in the CSF. (Methenamine silver stain.)

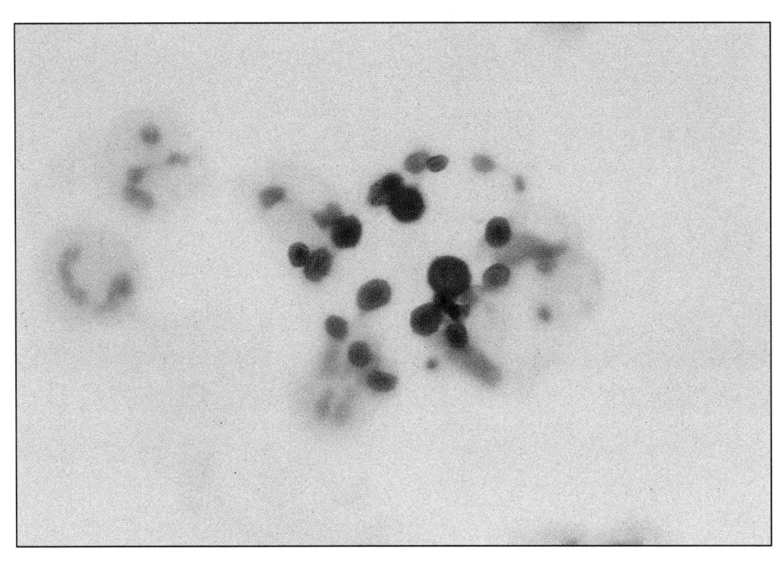

FIGURE 2-61 *Cryptococcus neoformans* in the CSF. (Mucicarmine stain.) The cryptococcal capsule contains a generous number of mucopolysaccharides. The presence of mucopolysaccharide confers mucicarmine positivity and, in part, accounts for the relative lack of inflammatory response often noted in the CSF and gross brain in patients with cryptococcal meningitis.

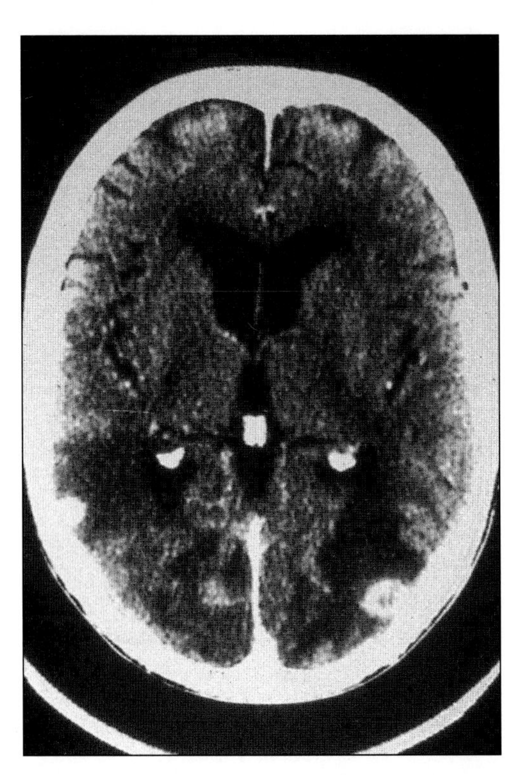

FIGURE 2-62 CT scan showing multiple enhancing lesions in the brain surrounded by edema. Although the most common CNS presentation of cryptococcal infection is that of meningitis, occasional cases also involve the brain parenchyma. (From *Infectious Diseases: Text and Color Atlas*, 2nd ed. by WE Farrar, MJ Wood, JA Innes, H Tubbs. Gower Medical Publishing; an imprint of Times Mirror International Publishers Ltd., London, UK, 1992; with permission. *Courtesy of* Dr. J Cure.)

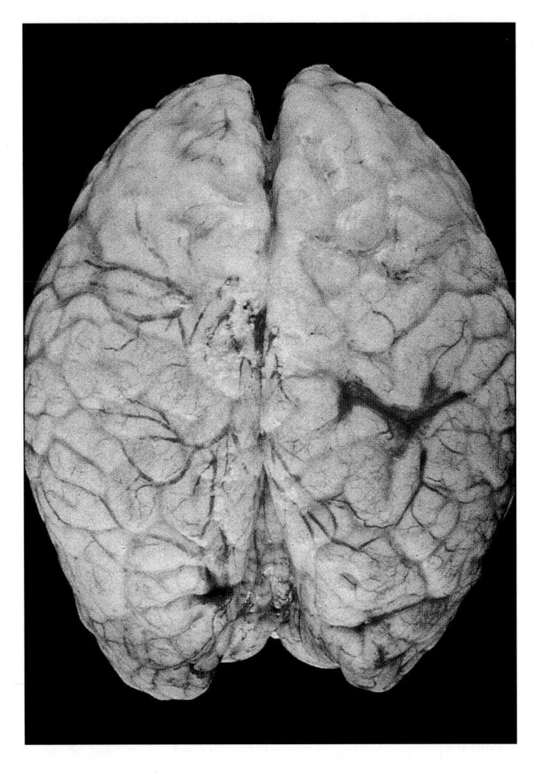

FIGURE 2-63 Leptomeningitis in cryptococcal meningitis. The leptomeningitis that regularly occurs in patients with cryptococcal meningitis is usually devoid of the thick exudation of purulent bacterial meningitis. Slight clouding of the leptomeninges may be the only indication of infection, as seen in this dorsal view of the cerebral hemispheres. (*From* Okazaki H, Scheithauer BW (eds.): *Atlas of Neuropathology*. London: Gower Medical Publishing; 1988:46; with permission.)

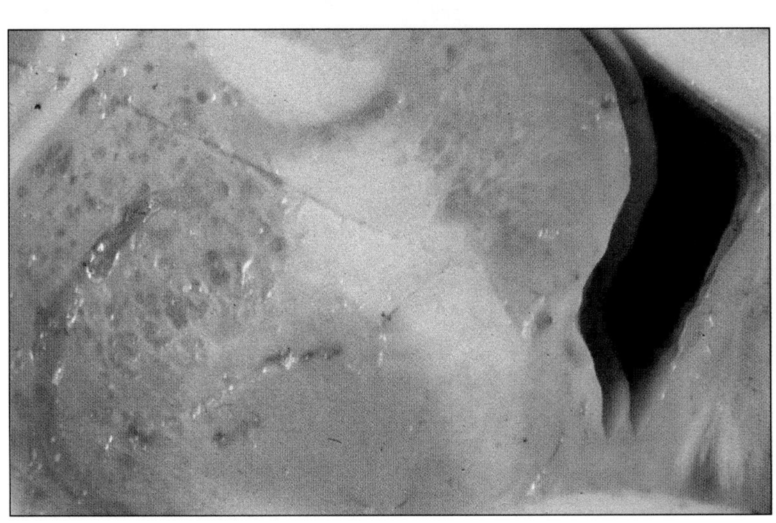

FIGURE 2-64 Brain parenchymal involvement in cryptococcal meningitis. A characteristic feature of cryptococcal meningitis is its extension into the brain parenchyma along the Virchow-Robin spaces, most noticeably in the basal ganglia and less prominently in the cerebral cortex where multiple, minute-to-small "bubbles" can be seen with the naked eye. (*From* Okazaki H, Scheithauer BW (eds.): *Atlas of Neuropathology*. London: Gower Medical Publishing; 1988:47; with permission.)

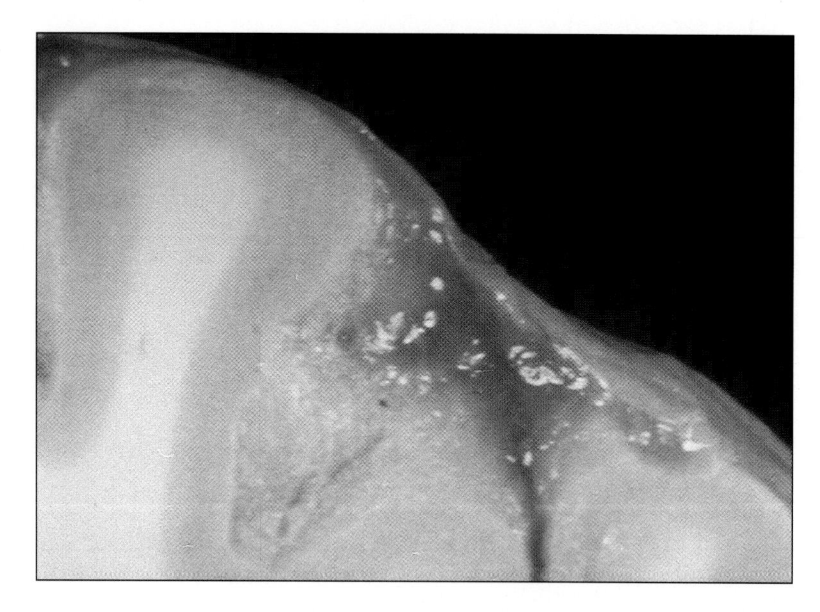

FIGURE 2-65 Cross-section of the frontal cortex revealing gelatinous material, which is the capsular material of the cryptococcal organism, in the sulci. (From *Infectious Diseases: Text and Color Atlas*, 2nd ed. by WE Farrar, MJ Wood, JA Innes, H Tubbs. Gower Medical Publishing; an imprint of Times Mirror International Publishers Ltd., London, UK, 1992; with permission.)

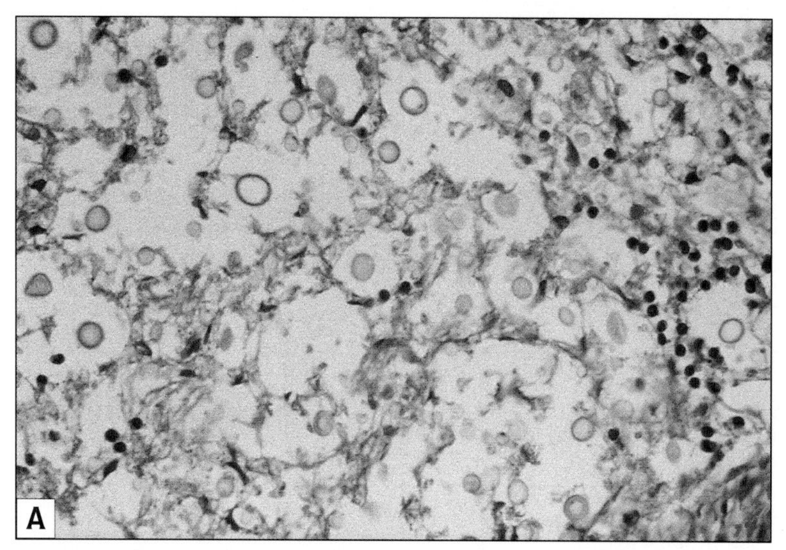

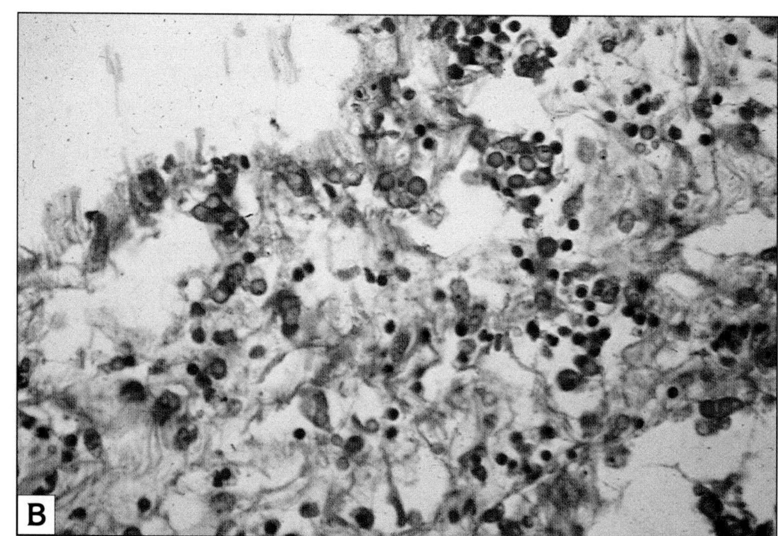

FIGURE 2-66 Microscopically, fungi in the form of budding yeasts can be seen free in the leptomeningeal space or engulfed by macrophages. **A**, Hematoxylin-eosin stain does not reveal the characteristic capsule of *Cryptococcus neoformans*. (*From* Okazaki H, Scheithauer BW (eds.): *Atlas of Neuropathology*. London: Gower Medical Publishing; 1988:46; with permission.) **B**, Mucicarmine stain reveals the capsule of *C. neoformans*.

Coccidioidal Meningitis

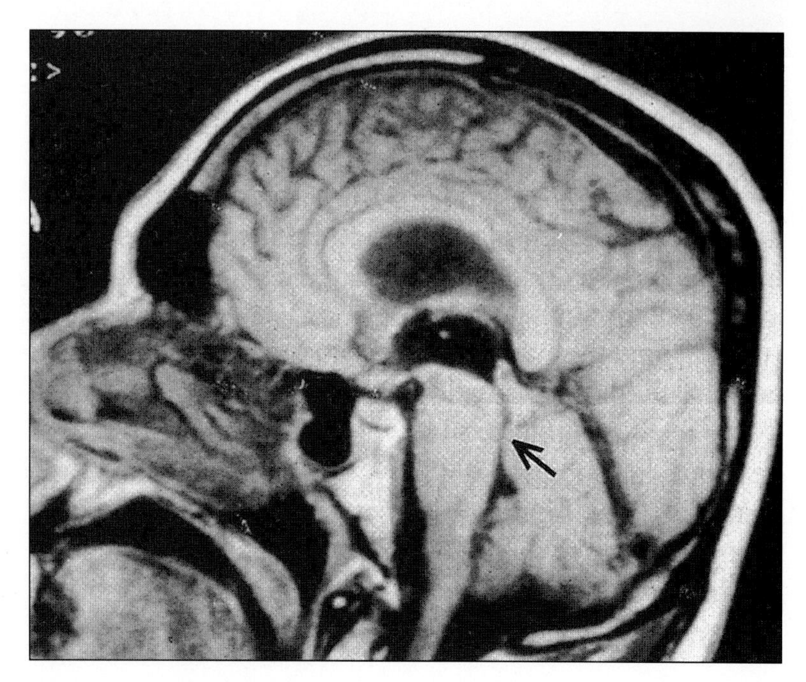

FIGURE 2-67 Hydrocephalus in coccidioidal meningitis. An MRI of the brain in a patient with coccidioidal meningitis complicated by hydrocephalus shows that the third ventricle is enlarged, but the aqueduct of Sylvius is patent (*arrow*). Hydrocephalus is a common complication of coccidioidal meningitis, and in children it is usually present at the time of diagnosis. Often the hydrocephalus is of the communicating type, as observed in this case. (*From* Galgiani JN: Coccidioidomycosis. *West J Med* 1993, 159:153–171; with permission.)

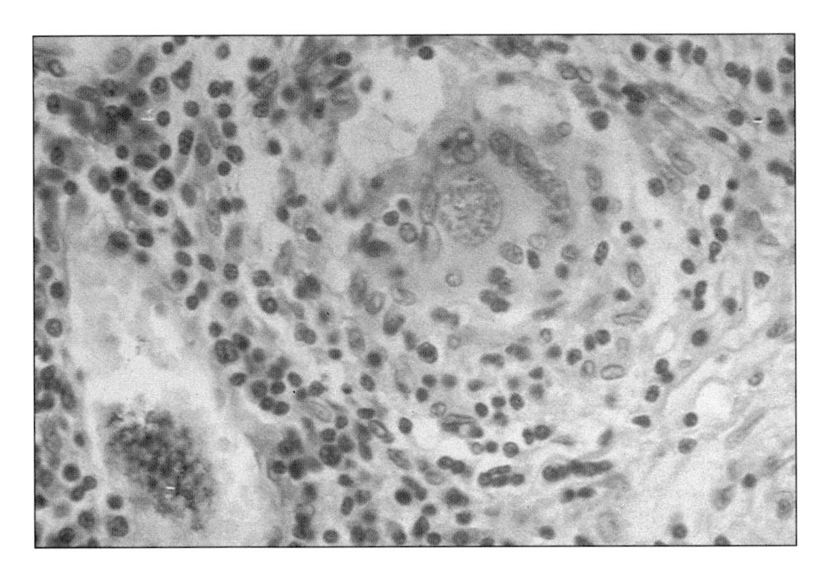

FIGURE 2-68 Granulomatous meningitis showing a multinucleated giant cell containing a spherule of the coccidioidal organism with many endospores. (Periodic acid–Schiff stain.) (From *Infectious Diseases: Text and Color Atlas*, 2nd ed. by WE Farrar, MJ Wood, JA Innes, H Tubbs. Gower Medical Publishing; an imprint of Times Mirror International Publishers Ltd., London, UK, 1992; with permission.)

Other Fungal Meningitides

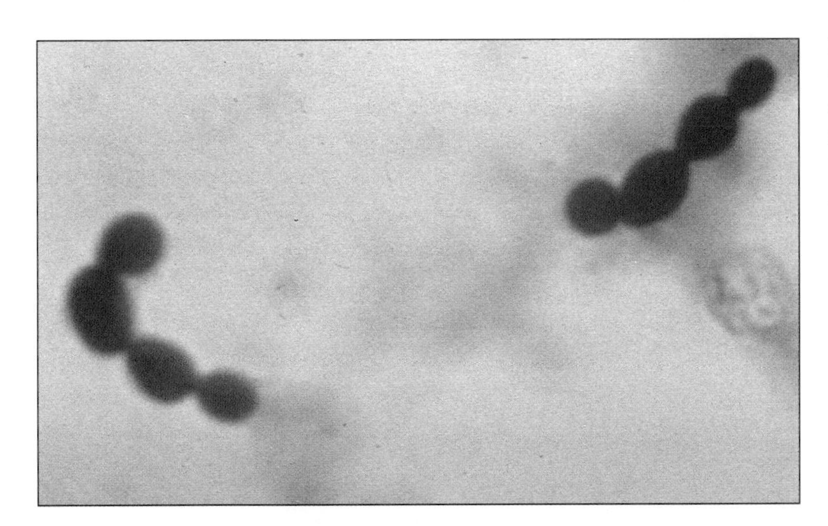

FIGURE 2-69 Candidal meningitis. Gram's stain of CSF shows the typical morphology of *Candida albicans* in a patient with disseminated candidiasis. (From *Infectious Diseases: Text and Color Atlas*, 2nd ed. by WE Farrar, MJ Wood, JA Innes, H Tubbs. Gower Medical Publishing; an imprint of Times Mirror International Publishers Ltd., London, UK, 1992; with permission. *Courtesy of* AE Prevost.)

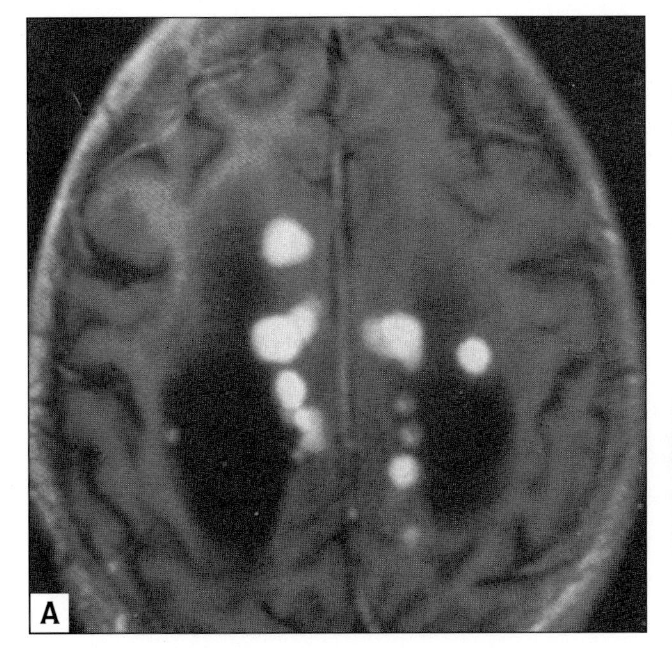

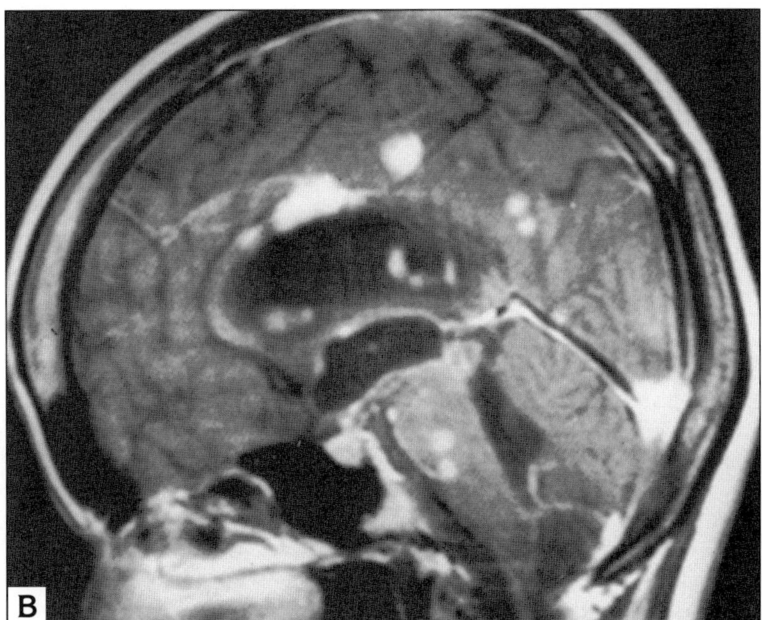

FIGURE 2-70 Central nervous system histoplasmosis. MRI of the head (T1-weighted with gadolinium enhancement) in a patient with CNS histoplasmosis demonstrates parenchymal granulomas, meningitis, and hydrocephalus. Note the presence of subependymal masses with marked, homogeneous enhancement. **A**, Axial view; **B**, midsagittal view. (*From* Bowen BC, Donovan Post MJ: Intracranial infection. *In* Atlas SW (ed.): *Magnetic Resonance Imaging of the Brain and Spine*. New York: Raven Press; 1991:501–538; with permission.)

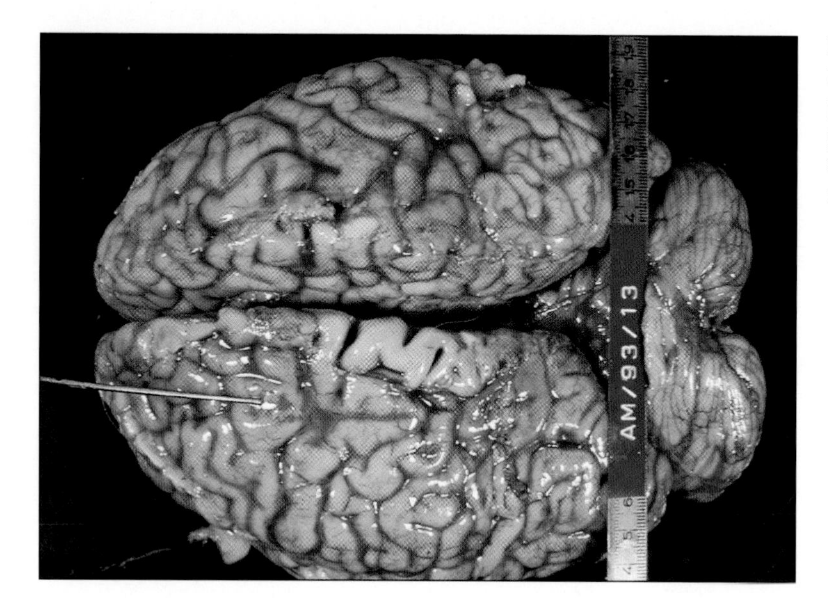

FIGURE 2-71 Aspergillus meningitis. An autopsy specimen of the brain shows marked congestion of the meninges. The probe points to one of the clear lesions that is circumscribed, yellow-green, and softened. This probably represents an *Aspergillus* abscess caused by embolic dissemination in a patient with systemic disease.

AMEBIC MENINGOENCEPHALITIS

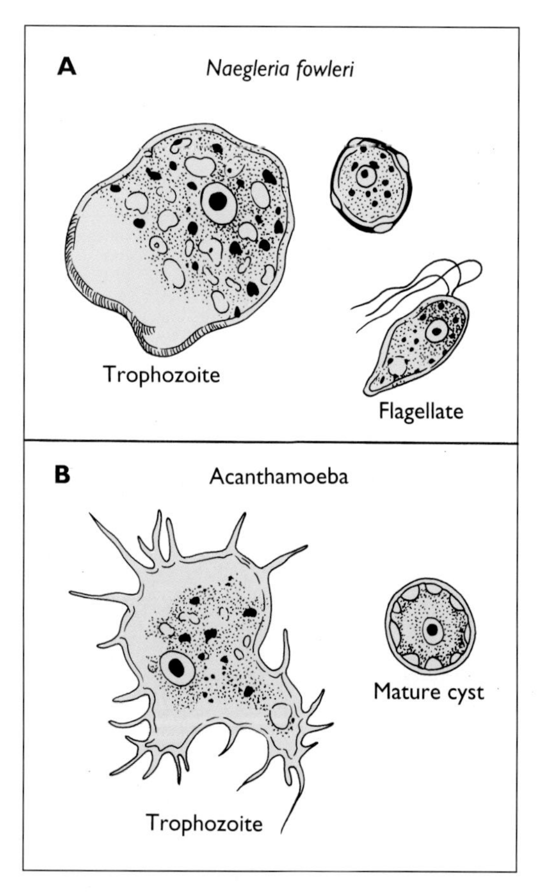

FIGURE 2-72 *Naegleria fowleri* and *Acanthamoeba* species. **A**, On *N. fowleri*, note the lobose pseudopodium, circular cyst, flagellate stage, and large single karyosome. **B**, The *Acanthamoeba* shows the acanthapodia, stellate cyst, absence of a flagellate stage, and large single karyosome. (*From* Duma RJ: Primary amebic meningoencephalitis: infection by free-living amebae. *In* Lambert HP (ed.): *Infections of the Central Nervous System*. Philadelphia: B.C. Decker; 1991: 255; with permission.)

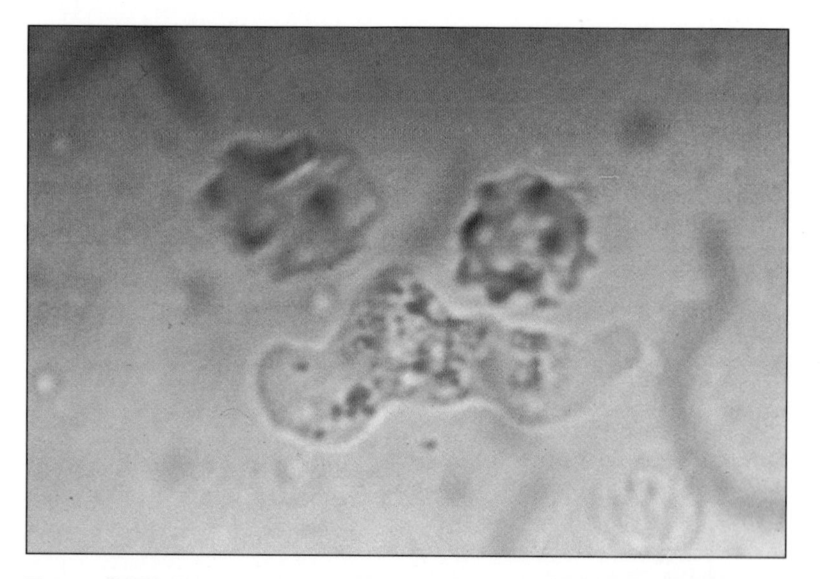

FIGURE 2-73 Wet mount of CSF revealing motile *Naegleria fowleri*. This organism is found worldwide in fresh warm water; most patients have a history of swimming in freshwater shortly before the onset of illness. CSF examination reveals a neutrophilic pleocytosis, decreased glucose, and increased protein. Wet mount of an unstained preparation of CSF can demonstrate motile trophozoites of *N. fowleri*. (From *Infectious Diseases: Text and Color Atlas*, 2nd ed. by WE Farrar, MJ Wood, JA Innes, H Tubbs. Gower Medical Publishing; an imprint of Times Mirror International Publishers Ltd., London, UK, 1992; with permission. *Courtesy of* AE Prevost.)

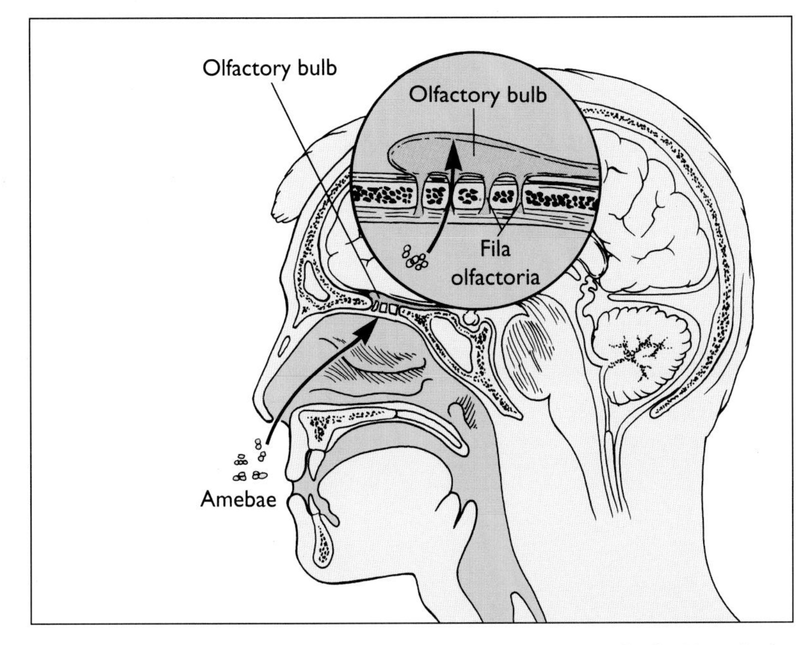

FIGURE 2-74 Invasion pathway of amebae into the CNS. *Naegleria*, and occasionally *Acanthamoeba*, invade the human olfactory nasal mucosa, migrate along the fila olfactoria, and directly invade the olfactory bulbs, tracts, and frontotemporal lobes. (*From* Niu MT, Duma RJ: Meningitis due to protozoa and helminths. *Infect Dis Clin North Am* 1990; 4:809–844; with permission.)

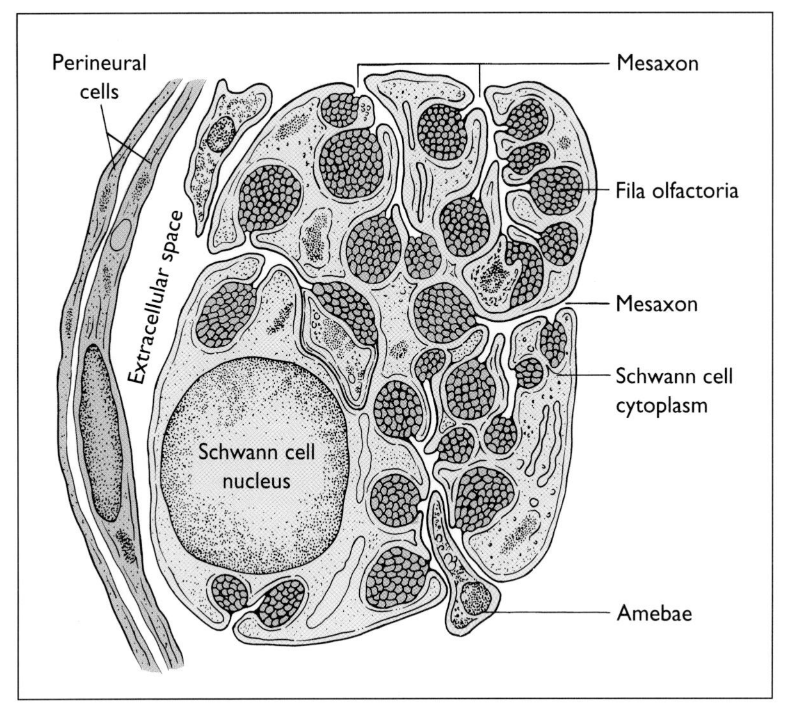

FIGURE 2-75 The olfactory submucosal nerve plexus showing fila olfactoria and invasion by several amebae located in the mesaxon and extracellular space. In this way, amebae reach the meninges surrounding the frontal lobes, where they multiply, spread, and destroy CNS tissue. (*From* Martinez AJ, Duma RJ, Nelson EC, Moretta FL: Experimental *Naegleria* meningoencephalitis in mice. *Lab Invest* 1973, 29:121–133; with permission.)

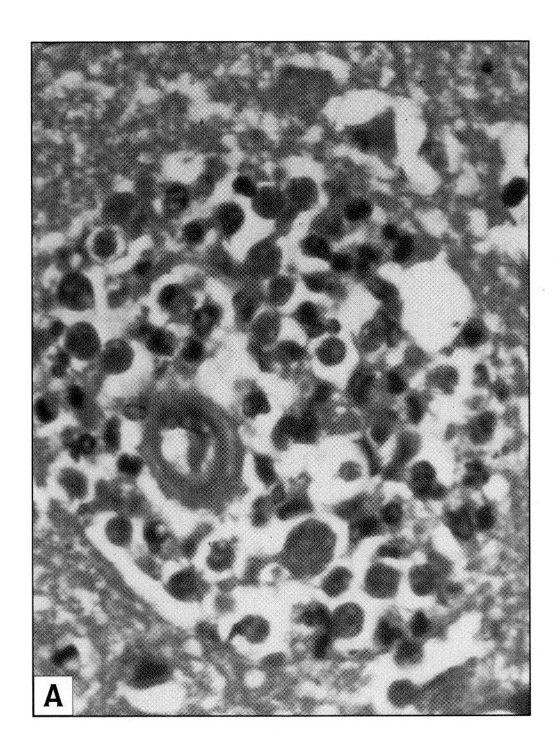

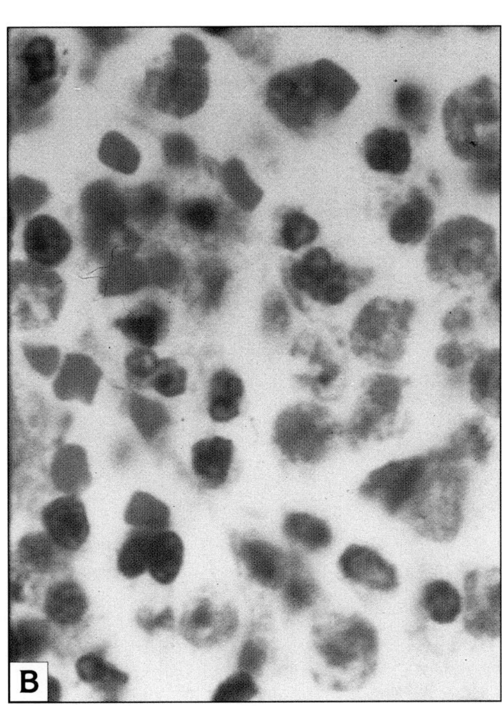

FIGURE 2-76 *Naegleria fowleri* enters the CNS by invasion of the nasal mucosa at the level of the cribriform plate, followed by passage along the fila olfactoria and olfactory nerve tracts. The trophozoites of *N. fowleri* are found in the olfactory nerves and around blood vessels in the brain. **A**, Section of brain reveals trophozoites of *N. fowleri* and inflammatory cells in the Virchow-Robin space. **B**, Higher power view reveals the large trophozoites scattered among inflammatory cells. (From *Infectious Diseases: Text and Color Atlas*, 2nd ed. by WE Farrar, MJ Wood, JA Innes, H Tubbs. Gower Medical Publishing; an imprint of Times Mirror International Publishers Ltd., London, UK, 1992; with permission. *Courtesy of* S. Conradi.)

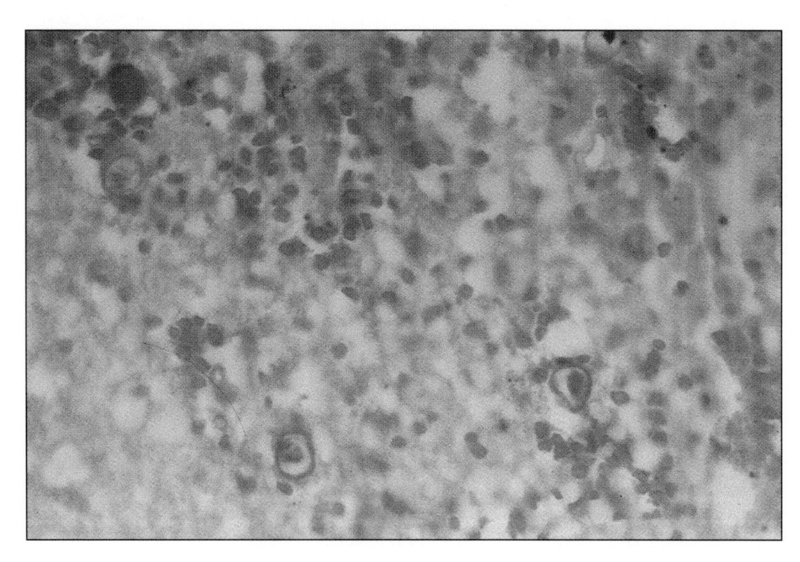

FIGURE 2-77 Brain specimen in a patient with acanthamoebic meningoencephalitis revealing hemorrhagic necrosis. Organisms have a thick irregular capsule and a central basophilic nucleus. In contrast to amebic meningoencephalitis caused by *Naegleria fowleri*, infection caused by *Acanthamoebae* is usually subacute to chronic and the olfactory bulbs are usually spared. Wet preparations of CSF are negative and the characteristic cysts must be identified in tissue biopsy specimens for definitive diagnosis. (*From* Farrar WE: The nervous system. From *Infectious Diseases: Text and Color Atlas*, 2nd ed. by WE Farrar, MJ Wood, JA Innes, H Tubbs. Gower Medical Publishing; an imprint of Times Mirror International Publishers Ltd., London, UK, 1992; with permission. *Courtesy of* Dr. P. Garen.)

A. Clinicopathologic characteristics of primary amebic meningoencephalitis: epidemiologic characteristics

Characteristic	Acute amebic meningoencephalitis	Granulomatous amebic encephalitis
Etiologic agent	*Naegleria fowleri* Rarely *Acanthamoeba* spp.	*Acanthamoeba* spp.
Sex	Males predominate	No sexual preponderance
Age	Children and young adults	Any age
Epidemiology	Recent intimate contact with fresh/brackish water Seasonal: warm weather May occur in epidemics Endemic areas exist Patient previously healthy	Preexisting extracerebral free-living ameba infection (*eg*, skin, eye, lung, ear) Often occurs in immunodeficient or debilitated persons Sporadic
Incubation period	5–7 days	Weeks to months

B. Clinicopathologic characteristics of primary amebic meningoencephalitis: clinical findings

Characteristic	Acute amebic meningoencephalitis	Granulomatous amebic encephalitis
Presenting clinical picture	Acute pyogenic meningitis	Subacute or chronic meningitis Brain abscess
CSF	Usually > 500 WBC/mm^3 PMNs predominate RBCs present Glucose low Trophozoites seen and cultured	Usually < 500 WBC/mm^3 Round cells usually predominate RBCs usually absent Glucose normal or low normal Trophozoites not usually seen or cultured
Areas of brain involved	Principally gray areas of olfactory, temporal, frontal, and cerebellar lobes	Principally deep posterior structures and white matter of brainstem, midbrain, corpus callosum, basal ganglia, etc.
Histopathology	Meningoencephalitis with acute hemorrhagic necrosis with preponderance of PMNs Only trophozoites seen	Principally encephalitis/brain abscesses with subacute or chronic granulomatous reaction and giant cells Trophozoites and cysts present
Course (untreated)	Usually fatal in 2–5 days	Usually fatal in days to weeks

FIGURE 2-78 Clinicopathologic characteristics of primary amebic meningoencephalitis. **A**, Epidemiologic characteristics. **B**, Clinical findings. PMN—polymorphonuclear leukocyte; RBC—red blood cell; WBC—white blood cell. (*From* Duma RJ: Primary amebic meningoencephalitis: infection by free-living amebae. *In* Lambert HP (ed.): *Infections of the Central Nervous System*. Philadelphia: B.C. Decker; 1991:256; with permission.)

Differential diagnoses of primary amebic meningoencephalitis
Acute amebic meningoencephalitis
Acute purulent (esp. bacterial) meningitis
Herpes meningoencephalitis
Granulomatous amebic encephalitis
Tuberculous meningitis
Cryptococcal or coccidioidomycotic meningoencephalitis
Viral meningoencephalitis (esp. herpetic, arboviral)
Spirochetal meningitis
Tumors and malignancy
Neurocysticercosis
Brain abscesses

FIGURE 2-79 Differential diagnosis of primary amebic meningoencephalitis. The major differential diagnoses of acute amebic meningoencephalitis are acute bacterial meningitis and meningoencephalitis caused by herpes simplex virus. (*From* Duma RJ: Primary amebic meningoencephalitis: infection by free-living amebae. *In* Lambert HP (ed.): *Infections of the Central Nervous System*. Philadelphia: B.C. Decker; 1991:257; with permission.)

Treatment of primary amebic meningoencephalitis
Amphotericin B
Miconazole
Rifampin
Sulfisoxazole
Tetracycline
Phenothiazine
Qinghaosu

FIGURE 2-80 Treatment of primary amebic meningoencephalitis. The optimal drug regimen for primary amebic meningoencephalitis is currently unknown. It has been suggested to use amphotericin B, parenterally together with intracisternal injection of amphotericin B, and concomitant administration of rifampin and tetracycline. Addition of experimental therapies, such as phenothiazines or qinghaosu, may be justified on the grounds that no effective regimen has been established.

SELECTED BIBLIOGRAPHY

Farrar WE: The nervous system. *In* Farrar WE, Wood MJ, Innes JA, Tubbs H (eds.): *Infectious Diseases Text and Color Atlas*. London: Gower Medical Publishing; 1992.

Okazaki H, Scheithauer BW (eds.): *Atlas of Neuropathology*. London: Gower Medical Publishing; 1988.

Scheld WM, Whitley RJ, Durack DT (eds.): *Infections of the Central Nervous System*. New York: Raven Press; 1991.

Tunkel AR, Scheld WM: Central nervous system infection in the compromised host. *In* Rubin RH, Young LS (eds.): *Clinical Approach to Infection in the Compromised Host*, 3rd ed. New York: Plenum; 1994:163–210.

Tunkel AR, Scheld WM: Acute meningitis. *In* Mandell GL, Bennett JE, Dolin R (eds.): *Principles and Practice of Infectious Diseases*, 4th ed. New York: Churchill-Livingstone; 1994:831–865.

Chapter 3

Viral Encephalitis and Related Conditions

Daniel F. Hanley
Jonathan D. Glass
Justin C. McArthur
Richard T. Johnson

Etiology and Epidemiology

Viral causes of encephalitis	
Togaviridae: alphaviruses	Rhabdoviridae: rabies
Eastern equine	Reoviridae: Colorado tick fever
Western equine	Orthomyxoviridae
Venezuelan equine	Mumps
Flaviviridae	Measles
St. Louis	Picornaviridae: enteroviruses
Japanese	Poliovirus
Murray Valley	Coxsackievirus
West Nile	Echovirus
Tick-borne complex	Herpesviridae
Bunyaviridae	Herpes simplex 1 and 2
California/La Crosse	Epstein-Barr
Rift Valley	Varicella-zoster
Adenovirus	Cytomegalovirus
Arenavirus	Retroviridae: HIV

Figure 3-1 Viral causes of encephalitis. A wide variety of viruses may cause encephalitis, but four families contain most of these: Flaviviridae, Togaviridae, Bunyaviridae, and Herpesviridae. The illnesses caused by these various agents may be clinically indistinguishable without laboratory testing, although epidemiologic features of the illnesses, including seasonality, geographic occurrence (or travel), patient age, and recent animal or insect bites, may aid in the diagnosis. (*Adapted from* Griffin DE: Encephalitis, myelitis, and neuritis. *In* Mandell GL, Bennett JE, Dolin R (eds.): *Principles and Practice of Infectious Diseases*, 4th ed. New York: Churchill Livingstone; 1995:877; with permission.)

Postinfectious viral encephalitis
Varicella-zoster
Mumps
Measles
Rubella
Influenza A and B

Figure 3-2 Postinfectious viral encephalitides. Postinfectious encephalitides typically develop 2 to 12 days after the onset of the primary illness and are characterized by a sudden recrudescence of fever and obtundation, with a perivascular demyelination of the brains of patients. Virus is rarely isolated from the brain, and the condition may represent an autoimmune or allergic response. Mumps can cause both primary and postinfectious central nervous system (CNS) involvement.

A. Nonviral conditions causing or simulating encephalitis: infectious causes	
Bacterial	Brain abscess
	Subacute bacterial endocarditis
	Tuberculosis, *Mycoplasma* pneumonia, brucellosis, listeriosis, cat scratch fever
	Syphilis, relapsing fever, Lyme disease, leptospirosis
Fungal	Cryptococcosis, coccidioidomycosis, histoplasmosis, candidiasis, nocardiosis, blastomycosis, actinomycosis
Rickettsial	Rocky Mountain spotted fever, typhus, *Ehrlichia canis*, Q fever
Parasitic	Amebic meningoencephalitis, malaria, toxoplasmosis, cysticercosis, trichinosis, trypanosomiasis

B. Nonviral conditions causing or simulating encephalitis: noninfectious causes	
Toxins/drugs	Heavy metals, salicylates, barbiturates, phencyclidine
Metabolic diseases	Electrolyte imbalances, hyperglycemia, hypoglycemia, acute porphyria, pheochromocytoma
Systemic diseases	Sarcoidosis, collagen disease, neoplasms, vasculitis, Whipple's disease, Behçet's disease
Others	Subdural empyema, subdural hematoma, cerebral infarction, demyelinating diseases, acute psychosis

Figure 3-3 Nonviral conditions causing or simulating encephalitis. Most nonviral causes of encephalitis are treatable and should be ruled out when evaluating a patient. **A**, Infectious causes of encephalitis include bacterial, rickettsial, fungal, and parasitic diseases. **B**, Many noninfectious conditions may have clinical presentations that mimic that of viral encephalitis. (*Adapted from* Mateos-Mora M, Ratzan KR: Acute viral encephalitis. *In* Schlossberg D (ed.): *Infections of the Nervous System*. New York: Springer-Verlag; 1990:106; with permission.)

Causes of encephalopathy in immunodeficient persons

Viral	Other
HIV	*Acanthamoeba*
CMV	*Toxoplasma*
HSV	*Cryptococcus*
Enteroviruses	*Nocardia*
Adenoviruses	*Histoplasma*
Measles	Primary CNS lymphoma
Papovavirus (PML)	

FIGURE 3-4 Causes of encephalopathy in immunodeficient persons. The causes of encephalitis are different in immunodeficient patients. In those with AIDS, various unusual agents may cause CNS disease, either singly or in combination. CMV—cytomegalovirus; HSV—herpes simplex virus; PML—progressive multifocal leukoencephalopathy.

Relative frequency of viral causes of encephalitis

Common	Less common	Rare
HSV-1	CMV	Adenovirus
Arboviruses	EBV	Colorado tick fever virus
Enteroviruses	HIV	Influenza A
Mumps virus	Measles virus	Lymphocytic choriomeningitis virus
	VZV	Parainfluenza virus
		Rabies
		Rubella

FIGURE 3-5 Relative frequency of viral causes of encephalitis. Each year, approximately 20,000 cases of encephalitis are reported in the United States. Herpes simplex virus type 1 (HSV-1) is the most common cause in the US, whereas worldwide most cases are probably due to the arboviruses. EBV—Epstein-Barr virus; VZV—varicella-zoster virus. (*From* Tyler KL: Viral and prion diseases of the nervous system. *In* Isselbacher KJ, *et al.* (eds.): *Harrison's Principles of Internal Medicine*, 13th ed. New York: McGraw-Hill; 1994:2313; with permission.)

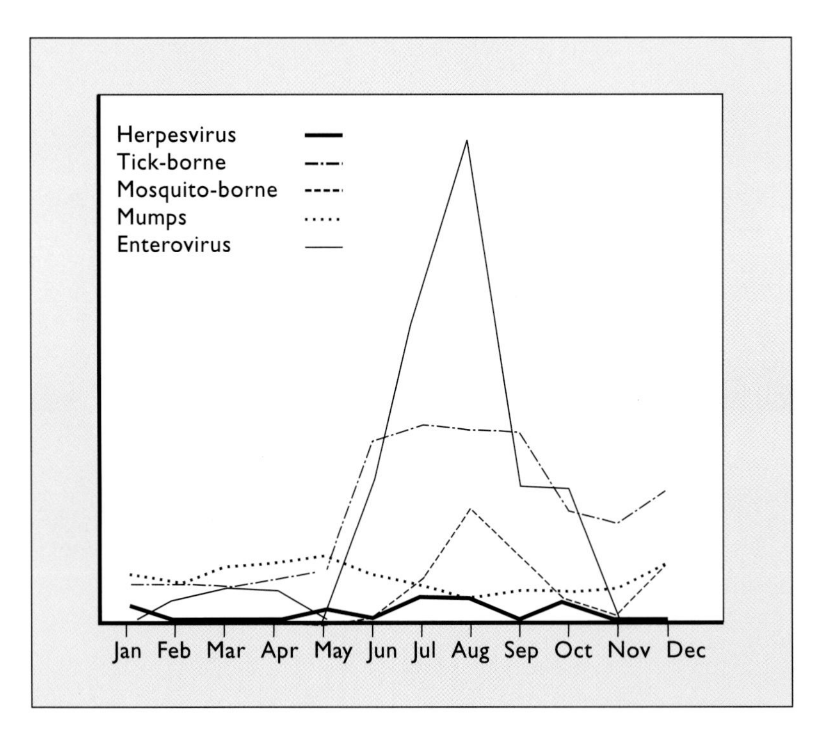

FIGURE 3-6 Seasonal variation of infections capable of causing viral encephalitis. In temperate climates of the northern hemisphere, the viral encephalitides have distinct seasonal occurrences that may be helpful in the differential diagnosis. Encephalitis caused by the mosquito-borne and tick-borne arboviruses peaks in the spring and summer, paralleling the periods of activity for their insect vectors. Others, such as the herpesvirus infections, may occur year-round. (*From* Griffin DE: Encephalitis, myelitis, and neuritis. *In* Mandell GL, Bennett JE, Dolin R (eds.): *Principles and Practice of Infectious Diseases*, 4th ed. New York: Churchill Livingstone; 1995:877; with permission.)

A. Geographical distribution of the major viral encephalitides

Virus	Geographic distribution
Japanese encephalitis	Eastern Asia, India
St. Louis encephalitis	US, Caribbean
California group encephalitis	North America
Eastern equine encephalitis	US Atlantic and Gulf coasts, Caribbean, South America
Western equine encephalitis	Western US and Canada, Central and South America
Venezuelan equine encephalitis	Texas, Florida, Central and South America
Murray Valley encephalitis	Australia, New Guinea
Rocio	Brazil
Tick-borne encephalitis complex	Worldwide
Lymphocytic choriomeningitis	Americas, Europe, Africa
Mumps	Worldwide
Measles	Worldwide
Rabies	Worldwide (except UK and Japan)
Herpes simplex encephalitis	Worldwide
Epstein-Barr encephalitis	Worldwide
Varicella-zoster encephalitis	Worldwide
HIV	Worldwide

B. Major causes of viral encephalitis in the United States

Virus	Geographical distribution
Herpes simplex	Nationwide
Mumps	Nationwide
St. Louis	Nationwide (esp. south and central)
California/La Crosse	Central and eastern US
Western equine	Western US
Eastern equine	Atlantic and Gulf coasts
Colorado tick fever	Western US
Venezuelan equine	Texas and Florida
Rabies	Nationwide

FIGURE 3-7 Geographical distribution of the major encephalitides. Geographic occurrence and travel histories may help in the diagnosis of the insect-borne encephalopathies, as each of the encephalitogenic arboviruses has a characteristic geographic distribution. For nonarthropod-borne viruses, occurrence can be worldwide, but seasonal occurrence and the presence of epidemic disease in the community may help identify the etiology. **A**, Major causes of viral encephalitis worldwide. **B**, Major causes of viral encephalitis in the United States.

Epidemiologic features of the major viral encephalitides

Virus	Age/Sex	Season	Transmission
Alphavirus group			
Eastern equine	< 10, > 55 yrs	Summer	Mosquito
Western equine	Infants, elderly	Summer	Mosquito
Venezuelan equine	Any age	Rainy months	Mosquito
Flavivirus group			
St. Louis	> 50 yrs	Summer	Mosquito
Japanese	< 10, > 65 yrs	Spring–summer	Mosquito
Tick-borne complex	Any	Summer	Tick
Bunyavirus			
California group	Children, M > F	Summer–fall	Mosquito
Orthomyxovirus			
Mumps	Children	Winter–spring	Respiratory
Measles	Children	Winter	Respiratory
Rhabdovirus			
Rabies	Any	Year round	Animal bites
Herpesvirus			
Herpes simplex 1	Any	Year round	Unknown
Epstein-Barr	Young adult	—	Respiratory/oral
Varicella-zoster	Any	—	Respiratory/latent

FIGURE 3-8 Epidemiologic features of the major viral encephalitides. Patient age and sex as well as seasonality may help in the diagnosis.

Approach to the Patient

Signs and symptoms of acute encephalitis	
Common	Fever
	Headache, nausea, vomiting
	Mental changes (confusion, delirium, lethargy, stupor, coma)
	Seizures (generalized or focal)
	Hyperreflexia, Babinski's sign, spasticity
	Mild stiff neck
Rare	Tremor, dysarthria
	Hemiparesis, cranial nerve palsies
	Aphasia, ataxia, blindness

Figure 3-9 Signs and symptoms of acute encephalitis. Acute encephalitis is a febrile illness characterized by the abrupt onset of headache and mental obtundation. Encephalitis differs from meningitis primarily in that patients with encephalitis present with prominent mental changes and less prominent meningeal signs. Headache and neck pain are the only localizing signs in viral meningitis.

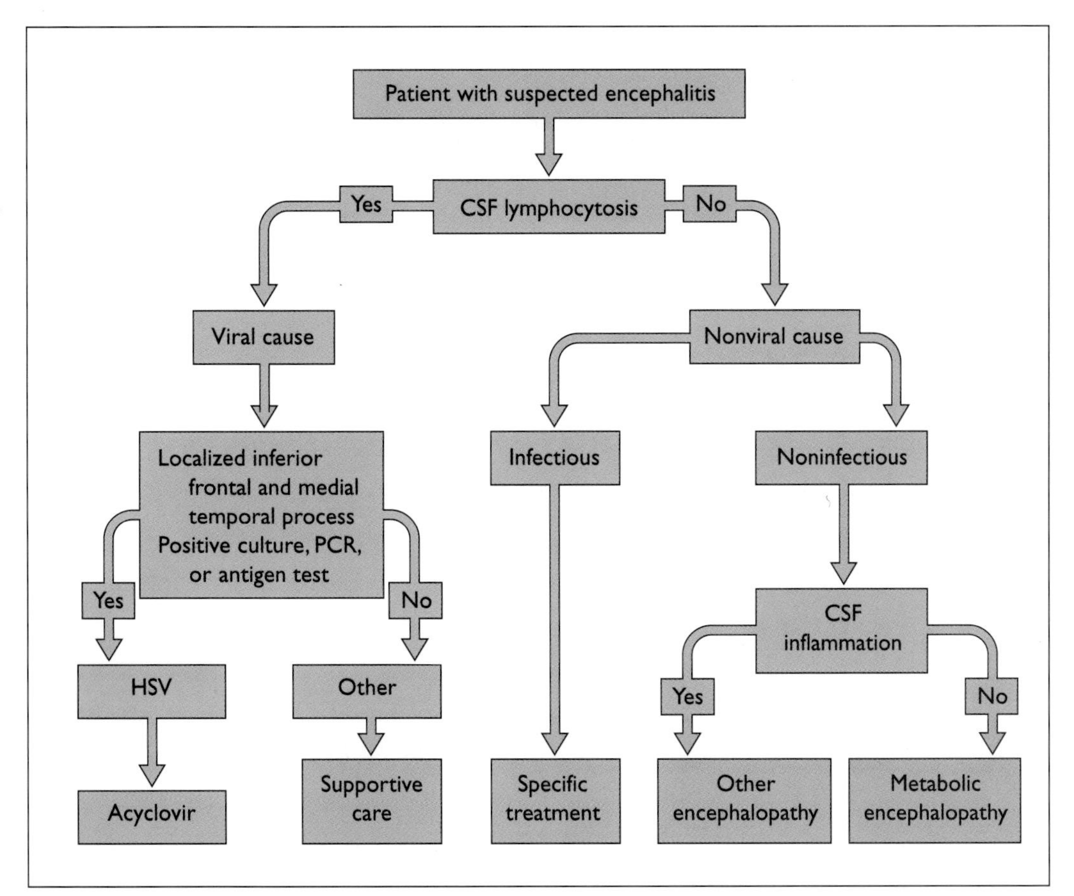

Figure 3-10 General approach to the patient with suspected encephalitis. In the febrile patient with depressed mental status, nonviral causes of encephalitis must first be considered and excluded, as treatment is available for many. Epidemiologic, clinical, and laboratory data are important in the differential diagnosis. If a viral encephalitis is suspected, a diagnosis of HSV encephalitis should next be considered. For HSV encephalitis, early treatment with acyclovir may be beneficial, whereas for most other viral encephalitides, treatment is supportive. CSF—cerebrospinal fluid; PCR—polymerase chain reaction.

Laboratory diagnosis of viral encephalitis	
CSF examination/ELISA	Neutralizing antibody (NA)
CSF culture	Immunofluorescence (IF)
Brain biopsy	PCR/nucleic acid amplification
Serologic studies/antigen detection	CT, MRI
Hemagglutination inhibition (HI)	EEG
Complement fixation (CF)	

Figure 3-11 Laboratory diagnosis of viral encephalitis. A range of diagnostic tests is available to help in the evaluation of the patient with suspected encephalitis, and their use is guided by the clinical situation. CSF examination is a key part of the evaluation of every patient, and assays for CSF virus-specific IgM (ELISA [enzyme-linked immunosorbent assay]) can aid in the rapid diagnosis of arbovirus infection. CSF cultures usually are negative for viruses but may be positive in bacterial infection. Serologic studies are useful in selected infections. Brain biopsy is usually necessary to diagnose HSV encephalitis definitively, although PCR holds promise as a substitute for biopsy. Computed tomography (CT), magnetic resonance imaging (MRI), and electroencephalography (EEG) are used to identify or help exclude alternative diagnoses and to help establish the presence of a focal encephalitic process.

CSF profile in viral encephalitis	
Opening pressure	Normal or elevated up to 300 mm H_2O
WBC count	0–500 lymphocytes/mm^3
Glucose	Normal
Protein	50–100 mg/dL
RBCs	Occasionally; presence suggests HSV
Demonstration of organism	Virus usually not recovered from CSF
Antibody detection	Positive after 7–14 days of infection or inflammation

FIGURE 3-12 Cerebrospinal fluid profile in viral encephalitis. The major distinction between encephalitis and encephalopathies is the presence of white blood cells (WBCs) in the CSF. Thus, CSF examination should be performed immediately in all patients with suspected viral infection of the CNS (unless contraindicated by mass effect and increased intracranial pressure). The CSF profile is indistinguishable from that of viral meningitis and consists of lymphocytic pleocytosis, mildly elevated protein, and a normal glucose. Occasionally, red blood cells (RBCs) will be present, especially in HSV encephalitis. Viral cultures may be positive in enterovirus, mumps, and occasionally arbovirus infections, but rarely in HSV infection. ELISA for CSF virus-specific IgM is key to the rapid diagnosis of many arboviral infections.

Virologic and serologic studies in viral encephalitis

Agent	Virologic studies	Serologic studies
HSV	Brain biopsy, PCR of CSF	Acute/convalescent sera CSF antibody detection
Arboviruses	Blood	IgM antibody capture ELISA of CSF or serum Acute/convalescent sera
Cytomegalovirus	Urine, saliva, circulating leukocytes; PCR	Acute/convalescent sera
Epstein-Barr virus	Rarely cultured	Acute sera for antibody profile
Varicella-zoster virus	Skin vesicles, CSF	Acute/convalescent sera
Rabies	Saliva, CSF	Serum after day 15
Adenovirus	Urine, nasal or conjunctival swab	Acute/convalescent sera
Enteroviruses	Throat washing, rectal swab PCR of CSF	Acute/convalescent sera
Influenza	Throat washing	Acute/convalescent sera

FIGURE 3-13 Virologic and serologic studies in viral encephalitis. Culture of skin and secretions is often helpful in establishing a diagnosis of viral infection. PCR is an investigational technique for detecting virus in CSF. (*Adapted from* Bale JF Jr: Viral encephalitis. *Med Clin North Am* 1993, 77(1):25–40; with permission.)

Antiviral chemotherapy for viral encephalitis

Virus	Drug	Dosage
HSV	Acyclovir	10 mg/kg q8h iv X 10–14 d
	Vidarabine	15 mg/kg/d X 10 d as 12-hr continuous iv infusion
VZV	Acyclovir	10–15 mg/kg q8h iv X 10 d
CMV	Ganciclovir	5 mg/kg q12h iv X 14–21 d
	Foscarnet	60 mg/kg q8h X 14–21 d (retinitis)
Influenza	Amantadine	200 mg/d po X 5–7 d
Rabies	HRIG	20 U/kg, *plus*
	HDCV	Five 1-mL doses given im over 28 d

FIGURE 3-14 Antiviral chemotherapy for viral encephalitis. Acyclovir significantly alters the course of HSV encephalitis, but therapy in most other viral encephalitides is limited to supportive care. Doses given are for patients with normal renal function. HDCV—human diploid cell vaccine; HRIG—human rabies immune globulin; IM—intramuscular; IV—intravenous; PO—oral. (*Adapted from* Bale JF Jr: Viral encephalitis. *Med Clin North Am* 1993, 77(1):25–40; with permission.)

Prognosis of selected encephalitides

	Mortality	Moderate to severe morbidity
HSV-1	Up to 80% untreated; 20% treated	30%–40%
Eastern equine encephalitis	Up to 70%	Up to 30%
St. Louis encephalitis	2%–20%	Rare
Measles virus (postinfectious)	15%	25%
Western equine encephalitis	< 5%	Low in adults, up to 50% in children
Enteroviruses	Rare	Low in general, but higher in areas of poliomyelitis under-vaccination
California encephalitis	Rare	Low in adults; sequelae in 15% of children

Figure 3-15 Prognosis of selected viral encephalitides. Although most patients with viral encephalitis have a benign outcome, a substantial number will have significant morbidity and sequelae. HSV causes only 10% of cases but is responsible for 50% of deaths in viral encephalitis. (*From* Kachuck N, Weiner LP: Viral meningitis and encephalitis. *In* Rakel RE (ed.): *Conn's Current Therapy 1993*. Philadelphia: W.B. Saunders; 1993:888; with permission.)

Herpes Simplex Encephalitis

Clinical and neurologic signs in herpes simplex encephalitis

Signs	%
Altered consciousness	97
CSF pleocytosis	93
Fever	85–87
Headache	79
Personality changes	70–80
Dysphasia	71
Autonomic dysfunction	58
Seizures (focal and generalized)	42–64
Vomiting	51
Ataxia	40
Hemiparesis	30–41
Cranial nerve defects	33
Memory loss	22
Visual field loss	13
Papilledema	13

Figure 3-16 Clinical and neurologic signs in herpes simplex encephalitis. A history of personality changes, bizarre behavior, hallucinations, focal seizures, or focal signs suggesting a temporal lobe lesion are common in HSV encephalitis, as this viral encephalitis usually is localized to the medial temporal and orbitofrontal areas and is often unilateral or asymmetrical. Signs do not differ significantly between patients with positive or negative cultures of brain biopsy material. (Whitley RJ, *et al.*: Herpes simplex encephalitis: clinical assessment. *JAMA* 1982, 247:317–320.)

Diseases that mimic herpes simplex encephalitis

Treatable ($n = 38$)		Nontreatable ($n = 57$)	
Infection		Nonviral ($n = 17$)	
Abscess/subdural empyema		Vascular disease	11
Bacterial	5	Toxic encephalopathy	5
Listeria	1	Reye's syndrome	1
Fungal	2	Viral ($n = 40$)	
Mycoplasma	2	St. Louis encephalitis	7
Tuberculosis	6	Western equine encephalitis	3
Cryptococcal	3	California encephalitis	4
Rickettsial	2	Eastern equine encephalitis	2
Toxoplasmosis	1	Epstein-Barr virus	8
Mucormycosis	1	Cytomegalovirus	1
Meningococcal meningitis	1	Echovirus	3
Tumor	5	Influenza A	4
Subdural hematoma	2	Mumps	3
Systemic lupus erythematosus	1	Adenovirus	1
Adrenal leukodystrophy	6	PML	1
		Lymphocytic choriomeningitis	2
		SSPE	2

FIGURE 3-17 Diseases that mimic herpes simplex encephalitis. PML—progressive multifocal leukoencephalopathy; SSPE—subacute sclerosing panencephalitis. (*From* Whitney RJ, Schlitt M: Encephalitis caused by herpesviruses, including B virus. *In* Scheld RJ, Whitley RJ, Durack DT (eds.): *Infections of the Central Nervous System*. New York: Raven Press; 1991:53; with permission.)

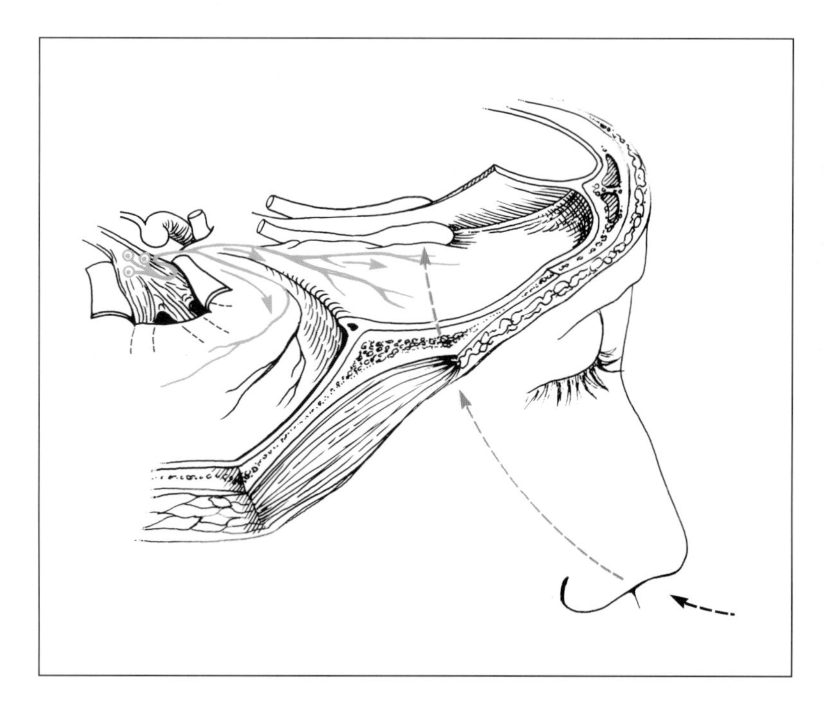

FIGURE 3-18 Route of infection in herpes simplex encephalitis. Anatomical pathways may explain the orbital-frontal and temporal localization of HSV encephalitis. Direct invasion of the olfactory bulb (*right*) could produce orbital-frontal infection, with spread to adjacent temporal lobes. Small sensory fibers from the trigeminal ganglia (*left*) project to the basilar dura of the anterior and middle fossae. (*From* Johnson RT: *Viral Infections of the Nervous System*. New York: Raven Press; 1984:137; with permission.)

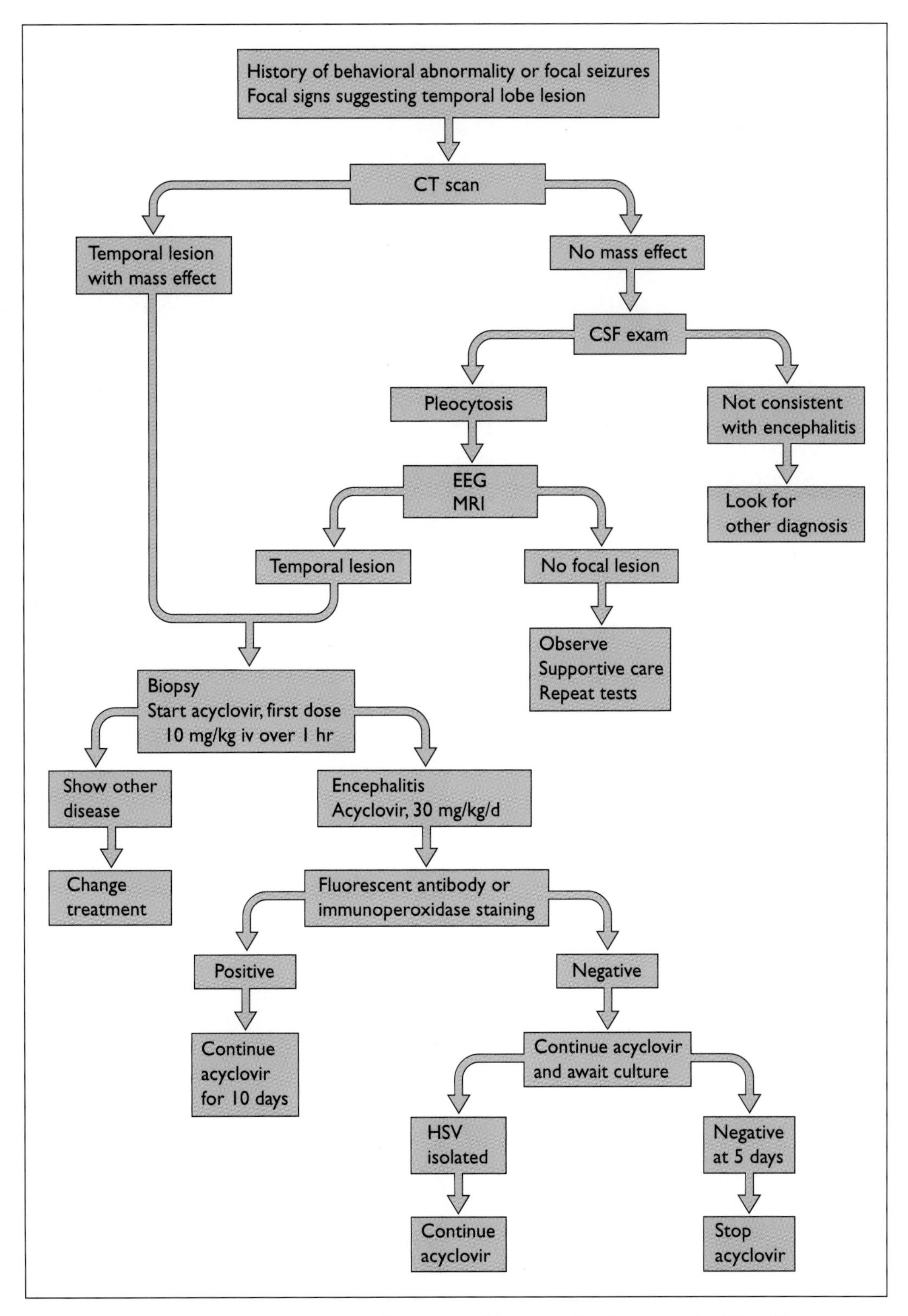

FIGURE 3-19 Steps in management of suspected herpes simplex encephalitis. (*From* Johnson RT: *Current Therapy in Neurologic Disease-2*. Philadelphia: B.C. Decker; 1987:126; with permission.)

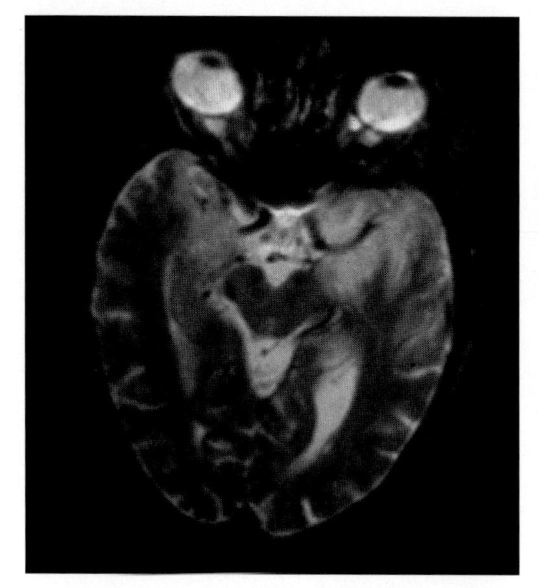

FIGURE 3-20 Brain edema in herpes simplex encephalitis. An MRI shows signal intensity in the bilateral anterior temporal lobes, consistent with brain edema. This MRI finding is commonly seen after 5 to 10 days of symptoms. Note the absence of compartment shift.

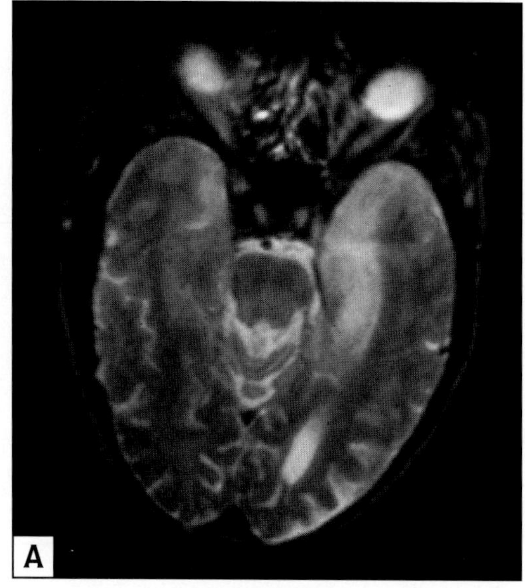

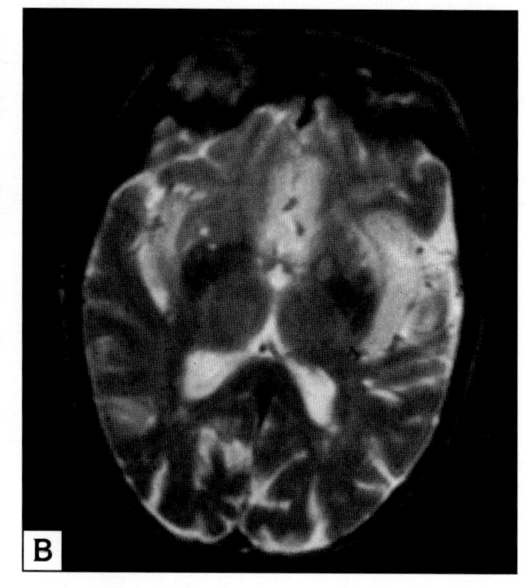

FIGURE 3-21 Brain edema in herpes simplex encephalitis. **A**, A rostral MRI section, from the patient seen in Fig. 3-20, demonstrates contiguous medial and temporal extension of brain edema. The presence of medial and temporal findings suggests contiguous spread from the trigeminal ganglia, across the meningeal space to the inferior space of the temporal lobe, and then direct rostral extension. **B**, The most rostral MRI section demonstrates direct extension to the insular cortex from the medial aspect of the temporal lobe.

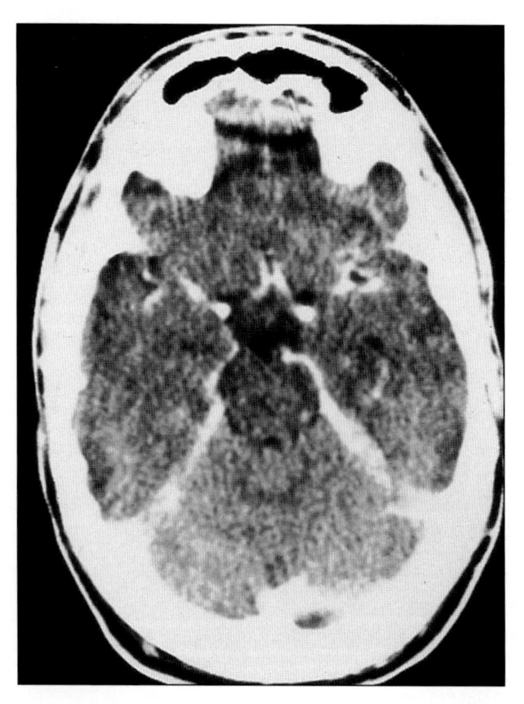

FIGURE 3-22 Temporal lucency and surface vessels on CT scan. A contrast-enhanced CT scan shows a medial temporal lucency and small linear enhancement suggestive of a cortical surface vessel. Dilation of surface vessels, increased number of surface vessels, and small areas of lucent tissue are early positive CT findings. However, the most common early CT picture in the first week of symptoms of HSV encephalitis is that of a normal CT.

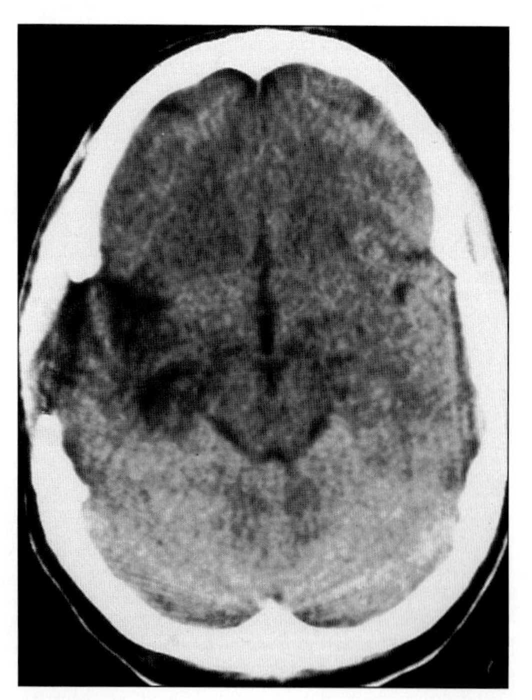

FIGURE 3-23 Temporal atrophy on CT scan. A post-biopsy CT scan demonstrates anterior and medial temporal atrophy. The absence of mass effect suggests that this CT was taken a month or more after the onset of HSV encephalitis and biopsy.

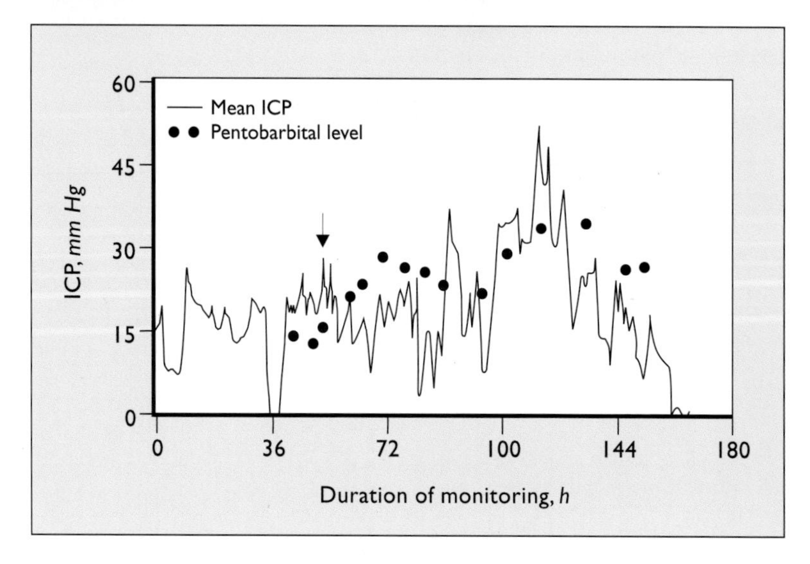

FIGURE 3-24 Time course of intracranial hypertension in herpes simplex encephalitis. Time course of intracranial hypertension is seen in a patient who underwent an unsuccessful attempt at high-dose barbiturate treatment of brain swelling. The *arrow* designates the time at which the patient experienced uncal herniation; the herniation appeared to occur without a severe alteration of intracranial pressure.

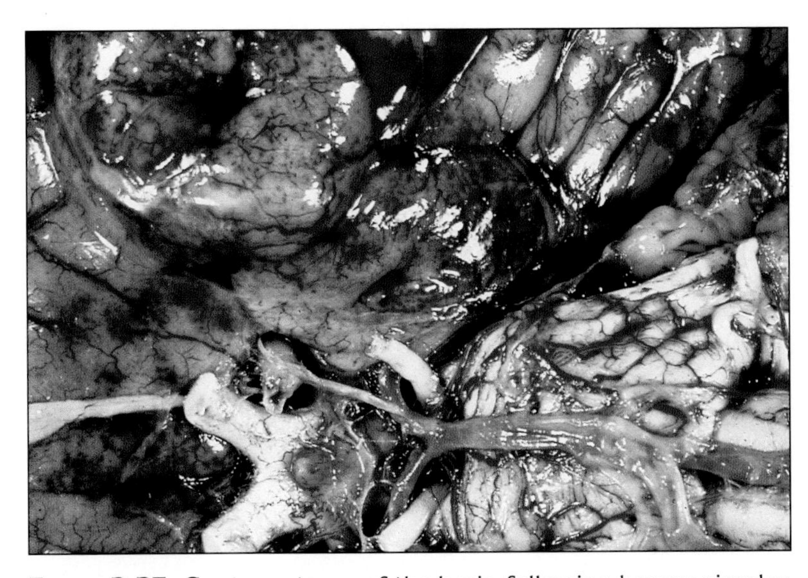

FIGURE 3-25 Gross anatomy of the brain following herpes simplex encephalitis. Note the marked frontal and temporal hemorrhages. Multiple petechial hemorrhages are seen on the medial temporal cortex surface. A lesser degree of hemorrhage is seen on the inferior surface of the orbitofrontal cortex.

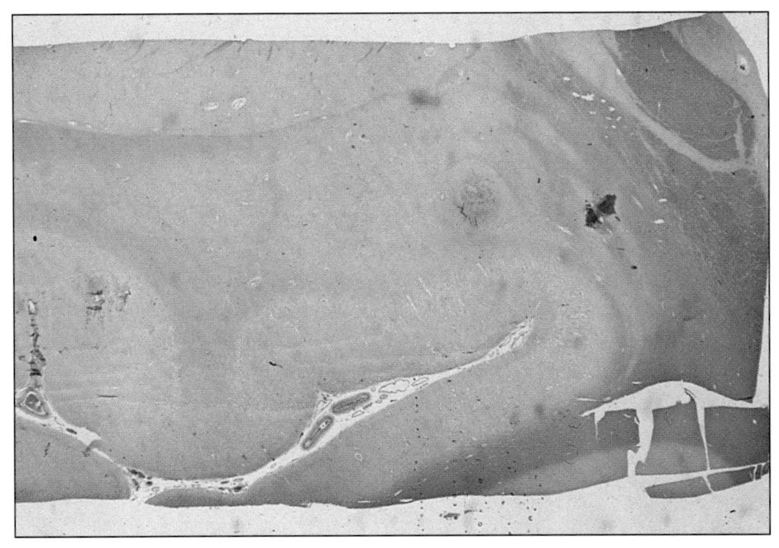

FIGURE 3-26 Temporal cortex from a patient with herpes simplex encephalitis. A low-power photomicrograph shows white matter and cortical involvement with hemorrhage. This bleeding is frequently punctate and can involve superficial cortex, white matter, or meningeal spaces.

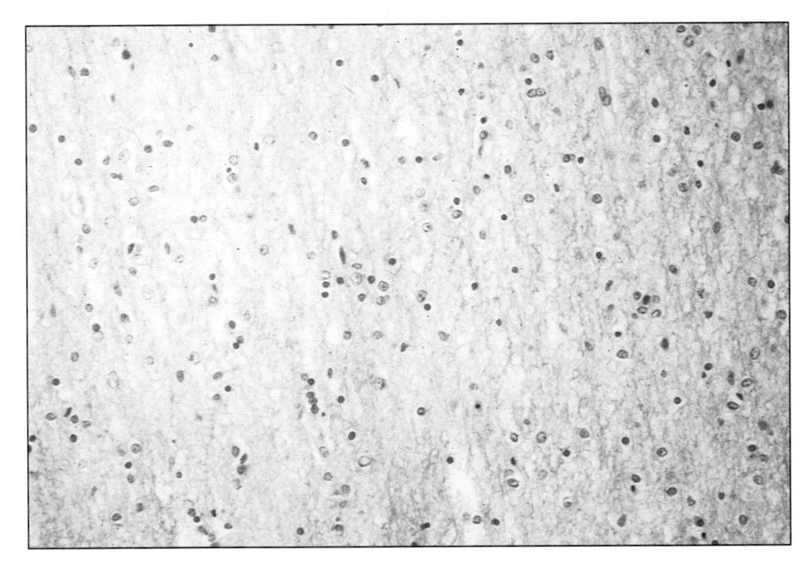

FIGURE 3-27 Herpes simplex inclusion bodies. A high-power photomicrograph from the specimen shown in Fig. 3-26 demonstrates inclusion bodies in both neurons and glia. Herpes simplex inclusion bodies can occur in vascular tissue as well.

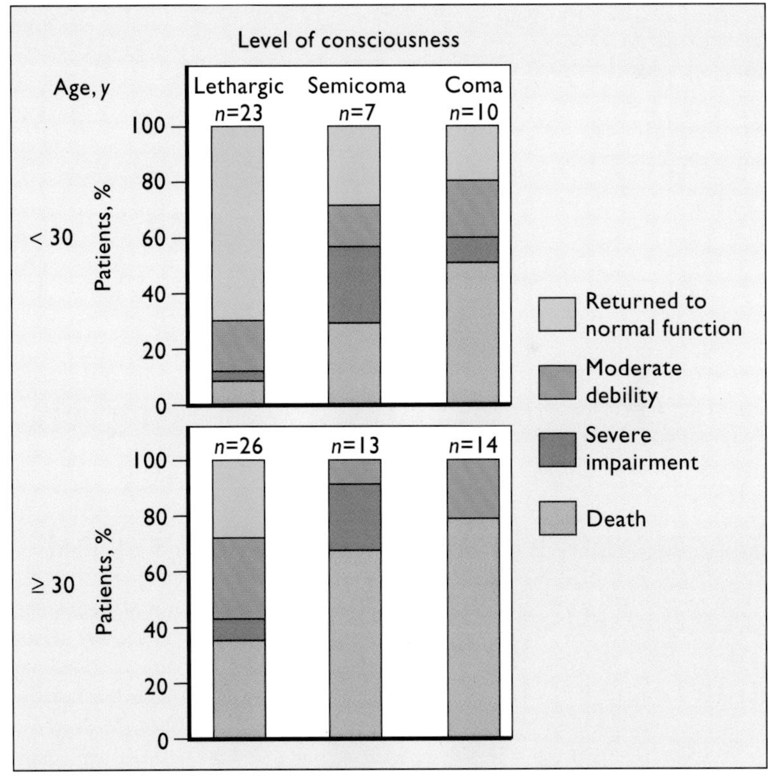

FIGURE 3-28 Prognostic factors in herpes simplex encephalitis (HSE). The level of consciousness and age are proven major determinants of clinical outcome in HSV encephalitis. Patients < 30 years of age and with a more normal level of consciousness (lethargic vs comatose) are more likely to return to normal functioning after HSE than older patients, especially those who are semicomatose or comatose. Mortality rates approach 70% in patients > 30 years of age, whether comatose or semicomatose, but are 25% in those < 30 years of age. (*From* Whitney RJ, Schlitt M: Encephalitis caused by herpesviruses, including B virus. *In* Scheld RJ, Whitley RJ, Durack DT (eds.): *Infections of the Central Nervous System*. New York: Raven Press; 1991:54; with permission.)

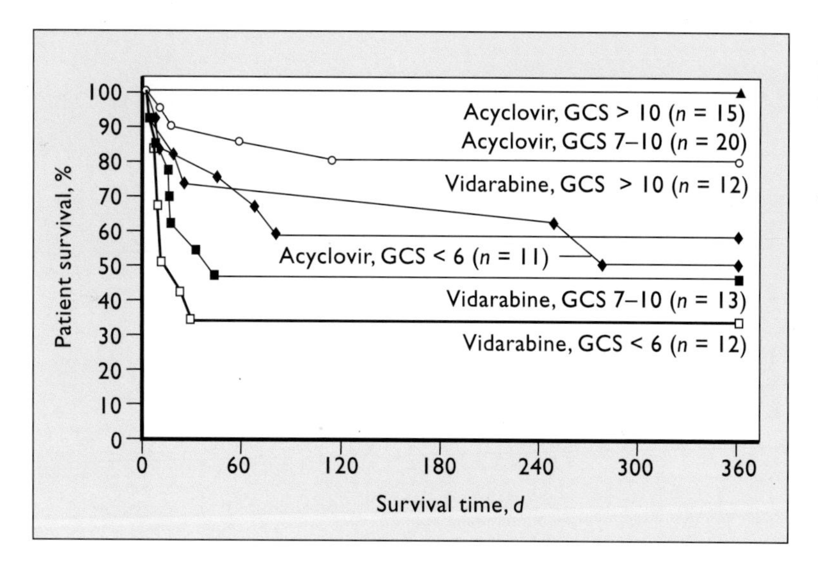

FIGURE 3-29 Survival of patients with biopsy-proven HSE: vidarabine vs acyclovir. Glasgow coma scores (GCS) which approached normal predicted improved survival. (*From* Whitney RJ, Schlitt M: Encephalitis caused by herpesviruses, including B virus. *In* Scheld RJ, Whitley RJ, Durack DT (eds.): *Infections of the Central Nervous System*. New York: Raven Press; 1991:55; with permission.)

POSTINFECTIOUS ENCEPHALITIDES

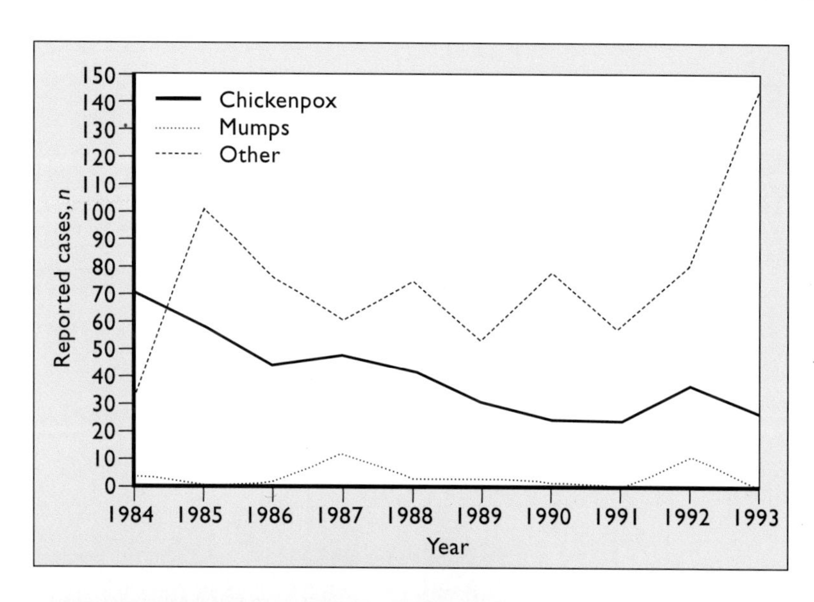

FIGURE 3-30 Frequency of postinfectious encephalitis, United States, 1984–1993. (*From* Centers for Disease Control and Prevention: Summary of notifiable diseases, United States, 1993. *MMWR* 1993, 42(53):27.)

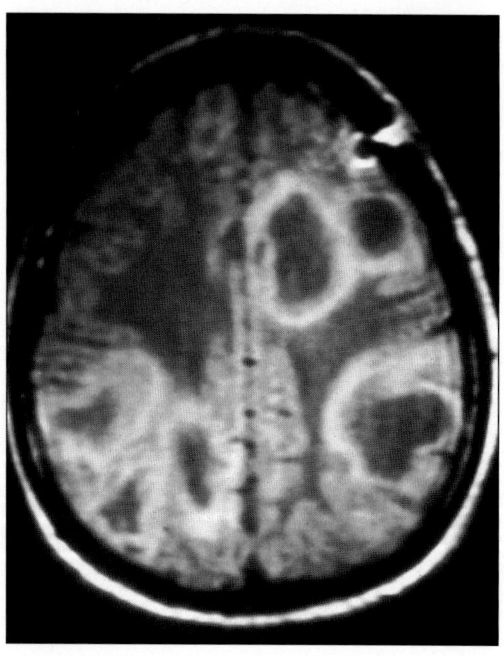

FIGURE 3-31 Ring-enhancing lesions on MRI in postmeasles encephalitis. An MRI scan with contrast demonstrates multiple ring-enhancing lesions of white matter occurring after measles infection. This condition is typically a postinfectious demyelinating disorder which presents 2 to 7 days after the initial rash. Usually the child is returning to normal activities when there is a sudden return of fever and depressed consciousness.

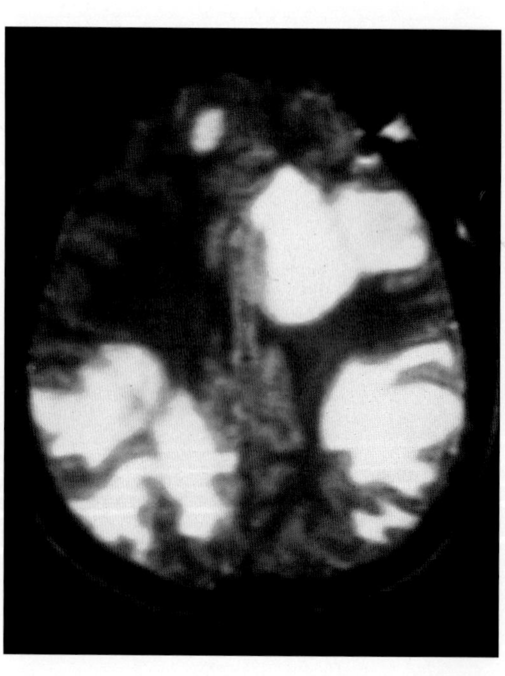

FIGURE 3-32 T2-weighted MRI of brain in post-measles demyelination syndrome. The MRI scan, from the patient shown in Fig. 3-31, suggests widespread edema or demyelination occurring in the entire subcortical white matter.

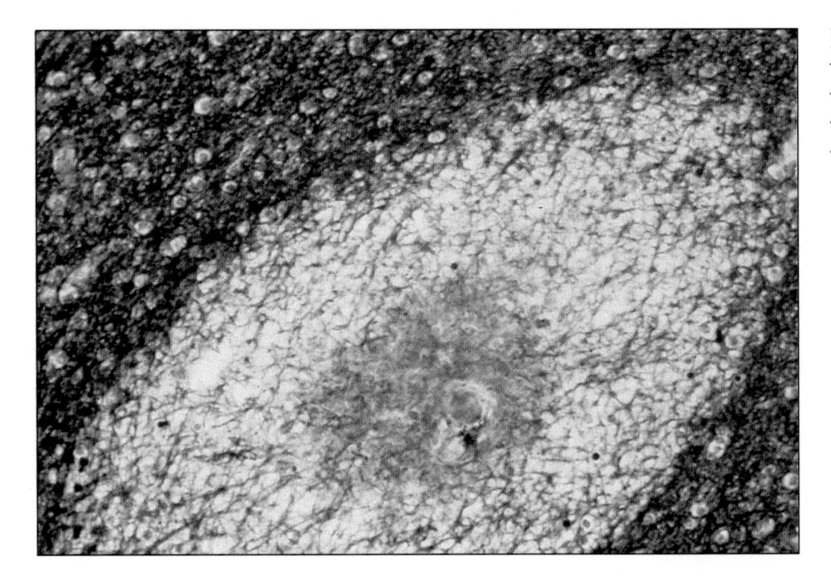

FIGURE 3-33 Perivascular demyelination in postmeasles encephalitis. A photomicrograph of brain tissue taken after measles infection shows a perivascular demyelination. Note the central blood vessel; this thin-walled vessel has a large lumen and represents a venule with circumferential demyelination.

ARBOVIRUS INFECTIONS

A. Major arboviral encephalitides: mosquito-borne viruses

Virus	Distribution
Togaviridae (alphaviruses)	
Eastern equine encephalitis	US Atlantic and Gulf coasts, Caribbean
Venezuelan equine encephalitis	Texas, Florida, Central and South America
Western equine encephalitis	Western US and Canada, Central and South America
Flaviviruses	
St. Louis encephalitis	US, Caribbean
Japanese encephalitis	Eastern Asia, India
Murray Valley encephalitis	Australia, New Guinea
Rocio	Brazil
West Nile	Africa and Mideast
Ilheus	Central and South America
Bunyaviruses	
California	Western US
La Crosse	Central and eastern US
Tahyna	Central and southern Europe
Rift Valley fever	Eastern and South Africa

B. Major arboviral encephalitides: tick-borne viruses

Virus	Distribution
Flavivirus	
Tick-borne complex	
Far Eastern	Eastern Russia
Central European	Eastern Europe, Scandinavia, France, Switzerland
Russian spring-summer	Eastern Europe, Asia
Kyasanur Forest disease complex	India
Negishi	Japan
Powassan	Northcentral US, eastern Canada
Louping ill	Great Britain
Reoviridae (orbivirus)	
Colorado tick fever	US and Canadian Rocky Mountains

FIGURE 3-34 Major arboviral encephalitides. Over 20 arthropod-borne viruses cause encephalitis worldwide; in addition, other members of these genuses occasionally cause encephalitis but are usually associated with febrile illness or hemorrhagic fevers. The arboviral causes of encephalitis are, for the most part, geographically and seasonally restricted. **A**, The mosquito-borne arboviruses. **B**, Tick-borne arboviruses.

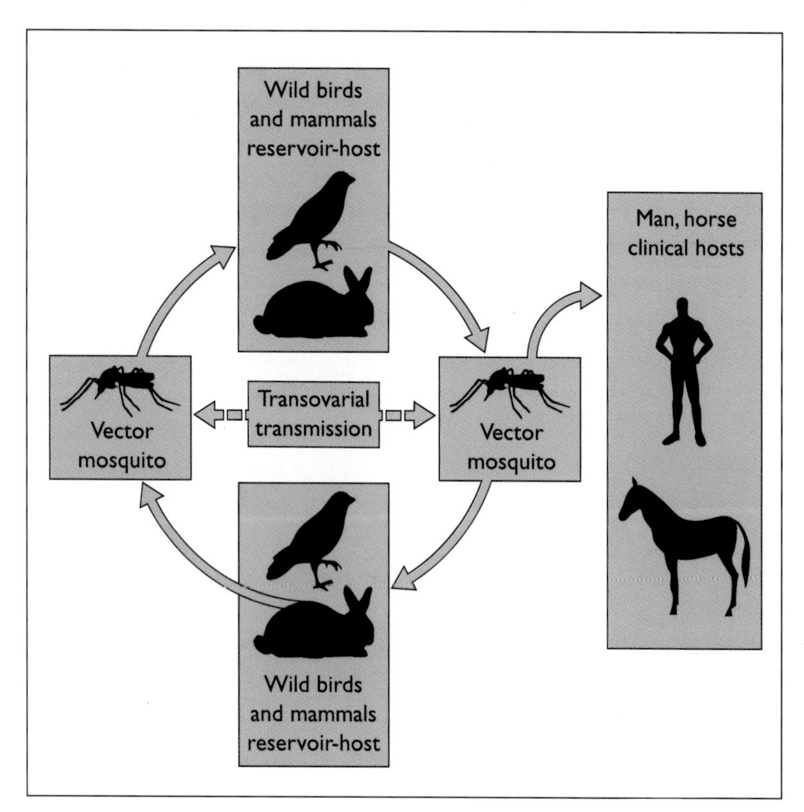

FIGURE 3-35 Generalized transmission cycle of mosquito-borne encephalitogenic viruses in North America. For all pathogenic viruses, humans are not natural reservoirs or amplifying hosts but only accidental "dead-end" hosts. The viruses are transmitted by mosquito vectors to birds and small mammals or rodents, in which they are amplified. The mosquitoes and reservoir hosts show no adverse effects from the virus. When viral infections occur in a large percentage of birds and small mammals in a region, coincidental infections and epidemics occur in larger animals (*eg*, horses and humans).

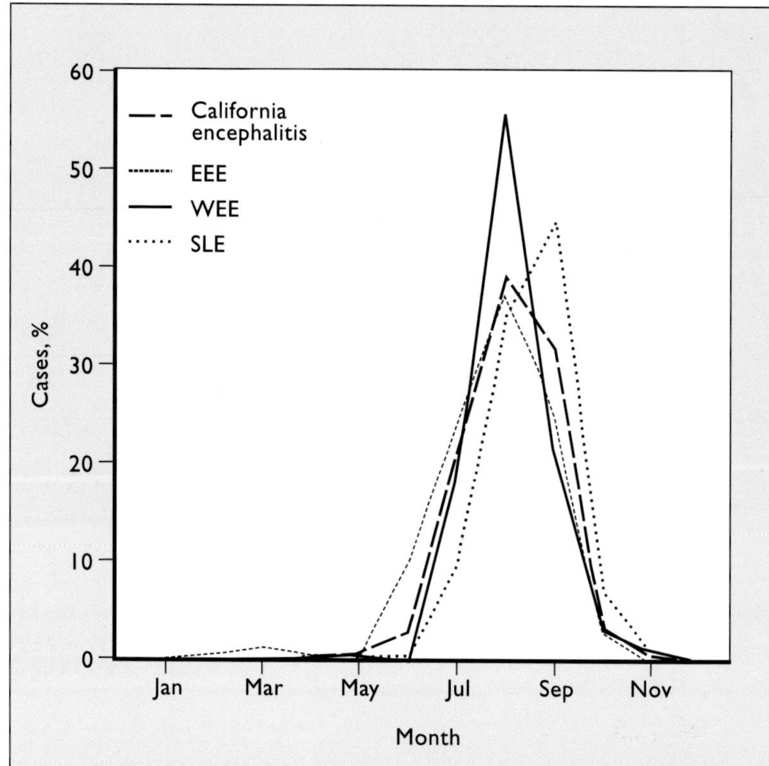

FIGURE 3-36 Seasonal distribution of arboviral encephalitides in the United States, 1972–1989. EEE—eastern equine encephalitis; SLE—St. Louis encephalitis; WEE—western equine encephalitis. (*From* Tsai TF: Arboviral infections in the United States. *Infect Dis Clin North Am* 1991, 5(1):73–103; with permission.)

Alphaviruses

Western Equine Encephalitis

Epidemiologic and clinical features of western equine encephalitis

Region	Western US and Canada, Central and South America
Environment	Rural
Season	June–September
Vector	Mosquitoes
Animal host	Birds, small mammals
Diagnosis	Acute/convalescent sera
Patient age	Infants, > 55 yrs
Unique clinical features	None
Mortality	3%
Sequelae	Low–moderate (esp. in young children)

FIGURE 3-37 Epidemiologic and clinical features of western equine encephalitis. WEE occurs primarily in rural agricultural areas of the western United States and Canada, with the central valley of California being an important endemic area; the virus also has been isolated from mosquitoes in the eastern United States. The severity of illness ranges from a mild, febrile, systemic illness lasting 5 to 10 days to severe neurologic illness with seizures, coma, and paralysis (in 5% to 10% of cases). Infants comprise approximately 25% of patients, but the highest attack rate is in those older than age 55 years. There is no sex predominance. Sequelae, including behavioral problems and convulsions, are frequent in very young children but diminish rapidly after 1 year of age.

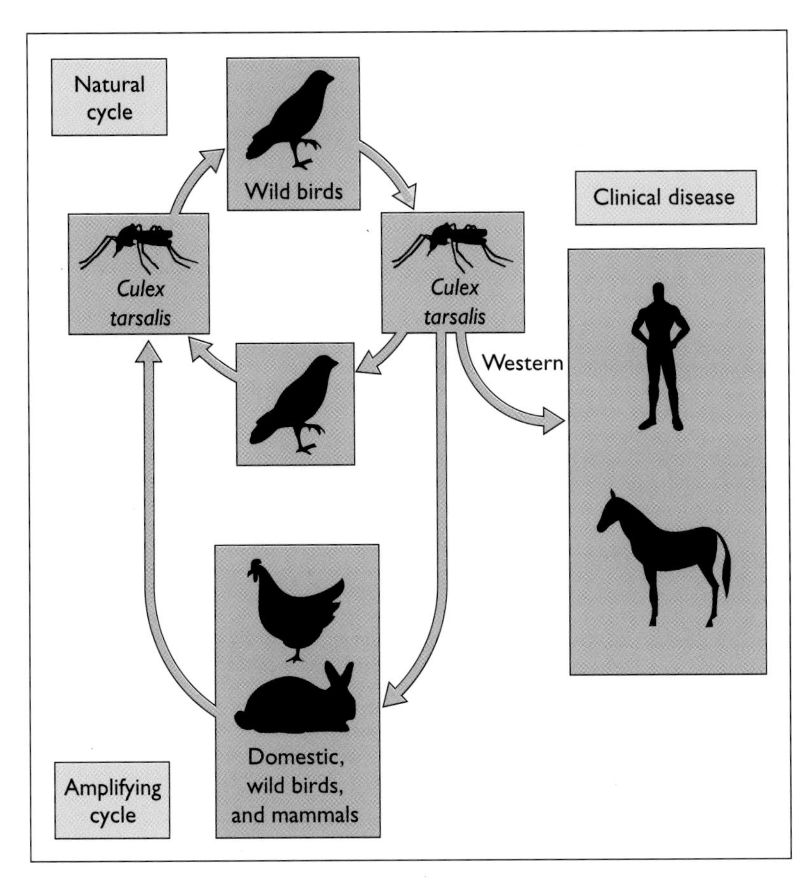

FIGURE 3-38 Transmission cycle of western equine encephalitis virus. The natural cycle is between *Culex tarsalis* and nesting and juvenile birds, but this cycle may be amplified by infection of domestic birds and wild and domestic animals. WEE virus can replicate in the mosquito at cooler temperatures, allowing epidemic disease in horses and humans to occur in early summer and north into Canada. (*From* Johnson RT: *Viral Infections of the Nervous System*. New York: Raven Press; 1984:113; with permission.)

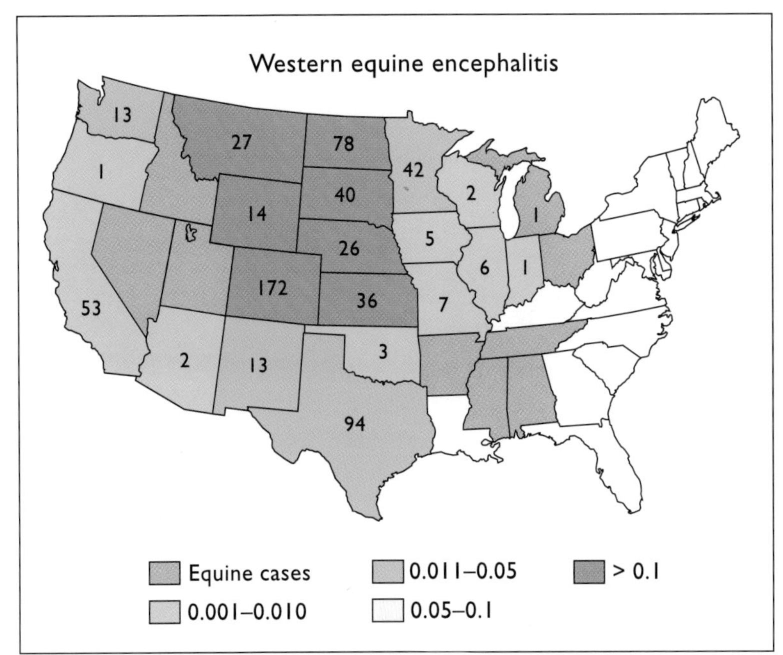

FIGURE 3-39 Geographic distribution of western equine encephalitis. Large equine epizootics were prevalent in the western United States in the 1930s. The largest WEE epidemic occurred in the central and northern plain states and western Canada in 1949, with > 3000 human cases. Currently, < 20 cases/yr are reported in the United States, although occasional outbreaks occur. The numbers represent cases reported from 1964 to 1989. (*From* Tsai TF: Arboviral infections in the United States. *Infect Dis Clin North Am* 1991, 5(1):73–103; with permission.)

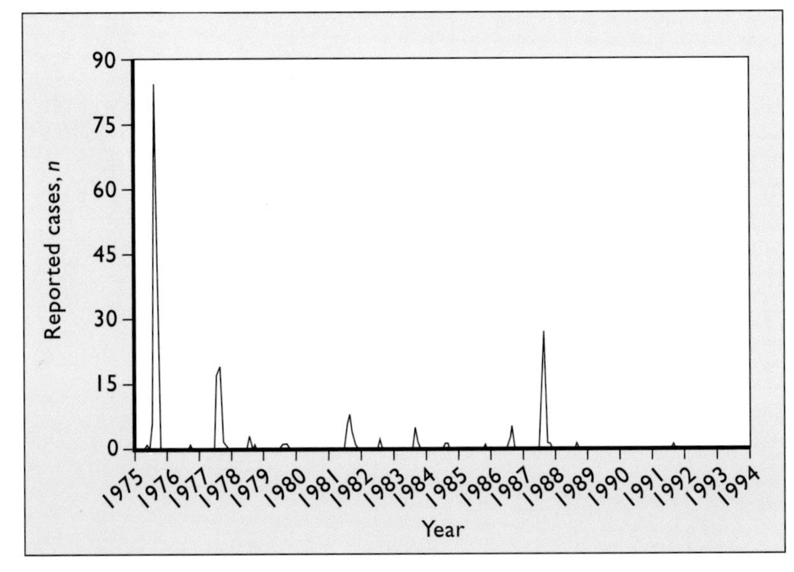

FIGURE 3-40 Frequency of western equine encephalitis, United States, 1975–1993. The incidence of WEE is decreasing with < 20 cases reported per year (no human cases were reported in 1993). In 1975, 300 cases were reported in an outbreak in the Red River Valley of Minnesota and the Dakotas. In 1987, 30 cases were reported in Colorado. (*From* Centers for Disease Control and Prevention: Summary of notifiable diseases, United States, 1993. *MMWR* 1993, 42(53):21.)

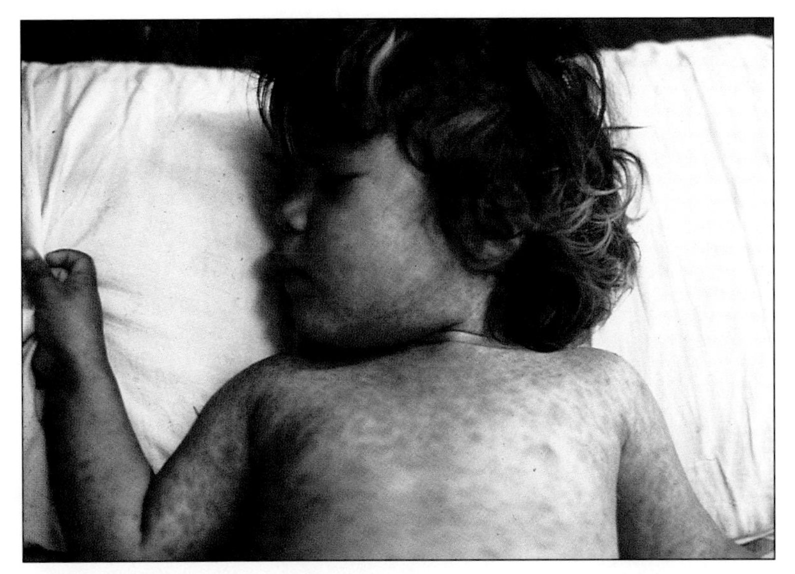

FIGURE 3-41 Macular rash of western equine encephalitis. A macular rash is evident on a child with WEE. The reason for a higher disease occurrence in children is not known.

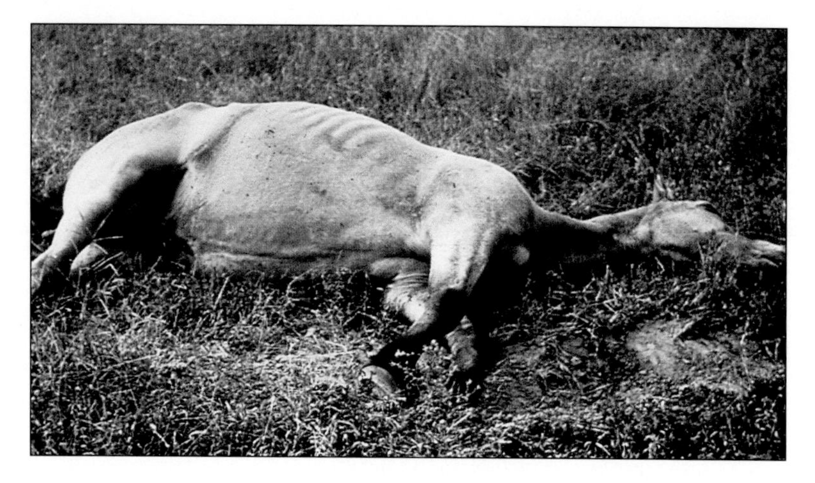

Figure 3-42 Dead horse. Human outbreaks of WEE are always preceded by an epidemic of infection in horses. The number of cases is dependent on the effect of rainfall on mosquito breeding, and the spread of virus from its 10 host birds into other animals, such as horses, is a marker for the spread of disease into the human population. (*From* CDC Teaching Collection, 3-42.)

Eastern Equine Encephalitis

Epidemiologic and clinical features of eastern equine encephalitis

Region	US Atlantic and Gulf coasts, Caribbean, South America
Environment	Coastal marshes
Season	June, July, August
Vector	Mosquitoes
Animal host	Birds
Diagnosis	Acute/convalescent sera
Age	< 10, > 55 yrs
Unique clinical features	CSF WBC > 1000/µL
Mortality	50%–70%
Sequelae	80% (esp. children < 10 yrs)

Figure 3-43 Epidemiologic and clinical features of eastern equine encephalitis. EEE is one of the most virulent forms of encephalitis in North America. Although it accounts for < 1% of human cases of viral encephalitis, it has an abrupt onset and rapid progression, with coma and death ensuing within 48 hours in many patients. A prodrome of intense headache, fever, myalgias, chills, and nausea and vomiting is quickly followed by rapid deterioration of mental status, seizures, and focal neurologic signs, leading to coma and death. Human infections occur sporadically and epidemically along the freshwater marshes of the East coast, Gulf coast, and Great Lakes region of the United States. Young children and the elderly are most susceptible and most often develop fulminant forms of encephalitis; young children have the most severe permanent sequelae, including emotional lability, retardation, and convulsions.

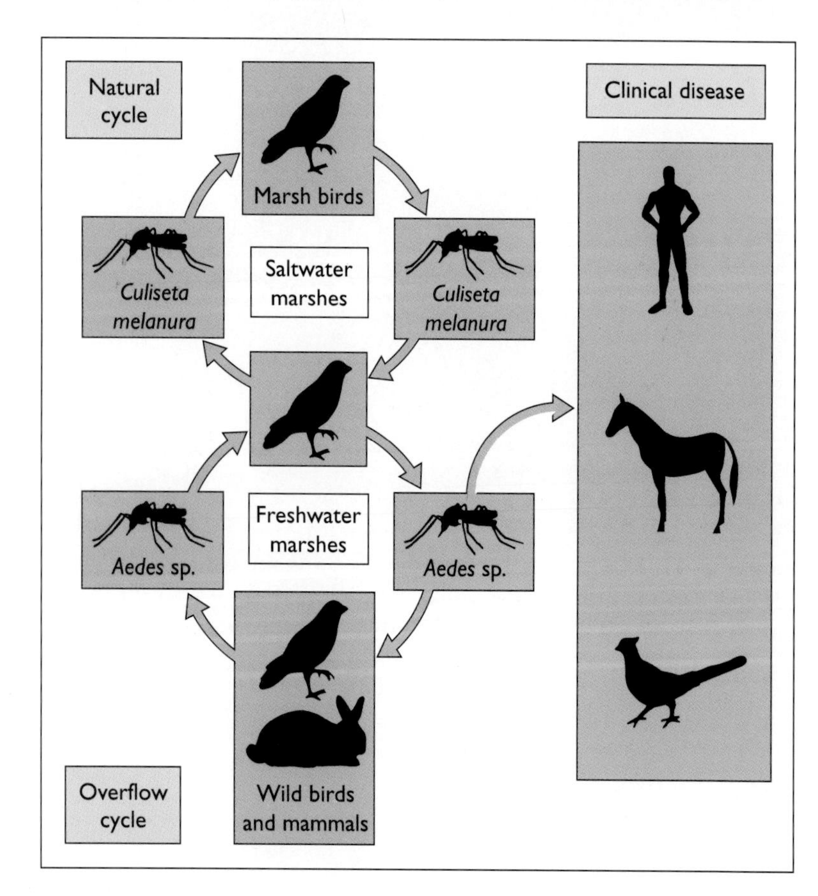

Figure 3-44 Transmission cycle of eastern equine encephalitis virus. The natural inapparent cycle is between small birds and *Culiseta melanura*, a saltwater marsh mosquito that does not bite large birds or mammals. Overflow of the cycle into *Aedes* mosquitoes, which inhabit freshwater marshes, can amplify the virus into other wild birds and mammals, and *Aedes* species may bite humans, horses, and pheasants which can develop clinical encephalitis. (*From* Johnson RT: *Viral Infections of the Nervous System.* New York: Raven Press; 1984:112; with permission.)

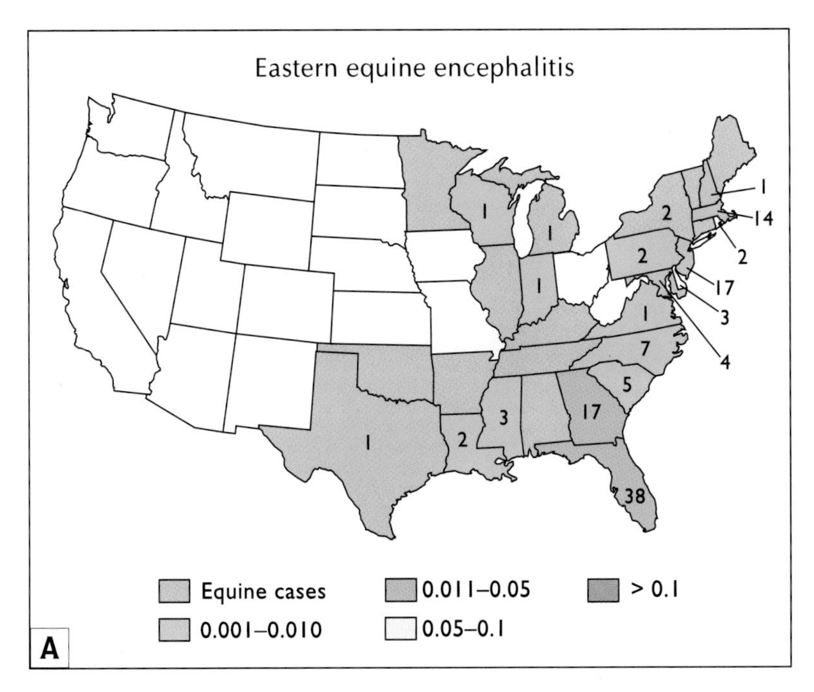

FIGURE 3-45 Geographic distribution of eastern equine encephalitis. **A**, In the United States, EEE occurs in areas of coastal marshes along the eastern and Gulf coasts, as well as the Great Lakes region. Numbers of cases reported are for the years 1964 to 1989. (*From* Tsai TF: Arboviral infections in the United States. *Infect Dis Clin North Am* 1991, 5(1):73–103; with permission.)

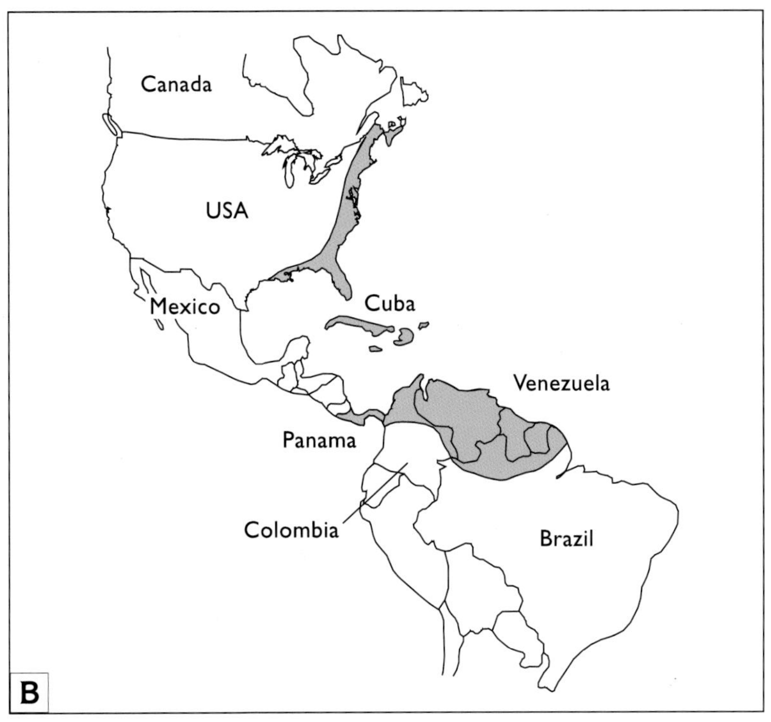

B, The range of EEE extends from the United States, though the Caribbean, and into northern South America. (*From* Wood M, Anderson M: *Neurological Infections*. Philadelphia: W.B. Saunders; 1988:392; with permission.)

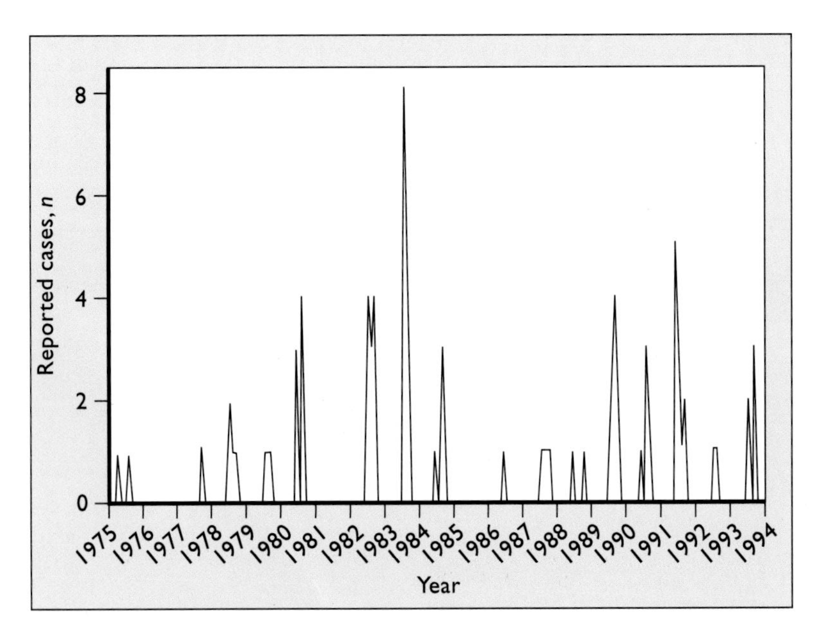

FIGURE 3-46 Frequency of eastern equine encephalitis, United States, 1975–1993. Less than five cases of EEE occur annually in the United States, and in 1993, there were five human cases reported from four states. The largest reported epidemic led to 32 cases in New Jersey in 1959. (*From* Centers for Disease Control and Prevention: Summary of notifiable diseases, United States, 1993. *MMWR* 1993, 42(53):21.)

Venezuelan Equine Encephalitis

Epidemiologic and clinical features of Venezuelan equine encephalitis

Region	Central and South America, Texas, Florida
Environment	Rural
Season	Rainy months (May–Dec in Northern Hemisphere)
Vector	Mosquitoes
Animal host	Horse, small animals
Diagnosis	Acute/convalescent sera
Age/sex	Any, increased severity in young
Unique clinical features	—
Mortality	< 1%
Sequelae	Rare

FIGURE 3-47 Epidemiologic and clinical features of Venezuelan equine encephalitis (VEE). VEE is principally an epizootic disease of horses in South America. Human infection is usually mild, encephalitis is uncommon, and mortality is < 1%. The disease usually presents as a mild febrile illness of 2 to 3 days' duration with no neurologic involvement. A second syndrome consists of a generalized systemic febrile illness; encephalitis, the third and least common pattern, occurs in < 10% of cases and is usually mild.

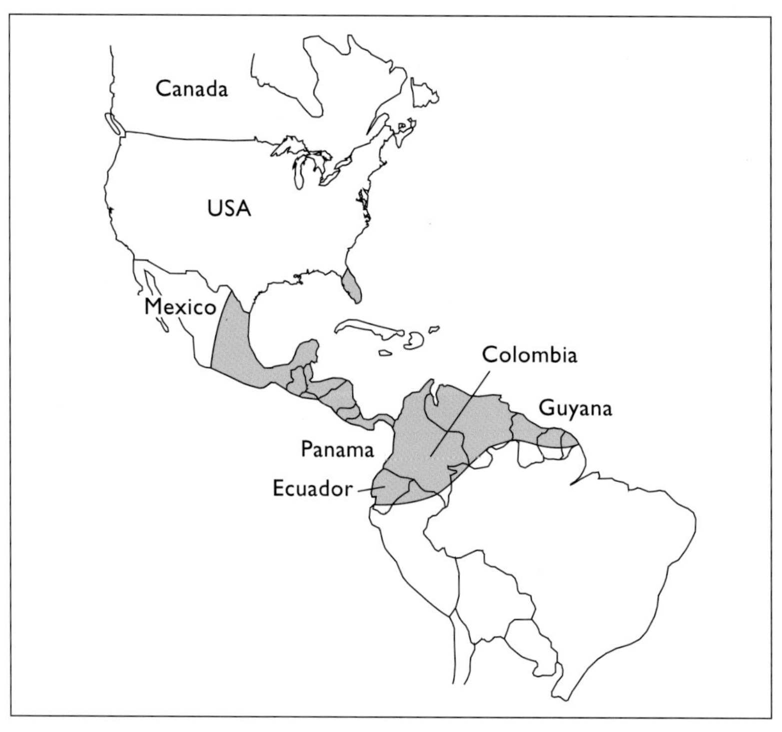

FIGURE 3-48 Geographic distribution of Venezuelan equine encephalitis. Epidemics occur regularly in northern South America and may extend to Texas and Florida. In the 1971 Texas epidemic, 88 cases were confirmed, though none developed encephalitis or died. (*From* Wood M, Anderson M: *Neurological Infections.* London: W.B. Saunders; 1988:395; with permission.)

Flaviviruses

Major flavivirus encephalitides

Mosquito-borne	
St. Louis	US (esp. south and central)
Japanese	Asia
Murray Valley	Australia, New Guinea
Rocio (São Paulo)	Brazil
West Nile	Africa and Mideast
Ilheus	South and Central America
Tick-borne	
Tick-borne complex	Worldwide
Powassan	US, Canada

FIGURE 3-49 Major flavivirus encephalitides. The family Flaviviridae contains 66 viruses, approximately 30% of which cause human disease. Several viruses in this family produce extremely severe and widespread viral illness, including yellow fever. Flaviviruses are transmitted by mosquitoes or ticks.

St. Louis Encephalitis

Epidemiologic and clinical features of St. Louis encephalitis	
Region	US (esp. south and central), Canada, Caribbean
Environment	Urban (eastern US), rural (western US)
Season	June, July, August
Vector	Mosquitoes
Animal host	Birds
Diagnosis	Acute/convalescent sera
Age/sex	Adults > 50 yrs, F > M
Unique clinical features	Dysuria
Mortality	2%–20%
Sequelae	25%

FIGURE 3-50 Epidemiologic and clinical characteristics of St. Louis encephalitis. St. Louis encephalitis is the leading cause of epidemic viral encephalitis in the United States. Numerous outbreaks have been reported since the 1930s, with the greatest activity in Texas, the Ohio-Mississippi River valleys, and Florida. In the western United States, the disease occurs sporadically in rural areas, but in the east, it affects primarily urban areas, causing widespread outbreaks that are especially severe among elderly residents. Unlike many other viral diseases, rates of infection and mortality increase with age. Most infections are clinically inapparent, but 75% of symptomatic patients develop encephalitis.

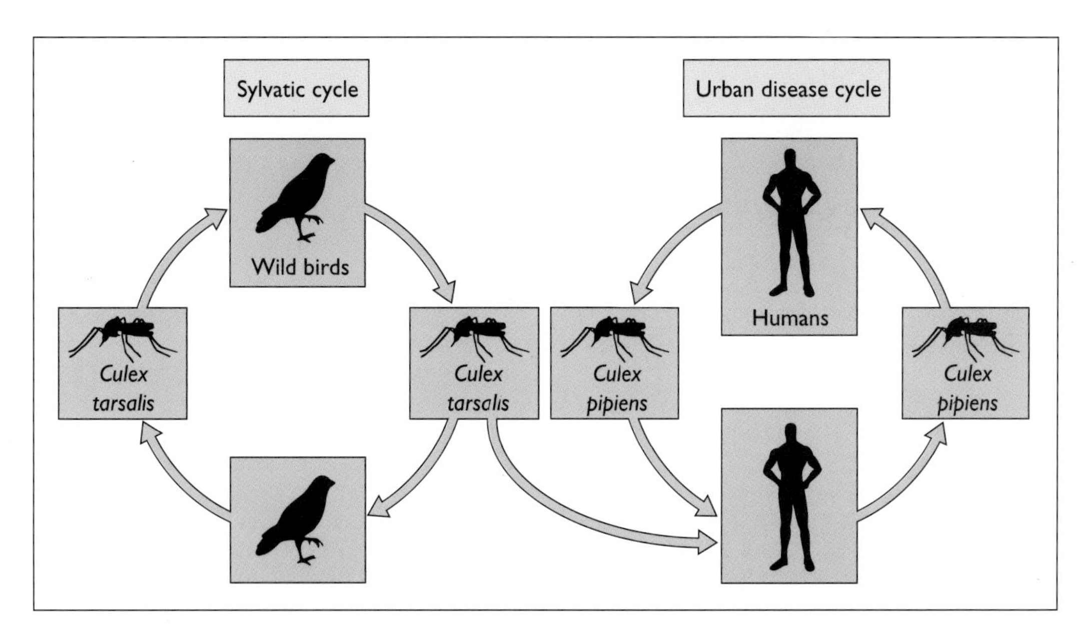

FIGURE 3-51 Transmission cycle of St. Louis encephalitis virus. The sylvatic cycle is repeated inapparently. The urban cycle can develop with city-breeding *Culex pipiens* transmitting virus directly from human to human (in this case, humans serve as active intermediate hosts). (*From* Johnson RT: *Viral Infections of the Nervous System.* New York: Raven Press; 1984:114; with permission.)

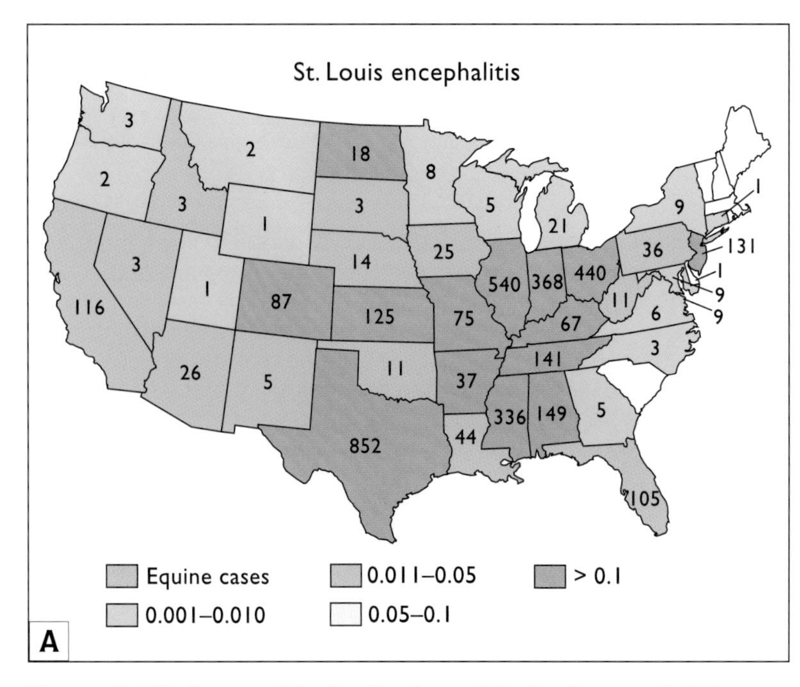

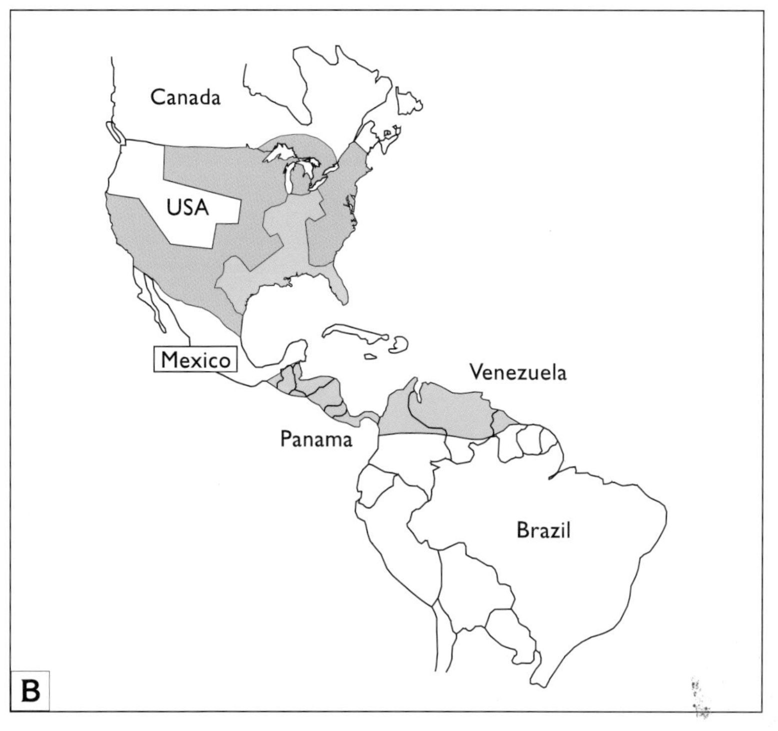

FIGURE 3-52 Geographic distribution of St. Louis encephalitis. **A**, In the United States, regions of most intense activity have been Texas, the Ohio-Mississippi River valleys, and Florida. The numbers represent cases reported for the years 1964 to 1989. (*From* Tsai TF: Arboviral infections in the United States. *Infect Dis Clin North Am* 1991, 5(1):73–103; with permission.) **B**, St. Louis encephalitis is most prevalent in the United States, but cases occur throughout the Caribbean and Central and South America. (*From* Wood M, Anderson M: *Neurological Infections.* Philadelphia: W.B. Saunders; 1988:397; with permission.)

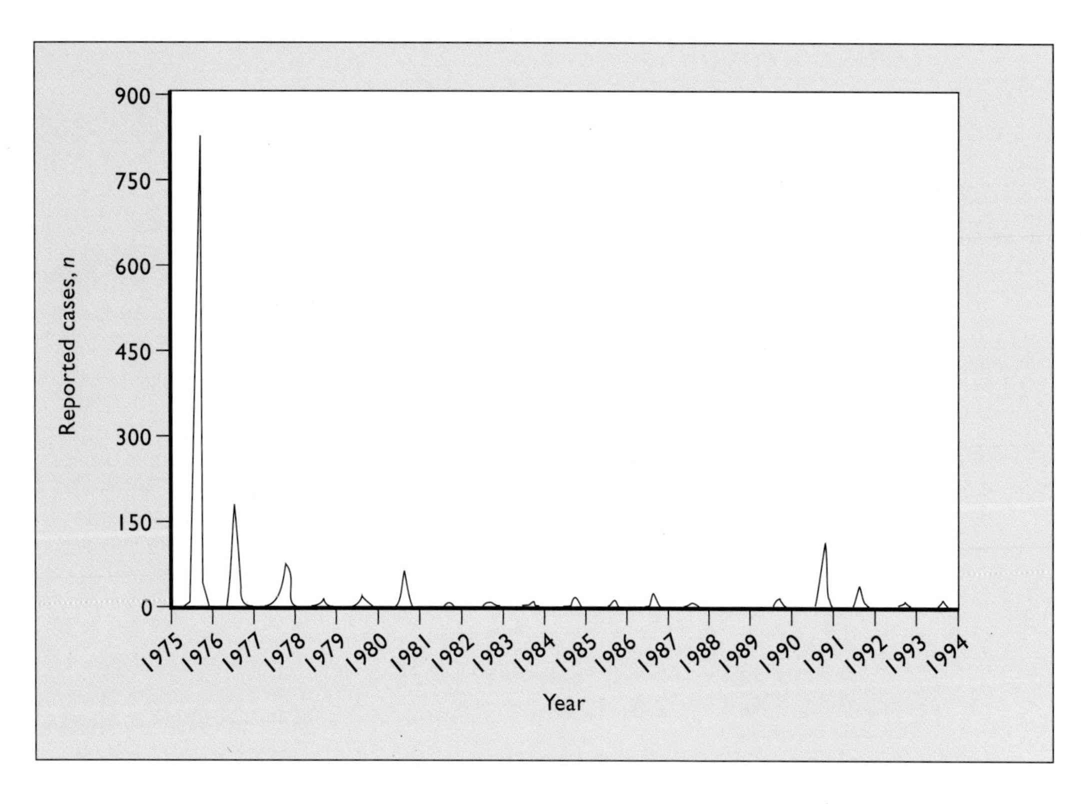

FIGURE 3-53 Frequency of St. Louis encephalitis, United States, 1975–1993. Intermittent epidemics of St. Louis encephalitis occur in urban areas of the east, affecting hundreds to thousands of people. Major multistate outbreaks occur at approximately 10-year intervals. The last great outbreak, in 1975, led to > 2800 cases in 31 states, with 171 deaths. In 1993, there were 18 cases reported from five states. (*From* Centers for Disease Control and Prevention: Summary of notifiable diseases, United States, 1993. *MMWR* 1993, 42(53):20.)

Japanese Encephalitis

Epidemiologic and clinical features of Japanese encephalitis

Region	East and southeast Asia, India
Environment	Rice fields
Season	May–September
Vector	Mosquitoes
Animal host	Wild birds, swine
Diagnosis	Acute/convalescent sera
Age/sex	< 10 yrs, > 65 yrs; M > F
Unique clinical features	Gastrointestinal symptoms (in some)
Mortality	7%–50%
Sequelae	30%–70% (esp. young children and the elderly)

FIGURE 3-54 Epidemiologic and clinical features of Japanese encephalitis. Japanese encephalitis is geographically the most widely distributed of all arthropod-borne encephalitides, occurring throughout Asia, and it is the most common cause of human viral encephalitis worldwide. It has been associated with frequent epidemics in Asia, causing as many as 50,000 cases annually. The ratio of inapparent to symptomatic infections is 200:1 to 300:1, but when encephalitis occurs, mortality is high and the neurologic sequelae significant. The infection has a 6- to 16-day incubation period, followed by the acute onset of nonspecific febrile illness lasting 2 to 4 days; the illness progresses with deterioration of mental function in up to 75% of cases. A gastrointestinal illness occurs in some patients. Seizures are more common in children than adults. Convalescence is prolonged; neurologic sequelae include seizures, ataxia, mental impairment, behavioral disorders, and tremulousness. An effective vaccine is available.

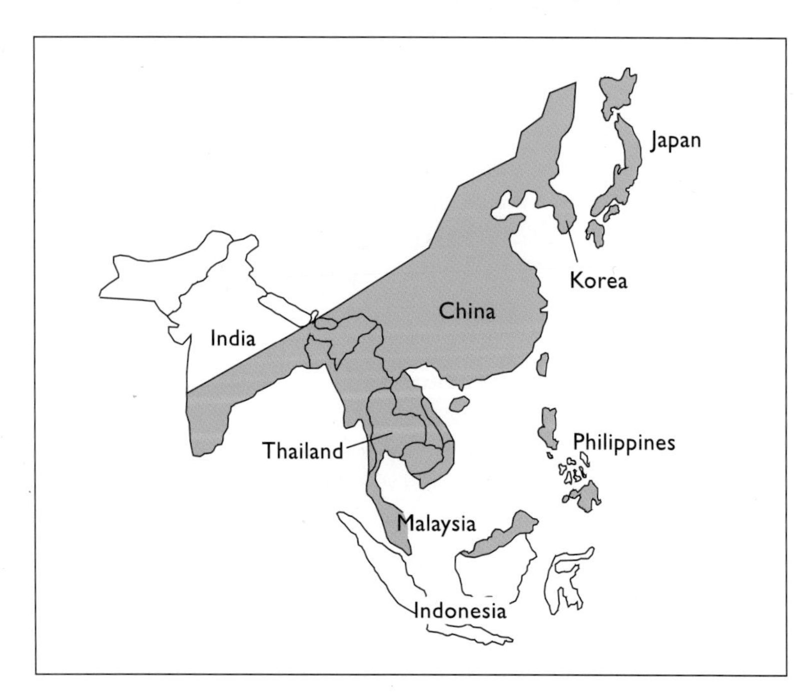

FIGURE 3-55 Geographic distribution of Japanese encephalitis. Japanese encephalitis is widespread throughout eastern and southern Asia and continues to cause > 10,000 cases/yr in China and Thailand. The *Culex* mosquito, primarily *C. tritaeniorhynchus*, which breeds in freshwater rice fields, is the main epidemic vector, with birds and pigs serving as amplifying hosts. In tropical climates, epidemics occur in the rainy monsoon months, and in temperate regions, the disease shows a late summer–early fall incidence. Since vaccination programs began in 1960, Japanese encephalitis has virtually disappeared in Japan (< 10 cases/yr); it is declining in frequency in China but continues to cause > 10,000 cases annually. (*From* Wood M, Anderson M: *Neurological Infections*. Philadelphia: W.B. Saunders; 1988:399; with permission.)

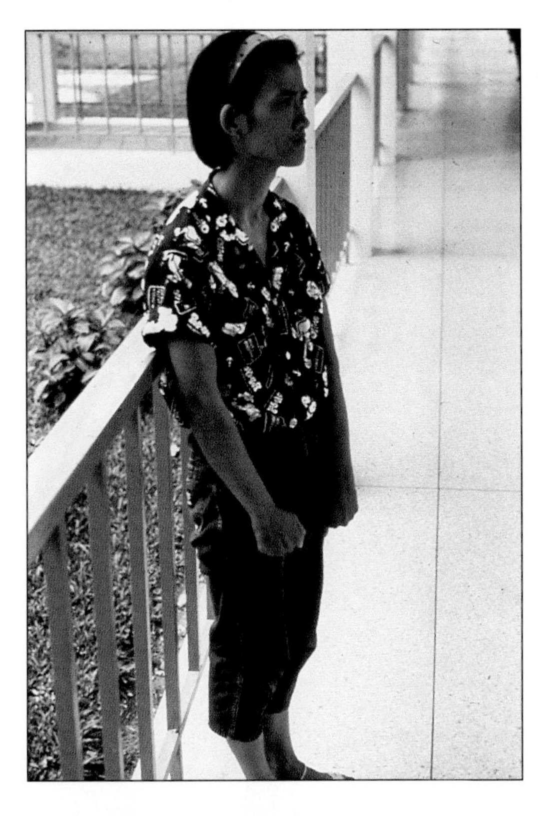

Figure 3-56 A patient chronically disabled from prior Japanese encephalitis. She has a dystonic posture and parkinsonian facies thought to be secondary to basal ganglion dysfunction.

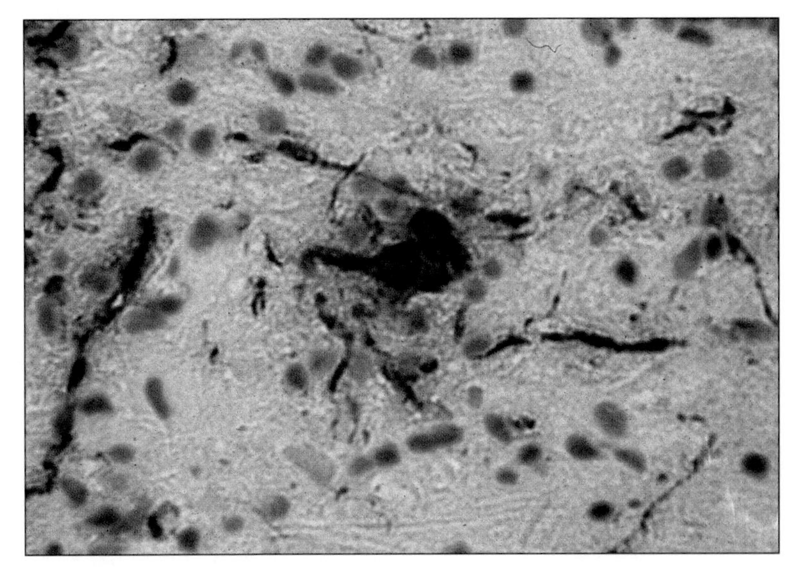

Figure 3-57 Medulla in Japanese encephalitis. A photomicrograph of the medulla from a patient with Japanese encephalitis demonstrates neuronophagia. The central body is a lipofuscin-containing neuron that is surrounded by glia and appears to be undergoing wallerian degeneration.

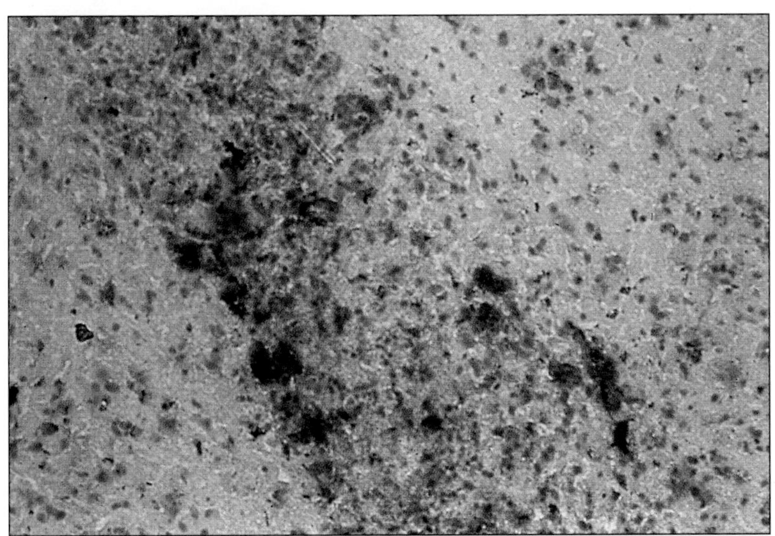

Figure 3-58 Basal ganglia in Japanese encephalitis. A photomicrograph of basal ganglia shows neuronal infection in Japanese encephalitis. This low-power view demonstrates gliosis, neuronal lipofuscin accumulation, and a decreased number of neurons.

Tick-Borne Flaviviruses

Tick-borne encephalitis complex

Virus	Tick genus	Geographical range
Far Eastern	*Ixodes*	Eastern USSR
Central European	*Ixodes*	Eastern Europe, Scandinavia, central Europe
Russian spring-summer	*Ixodes*	Eastern Europe, Asia
Powassan	*Ixodes, Dermacentor*	Northcentral US, Canada
Kyasanur Forest disease complex	*Haemaphysalis*	India
Negishi	Unknown	Japan
Louping ill	*Ixodes*	Great Britain

Figure 3-59 Tick-borne encephalitis complex. Tick-borne encephalitogenic flaviviruses comprise 14 antigenically related viruses that cause geographically isolated and clinically distinct syndromes worldwide. Ticks, primarily *Ixodes* spp., are the vector, and small wild mammals serve as natural hosts. Transmission in food, such as raw milk or cheese, also may occur. Powassan encephalitis is the only variant that has occurred in the United States and Canada, but human illness is very rare.

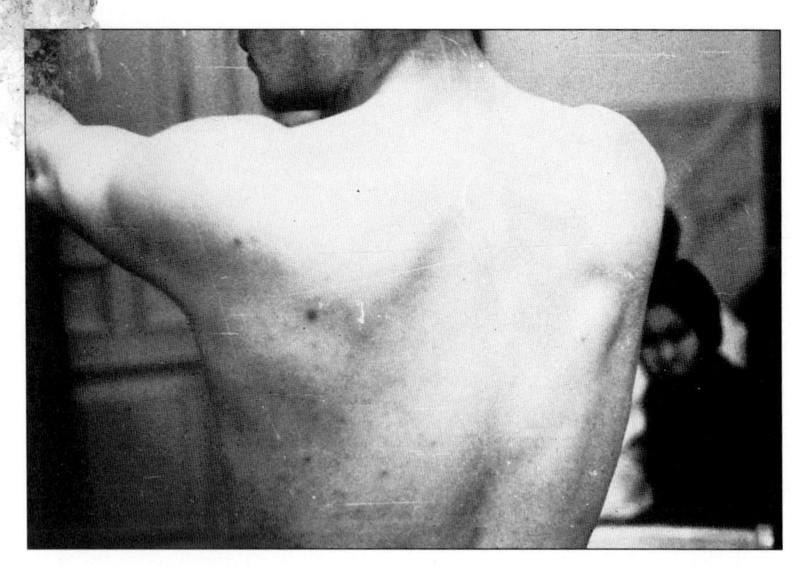

Figure 3-60 Scapular atrophy in tick-borne encephalitis complex. A Siberian man is shown with scapular atrophy several years after an episode of tick-borne encephalitis. This disorder demonstrates the propensity of some flaviviruses (tick-borne, St. Louis, and Japanese encephalitides) to infect the brain stem and upper cervical motor neurons. Note the outward displacement of the scapula and atrophy of the left trapezius.

Bunyaviridae

Bunyaviridae causing encephalitis

Virus	Mosquito genus	Geographical range
Bunyaviruses		
California serogroup		
California	*Aedes, Culex*	Western US
La Crosse	*Aedes*	Central and eastern US
Jamestown Canyon	*Culiseta, Aedes*	Michigan, New York, Ohio, Canada
Snowshoe hare	*Aedes*	Central Canada, northern US
Tahyna	*Aedes, Culiseta*	Central and southern Europe
Inkoo	Unknown	Finland
Phlebovirus		
Rift Valley fever	*Culex, Aedes*	Eastern and South Africa

Figure 3-61 Bunyaviridae causing encephalitis. Bunyaviridae comprises > 250 viruses, of which only a few cause significant human disease. These diseases include encephalitis, various hemorrhagic fevers (Congo-Crimean fever), as well as the 1993 Four-Corners hantavirus disease outbreak in the US southwest. These viruses are transmitted by arthropods, with the encephalitic viruses being transmitted by mosquitoes. La Crosse encephalitis, a member of the California encephalitis serogroup, is likely the second most prevalent mosquito-borne viral infection in the United States (following St. Louis encephalitis). Rift Valley fever, caused by a Phlebovirus, occasionally results in encephalitis and has been recognized recently in an Egyptian outbreak.

California Group Encephalitis

Epidemiologic and clinical features of California serogroup encephalitis

	La Crosse encephalitis
Region	US midwest and northeast, southern Canada
Environment	Woodlands
Season	June–September
Vector	Mosquitos (*Aedes*)
Animal host	Chipmunks, squirrels, small mammals
Diagnosis	Acute/convalescent sera
Age/sex	Children < 20 yrs, M > F
Unique clinical features	Seizures
Mortality	< 1%
Sequelae	Rare (< 2%)

Figure 3-62 Epidemiologic and clinical characteristics of California Group (La Crosse) encephalitis. The California encephalitis group consists of five antigenically related viruses, each of which has a distinct and narrow host range and geographic distribution. The La Crosse virus is considered the prototype of the group and is responsible for nearly all infections due to California group viruses in the United States. Less than 17% of La Crosse virus infections become apparent, manifesting as a simple febrile illness, encephalitis, or, most often, aseptic meningitis. In encephalitis, fever and somnolence are universal findings, and seizures occur in about 50% of cases.

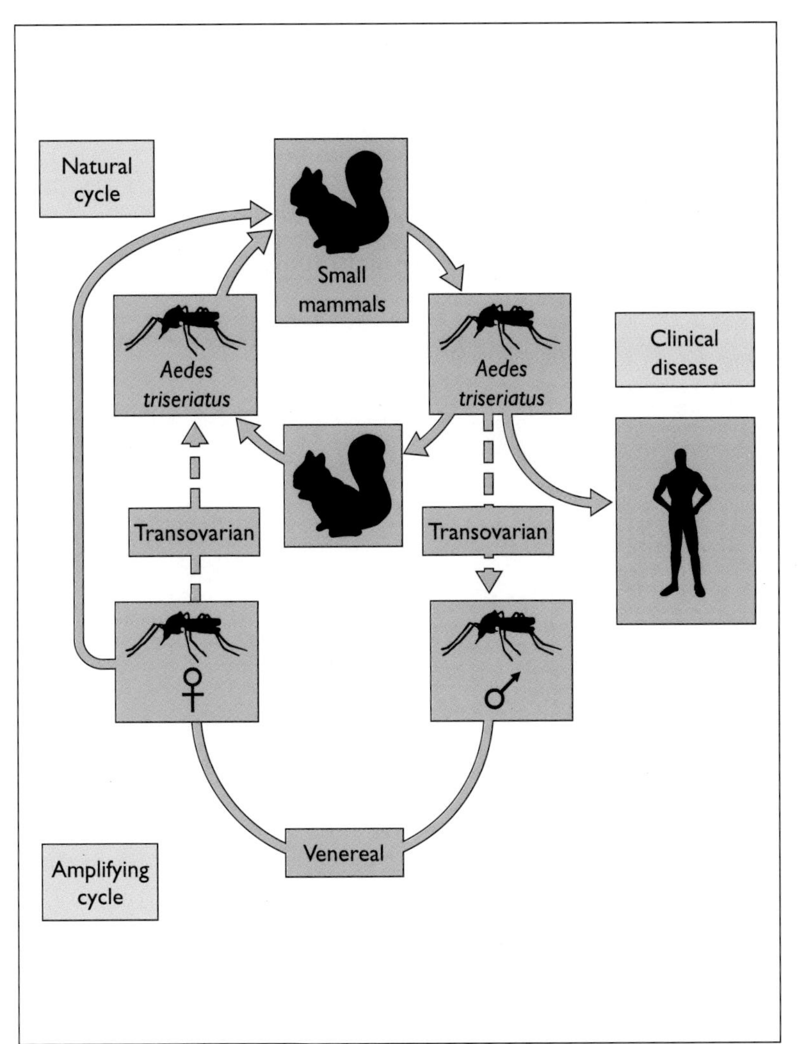

FIGURE 3-63 Transmission cycle of California (La Crosse) encephalitis virus. The inapparent cycle of the La Crosse virus is between *Aedes triseriatus*, a woodland mosquito, and chipmunks and tree squirrels. The virus is maintained over winters by transovarian transmission and is amplified by venereal transmission between the infected male nonbiting mosquito and the infected female. Humans are the only known hosts to develop clinical disease and are dead-end hosts for the virus. (*From* Johnson RT: *Viral Infections of the Nervous System*. New York: Raven Press; 1984:116; with permission.)

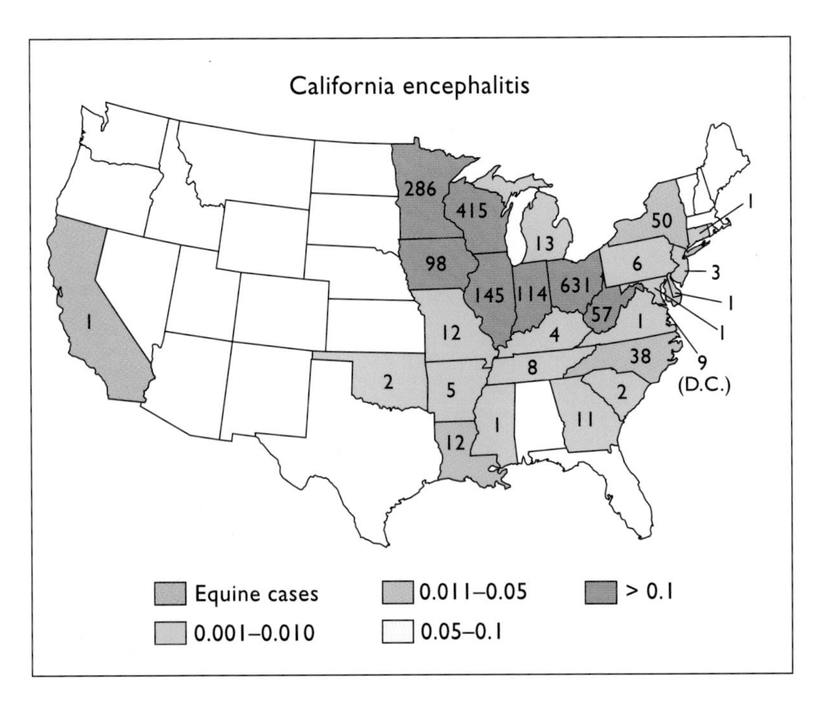

FIGURE 3-64 Geographic distribution of California group encephalitis. The highest incidence of cases occurs in the US midwest, and these are due mostly to the La Crosse virus. The annual incidence of La Crosse encephalitis is approximately five to 10 cases/100,000 population in endemic areas. The numbers represent cases reported for the years 1964 to 1989. (*From* Tsai TF: Arboviral infections in the United States. *Infect Dis Clin North Am* 1991, 5(1):73–103; with permission.)

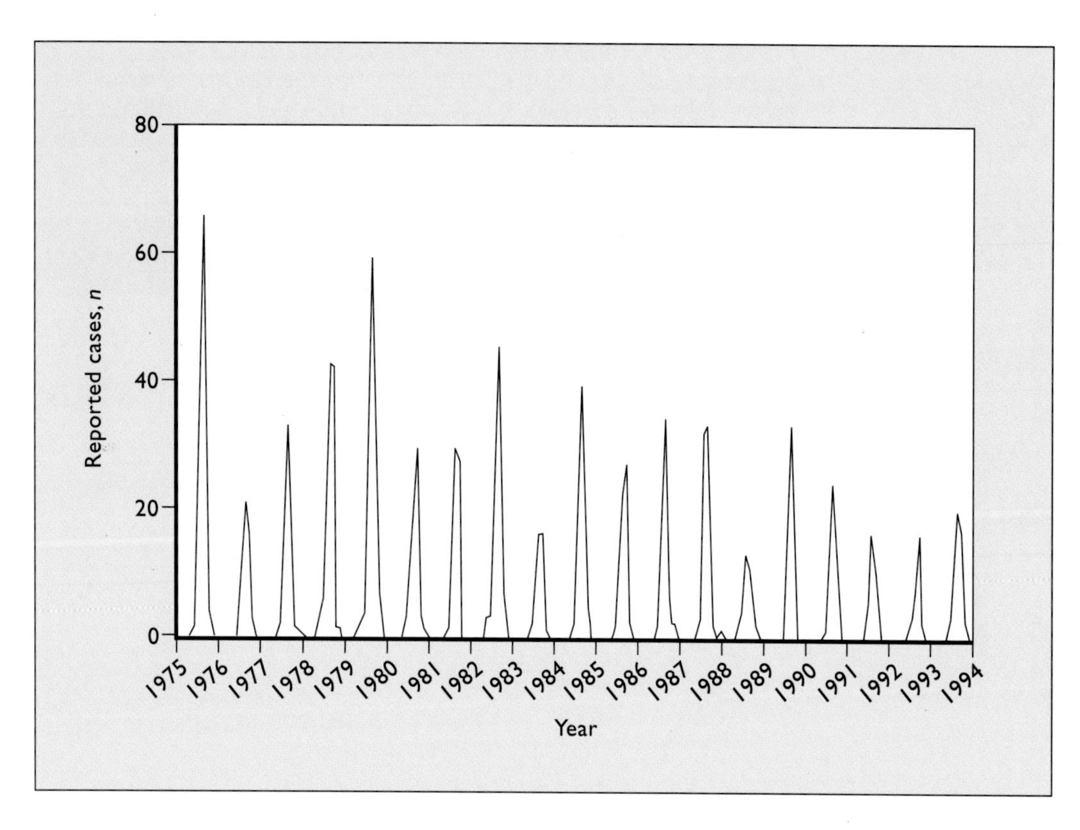

FIGURE 3-65 Frequency of California group encephalitis, United States, 1975–1993. Most cases occur in the late summer–early fall each year. In 1993, there were 55 human cases with two fatalities reported from 11 states. (*From* Centers for Disease Control and Prevention: Summary of notifiable diseases, United States, 1993. *MMWR* 1993, 42(53):20.)

ORBIVIRIDAE (COLORADO TICK FEVER)

Epidemiologic and clinical features of Colorado tick fever	
Region	Rocky Mountains (US and Canada)
Environment	Woodlands
Season	March–September
Vector	Ticks (*Dermacentor andersoni*)
Animal host	Ground squirrels, chipmunks, other rodents
Diagnosis	Acute/convalescent sera
Age/sex	Young adults, esp. males
Unique clinical features	Leukopenia, thrombocytopenia
Mortality	< 1%
Sequelae	Rare

FIGURE 3-66 Epidemiologic and clinical features of Colorado tick fever. Colorado tick fever is one of the two tick-borne viral diseases in the United States, with Powassan encephalitis being the other. Unlike Powassan and the tick-borne encephalitides of Eurasia, Colorado tick fever is an orbivirus rather than a togavirus. Colorado tick fever is generally a mild influenza-like illness that affects young adults, mostly males who are camping or hiking in woodlands. After an incubation of 3 to 6 days, there is an acute onset of chills, myalgia, fever, headache, photophobia, and malaise lasting 5 to 10 days. Encephalitis (as well as hemorrhagic findings) are rare complications (3% to 7%).

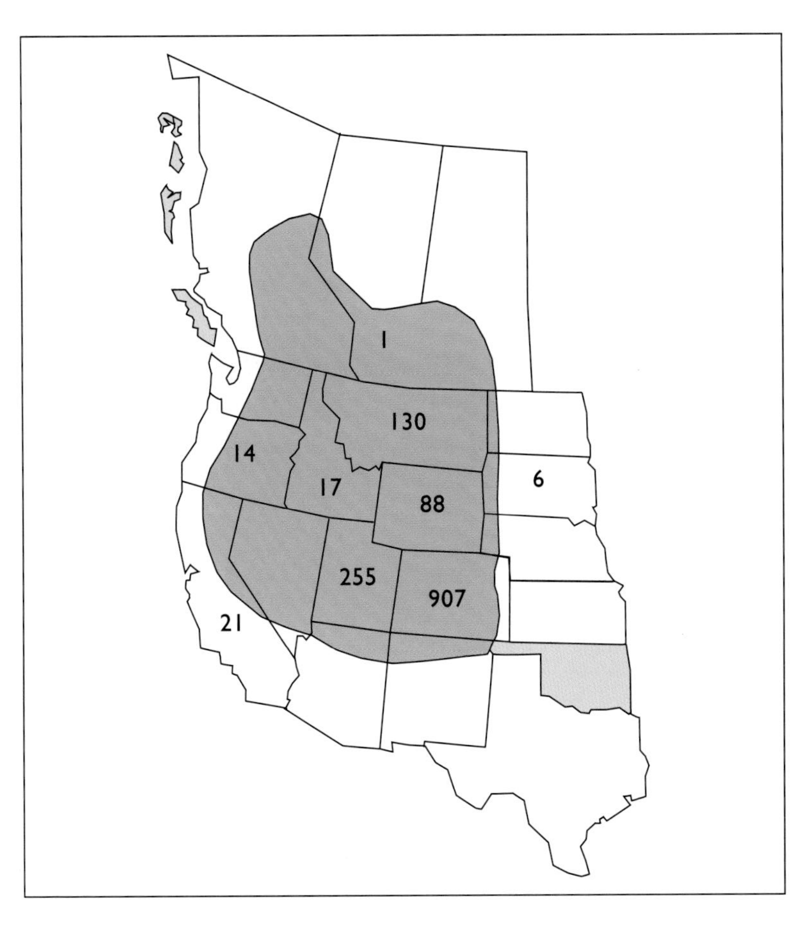

FIGURE 3-67 Geographic distribution of Colorado tick fever. Colorado tick fever is isolated to the forested Rocky Mountain regions of the United States and Canada, at altitudes of 4000 to 10,000 feet, corresponding to the endemic ranges for *Dermacentor andersoni* ticks. The numbers represent cases reported for the years 1980 to 1988. The illness is often misdiagnosed as Rocky Mountain spotted fever, which is 20-fold less common than Colorado tick fever in Colorado. The presence of rash is unusual in Colorado tick fever (5% to 12%) and suggests Rocky Mountain spotted fever. (*From* Tsai TF: Arboviral infections in the United States. *Infect Dis Clin North Am* 1991, 5(1):73–103; with permission.)

RHABDOVIRIDAE (RABIES)

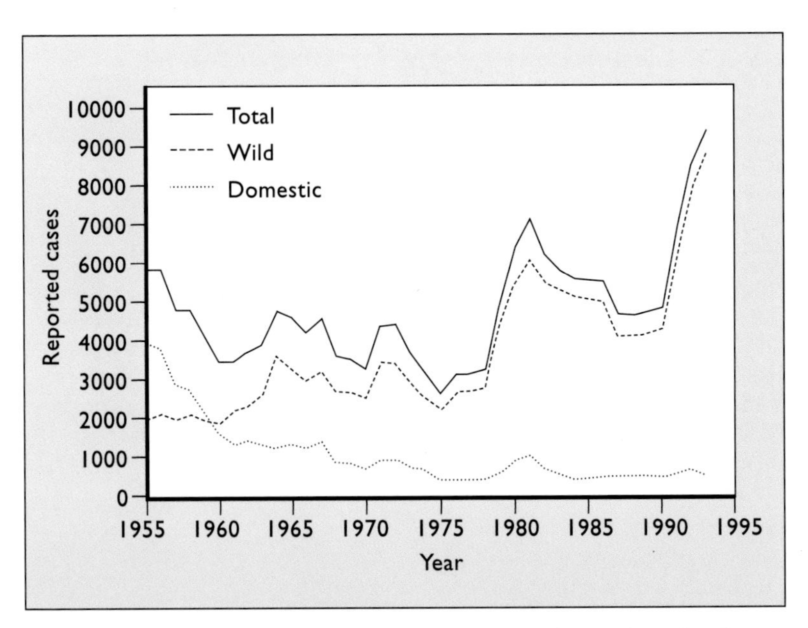

FIGURE 3-68 Frequency of rabies in wild and domestic animals, United States, 1955–1993. In the United States, rabies is extremely rare, despite a recent increase in annual incidence due to an outbreak among wild raccoons in the northeast. Wild animals account for 85% of infections. Worldwide, about 1000 deaths occur per year due to rabies. (*From* Centers for Disease Control and Prevention: Summary of notifiable diseases, United States, 1993. *MMWR* 1993, 42(53):46.)

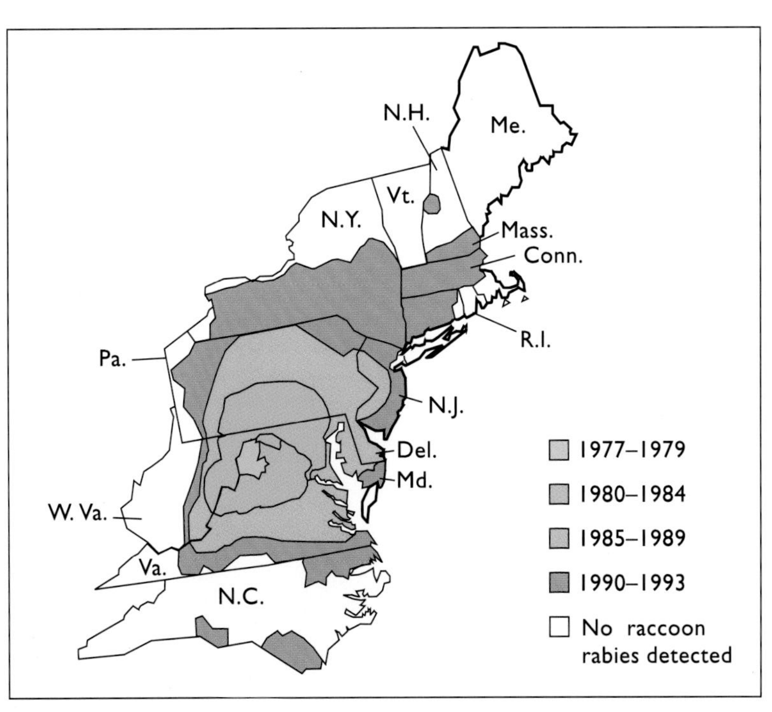

FIGURE 3-69 Spread of rabies in raccoons, United States, 1977–1993. Although the incidence of rabies is low among domestic animals in the United States, a recent increase in the occurrence of wildlife rabies in the mid-Atlantic and northeastern regions has increased the risk to humans. (*From* Centers for Disease Control and Prevention: Raccoon rabies epizootic—United States, 1993. *MMWR* 1994, 43(15):271.)

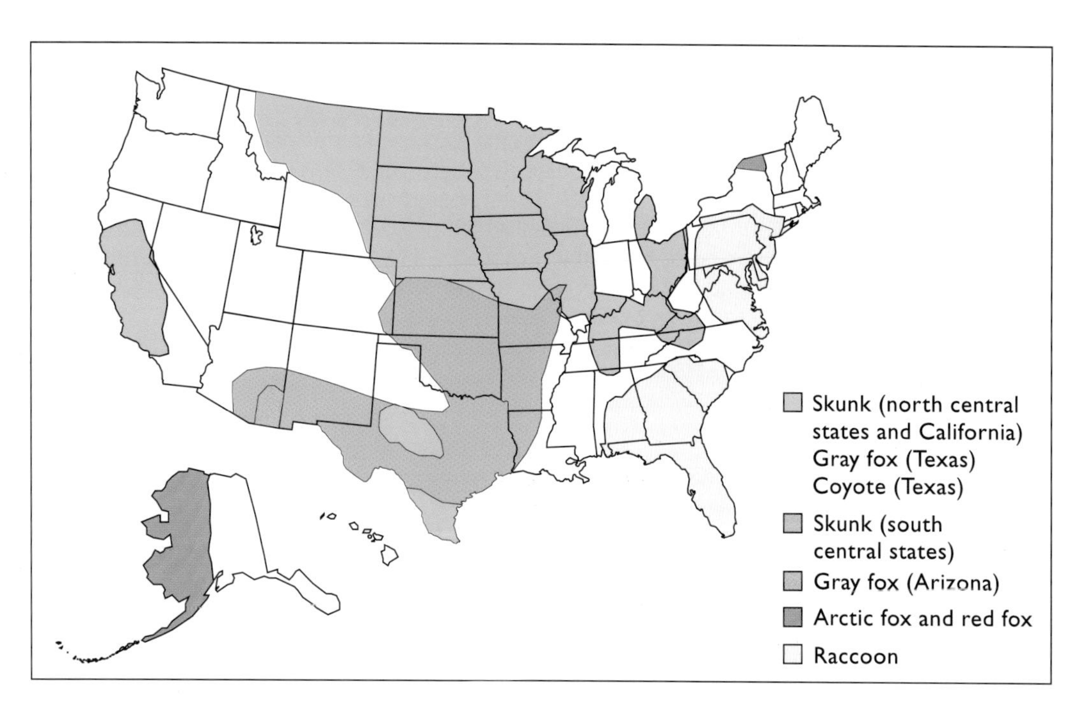

FIGURE 3-70 Distribution of rabies strains. In 1991, five antigenically distinct rabies virus strains, each infecting distinct wildlife species in discrete regions, were present in the United States. In clinical rabies, the severity of disease and the signs/symptoms do not vary among strains. There are no "healthy carriers" among animals, and all hosts express disease. (*From* Krebs JW, Holman RC, Hines U, *et al.*: Rabies surveillance in the United States during 1991. *J Am Vet Med Assoc* 1992, 201:1836–1848; with permission.)

Rabies in humans, United States, 1971–1990

Source	Indigenous exposure	Foreign exposure
Dogs	—	11
Bats	4	—
Cat	1	—
Laboratory aerosols	2	—
Corneal transplant	1	—
Unknown	8	5
Totals	16	16

FIGURE 3-71 Rabies in humans, United States, 1971–1990. In the two decades, only 16 indigenous cases of rabies were reported in the continental United States, with another 16 cases acquired in foreign exposures. (*From* Constantine DG: Rabies. *In* Hoeprich PD, Jordan MC (eds.): *Infectious Diseases: A Modern Treatise of Infectious Processes*, 4th ed. Philadelphia: J.B. Lippincott; 1989:1156; with permission.)

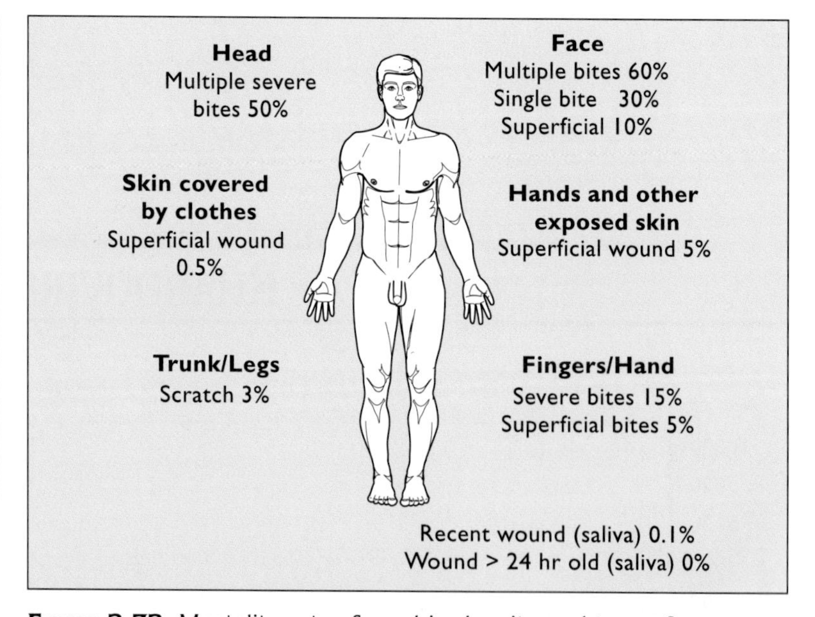

FIGURE 3-72 Mortality rates for rabies by site and type of exposure. During a bite from an infected animal, virus is transmitted with saliva into muscle, where it may multiply at the site of inoculation. The virus then travels along nerves to the CNS. The dense concentration of sensory nerve endings in the head, face, neck, and fingers explains the higher fatality rates associated with wounds in these areas. The severity of exposure (*ie*, multiple severe bites vs superficial wounds) also correlates with mortality rates.

Clinical progression of rabies in humans

Stage	Duration	Clinical association
Incubation	30–90 days (~ 50% of cases) <30 days (~ 25%)	No clinical findings
Prodrome and early clinical symptoms	2–10 d	Paresthesia and/or pain at site of bite Fever, malaise Anorexia, nausea, vomiting Headache
Acute neurologic disease	2–7 d	"Furious rabies" (80% of cases) Hallucinations, bizarre behavior, anxiety, agitation, biting Hydrophobia Autonomic dysfunction "Paralytic rabies" (20% of cases) Flaccid paralysis Paresis and plegias Ascending paralysis
Coma	0–14 d	SIADH Diabetes insipidus Multiorgan failure
Death or recovery (rare)	Variable	Respiratory cardiac

Figure 3-73 Clinical progression of rabies in humans. The clinical course following infection with rabies progresses through five stages. The incubation period is variable, ranging from < 30 days in 25% of cases to > 1 year in 5%. SIADH—syndrome of inappropriate secretion of antidiuretic hormone. (*From* Whitley RJ, Middlebrook M: Rabies. *In* Scheld WM, Whitley RJ, Durack DT (eds.): *Infections of the Central Nervous System*. New York: Raven Press; 1991:127–144; with permission.)

Common clinical presentations in rabies

Finding	%
Fever	73
Dysphagia	58
Altered mental state	55
Pain, paresthesias referable to site of exposure	45
Excitement, agitation	45
Paralysis, weakness	26
Hydrophobia	21
Hypersalivation	16
Nausea, vomiting	18.6
Malaise	16.3
Dyspnea	14.0
Headache	14.0
Convulsions, spasms	9.1
Coma	4.5
Miscellaneous (lethargy, dysuria, anorexia, hydrophobia)	16.3
No history of rabies exposure	16

Figure 3-74 Common clinical presentations in rabies. The approximate prevalence of clinical findings in rabies is shown. Fever, dysphagia (excluding hydrophobia-related symptoms), and altered consciousness are the most common presentations. Eighty-nine percent of patients develop at least one neurologic finding in the course of illness, and 71% usually develop two or more classic symptoms during the course of illness. (*Adapted from* Robinson P: Rabies. *In* Gorbach SL, Bartlett JG, Blacklow NR (eds.): *Infectious Diseases*. Philadelphia: W.B. Saunders; 1992:1272; with permission.)

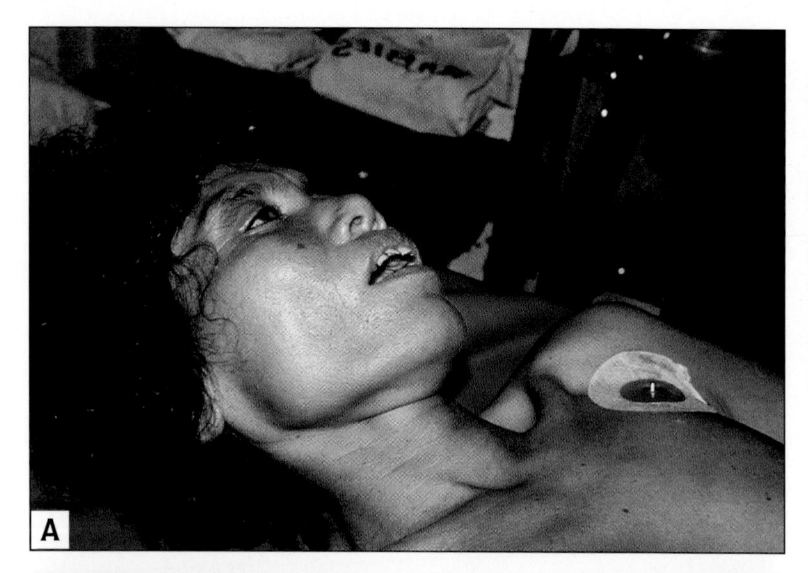

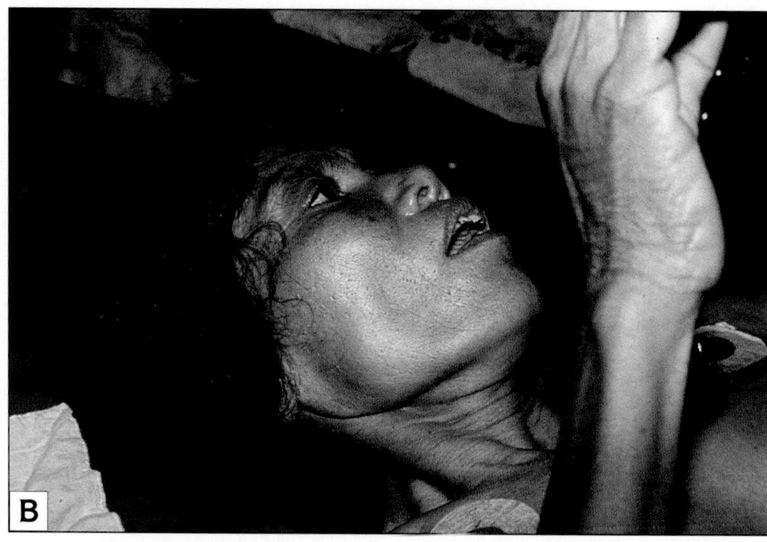

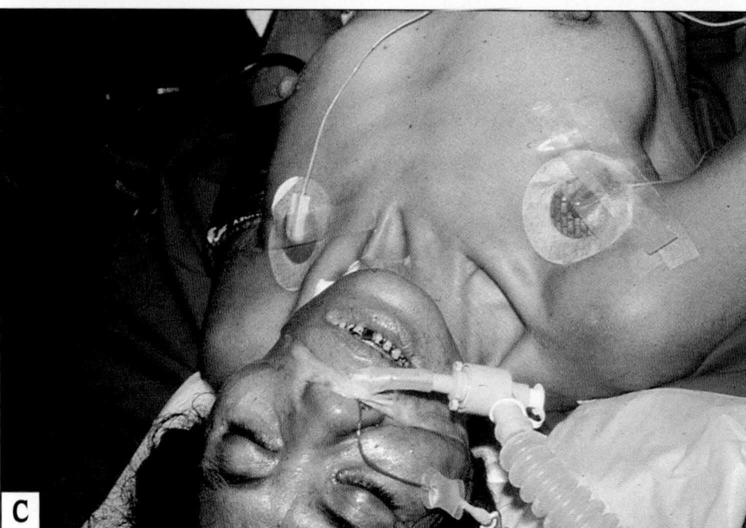

FIGURE 3-75 Classic clinical features of rabies encephalitis. The manifestations of brainstem dysfunction begin 2 to 10 days after the onset of the encephalitic phase (acute neurologic disease). **A**, A patient with hydrophobia. Note the grimace and stare that accompany pharyngeal spasms occurring when water is presented to drink. Such intermittent stimulus-sensitive behavior can be demonstrated in some rabies patients during the acute neurologic phase of their illness. **B**, The same patient shows aerophobia. As with hydrophobia, pharyngeal spasms may be provoked by fanning air across the patient's face. **C**, Inspiratory spasms. The patient, late in the course of infection, shows inspiratory spasms resulting from involvement of the respiratory center. Death often results at least partly from respiratory failure. (*Courtesy of* T. Hemachudha, MD.)

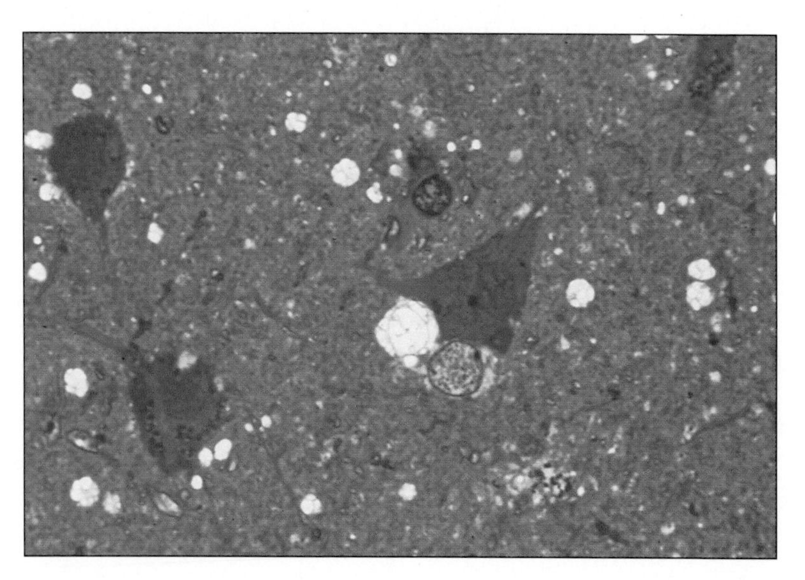

FIGURE 3-76 Negri body. The presence of these intracytoplasmic inclusion bodies is pathognomonic of rabies (though they are not seen in all cases). The Ammons' horn region and cerebellar Purkinje cells are commonly positive. Because rabies virus enters the CNS via intracellular axonal transport, it does not invoke an inflammatory response.

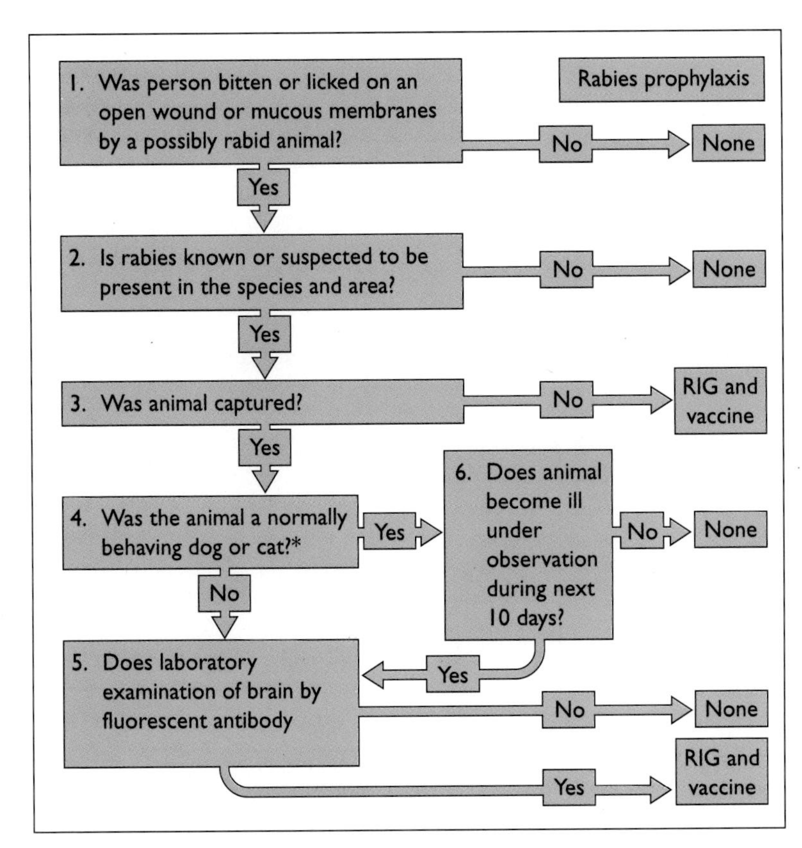

FIGURE 3-77 Decision-making in postexposure rabies prophylaxis. Each year, > 1 million Americans are bitten by animals, and in each incident, a decision must be made whether to initiate prophylaxis. In step 4, if the exposure was to livestock or a normally behaving unvaccinated dog or cat, the situation should be considered individually and local or state health officials consulted. RIG–rabies immune globulin. (*From* Corey L: Rabies, rhabdoviruses, and Marburg-like agents. *In* Isselbacher KJ, *et al.* (eds.): *Harrison's Principles of Internal Medicine*, 13th ed. New York: McGraw Hill; 1994:834; with permission.)

Postexposure rabies prophylaxis regimen	
1. Local wound care	Cleanse wound with soap and water Tetanus toxoid and antibiotics
2. Passive immunization with rabies antiserum	HRIG, 20 U/kg, one-half given by local infiltration into wound and one-half im in gluteus *or* ARS, 40 U/kg, one-half given by local infiltration into wound and one-half im in gluteus
3. Active immunization with antirabies vaccine	HDCV, 1-mL dose im in deltoid or thigh, X 5 doses (given on days 0, 3, 7, 14, and 28)

FIGURE 3-78 Postexposure rabies prophylaxis regimen. Human rabies immune globulin (HRIG) should be given as soon as possible after exposure. If HRIG is unavailable, the equine antirabies serum (ARS) can be substituted, but serum sickness may result. Human diploid cell vaccine (HDCV) should be started immediately, with four subsequent injections over the following 28 days. (Corey L: Rabies, rhabdoviruses, and Marburg-like agents. *In* Isselbacher KJ, *et al.* (eds.): *Harrison's Principles of Internal Medicine*, 13th ed. New York: McGraw Hill; 1994:834–835.)

POLIOMYELITIS

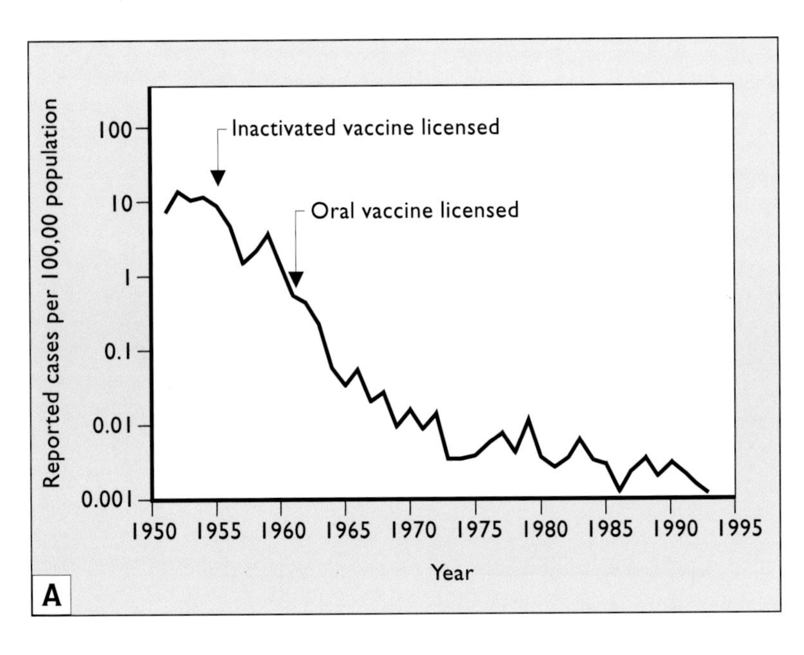

FIGURE 3-79 Incidence of poliomyelitis. **A**, Frequency of poliomyelitis (paralytic), United States, 1951–1993. (*From* Centers for Disease Control and Prevention: Summary of notifiable diseases, United States, 1993. *MMWR* 1993, 42(53):45.) (*continued*)

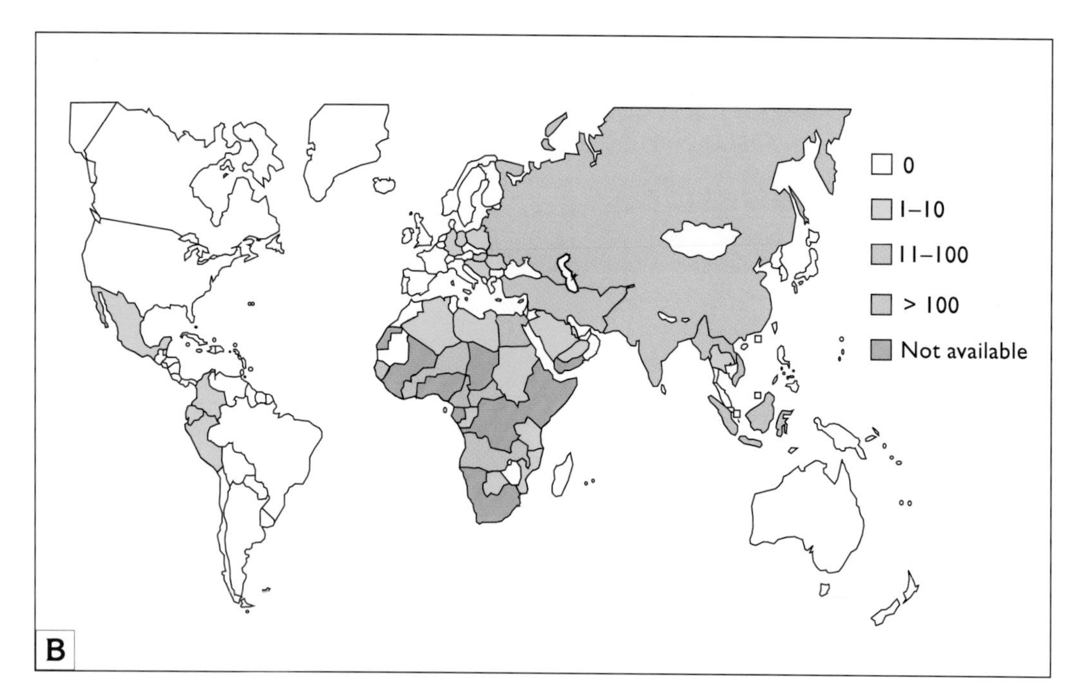

FIGURE 3-79 *(continued)* **B**, Reported incidence of poliomyelitis, worldwide, 1990. In 1990, approximately 150,000 cases of paralytic poliomyelitis occurred worldwide, although through vaccination programs, the rate of new cases is dropping. (*From* Hull HF, Ward NA: Progress towards the global eradication of poliomyelitis. *World Health Stat Q* 1992, 45:280–283; with permission.)

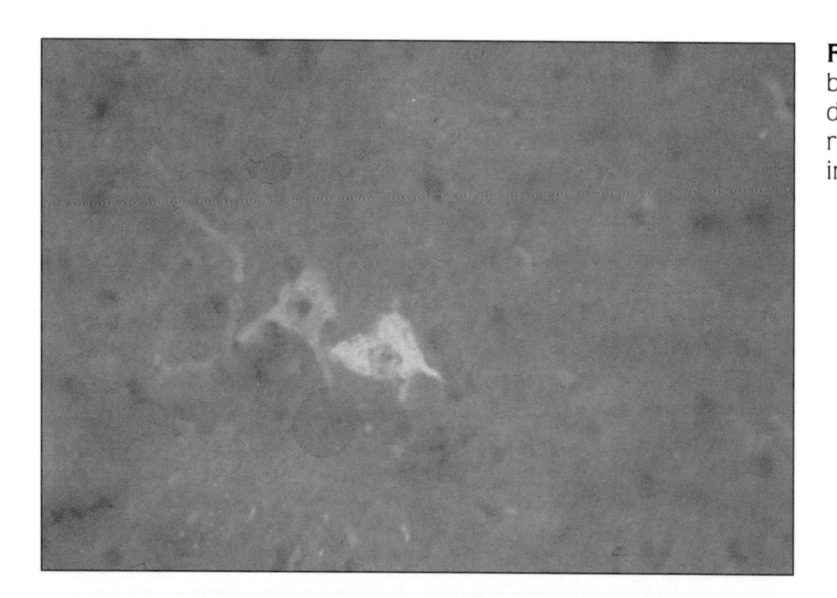

FIGURE 3-80 Immunofluorescence of antipoliovirus type 2 antibody from mouse spinal chord. This high-power photomicrograph demonstrates prominent immunofluorescence in somata in anterior horn cells of the mouse spinal chord. Note the selective involvement of these cells and their processes.

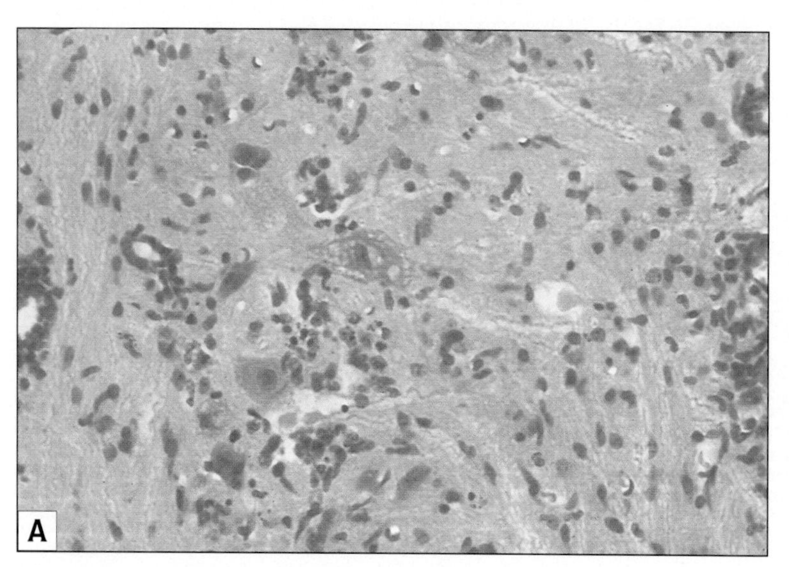

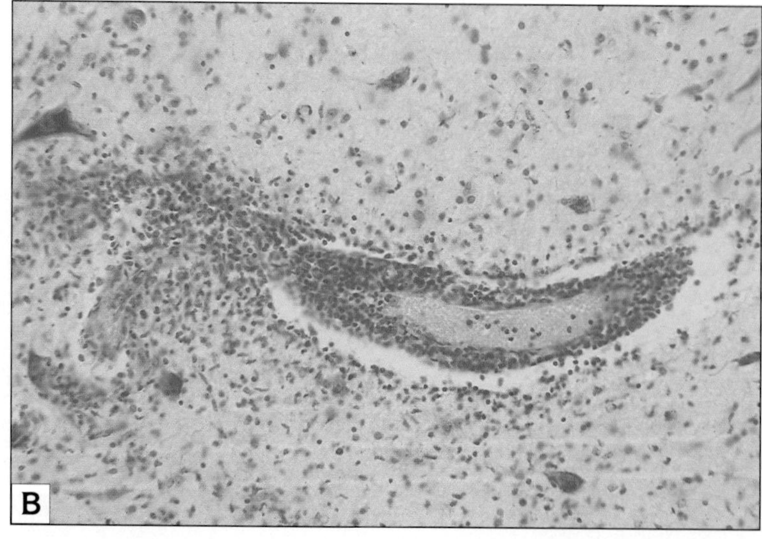

FIGURE 3-81 Poliomyelitis. **A**, Histologic section of spinal cord showing microglial nodules. **B**, Perivascular cuffing and infiltration of the brain by mononuclear cells are visible in the hypoglossal nucleus. (Nissl stain.) (*From* Hirano A (ed.): *Color Atlas of Pathology of the Central Nervous System*, 2nd ed. New York: Igaku-Shoin; 1988:194; with permission.)

AIDS-Related CNS Conditions

Major neurologic complications of HIV-1 infection

HIV-1-related conditions	Opportunistic processes
Acute aseptic meningitis	Cryptococcal meningitis*
Chronic meningitis	Toxoplasmosis*
HIV-1 encephalopathy*	CMV retinitis/encephalitis*
Vacuolar myelopathy	Other opportunistic CNS infections
Predominantly sensory neuropathy	Herpes encephalitis/radiculitis
Inflammatory demyelinating polyneuropathy	Progressive multifocal leukoencephalopathy (PML)*
Mononeuritis multiplex	Primary CNS lymphoma*
Myopathy	Systemic lymphoma*

*AIDS indicator diseases.

Figure 3-82 Major neurologic complications of HIV-1 infection. The nervous system is involved frequently in HIV-1 infection, sometimes before opportunistic infections and frank AIDS develop. It is estimated that 10% of all AIDS patients present with complaints related to the nervous system. These neurologic problems may be primary to the overall pathogenic process of HIV infection or secondary to opportunistic infections or neoplasms. Conditions that are considered AIDS-indicator diseases are indicated with *asterisks* in the table. (*Adapted from* McArthur JC: Neurologic complications of human immunodeficiency virus infection. *In* Gorbach SL, Bartlett JG, Blacklow NR (eds.): *Infectious Diseases*. Philadelphia: WB Saunders; 1992:956–972; with permission.)

Prevalence of neurologic manifestations of HIV infection

Source	CDC surveillance	UCSF all AIDS	JHH referrals	Other, autopsies
HIV-1 encephalopathy	3.0	8.0	16	66.0
Cryptococcal meningitis	5.4	5.3	6	12.4
Cerebral toxoplasmosis	2.7	3.8	8	30.8
PML	0.8	0.6	0.5	6.8
Primary CNS lymphoma	0.7	1.9	4	3.4

Figure 3-83 Prevalence of neurologic manifestations of HIV-1 infection. The frequency of different disorders varies with the geographic, racial, and age characteristics of the population. The Centers for Disease Control and Prevention (CDC) study included surveillance data on the first 23,307 cases of AIDS (through 1985). A retrospective study from the University of California San Francisco (UCSF) evaluated all 1286 AIDS cases at that institution. The Johns Hopkins Hospital (JHH) cases comprised 186 referrals. The autopsy data have documented pathologic abnormalities in up to 90% of cases, but many of these processes may have been clinically silent. PML—progressive multifocal leukoencephalopathy. (*Adapted from* McArthur JC: Neurologic complications of human immunodeficiency virus infection. *In* Gorbach SL, Bartlett JG, Blacklow NR (eds.): *Infectious Diseases*. Philadelphia: WB Saunders; 1992:956–972; with permission.)

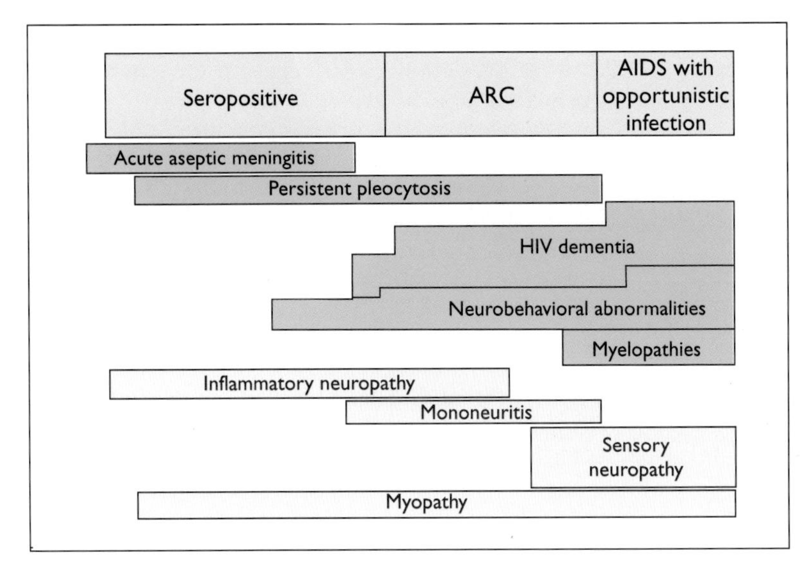

Figure 3-84 Onset of HIV-related neurologic diseases. Diseases that affect the CNS (*yellow*) and peripheral nervous system (*blue*) develop at different times in relation to the stage of HIV infection and at different frequencies (*vertical width of bands*). ARC—AIDS-related complex. (*Adapted from* Johnson RT, McArthur JC, Narayan O: The neurobiology of HIV infections. *FASEB J* 1988, 2:2970; with permission.)

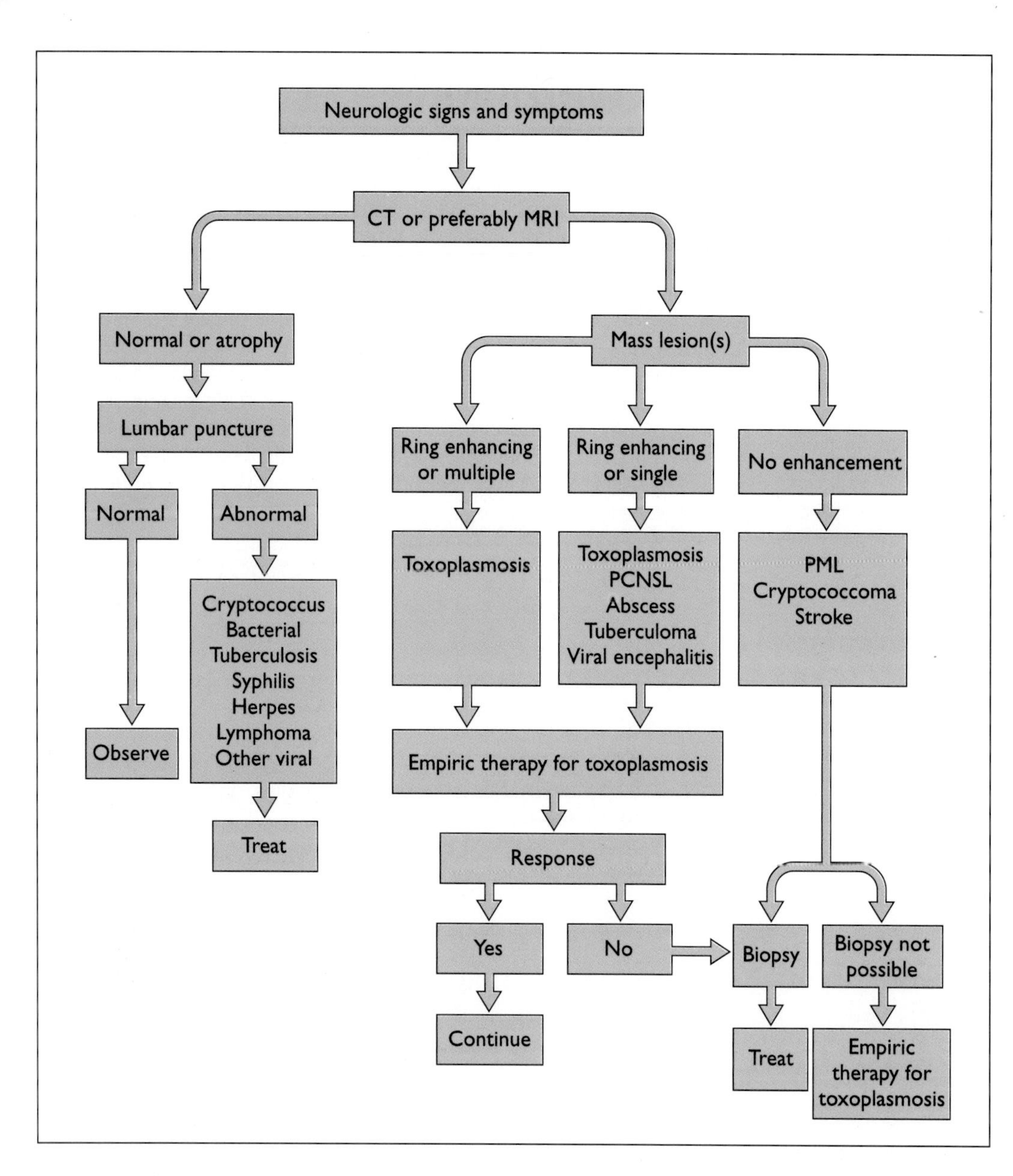

FIGURE 3-85 Evaluation of neurologic abnormalities in HIV infection. The neurologic examination serves to refine the localization and uncover additional symptomatic abnormalities. A neuroimaging study, either CT or, preferably, MRI, helps localize the disease process and narrow diagnostic possibilities. Findings on neuro-imaging studies may be suggestive, though not diagnostic, of various processes. If an initial CT scan does not show ring enhancement or multiple lesions, then an MRI should be performed. In cases with ring enhancement or multiple lesions, empiric anti-*Toxoplasma* therapy is often started, because of the high frequency of cerebral toxoplasmosis and its rapid response to therapy. PCNSL—primary CNS lymphoma. (*Adapted from* Chaisson RE, Volberding PA: Clinical manifestations of HIV infection. *In* Mandell GL, *et al.* (eds.): *Principles and Practice of Infectious Diseases*, 4th ed. New York: Churchill Livingstone; 1995:1238; with permission.)

Differential diagnosis of common CNS complications of AIDS

	Clinical		Neuroimaging		
Disorder	**Onset**	**Alertness**	**Lesions, *n***	**Type of lesions**	**Location of lesions**
Cerebral toxoplasmosis	Days	Reduced	Multiple	Spherical, enhancing, mass effect	Cortex, basal ganglia
Primary CNS lymphoma	Days to weeks	Variable	One or few	Diffuse enhancement, mass effect	Periventricular, white matter
PML	Weeks	Preserved	Multiple	Nonenhancing, no mass effect	White matter, adjacent to cortex
AIDS dementia complex	Weeks to months	Preserved	None, multiple or diffuse	Increased T2 signal, no enhancement or mass effect	White matter, basal ganglia

FIGURE 3-86 Differential diagnosis of common CNS complications of AIDS. (*Adapted from* Price RW, Brew BJ, Roke M: Central and peripheral nervous system complications of HIV-1 infections and AIDS. *In* DeVita VT Jr, Hellman S, Rosenberg SA, *et al.*, (eds.): *AIDS: Etiology, Diagnosis, Treatment, and Prevention.* Philadelphia: J.B. Lippincott; 1992:237–254; with permission.)

HIV Encephalopathy

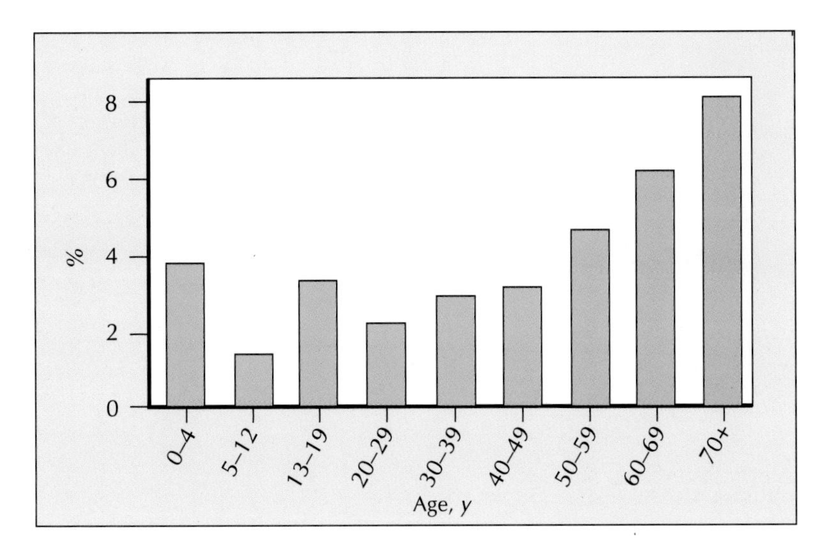

FIGURE 3-87 Surveillance incidence of HIV-1 encephalopathy, 1984–1988. HIV-1 encephalopathy has a bimodal distribution, being more frequent at the extremes of age. There is no predilection for sex, race, risk groups, or geographic regions. It is unclear if the increased incidence of HIV-1 encephalopathy with age might reflect the coexistence of other conditions, such as Alzheimer's disease or multiinfarct dementia. (*From* McArthur JC: Neurologic complications of human immunodeficiency virus infection. *In* Gorbach SL, Bartlett JG, Blacklow NR (eds.): *Infectious Diseases*. Philadelphia: W.B. Saunders; 1992:956–972; with permission.)

A. Clinical features of the AIDS dementia complex: early manifestations
Symptoms
Cognition
Impaired concentration
Forgetfulness
Mental slowing
Motor
Unsteady gait
Leg weakness
Loss of coordination, impaired handwriting
Tremor
Behavior
Apathy, withdrawal, personality change
Agitation, confusion, hallucinations
Signs
Mental status
Psychomotor slowing
Impaired serial 7s or reversals
Organic psychosis
Neurologic examination
Impaired rapid movements (limbs, eyes)
Hyperreflexia
Release reflexes (snout, glabellar, grasp)
Gait ataxia (impaired tandem gait, rapid turns)
Tremor (postural)
Leg weakness

B. Clinical features of the AIDS dementia complex: late manifestations
Mental status
Global dementia
Psychomotor slowing: verbal responses delayed, near or absolute mutism, vacant stare
Unawareness of illness, disinhibition
Confusion, disorientation
Organic psychosis
Neurologic signs
Weakness (legs, arms)
Ataxia
Pyramidal tract signs: spasticity, hyperreflexia, extensor plantar responses
Bladder and bowel incontinence
Myoclonus

FIGURE 3-88 Clinical features of HIV-related dementia complex. Precise criteria do not yet exist for diagnosing HIV encephalopathy, but dementia has been included as an AIDS-indicator condition by the CDC. **A**, Early manifestations. **B**, Late manifestations. (*From* Price RW, Brew BJ, Roke M: Central and peripheral nervous system complications of HIV-1 infections and AIDS. *In* DeVita VT Jr, Hellman S, Rosenberg SA, *et al.* (eds.): *AIDS: Etiology, Diagnosis, Treatment, and Prevention*. Philadelphia: J.B. Lippincott; 1992:237–254; with permission.)

Clinical staging of AIDS dementia complex	
Stage 0 (normal)	Normal mental and motor function
Stage 0.5 (equivocal/ subclinical)	Absent, minimal, or equivocal symptoms No impairment of work or ADLs Mild signs (snout response, slowed ocular or extremity movements) may be present Gait and strength normal
Stage 1 (mild)	Able to perform all but more demanding aspects of work or ADL Unequivocal evidence of functional, intellectual, or motor impairment Can walk without assistance
Stage 2 (moderate)	Able to perform basic activities of self-care Cannot work or maintain more demanding ADLs Ambulatory but may require a single prop
Stage 3 (severe)	Major intellectual incapacity or motor disability
Stage 4 (end stage)	Nearly vegetative Intellectual and social comprehension and output are at rudimentary level Nearly or absolutely mute Paraparetic or paraplegic with urinary and fecal incontinence

FIGURE 3-89 Clinical staging of HIV-related dementia complex. HIV encephalopathy or dementia develops in 20% of patients with AIDS and progresses in parallel with the later stages of AIDS. The early stages are subtle and may be overlooked or ascribed to depression or anxiety. ADL—activities of daily living. (Sidtis JJ, Price RW: Early HIV infection and the AIDS dementia complex. *Neurology* 1990, 40:197.)

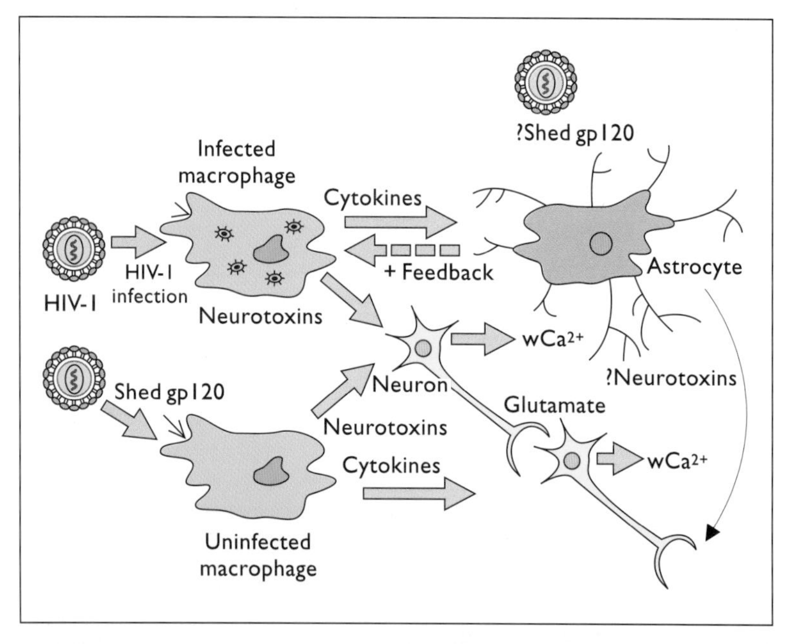

FIGURE 3-90 Model of HIV-related neuronal injury. Macrophages/ microglia infected by HIV-1 or activated by gp120 secrete potential neurotoxins and cytokines. Neurons are thereby excited, intracellular Ca^{2+} rises, and the excitatory neurotransmitter glutamate is released, leading to further neuronal injury in neighboring neuronal cells. Cytokines released from macrophages contribute to astrocytosis, and astrocytes may in turn send a feedback signal (*dashed arrow*) to increase macrophage secretions. Astrocytes may also be directly influenced by gp120 and release substances contributing to neurotoxicity. (*From* Lipton SA: HIV displays its coat of arms. *Nature* 1994, 367:113; with permission.)

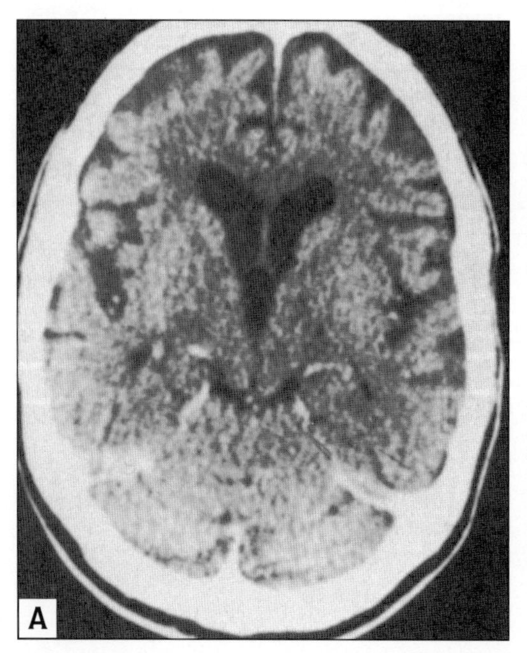

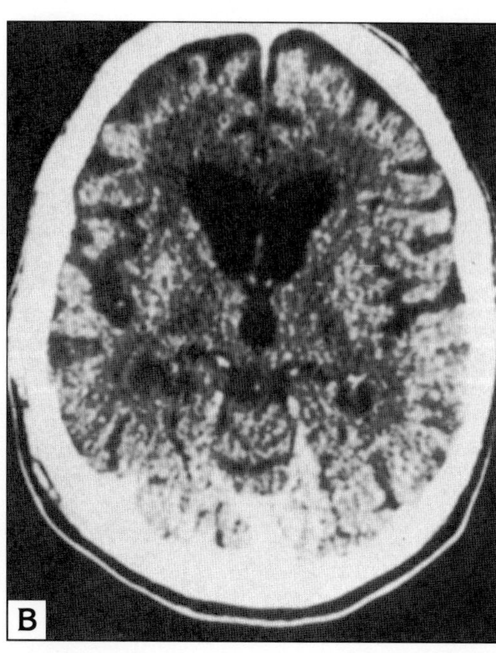

FIGURE 3-91 HIV encephalopathy on CT scanning. **A**, CT scan of a 36-year-old intravenous drug user with AIDS-related complex and early HIV encephalopathy. Mild frontotemporal atrophy and ventricular enlargement are seen. **B**, CT scan of same patient 3 months later with far-advanced HIV encephalopathy. Severe frontotemporal atrophy and ventriculomegaly are noted with attenuation of the periventricular white matter. (*From* McArthur JC: Neurologic complications of human immunodeficiency virus infection. *In* Gorbach SL, Bartlett JG, Blacklow NR (eds.): *Infectious Diseases*. Philadelphia: WB Saunders; 1992:956–972; with permission.)

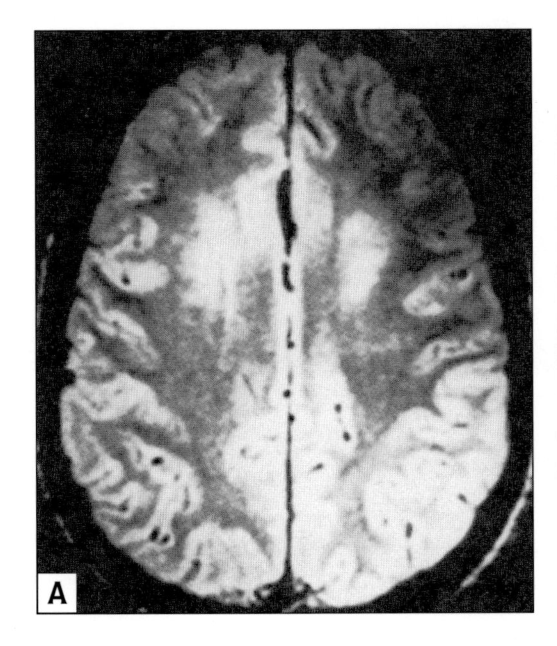

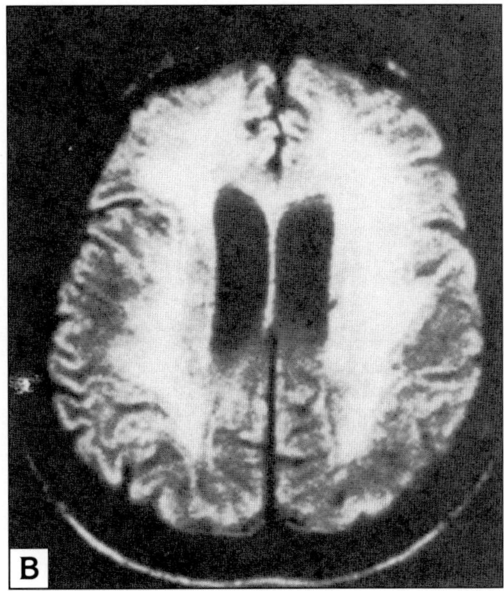

Figure 3-92 HIV encephalopathy on MRI scans. **A**, MRI scan (T2-weighted image) of a 33-year-old homosexual man shows large areas of abnormal signal intensity in the white matter. No mass effect is present. **B**, MRI scan (T2-weighted image) of a 38-year-old bisexual man with late HIV encephalopathy demonstrates enlargement of the ventricles, cerebral atrophy, and diffuse abnormalities throughout the white matter. (*From* McArthur JC: Neurologic complications of human immunodeficiency virus infection. *In* Gorbach SL, Bartlett JG, Blacklow NR (eds.): *Infectious Diseases*. Philadelphia: W.B. Saunders; 1992:956–972; with permission.)

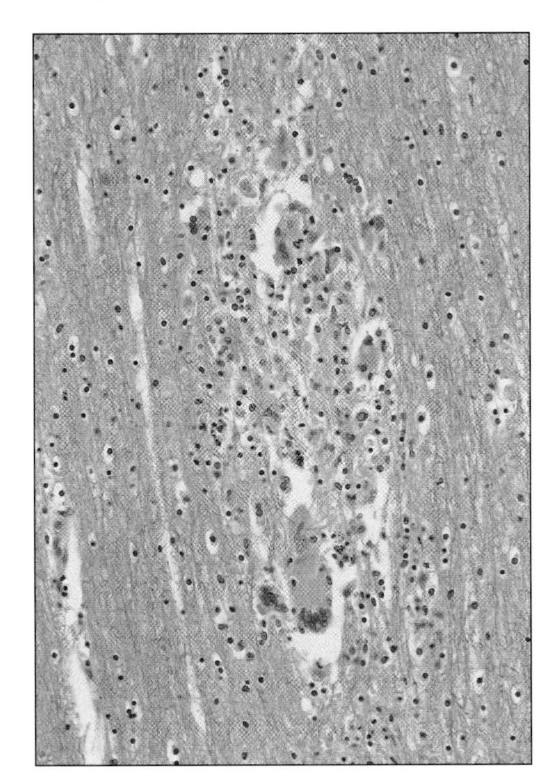

Figure 3-93 HIV encephalitis. Histologic examination shows a focal region of inflammation, tissue disruption, and a multinucleated giant cell. This lesion is composed mostly of macrophages and microglial cells. Macrophages, microglia, and multinucleated giant cells all may be infected with HIV. The correlation of this lesion to the clinical syndrome of HIV-related dementia, however, is unclear.

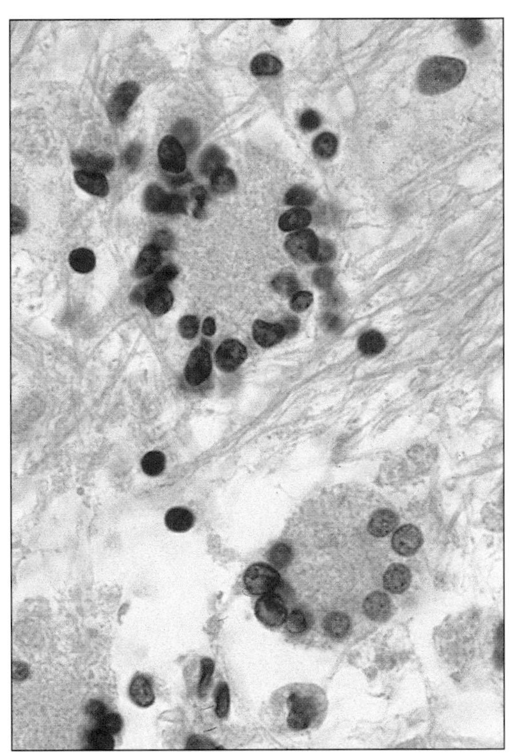

Figure 3-94 Multinucleated giant cells in HIV encephalitis. The cells are of macrophage origin and are produced by fusion of cells in response to HIV infection.

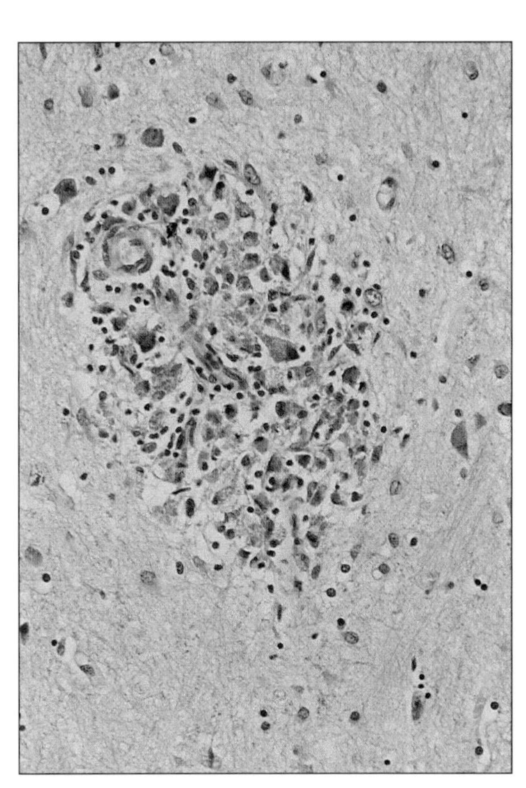

Figure 3-95 Microglial nodules in HIV encephalitis. These nodules consist of a focal collection of macrophages and microglia, many infected with HIV.

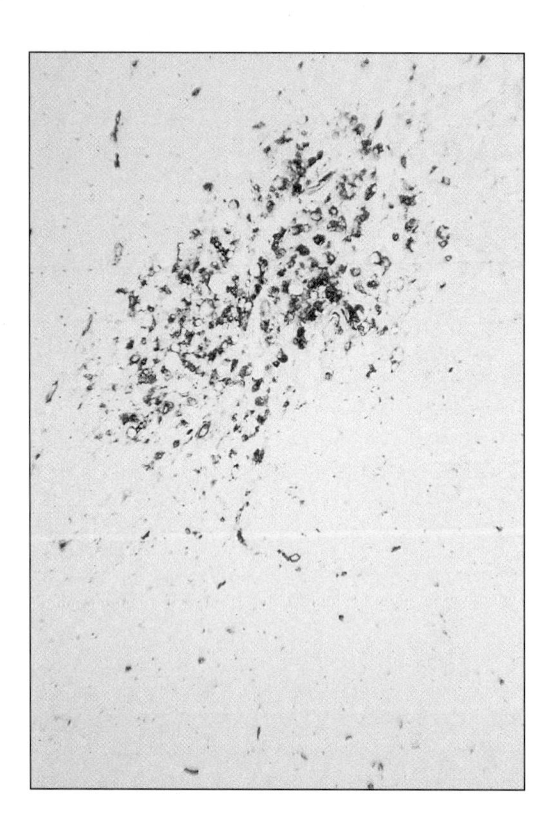

FIGURE 3-96 Microglial nodules in HIV encephalitis. A focal collection of macrophages and microglial cells is demonstrated with the immunocytochemical marker HAM-56, which stains activated macrophages. These microglial nodules may be abundant in cerebral cortex, and many contain cells with cytomegalovirus (CMV) inclusions.

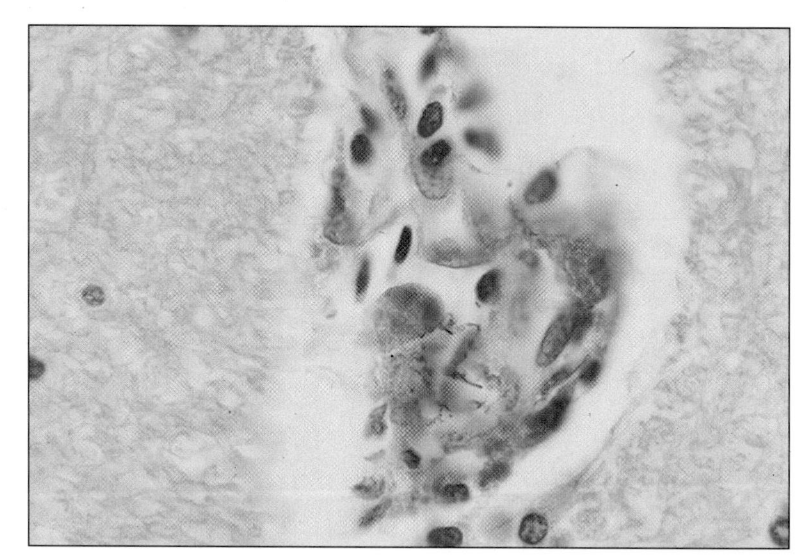

FIGURE 3-97 Immunocytochemical staining of subcortical white matter with anti-gp41. A monoclonal antibody against gp41, an HIV coat glycoprotein, is used to show cells infected with HIV. The infected cells show a perivascular location and are macrophages and microglia. Neuronal infection with HIV is extremely uncommon, and neurologic dysfunction is probably produced through indirect mechanisms of neuronal damage.

Treatment of HIV encephalopathy

Antiretroviral agents
- Zidovudine
- Didanosine (ddl)
- Zalcitabine (ddC)
- Stavudine (d4T)

Antimicrobials (for systematic prophylaxis)

Symptomatic treatment
- Methylphenidate (Ritalin)
- Tricyclic antidepressants
- Neuroleptics (if needed)

FIGURE 3-98 Treatment of HIV encephalopathy. In adult patients with HIV-1 infection, zidovudine has resulted in improved neuropsychological performance compared to placebo, although the optimal dosage is not established. Didanosine and other antiretroviral agents may be used as alternatives or, in some cases, in conjunction with zidovudine. In symptomatic management, patients should be given small or reduced dosages, because patients with HIV encephalopathy are very susceptible to adverse effects.

Progressive Multifocal Leukoencephalopathy

Clinical signs of progressive multifocal leukoencephalopathy

Occurs in 2%–4% of AIDS patients

Worsening focal neurologic deficits
- Hemiparesis
- Hemianopia
- Aphasia
- Hemisensory deficit
- Ataxia

No specific CSF or EEG abnormalities

Late mental status changes
- Confusion
- Personality change

Progression to death in weeks to months

FIGURE 3-99 Clinical signs of progressive multifocal leukoencephalopathy. Progressive multifocal leukoencephalopathy (PML) is a demyelinating disease of cerebral white matter, caused by JC virus. Diagnosis is usually by recognition of the typical clinical picture of progressive focal neurologic deficit and by neuroimaging studies, which show multiple, nonenhancing areas of subcortical white matter. Biopsy is needed for definitive diagnosis. There is no effective treatment, although several antiviral agents have shown limited success.

Pathologic features of progressive multifocal leukoencephalopathy

1. Multifocal areas of demyelination with macrophage infiltration
2. Enlarged "transformed" astrocytes with hyperchromatic bizarre nuclei
3. Intranuclear "ground-glass" viral inclusions in oligodendrocytes

FIGURE 3-100 Pathologic features of PML. PML is caused by infection of glial cells with the JC virus. Oligodendrocytes are productively infected and killed by the virus, leading to demyelination. Astrocytes are latently infected and "transformed" into cells with malignant potential. Survival after diagnosis rarely exceeds 6 months.

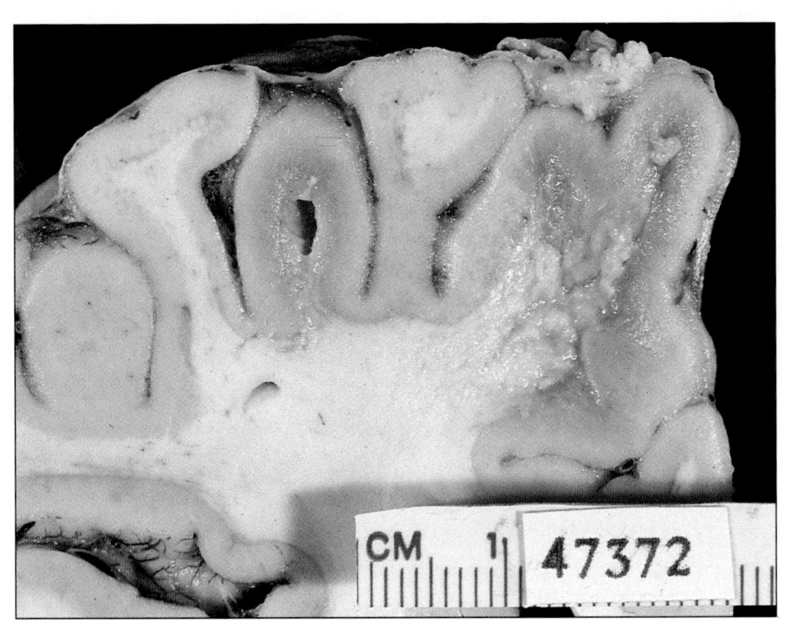

FIGURE 3-101 Gross postmortem specimen of brain from a patient with PML. Necrosis and cavitation are seen in the subcortical white matter, with relative sparing of the cortex. These regions are typically multifocal and may occur at all levels of the neuraxis.

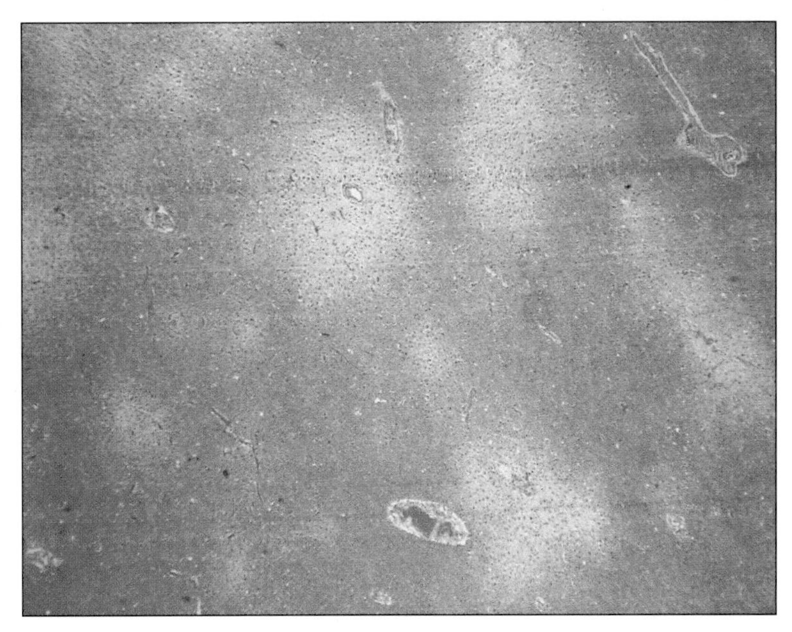

FIGURE 3-102 Low-power photomicrograph showing demyelination in PML. Multifocal regions of pallor indicating demyelination are evident. The demyelinated regions contain macrophages, astrocytes, and virally infected oligodendrocytes. (Hematoxylin-eosin stain.)

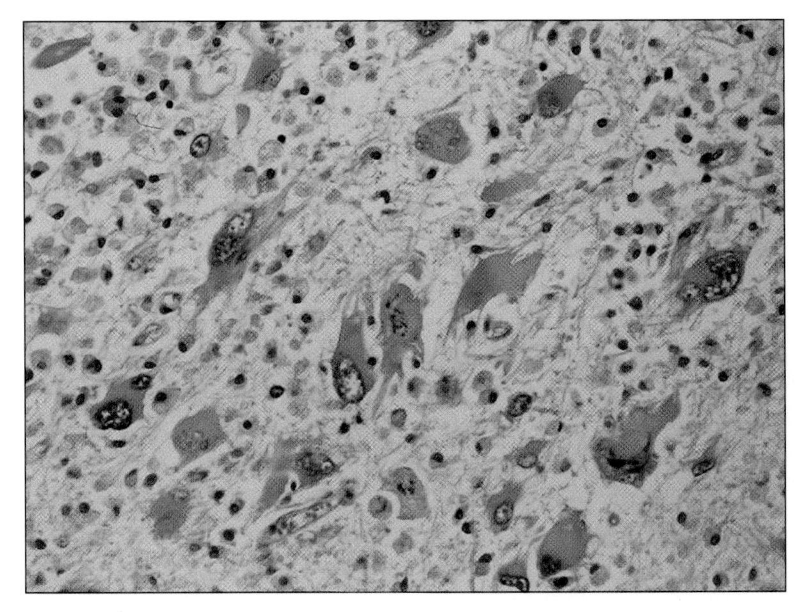

FIGURE 3-103 Bizarre, transformed astrocyte in the center of a PML lesion. There are large nuclei, abundant cytoplasm, and occasional multinucleated forms. These have malignant potential.

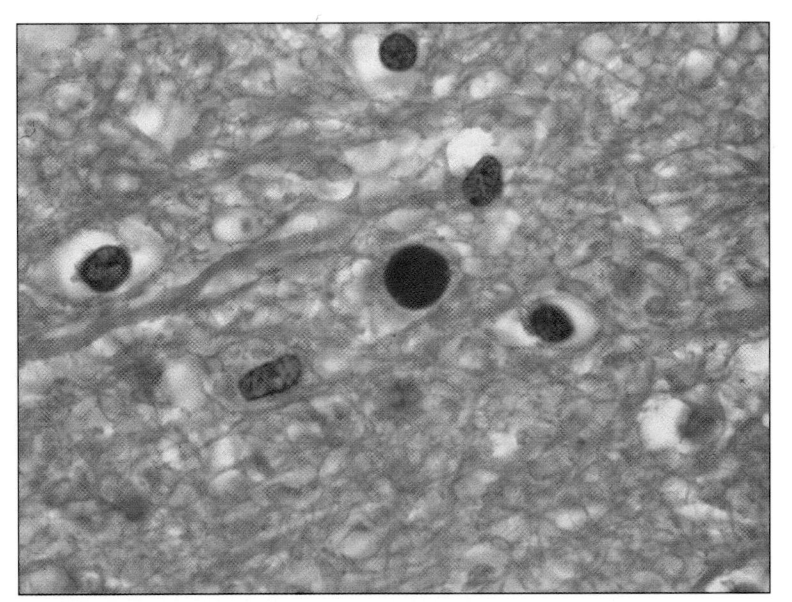

FIGURE 3-104 High-power photomicrograph of an intranuclear inclusion in oligodendrocytes. The roundness and ground-glass appearance of the inclusion are characteristic. (Hematoxylin-eosin stain.)

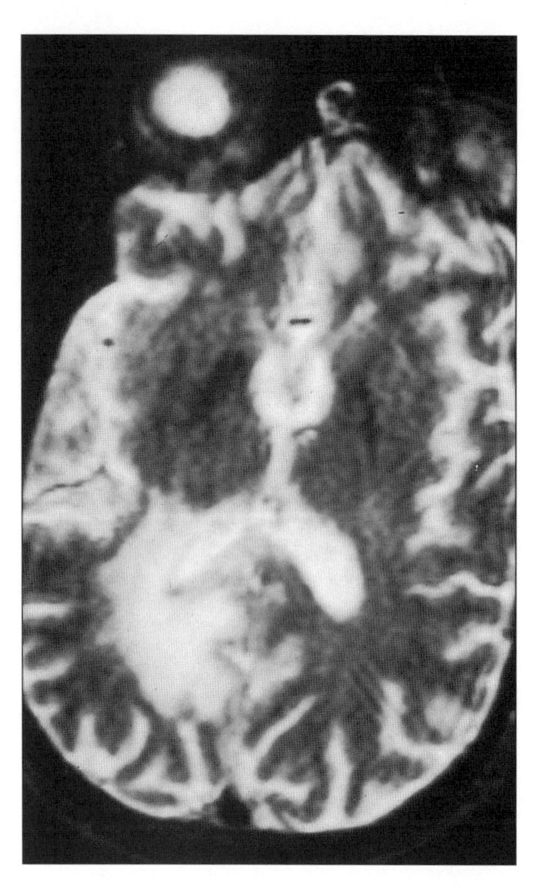

Figure 3-105 T2-weighted MRI in a patient with PML. The occipital white matter shows abnormal intensity suggestive of demyelination. The lesion typically involves subcortical white matter U-shaped fibers. These demyelinated regions are imaged best in T2-weighted sequences and rarely enhance.

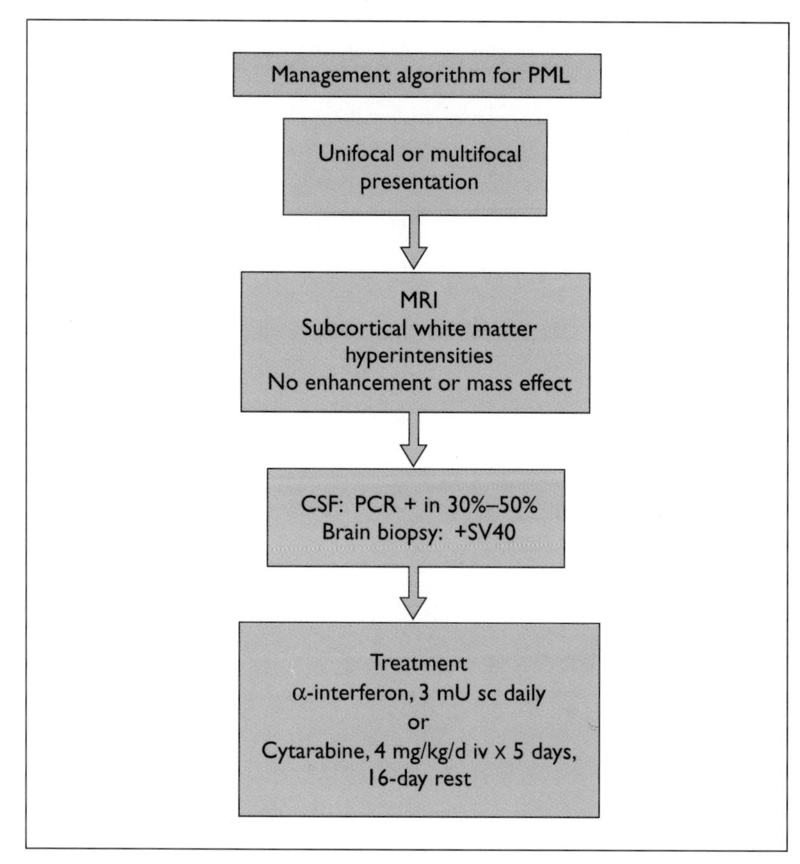

Figure 3-106 Management algorithm for PML.

Cytomegalovirus Infection

Neurologic effects of cytomegalovirus infection
Ventriculitis/encephalitis
Rapidly progressive mental status change
Periventricular white-matter "caps" on T2-weighted MRI
Polyradiculitis
Urinary retention, sacral anesthesia, paraparesis, pain
CSF findings:
↑ leukocytes with PMN predominance
High protein
Low glucose
CMV-positive by culture, PCR, and/or cytology

Figure 3-107 Neurologic effects of cytomegalovirus infection. CMV infects all levels and all cells of the nervous system. Most affected patients are in the late stages of AIDS ($CD4^+$ count <100 cells/mm3) and show evidence of CMV infection elsewhere, including retinitis, pneumonitis, and hepatitis. The clinical presentation of CMV polyradiculitis is stereotyped. Early therapy is essential to possible recovery. PMN—polymorphonuclear leukocytes; PCR—polymerase chain reaction.

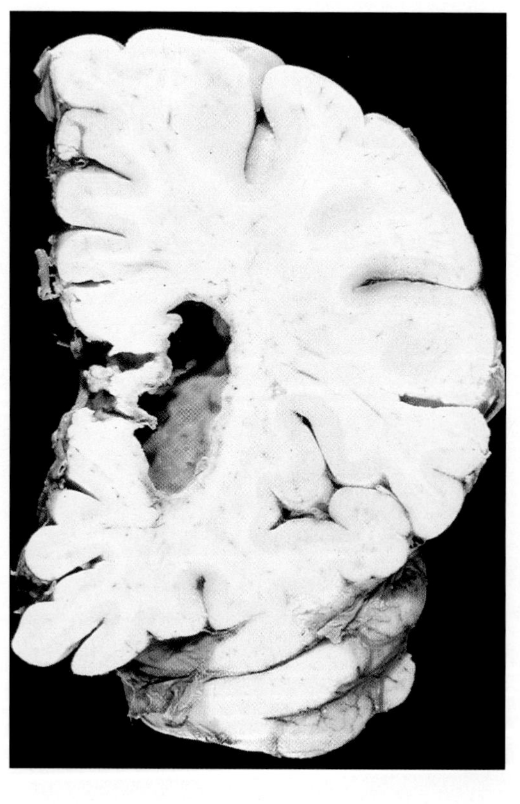

Figure 3-108 Gross pathologic specimen from a patient with CMV ventriculitis. An irregular border to the lateral ventricle can be seen, with discoloration and necrosis. This patient had a rapid course from onset to death.

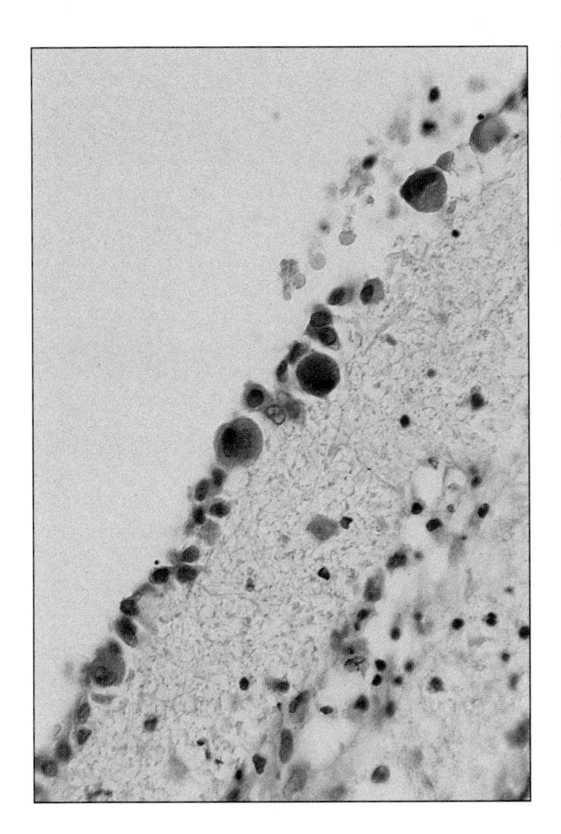

FIGURE 3-109 Photomicrograph of CMV inclusions. CMV inclusions are seen in the ependymal cells lining the lateral ventricle.

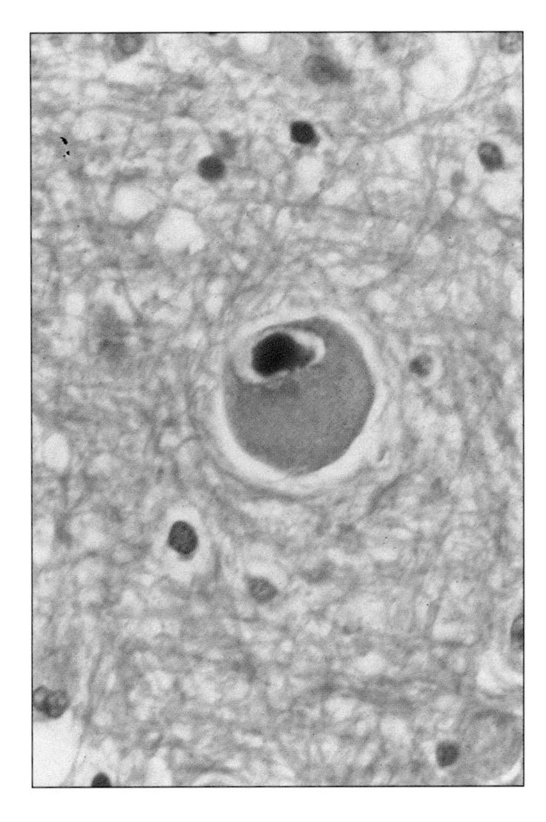

FIGURE 3-110 Typical CMV-infected cell with Cowdry type A intranuclear inclusion surrounded by a clear halo. Immunocytochemically, productive CMV infection is also found in the cytoplasm of many cells not bearing inclusions.

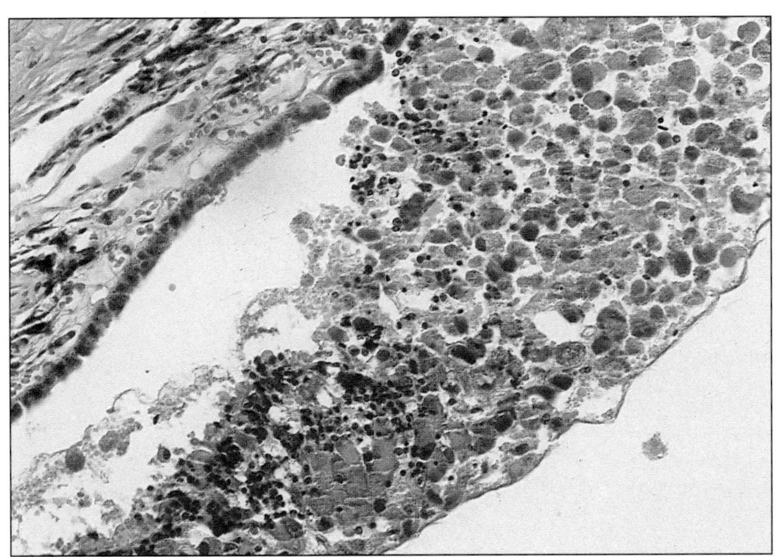

FIGURE 3-111 CMV retinitis. Masses of CMV-infected neurons and glial cells have replaced the normal retinal architecture at all levels above the retinal pigmented epithelial membrane. This disorder is treatable with antiviral agents but frequently leads to blindness.

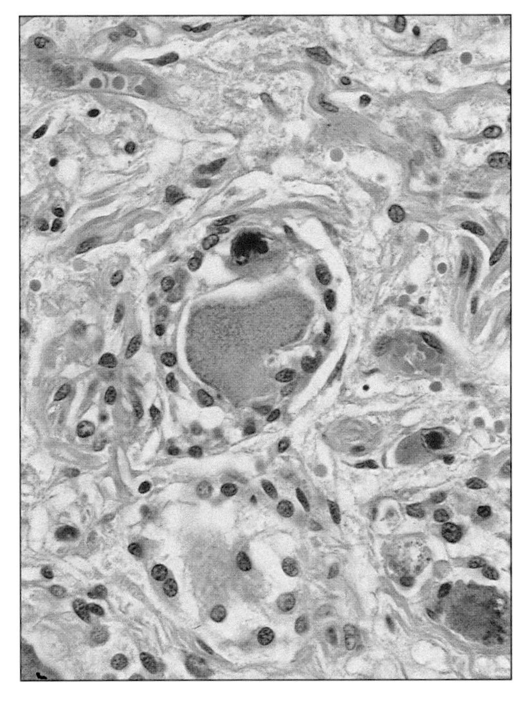

FIGURE 3-112 CMV dorsal root ganglionitis. A CMV-infected cell is seen among the satellite cells surrounding a dorsal root ganglion neuron. CMV may also infect Schwann cells in peripheral nerves, causing mixed demyelinating and axonal neuropathy.

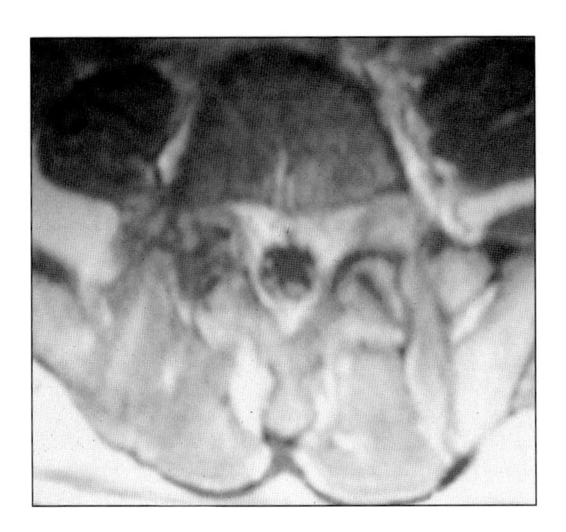

FIGURE 3-113 Gadolinium-enhanced MRI through the pelvis in a patient with CMV polyradiculitis. Enlargement and enhancement of the sacral nerve roots can be seen. This picture, along with urinary retention, sacral anesthesia, and CSF pleocytosis, is virtually diagnostic of this disorder.

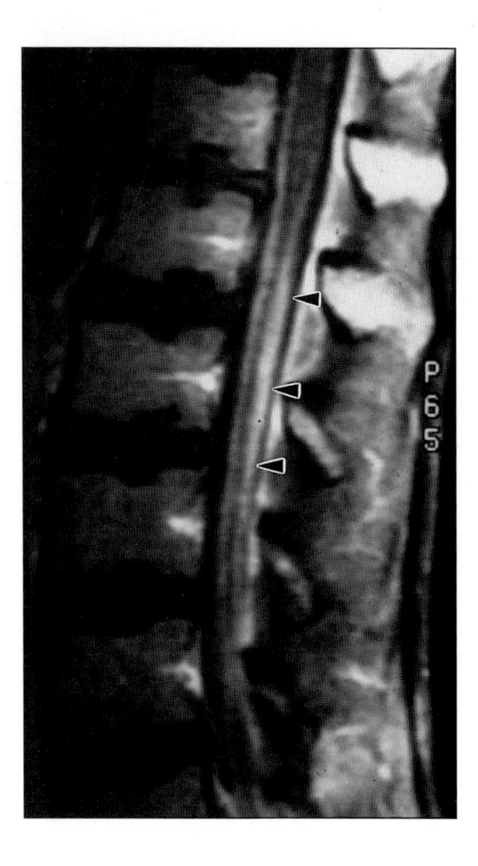

FIGURE 3-114 Contrast MRI of lumbar spinal chord in CMV radiculitis. *Arrowheads* indicate brightly enhancing nerve roots.

Treatment of cytomegalovirus retinitis	
Ganciclovir (first line)	
Induction	5 mg/kg bid × 2 wks
Maintenance	5 mg/kg qd for life
Foscarnet (second line)	
Induction	60–90 mg/kg q8h × 2 wks
Maintenance	90–120 mg/kg/d for life

FIGURE 3-115 Treatment of CMV retinitis. If CMV infection of the brain is suspected, specific antiviral therapy with ganciclovir should be considered, although its efficacy in CNS CMV infection (other than retinopathy) has not yet been proven. Ganciclovir usually cannot be given in conjunction with zidovudine or trimethoprim/sulfamethoxazole because of hematologic toxicity. Foscarnet may have significant toxicities, including nephrotoxicity.

Primary CNS Lymphoma

Pathologic features of primary CNS lymphoma
1. Mass lesions in deep gray structures
2. Pleomorphic, large blue cell perivascular infiltrate
3. "Diffusion" of malignant cells into parenchyma
4. Necrosis without macrophage infiltration or cavitation
5. Malignant cells of B-cell origin, positive for Epstein-Barr virus on in situ hybridization

FIGURE 3-116 Pathologic features of primary CNS lymphoma. Primary CNS lymphoma affects up to 10% of AIDS patients. The presence of Epstein-Barr virus (EBV) transcripts in malignant cells suggests that this is a virally induced disease.

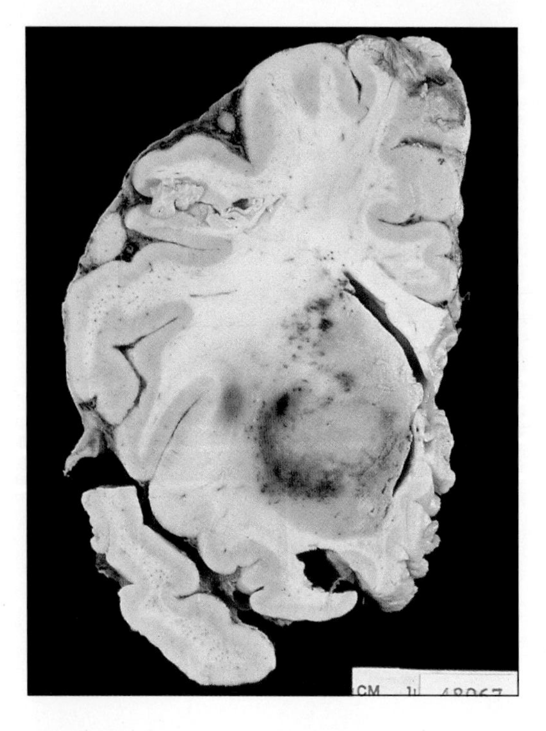

FIGURE 3-117 Gross postmortem specimen showing a hemorrhagic tumor mass in the region of the basal ganglia, a typical finding in primary CNS lymphoma. MRI scan may show enhancement, especially if necrosis is present.

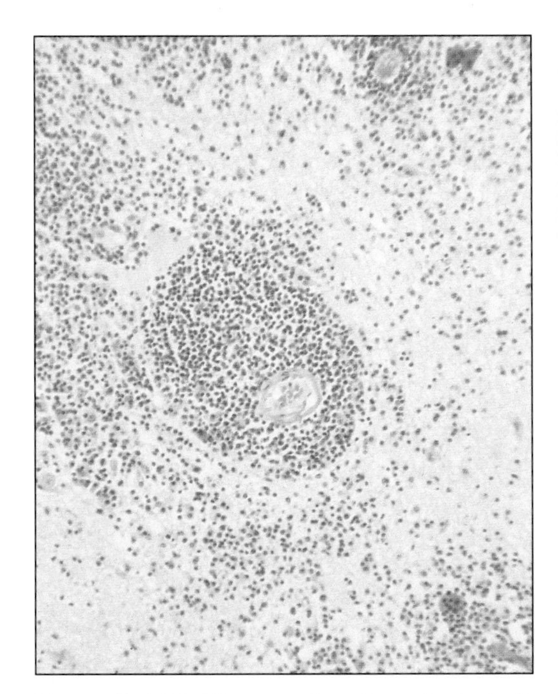

Figure 3-118 Microscopic pattern typical of primary CNS lymphoma. Perivascular malignant lymphocytes with infiltration of the surrounding brain parenchyma are seen. These malignant cells are usually B cells and have been demonstrated to be latently infected with EBV in patients with AIDS.

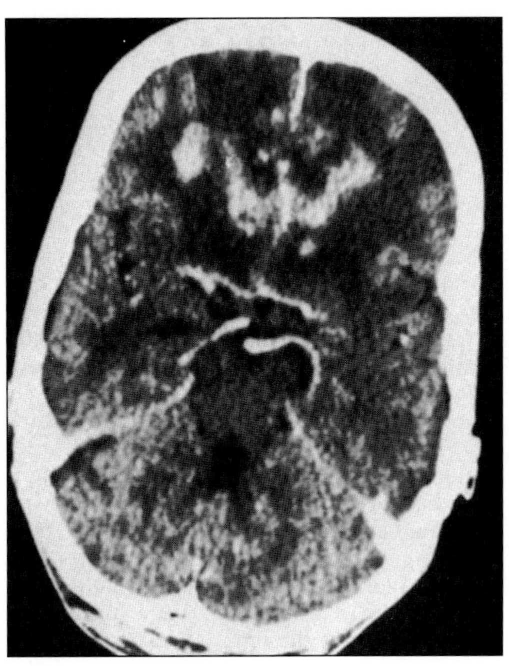

Figure 3-119 CT scan of primary CNS lymphoma. CT scan of a patient with autopsy-proven primary CNS lymphoma. There is a multicentric contrast-enhancing lesion in the frontal lobes with massive surrounding edema and posterior displacement of the middle cerebral arteries. (*From* McArthur JC: Neurologic complications of human immunodeficiency virus infection. *In* Gorbach SL, Bartlett JG, Blacklow NR (eds.): *Infectious Diseases*. Philadelphia: W.B. Saunders; 1992:956–972; with permission.)

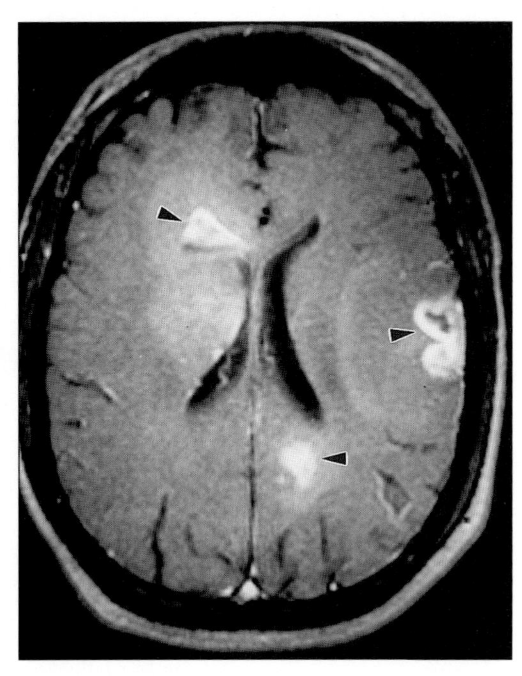

Figure 3-120 Contrast MRI scan showing multiple ring-enhancing lesions of primary CNS lymphoma. Multiple areas of dense contrast enhancement can be seen (*arrowheads*).

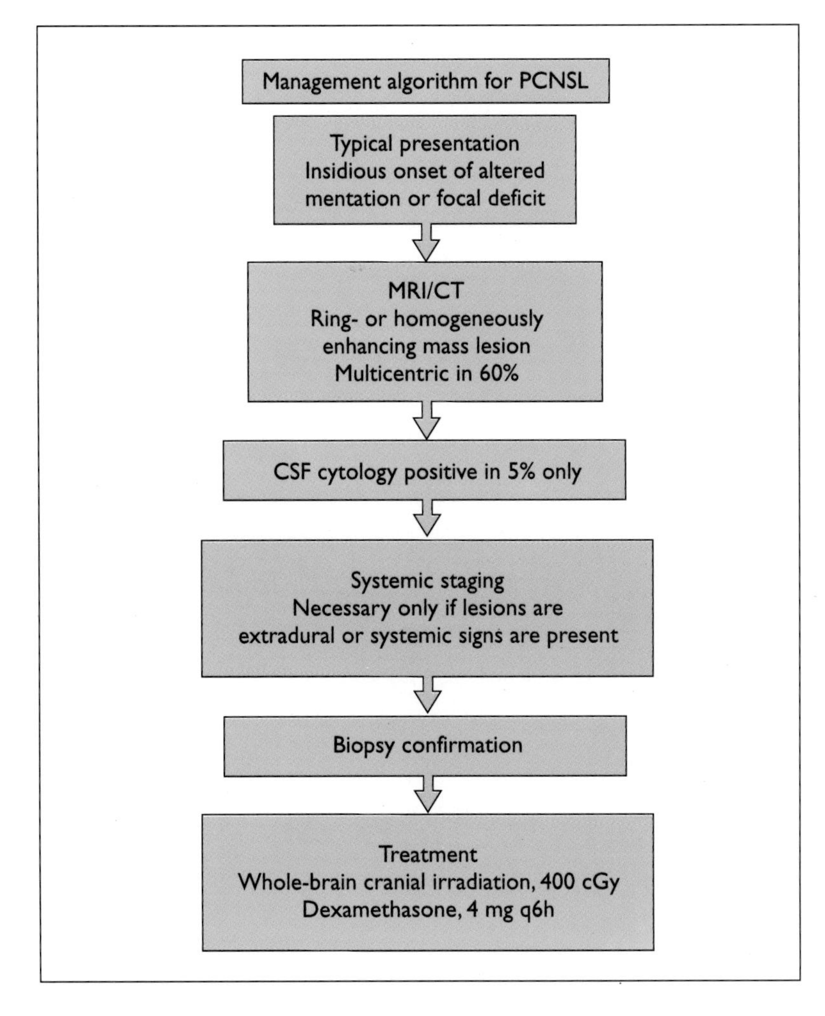

Figure 3-121 Management of primary CNS lymphoma. (*From* McArthur JC: Neurologic complications of human immunodeficiency virus infection. *In* Gorbach SL, Bartlett JG, Blacklow NR (eds.): *Infectious Diseases*. Philadelphia: W.B. Saunders; 1992:956–972.)

Selected Bibliography

Harrison MJG, McArthur JC (eds.): *AIDS and Neurology*. New York: Churchill Livingstone; 1995.

Johnson RT: *Viral Infections of the Nervous System*. New York: Raven Press; 1984.

Mandell GL, Bennett JE, Dolin R (eds.): *Principles and Practice of Infectious Diseases*, 4th ed. New York: Churchill Livingstone; 1995.

Scheld WM, Whitley RJ, Durack DT (eds.): *Infections of the Central Nervous System*. New York: Raven Press; 1991.

Whitley RJ: Viral encephalitis. *N Engl J Med* 1990, 323:242.

Chapter 4

Brain Abscesses

Brian Wispelwey

Pathology

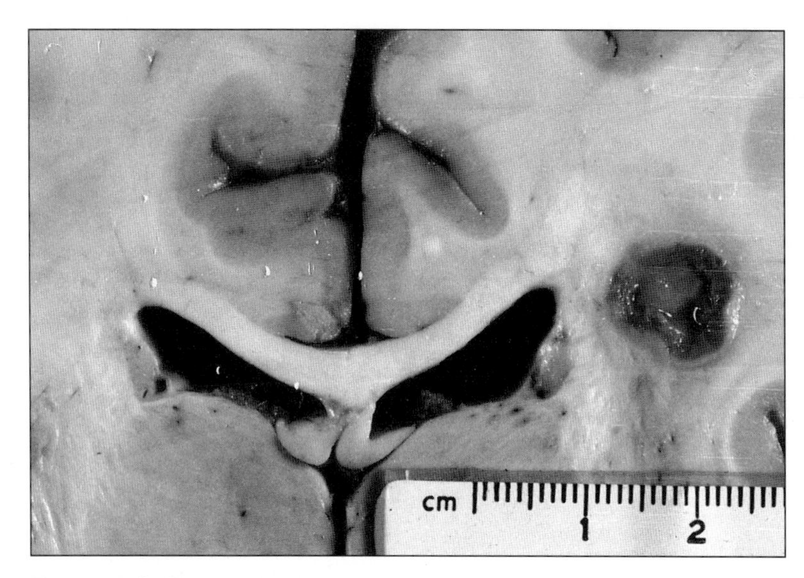

Figure 4-1 Deep white matter abscess adjacent to the body of the lateral ventricle. An abscess in this location is most consistent with hematogenous dissemination from a distant focus of infection. Chronic pyogenic lung diseases, especially lung abscess and bronchiectasis, are important diagnostic considerations and account for approximately one half of all hematogenous abscesses. (*From* Wispelwey B, Dacey R Jr, Scheld WM: Brain abscess. *In* Scheld WM, Durack D, Whitley R (eds.): *Infections of the Central Nervous System*. New York: Raven Press; 1991; with permission.)

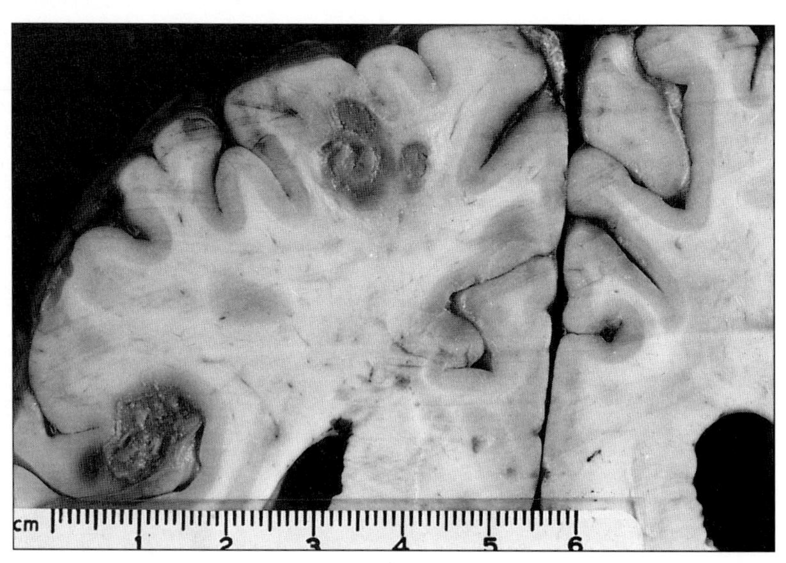

Figure 4-2 Multiple brain abscesses. These abscesses occur at the junction between gray and white matter and are consistent with hematogenous dissemination as a proximate cause. The incidence of multiple brain abscesses was only 1% to 15% in older series; however, with the advent of computed tomographic (CT) scanning, multiple lesions are now recognized in 10% to 50% of cases. Prior to recent therapeutic modalities, the mortality from multiple brain abscesses approached 100%. With the advent of CT-guided aspiration, this mortality can be decreased to < 10%. (*From* Wispelwey B, Dacey R Jr, Scheld WM: Brain abscess. *In* Scheld WM, Durack D, Whitley R (eds.): *Infections of the Central Nervous System*. New York: Raven Press; 1991; with permission.)

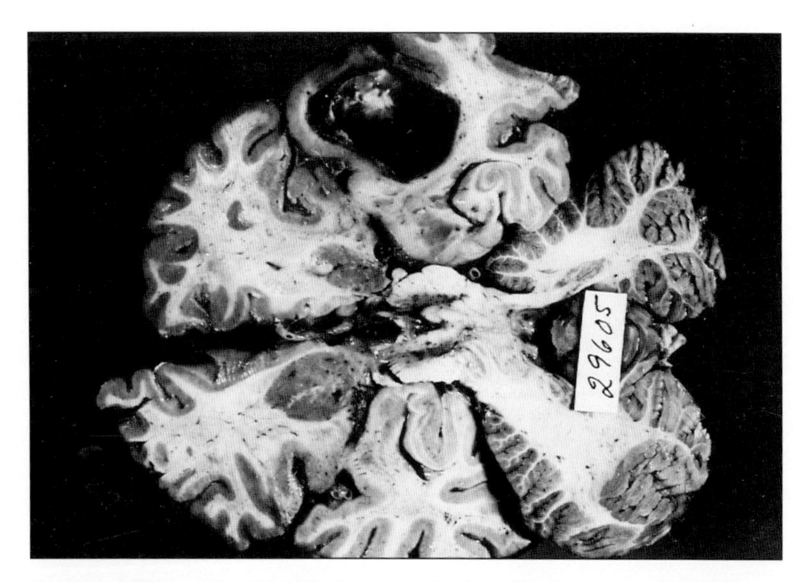

Figure 4-3 Large, chronic temporal lobe abscess secondary to chronic otitis media. The location of this abscess is immediately above the petrous temporal bone. About 50% to 75% of otogenic brain abscesses are located in the temporal lobe. The cerebellum is the next most commonly affected area in this setting. (*From* Wispelwey B, Dacey R Jr, Scheld WM: Brain abscess. *In* Scheld WM, Durack D, Whitley R (eds.): *Infections of the Central Nervous System*. New York: Raven Press; 1991; with permission.)

Pathologic stages of brain abscess development

Stage	Days
Early cerebritis	Days 1–3
Late cerebritis	Days 4–9
Early capsule formation	Days 10–13
Late capsule formation	Day 14+

Figure 4-4 Pathologic stages of brain abscess development. The four stages of brain abscess development (experimentally induced in animal models) include early cerebritis (days 1–3); late cerebritis (days 4–9), at which time a well-formed necrotic center reaches its maximum size; early capsule formation (days 10–13), when a well-developed layer of fibroblasts appears; and late capsule formation (day 14 on). This pattern is affected by local oxygen concentration, offending organism, and host immune response.

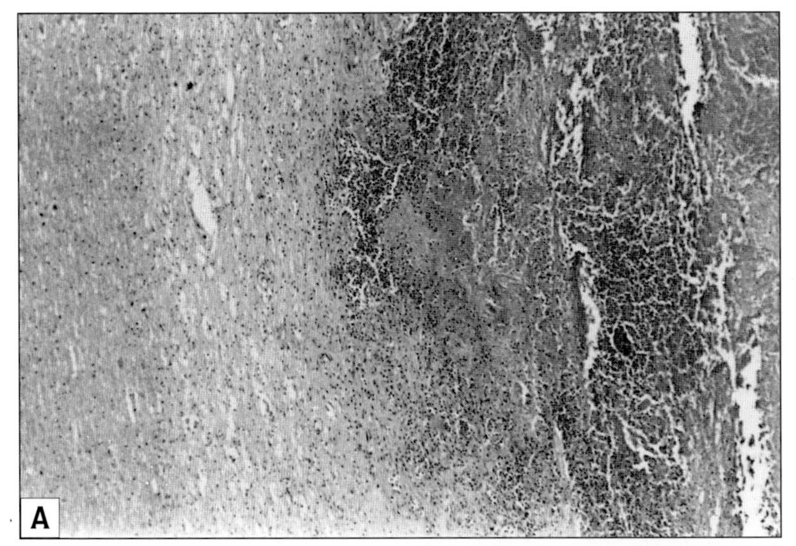

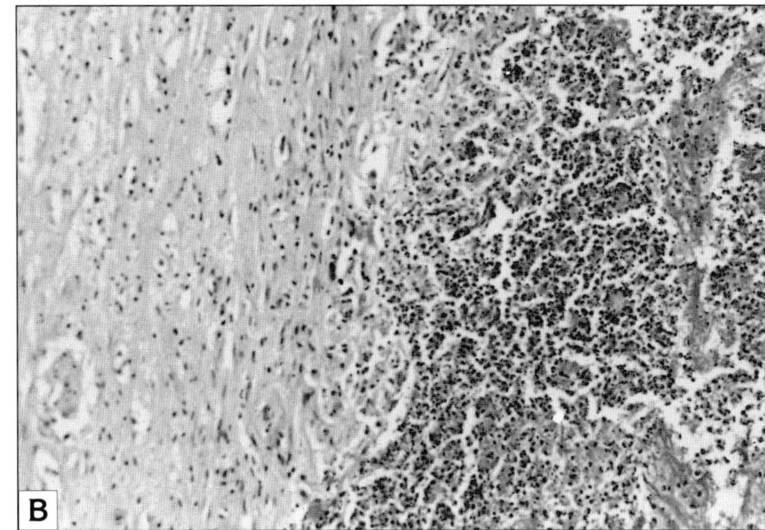

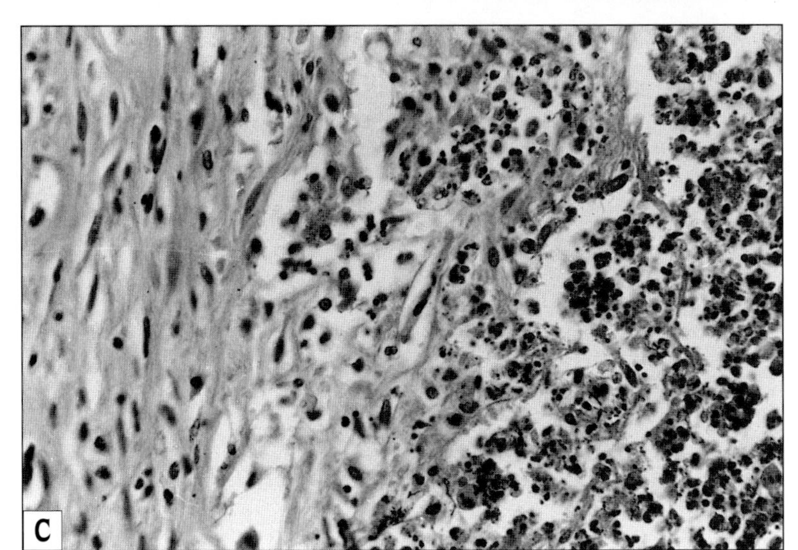

FIGURE 4-5 Wall of a brain abscess during early capsule formation. **A**, Normal white matter is seen to the left of the slide, with an intermediate area of edematous brain abscess adjacent to the abscess wall. This abscess is at the early stages of abscess development, at the very beginning of capsule formation. **B**, A higher magnification shows a periabscess inflammatory exudate. There is relatively little encapsulation at this early stage. **C**, Higher magnification of the abscess wall shows the combination of increased gliosis and inflammatory cells adjacent to the abscess. (*All panels*, Hematoxylin-eosin stain. *Panels A* and *B*, × 40; *C*, × 100.)

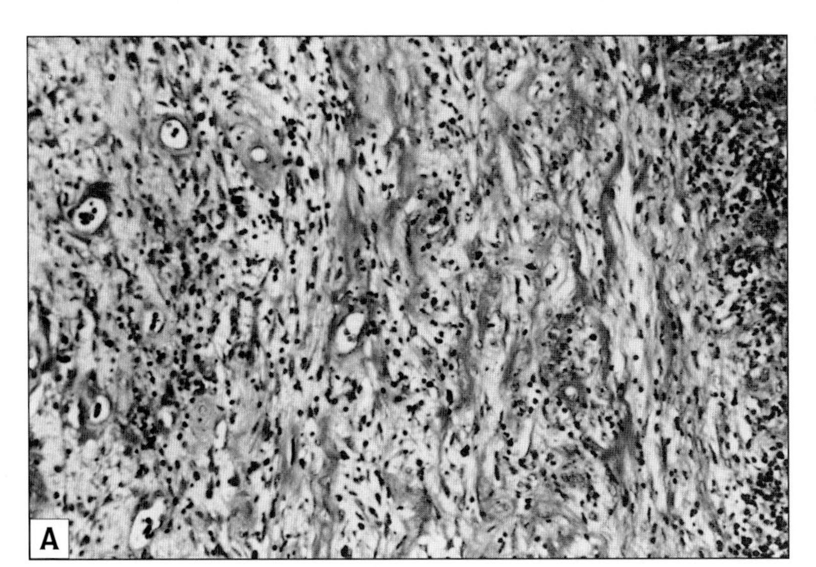

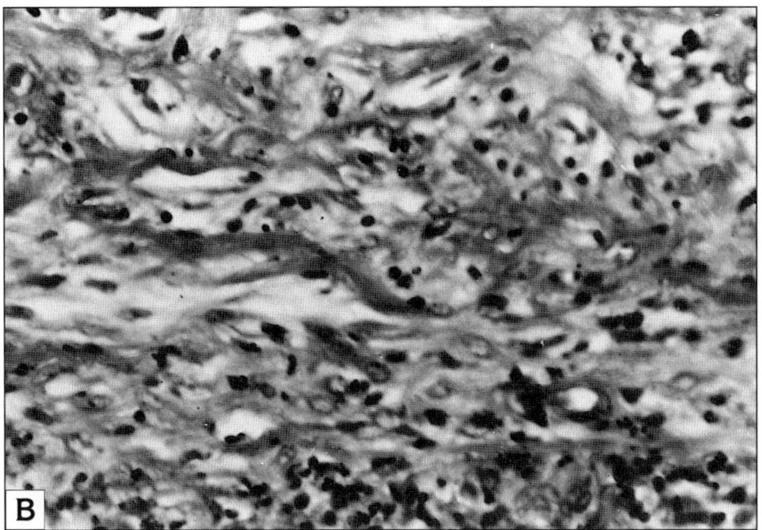

FIGURE 4-6 Abscess wall during later stage of abscess development. **A**, Thick collagen fibers are seen within the capsule wall. Experimentally, it takes approximately 2 weeks to reach this stage of abscess development. (Hematoxylin-eosin stains, × 40.) **B**, Trichrome staining of the abscess wall shows thick collagen fibers present above the inflammatory mass (× 100).

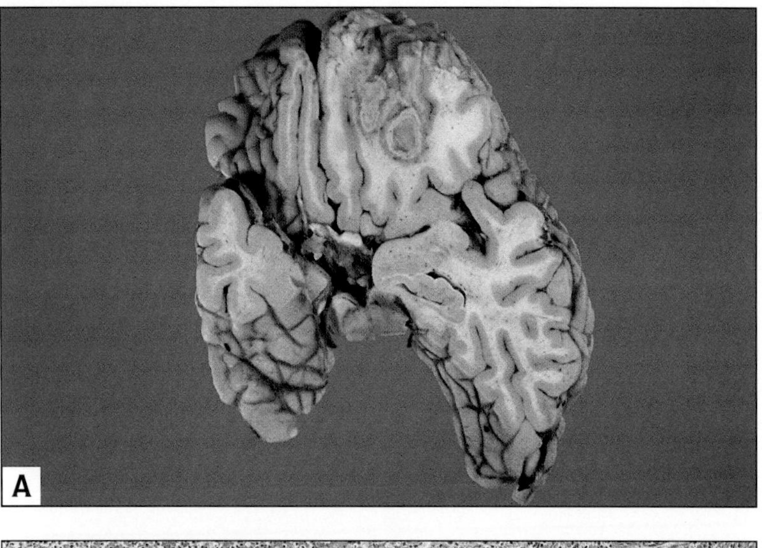

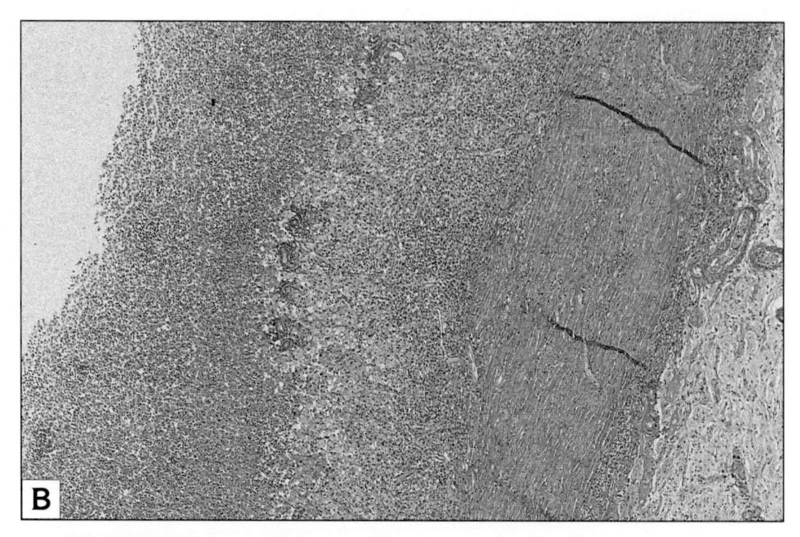

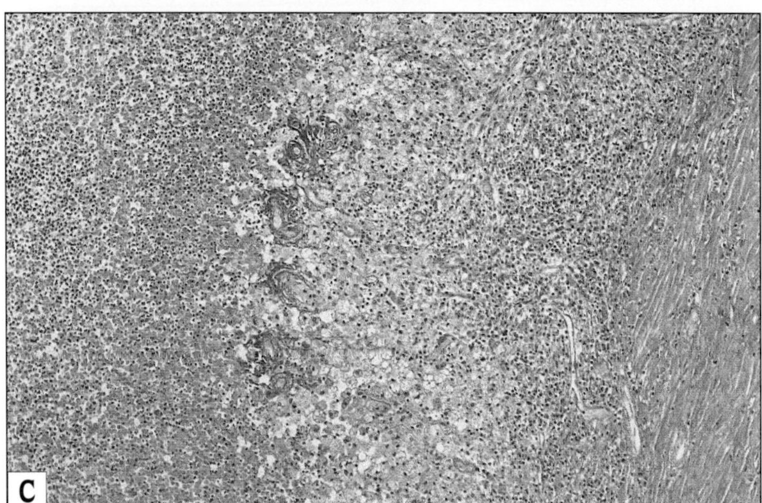

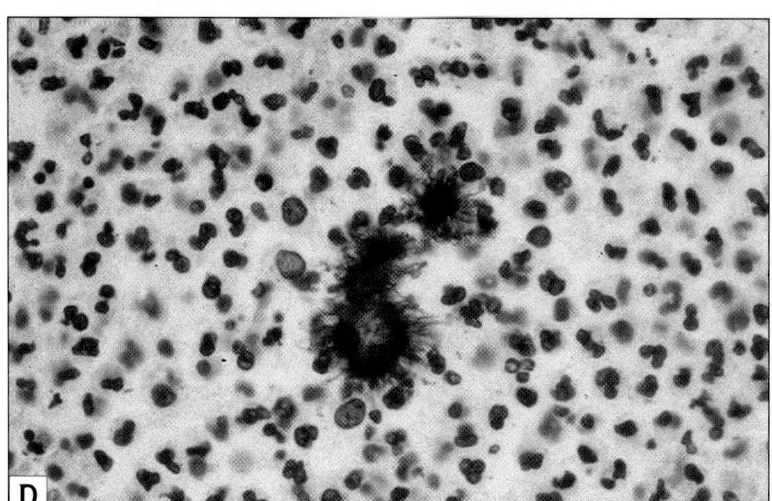

FIGURE 4-7 Brain abscess due to actinomycosis. **A**, On gross examination, two well-encapsulated abscesses can be seen. **B**, Low-power photomicrograph of a periodic acid–Schiff-stained section through the wall of a mature abscess. At the left is the necrotic inflammatory core with an intermediate edematous zone of neovascularity, macrophages, and lymphocytes surrounded by a layer of fibrosis in the collagenous capsule. **C**, A high-power photomicrograph through the abscess wall. **D**, Staining of the central necrotic region reveals sulfur granules consistent with cerebral actinomycosis.

PATHOGENESIS AND ETIOLOGY

Predisposing conditions for brain abscess

	Frequency, %
Adjacent focus of infection	30–50
Otitis media	
Mastoiditis	
Paranasal sinus infection	
Face or scalp infection	
Dental sepsis	
Osteomyelitis of skull	
Penetrating head injury	
Postsurgical (craniotomy) infection	
Hematogenous spread	~35
Lung abscess, empyema, bronchiectasis	
Congenital heart disease	
Bacterial endocarditis	
Compromised host	
Cryptogenic	20

FIGURE 4-8 Predisposing conditions for brain abscess. Brain abscesses develop in four clinical settings: 1) in association with a contiguous suppurative focus; 2) after hematogenous spread from a distant focus; 3) after trauma; and 4) cryptogenic. Most patients with brain abscesses will have a contiguous focus of infection, usually sinusitis or otitis. These infections spread to contiguous sites via direct extension through areas of infection, by retrograde thrombophlebitic spread along diploic or emissary veins, or via preexisting channels such as the internal auditory canal in otogenic infections. Abscesses due to hematogenous spread are more commonly multiple and multiloculated. They often occur in the area of distribution of the middle cerebral artery, occur initially at the gray-white matter junction where brain capillary flow is slowest, and show poor encapsulation.

Predisposing conditions, site of abscess, and usual microbial isolates

Predisposing condition	Site of abscess	Usual microbial isolates
Contiguous focus or primary infection		
Otitis media and mastoiditis	Temporal or cerebellar lobes	Streptococci (anaerobic or aerobic), *Bacteroides fragilis*, Enterobacteriaceae
Frontoethmoidal sinusitis	Frontal lobe	Predominantly streptococci (anaerobic or aerobic), *Bacteroides* spp., Enterobacteriaceae, *Staphylococcus aureus*, *Haemophilus* spp.
Sphenoidal sinusitis	Frontal or temporal lobe	Same as frontoethmoidal sinusitis
Dental sepsis	Frontal lobe	Mixed *Fusobacterium*, *Bacteroides*, and *Streptococcus* spp.
Penetrating head injury or postsurgical infection	Related to wound	*Staphylococcus aureus*, streptococci, Enterobacteriaceae, *Clostridium* spp.
Hematogenous spread/distant site of infection		
Congenital heart disease (CHD)	Multiple sites; middle cerebral artery distribution common but may occur at any site	Streptococci (*viridans*, anaerobic, or microaerophilic), *Haemophilus* spp.
Lung abscess, empyema, bronchiectasis	Same as CHD	*Fusobacterium*, *Actinomyces*, *Bacteroides*, *Streptococcus*, *Nocardia asteroides*
Bacterial endocarditis	Same as CHD	*Staphylococcus aureus*, *Streptococcus* spp.
Compromised host	Same as CHD	*Toxoplasma*, fungi, Enterobacteriaceae, *Nocardia*

FIGURE 4-9 Predisposing conditions, site of abscess, and usual microbial isolates. Understanding the predisposing condition in a brain abscess can suggest the likely infecting organism, which has important implications for therapy. (*From* Wispelwey B, Scheld WM: Brain abscess. *In* Mandell GL, Douglas RG Jr, Bennett JE (eds.): *Principles and Practice of Infectious Diseases*, 3rd ed. New York: Churchill Livingstone; 1990:778; with permission.)

Microbiologic etiology of brain abscesses

Organism	Percent
Staphylococcus aureus	10–15
Enterobacteriaceae	23–33
Streptococcus pneumoniae	< 1
Haemophilus influenzae	< 1
Streptococcus milleri group	60–70
Bacteroides spp.	20–40
Fungi	10–15
Protozoa, helminths	< 1

FIGURE 4-10 Microbiologic etiology of brain abscesses. In the pre-antibiotic era, *Staphylococcus aureus*, streptococci, and coliform bacteria were the most common isolates from brain abscesses. Currently, anaerobic organisms are seen as the predominant cause of such abscesses, especially those of otic origin. The Enterobacteriaceae usually occur in mixed culture, with *Proteus* spp., *Escherichia coli*, and *Pseudomonas* spp. appearing most often (in decreasing order of frequency). The *Streptococcus milleri* group (including *S. intermedius* and *S. anginosus*) has a predilection for causing focal suppurative disease, probably related to its group O III antigen, which is a potent virulence factor. *Bacteroides* spp., including *B. fragilis*, often occur in mixed cultures. Various protozoa or helminths are etiologic in certain geographic regions. (*From* Wispelwey B, Scheld WM: Brain abscess. *In* Mandell GL, Douglas RG Jr, Bennett JE (eds.): *Principles and Practice of Infectious Diseases*, 3rd ed. New York: Churchill Livingstone; 1990:780; with permission.)

Etiology of brain abscess in the compromised host

Abnormal cell-mediated immunity	Neutropenia or neutrophil defects
Toxoplasma gondii	Aerobic gram-negative bacteria
Nocardia asteroides	*Aspergillus* spp.
Cryptococcus neoformans	Zygomycetes
Listeria monocytogenes	*Candida* spp.
Mycobacterium spp.	

FIGURE 4-11 Etiology of brain abscess in the compromised host. The patient's immune status is an important determinant of the microbiology. Compromised hosts, including those on immunosuppressive therapy, with underlying malignancy, or with AIDS, are at increased risk for brain abscess, and the infecting organism can be predicted, or the differential diagnosis narrowed, depending on the arm of the immune system affected. Patients with T-lymphocyte or mononuclear phagocyte defects are commonly seen in hospital settings, and *Toxoplasma gondii* and *Nocardia asteriodes* are especially common pathogens. Neutrophil defects or neutropenia are often due to chemotherapy. Fungi and parasites are important diagnostic considerations in these patients.

Diagnosis

Clinical manifestations of brain abscess

Sign or symptom	Percent
Headache	70
Fever	40–50
Focal neurologic deficit	≈ 50
Triad of fever, headache, focal deficit	< 50
Nausea/vomiting	22–50
Seizures	25–45
Nuchal rigidity	≈ 25
Papilledema	≈ 25

Figure 4-12 Clinical manifestations of brain abscess. The clinical manifestations of brain abscess can vary greatly and depend on several interdependent factors, including the relative virulence of the infecting organism, host immune status, abscess location, number of lesions, and the presence or absence of associated meningitis or ventricular rupture.

Clinical manifestations according to abscess location

Temporal lobe abscesses
- Ipsilateral headache
- Aphasia
- Upper homonymous quadrant-anopsia

Parietal lobe abscesses
- Headache
- Visual field defects
- Endocrine disturbances

Frontal lobe abscesses
- Headache
- Drowsiness
- Inattention
- Mental function deterioration
- Hemiparesis
- Motor speech disorder

Cerebellar abscesses
- Nystagmus
- Ataxia
- Vomiting
- Dysmetria

Figure 4-13 Clinical manifestations according to abscess location. Symptoms and signs are dependent on abscess location. Neurologic findings in a patient with a predisposing condition mandate investigation to exclude a brain abscess and other intracranial complications of these disorders.

A. Differential diagnosis of brain abscesses

Subdural empyema	Epidural abscess
Pyogenic meningitis	Cerebral neoplasms
Viral encephalitis (esp. herpes simplex)	Hemorrhagic leukoencephalitis
Cysticercosis	Echinococcosis
Cerebral infarction	Cryptococcosis
Mycotic aneurysms	CNS vasculitis
	Chronic subdural hematoma

B. Differential diagnosis of focal CNS lesions in AIDS patients

Toxoplasmosis	*Listeria monocytogenes*
Primary CNS lymphoma	*Nocardia asteroides*
Mycobacterium tuberculosis	*Salmonella* group B
Mycobacterium avium complex	*Aspergillus* spp.
Progressive multifocal leukoencephalopathy	*Rhodococcus* spp.
Cryptococcus neoformans	*Acanthamoeba* spp.
Candida spp.	

Figure 4-14 Differential diagnosis of brain abscess. **A**, A broad list of differential diagnoses is possible in brain abscess. Often, computed tomography (CT) can detect these lesions but frequently is not sufficient for differentiation. **B**, Central nervous system (CNS) complications are increasingly recognized in AIDS patients, and multiple pathologic processes may coexist. The table represents a partial list of the most frequently described etiologies. In one series, CNS toxoplasmosis was recognized in 28% of AIDS patients with CNS complications and primary CNS lymphoma was recognized in 11%. The other conditions are less common causes of mass lesions in this population. (*Panel B adapted from* Wispelwey B, Scheld WM: Brain abscess. *In* Mandell GL, Douglas RG Jr, Bennett JE (eds.): *Principles and Practice of Infectious Diseases*, 3rd ed. New York: Churchill Livingstone; 1990:780; with permission.)

Diagnostic work-up

- Laboratory findings often not helpful
- Lumbar puncture contraindicated
- Skull roentgenograms usually normal
- CT scan with contrast enhancement is 95% sensitive
- MRI is more sensitive at earlier stages and is the procedure of choice
- Biopsy or aspiration usually needed

Figure 4-15 Diagnostic work-up for patients with suspected brain abscess. A patient with clinical manifestations suggestive of an abscess should undergo tests to verify the presence of an abscess and to exclude other conditions. Laboratory studies are often not helpful. A moderate leukocytosis may be present but exceeds > 20,000 cells/mL in only 10% of patients, and the erythrocyte sedimentation rate is usually increased to 45–50 mm/hr. Lumbar puncture is contraindicated because the diagnostic yield is poor and because the procedure may result in herniation. Skull films are usually normal in patients with abscesses. CT is quickly and safely performed and has a high sensitivity for brain abscesses, especially with contrast enhancement. MRI is more sensitive, showing abscesses at earlier stages of development, and is the procedure of choice where available. Biopsy or aspiration is almost always required to differentiate these abscesses from malignant lesions as well as to identify the pathologic organism.

Radiologic Evaluation

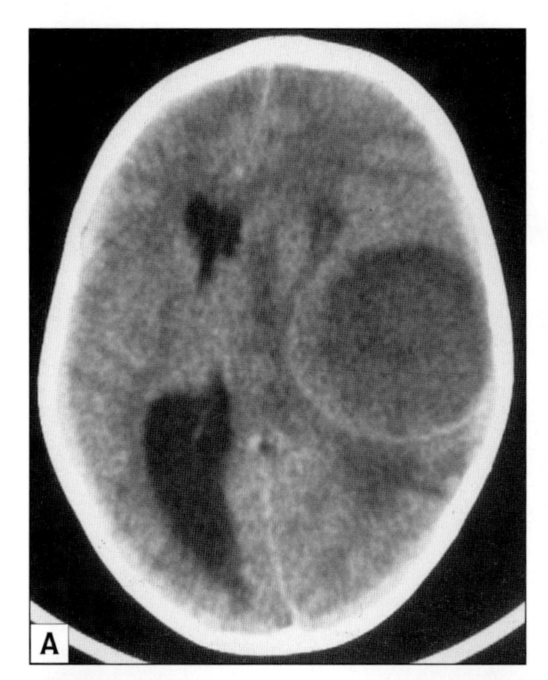

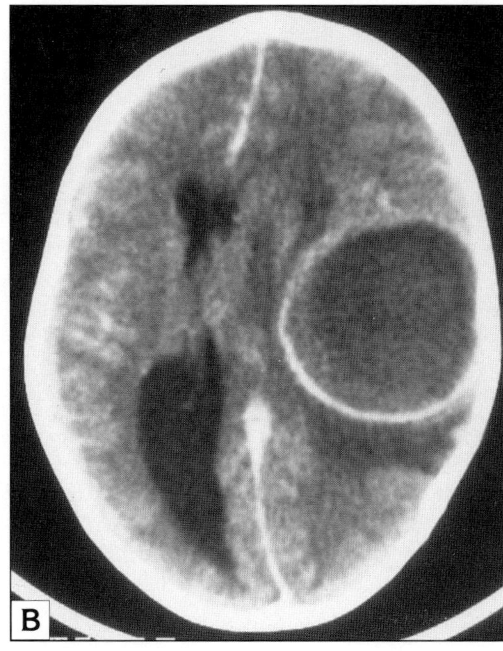

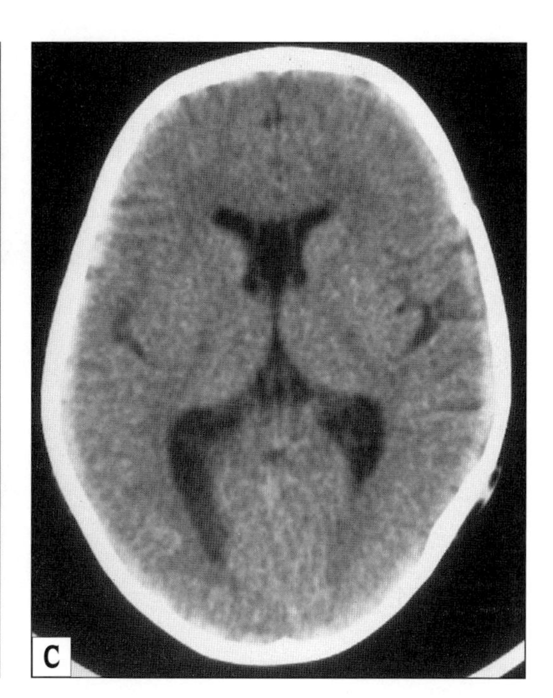

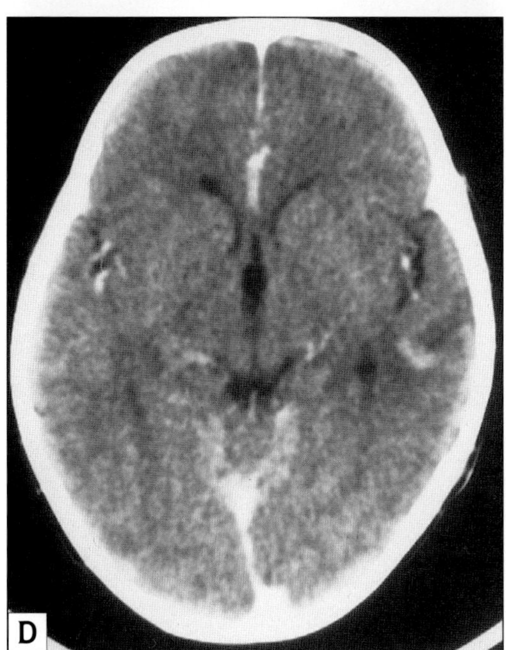

Figure 4-16 Temporal abscess due to presumed otogenic infection. **A**, Unenhanced CT scan shows a large, right, frontotemporoparietal brain abscess which is causing marked right-to-left shift of midline structures and effacement of the ipsilateral lateral ventricle. **B**, On contrast enhancement, the CT scan shows a thin-rimmed, homogeneous enhancement surrounding an area of decreased attenuation within the center of the abscess. **C**, An unenhanced CT scan, done 6 weeks after surgical aspiration of the abscess and antibiotic therapy, shows resolution of the mass effect. **D**, A follow-up enhanced CT scan shows minimal contrast enhancement in the temporal lobe. A cured brain abscess, however, may continue to exhibit contrast enhancement on CT for 4 to 10 weeks to up to 6 to 9 months. (*From* Wispelwey B, Dacey R Jr, Scheld WM: Brain abscess. *In* Scheld WM, Durack D, Whitley R (eds.): *Infections of the Central Nervous System.* New York: Raven Press; 1991; with permission.)

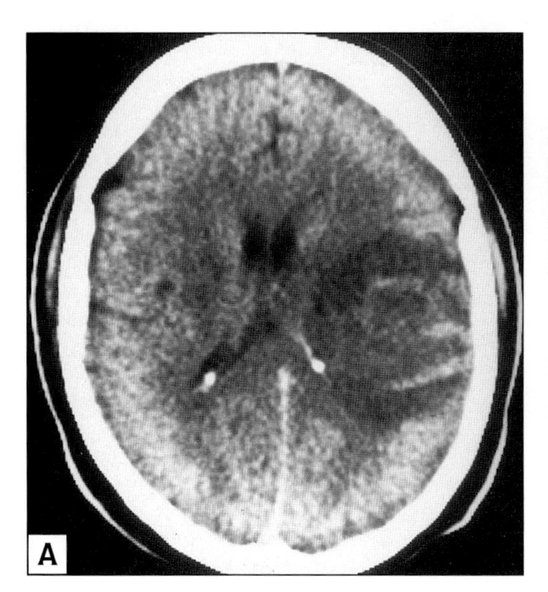

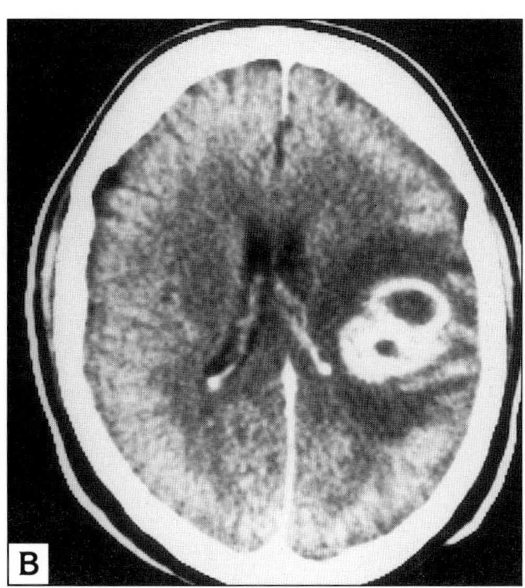

Figure 4-17 Unenhanced and enhanced axial CT scans. **A**, Unenhanced axial CT scan shows irregular areas of high and low attenuation producing effacement of the sylvian cistern and ipsilateral lateral ventricle on the left. **B**, After contrast enhancement, somewhat thick, irregular, ring-enhancing lesions with multiple loculi are seen to be surrounded by an area of decreased attenuation, indicating cerebral edema. (*From* Wispelwey B, Dacey R Jr, Scheld WM: Brain abscess. *In* Scheld WM, Durack D, Whitley R (eds.): *Infections of the Central Nervous System.* New York: Raven Press; 1991; with permission.)

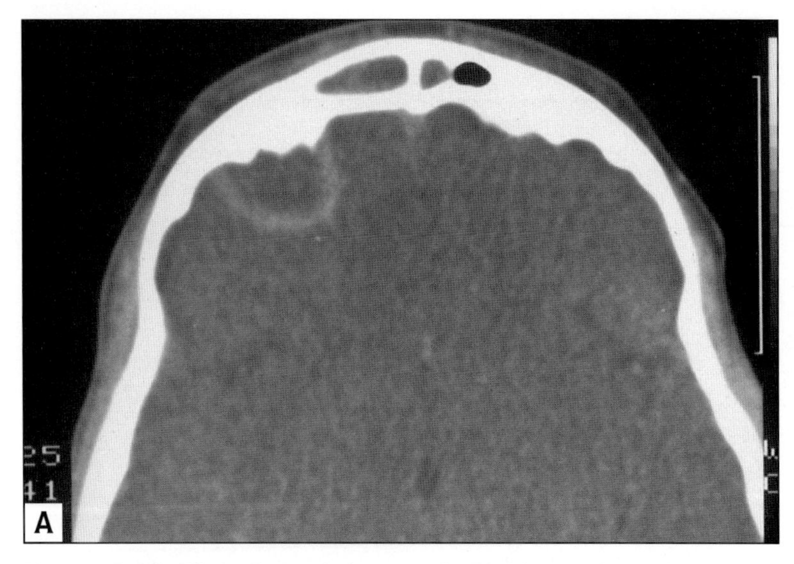

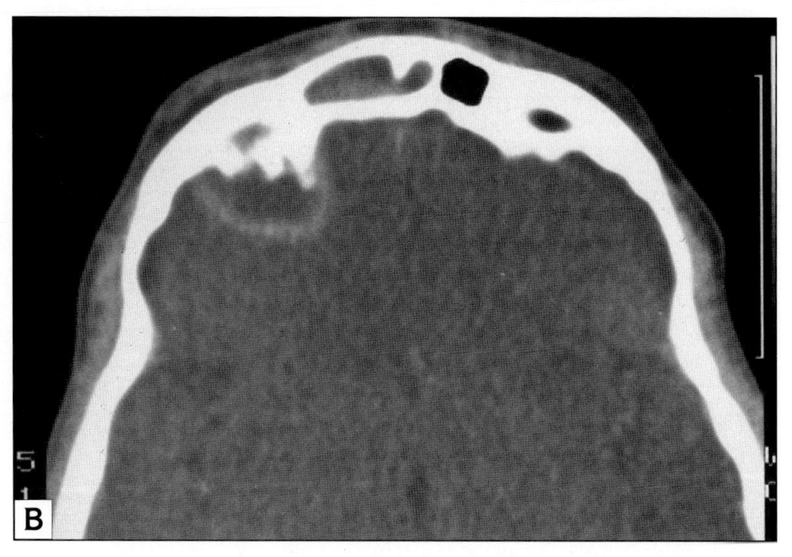

Figure 4-18 Right frontal abscess. **A**, Right anterior inferior frontal brain abscess immediately contiguous to an opacified right frontal sinus. **B**, Thin, homogeneous contrast enhancement is characteristic in this abscess. Direct spread of the infection from the contiguous frontal sinus, probably by thrombosed emissary veins, is the presumed route of entry of the pathogen into brain in cases such as this. (*From* Wispelwey B, Dacey R Jr, Scheld WM: Brain abscess. *In* Scheld WM, Durack D, Whitley R (eds.): *Infections of the Central Nervous System.* New York: Raven Press; 1991; with permission.)

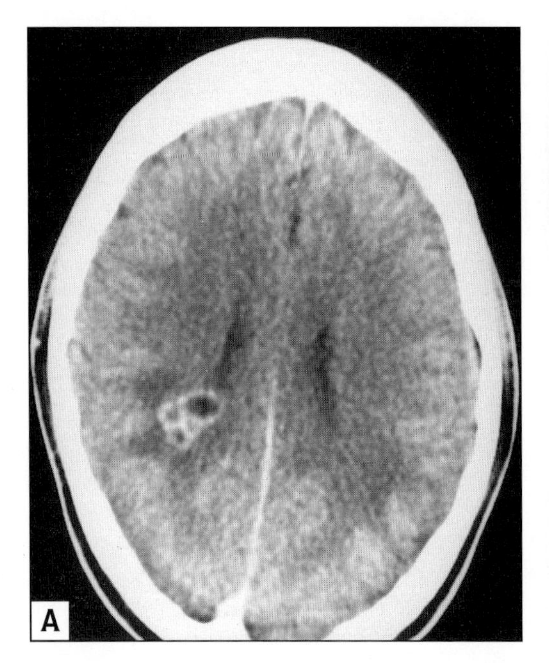

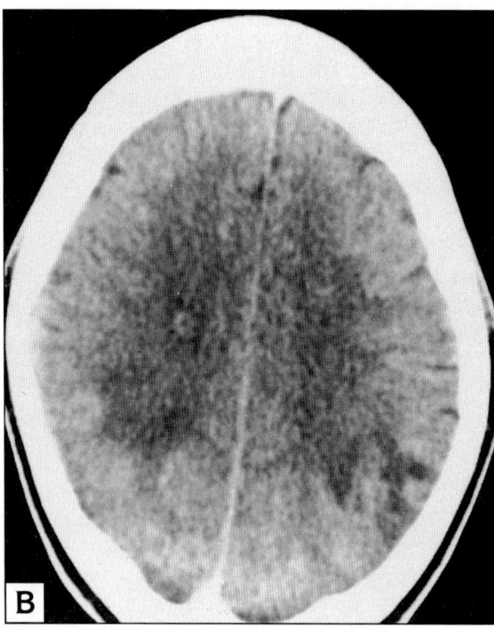

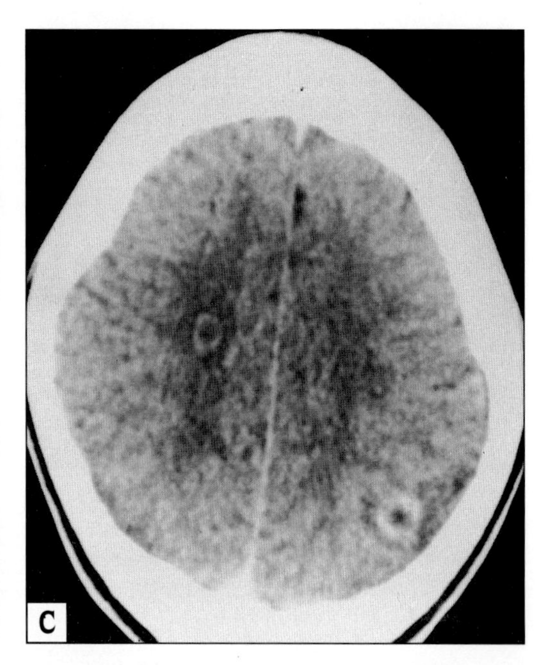

Figure 4-19 Hematogenous spread leading to brain abscess. **A**, **B**, and **C**, Multiple cerebral abscesses are presumably due to hematogenous spread of *Staphylococcus aureus* in a patient with septicemia. Lesions are seen in periventricular locations (*panel A*), centrum semiovale (*panel B*), and the junction between gray and white matter (*panel C*). Brain abscess secondary to endocarditis is surprisingly rare but is more likely in cases of *S. aureus* endocarditis. (*From* Wispelwey B, Dacey R Jr, Scheld WM: Brain abscess. *In* Scheld WM, Durack D, Whitley R (eds.): *Infections of the Central Nervous System.* New York: Raven Press; 1991; with permission.)

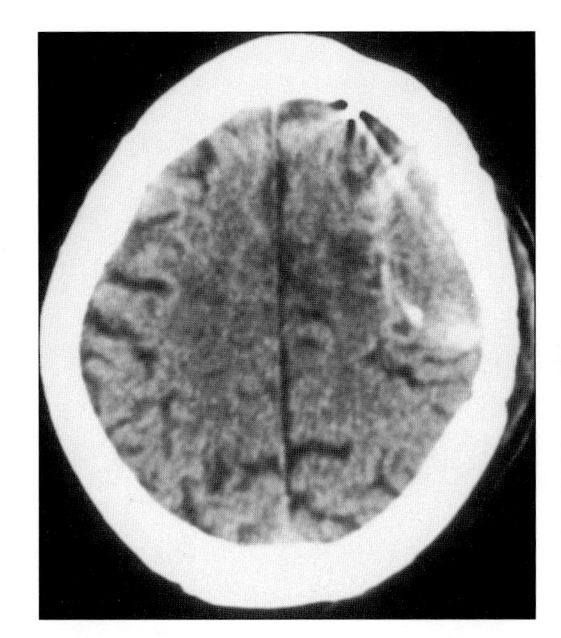

FIGURE 4-20 Abscess secondary to penetrating trauma. Ring-enhancing lesion around an area of increased attenuation is seen in a patient with brain abscess subsequent to penetrating intracranial injury. The risk of a brain abscess has been observed to be as high as 3% to 17% in this setting. Increased risk is associated gunshot wounds, multilobe injuries, wound complications, and retained bone fragments. (*From* Wispelwey B, Dacey R Jr, Scheld WM: Brain abscess. *In* Scheld WM, Durack D, Whitley R (eds.): *Infections of the Central Nervous System*. New York: Raven Press; 1991; with permission.)

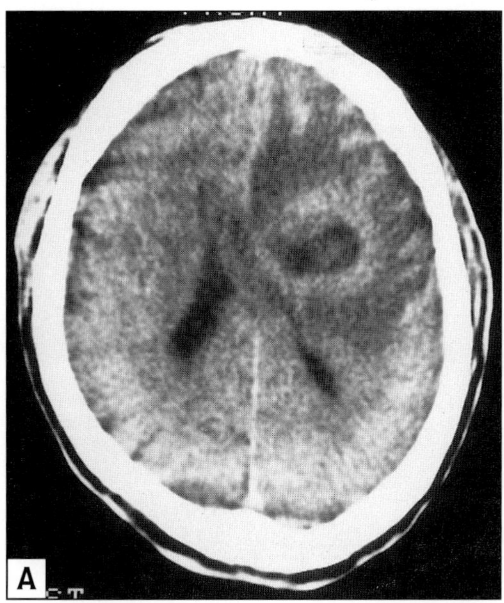

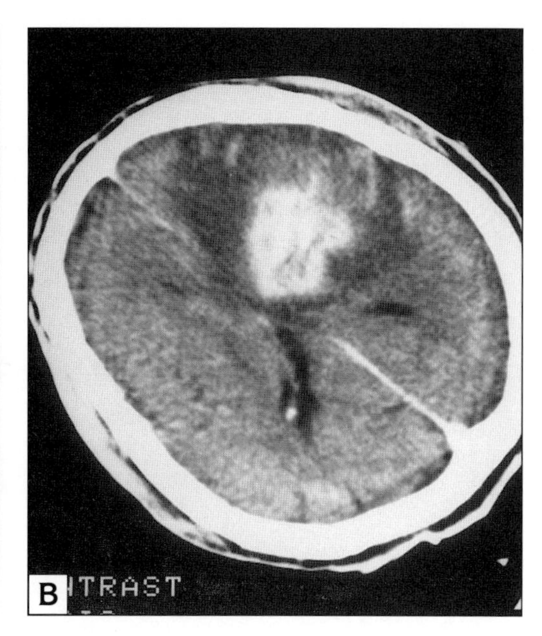

FIGURE 4-21 Unenhanced and enhanced CT scans in a patient with a brain abscess. **A**, Unenhanced scan done after angiography shows minimal contrast enhancement around a central area of decreased attenuation, producing mass effect on the ipsilateral lateral ventricle with surrounding edema. It is impossible to differentiate between an abscess and a malignancy on this study. **B**, Thick, irregular contrast enhancement without a prominent ring-enhancing pattern might suggest a primary or metastatic malignancy in this patient who was found to have a brain abscess. (*From* Wispelwey B, Dacey R Jr, Scheld WM: Brain abscess. *In* Scheld WM, Durack D, Whitley R (eds.): *Infections of the Central Nervous System*. New York: Raven Press; 1991; with permission.)

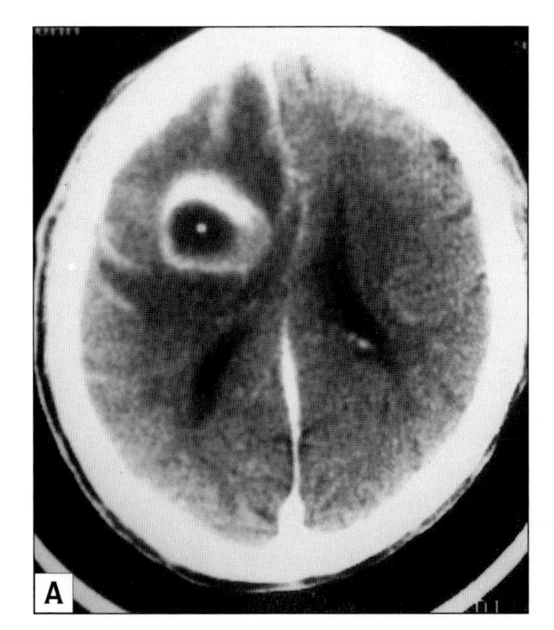

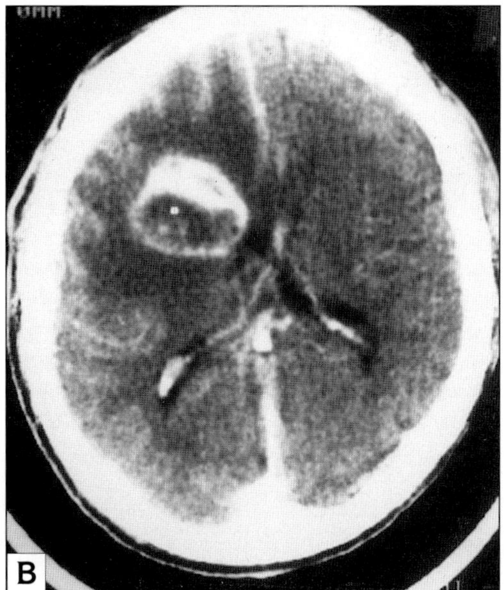

FIGURE 4-22 Irregular contrast enhancement around an abscess. These scans demonstrate that contrast enhancement may be irregular around an abscess and that the thinnest portion of the capsule is usually adjacent to the ventricle due to decreased capsule formation on the ventricular side relative to the cortical side of an abscess. **A**, Right posterior frontal abscess with irregular but homogenous ring contrast enhancement around an area of decreased attenuation. **B**, At a slightly lower axial level, irregular contrast enhancement is seen in a "target" pattern. (*From* Wispelwey B, Dacey R Jr, Scheld WM: Brain abscess. *In* Scheld WM, Durack D, Whitley R (eds.): *Infections of the Central Nervous System*. New York: Raven Press; 1991; with permission.)

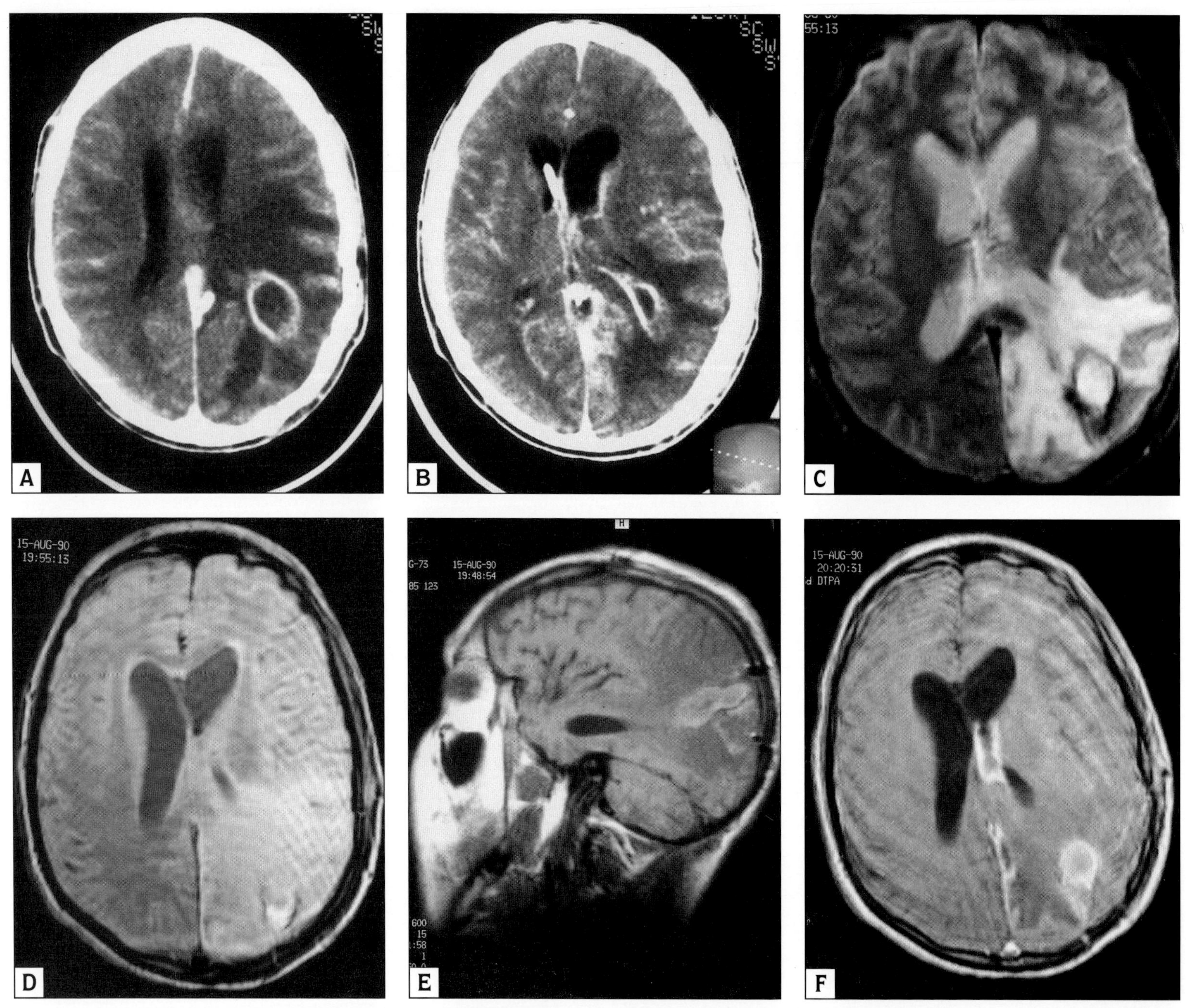

FIGURE 4-23 Left parietal abscess. **A**, Left parietal brain abscess with thin, right-enhancements surrounded by edematous white matter, causing midline shift and effacement of the lateral ventricle. **B**, Despite aspiration and antibiotic treatment, the abscess ruptured into the ventricle, producing contrast-enhancement of the ependymal surface. Ependymal enhancement, when present, is an indication of associated ventriculitis. It favors the diagnosis of a brain abscess and may suggest the devastating complication of ventricular rupture. (A ventriculostomy catheter has been placed in the anterior horn of the right lateral ventricle). **C**, T2-weighted image shows symmetrical ventricular enlargement. The marked edema in the parieto-occipital region is noted surrounding the abscess. Regions of decreased signal intensity in the abscess wall are due to paramagnetic hemoglobin degradation products in the area immediately around the wall. **D**, Proton density images of the parieto-occipital abscess. **E**, Parasagittal images of the left parietal abscess show the lesion tracking toward the trigone of the lateral ventricle. **F**, Gadolinium-enhanced T1-weighted image shows enhancement around the abscess and the ependymal surface of the body of the lateral ventricle. Magnetic resonance images' (MRI) lack of ionizing radiation, greater tissue characterization, and lack of bone artifact (which improves sensitivity in posterior fossa lesions), as well as the lack of toxicity of gadolinium compared to CT contrast agents, make it the procedure of choice in the evaluation of a brain abscess. (*From* Wispelwey B, Dacey R Jr, Scheld WM: Brain abscess. *In* Scheld WM, Durack D, Whitley R (eds.): *Infections of the Central Nervous System*. New York: Raven Press; 1991; with permission.)

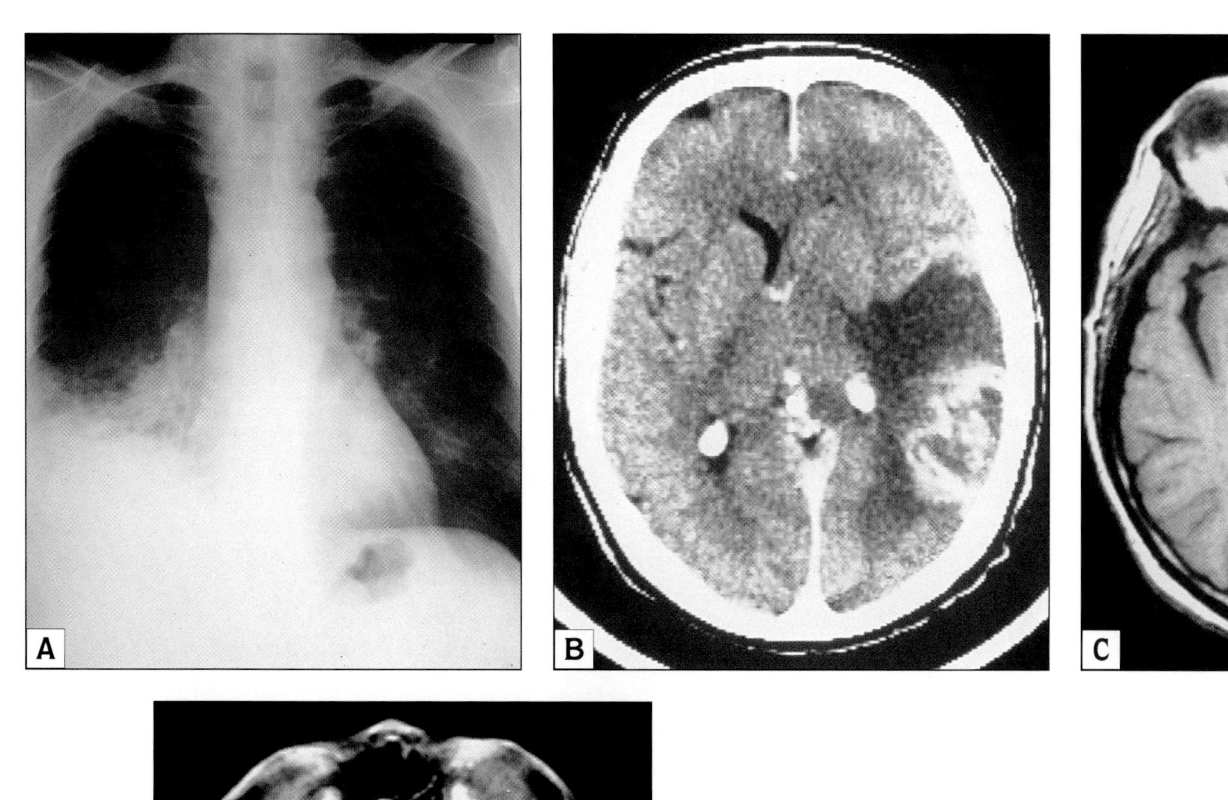

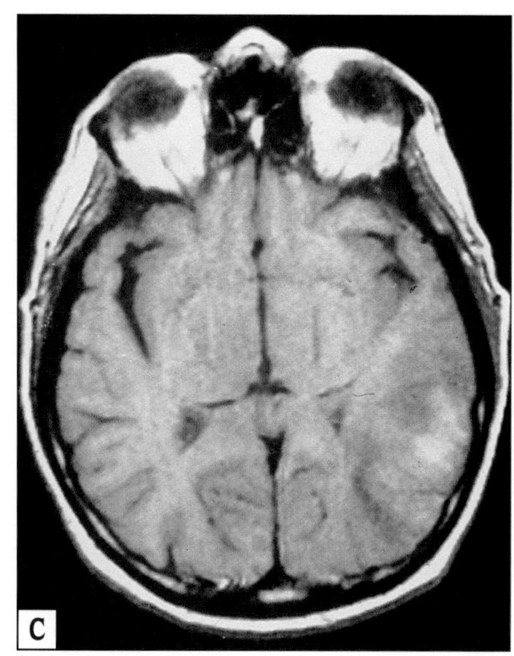

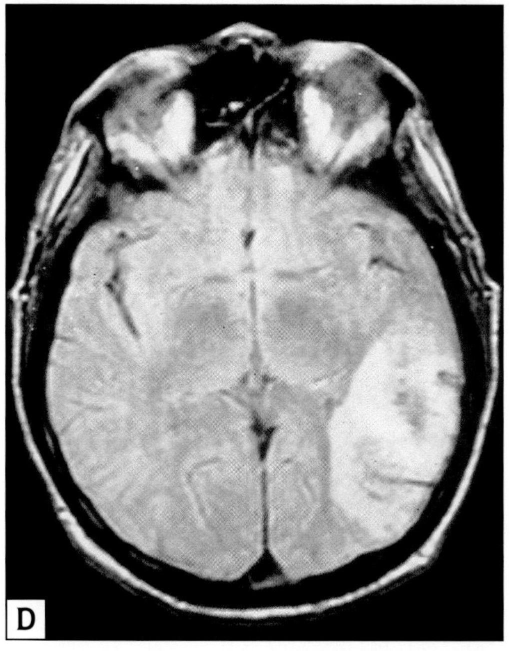

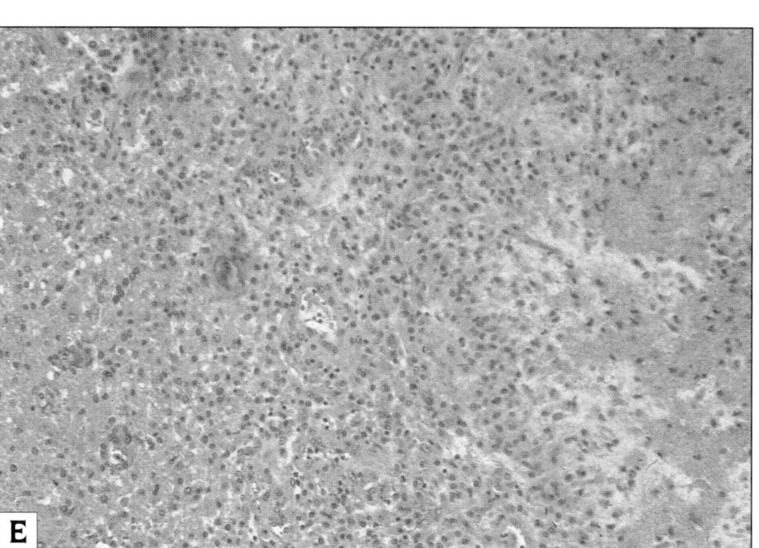

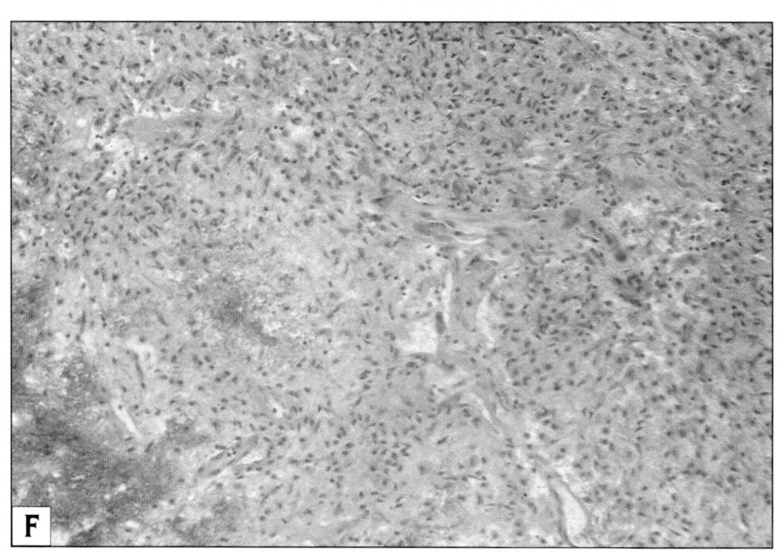

Figure 4-24 Septic pulmonary emboli leading to brain abscess. **A**, A 60-year-old man presented to the hospital with respiratory symptoms and fevers of 2 weeks' duration and with a chest radiograph consistent with the diagnosis of aspiration pneumonia. **B**, A head CT scan was obtained due to his associated mental status changes and revealed a mass consistent with an abscess or tumor. **C**, An MRI was obtained, and the T1-weighted image revealed a lesion with inhomogeneous enhancement. **D**, The T2-weighted image better defined the degree of surrounding edema. **E**, A biopsy revealed a central core of necrotic brain tissue with a significant inflammatory infiltrate. **F**, Trichrome staining revealed significant collagen deposition consistent with the diagnosis of a mature abscess. In this setting, the brain abscess was presumed to be secondary to septic thrombosis of a pulmonary vein with subsequent embolization.

Abscesses in Compromised Hosts

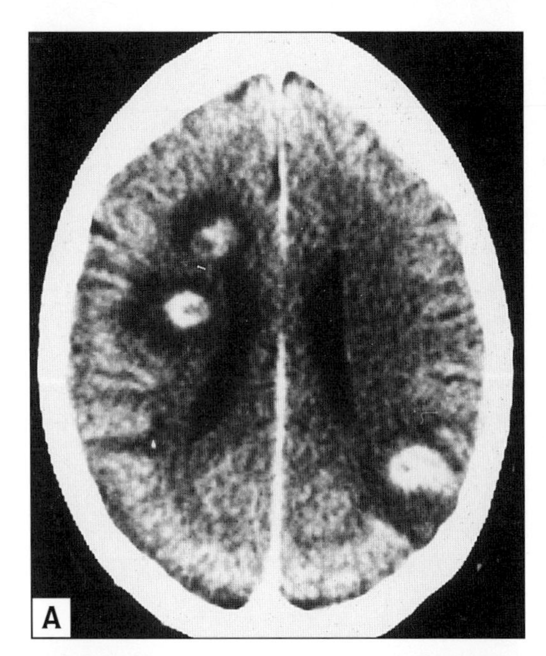
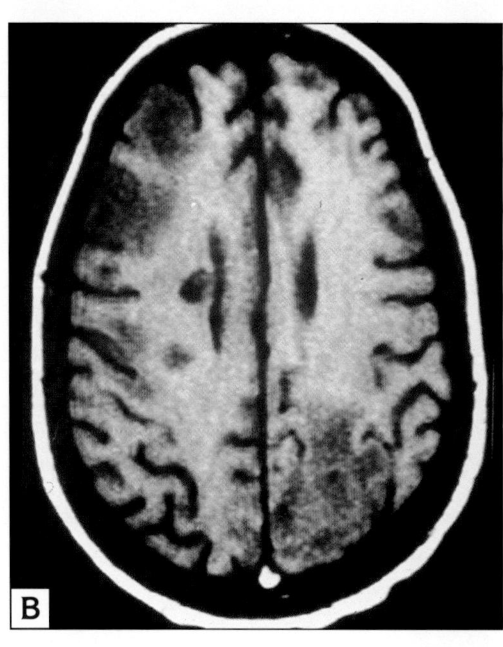
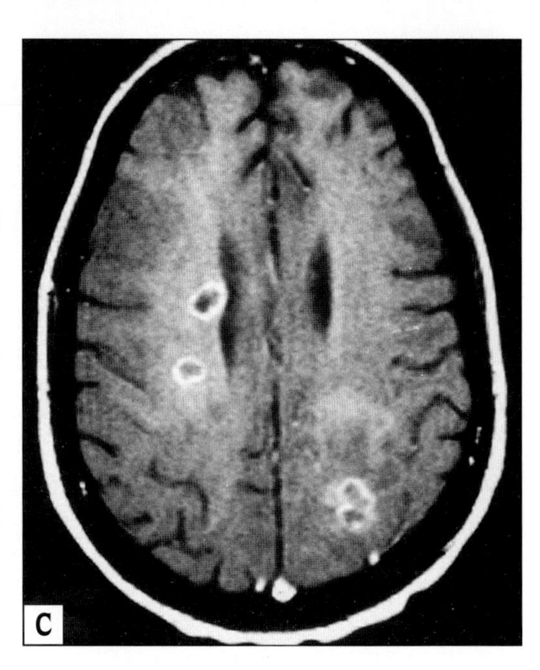
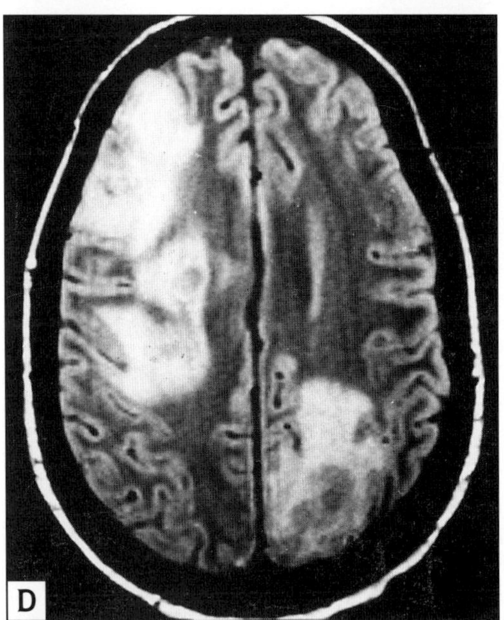

Figure 4-25 Cerebral toxoplasmosis in AIDS. **A**, An axial CT scan shows multiple areas of contrast enhancement in a patient with AIDS and cerebral toxoplasmosis. **B**, T1-weighted images show periventricular and gray-white junction lesions consistent with hematogenous dissemination. **C**, After gadolinium administration, contrast enhancement is seen on the T1-weighted image corresponding to that in *panel B*. **D**, Axial T2-weighted images show edema surrounding multiple cortical and subcortical lesions, further illustrating the increased information attainable by MRI relative to CT. (*From* Wispelwey B, Dacey R Jr, Scheld WM: Brain abscess. *In* Scheld WM, Durack D, Whitley R (eds.): *Infections of the Central Nervous System*. New York: Raven Press; 1991; with permission.)

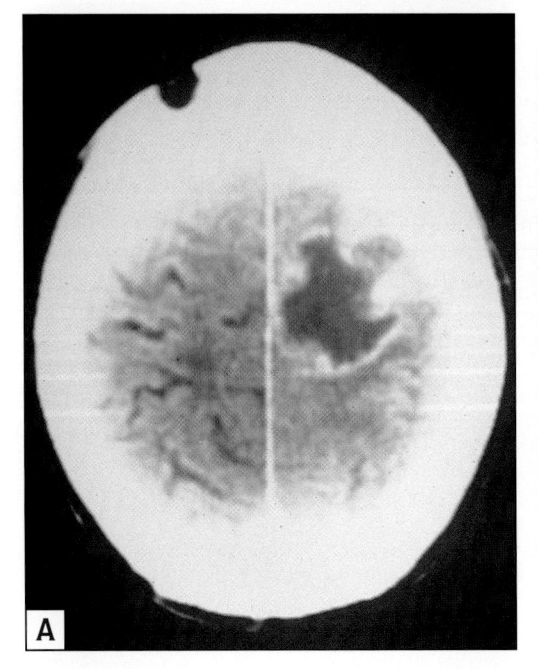
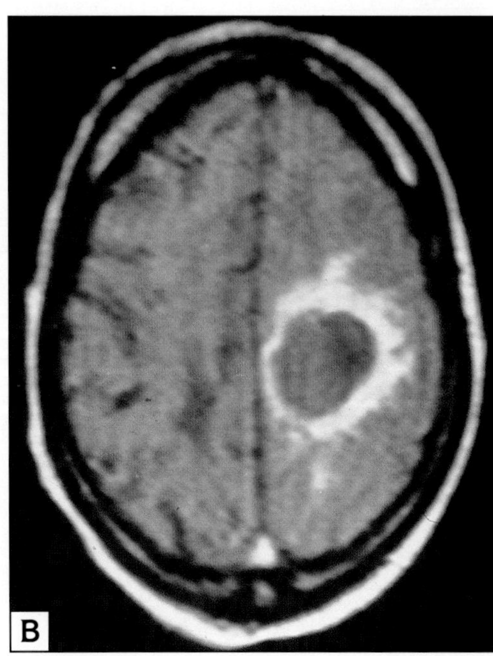

Figure 4-26 *Listeria* abscess. **A**, A 50-year-old man with multiple sclerosis and a cerebellar arteriovenous malformation who was on long-term high-dose corticosteroids presented with fever, headache, and mental status changes. The enhanced head CT scan revealed a large mass lesion. **B**, The gadolinium-enhanced MRI study was similar, except for evidence of an early associated satellite lesion. (*continued*)

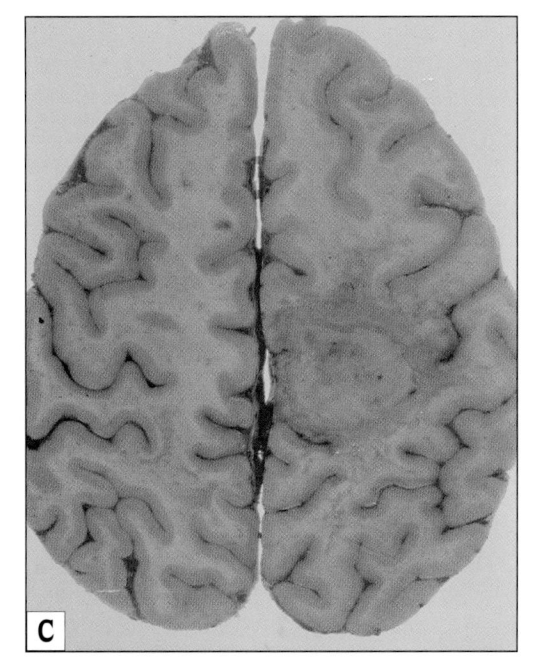

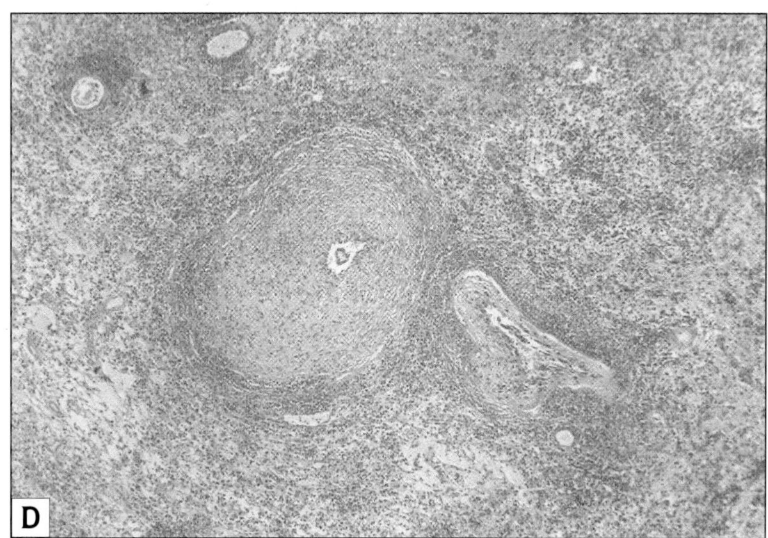

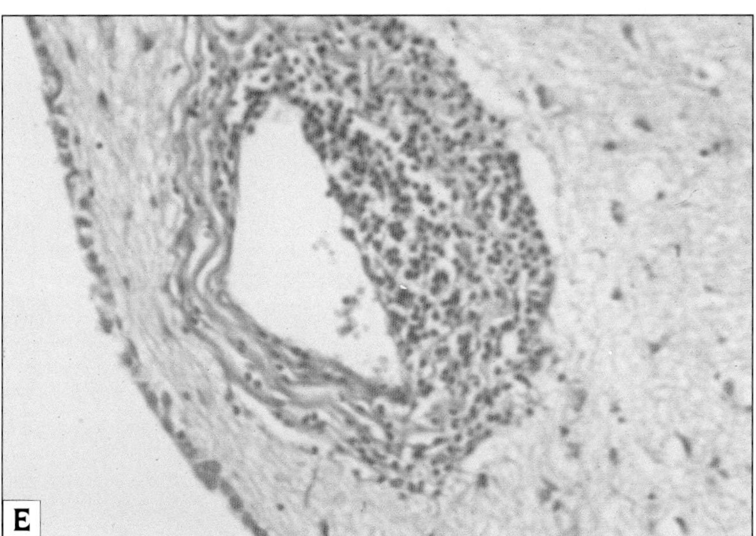

FIGURE 4-26 (*continued*) **C**, Both blood cultures and aspirate cultures grew *Listeria monocytogenes*. Despite aggressive therapy, the patient died. Gross pathologic examination revealed a large temporoparietal abscess. **D** and **E**, Histopathologic studies revealed acute and chronic inflammatory cells and vasculitis, with perivascular cuffing seen on higher magnification. *Listeria* spp. more commonly cause a meningitis or meningoencephalitis, but mass lesions will occur, particularly in patients with impaired cell-mediated immunity, including AIDS.

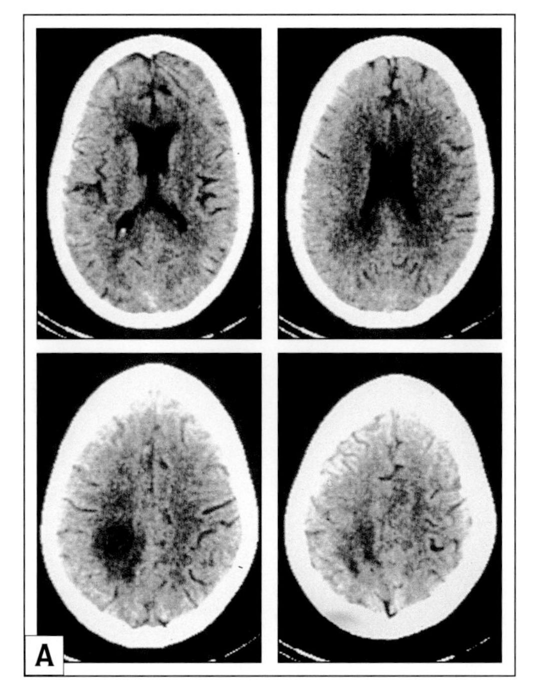

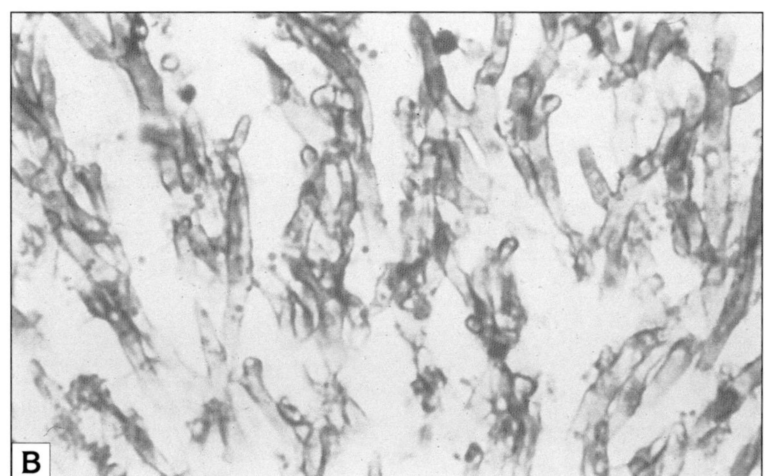

FIGURE 4-27 *Aspergillus* abscess. A 20-year-old woman with leukemia developed a headache with focal neurologic findings while neutropenic from her induction chemotherapy regimen. **A**, An unenhanced CT scan revealed several areas of hypoattenuation. **B**, The aspirate grew *Aspergillus fumigatus*. The patient died despite amphotericin therapy. (*continued*)

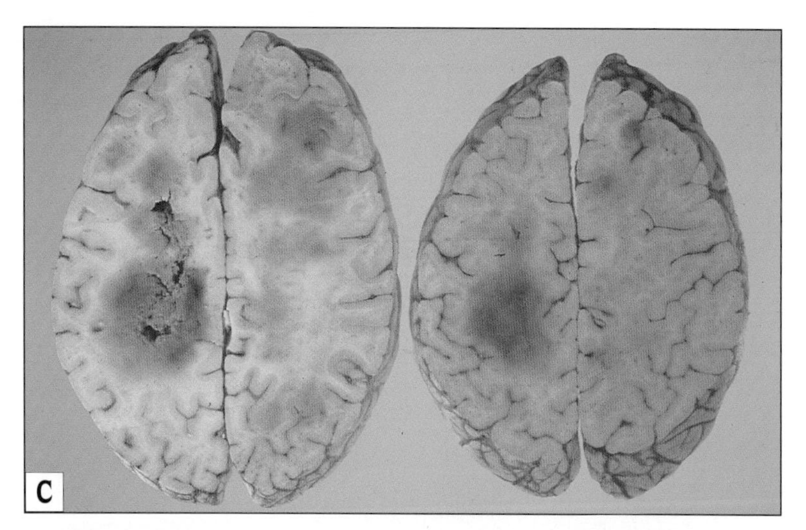

FIGURE 4-27 (*continued*) **C**, Gross pathologic examination revealed several areas of infarction and necrosis consistent with this organism's predilection to invade blood vessels. *Aspergillus* species most commonly invade the central nervous system in the setting of neutropenia, and survival has been rare. Total excision combined with maximal antifungal therapy has been advocated as the therapy of choice.

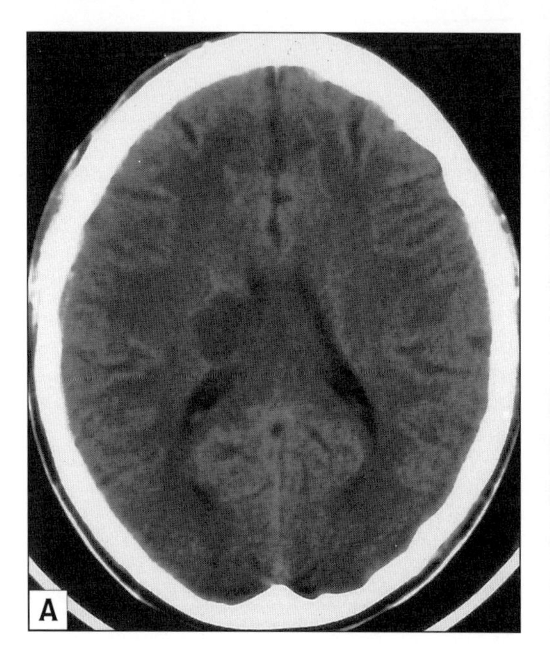

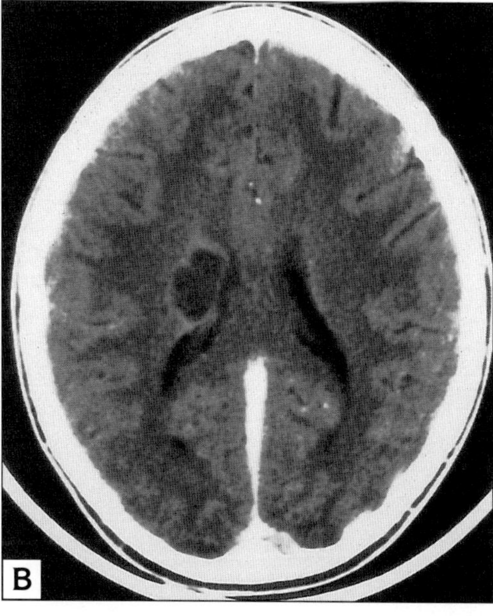

FIGURE 4-28 Cryptococcoma. A 15-year-old hemophiliac with AIDS and a fever of 2 weeks' duration developed a slowly progressive headache without focal findings. **A** and **B**, The unenhanced (*panel A*) and enhanced (*panel B*) CT scans revealed a large cystic-appearing periventricular mass with only minimal enhancement. Aspirate cultures revealed numerous budding yeast, and culture and antigen studies confirmed *Cryptococcus neoformans* as the etiologic agent. Cryptococcomas in the brain parenchyma are much less common than meningeal disease. Intraventricular cryptococcomas, as seen in this case, have been previously described and may originate in the choroid plexus. In AIDS patients, a ring-enhancing brain lesion, even in the setting of cryptococcal meningitis, could still represent a second etiologic agent such as toxoplasmosis.

MANAGEMENT

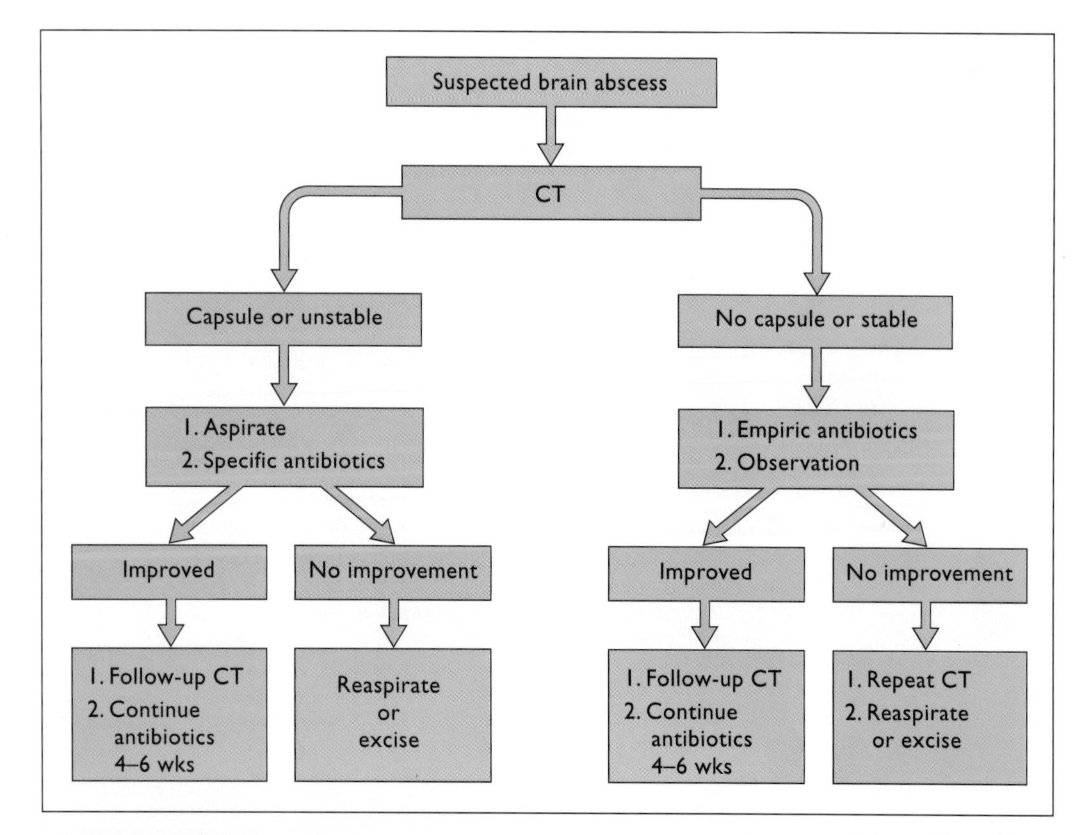

FIGURE 4-29 Management of a brain abscess. No general management guidelines can be formulated to ensure optimal results in the individual patient with a brain abscess. However, rational management is dependent on the initial imaging assessment, and operative therapy remains the definitive approach for most brain abscesses.

Empiric antimicrobial therapy for brain abscess

Predisposing condition	Usual bacterial isolates	Antimicrobial regimen
Otitis media or mastoiditis	Streptococci (anaerobic or aerobic) *Bacteroides* spp. Enterobacteriaceae	Penicillin + metronidazole + third-generation cephalosporin
Sinusitis (frontoethmoidal or sphenoidal)	Streptococci *Bacteroides* spp. Enterobacteriaceae *Staphylococcus aureus* *Haemophilus* spp.	Vancomycin + metronidazole + third-generation cephalosporin
Dental sepsis	Mixed *Fusobacterium* *Bacteroides* spp. *Streptococcus* spp.	Penicillin + metronidazole
Penetrating trauma or postneurosurgical	*Staphylococcus aureus* Streptococci Enterobacteriaceae *Clostridium*	Vancomycin + third-generation cephalosporin
Congenital heart disease	Streptococci *Haemophilus* spp.	Penicillin + third-generation cephalosporin
Lung abscess, empyema, bronchiectasis	*Fusobacterium* *Actinomyces* *Bacteroides* spp. *Nocardia asteroides* Streptococci	Penicillin + metronidazole (+ trimethoprim-sulfamethoxazole)
Bacterial endocarditis	*Staphylococcus aureus* Streptococci	Vancomycin + gentamicin

FIGURE 4-30 Empiric antimicrobial therapy for brain abscess. When a diagnosis of brain abscess is made either presumptively by radiologic studies or by aspiration of the abscess, empiric antimicrobial therapy should be initiated based on knowledge of the likely etiologic agent associated with a given predisposing condition.

Criteria for nonoperative management (antibiotics alone)

- Cerebritis, neurologically stable
- Medical conditions increasing the risk of surgery (*eg*, bleeding disorders, unstable cardiac status)
- Multiple abscesses, especially if distant
- Deep or dominant location of abscess
- Concomitant meningitis or ependymitis
- Early abscess reduction or improvement on empiric therapy
- Abscess size < 3 cm

FIGURE 4-31 Criteria for nonoperative management (antibiotics alone). Antibiotic therapy alone, when given early, can result in successful resolution of bacterial cerebritis. With the availability of CT-guided aspiration, however, the tendency is toward intervention whenever possible.

Factors associated with poor prognosis

- Delayed or missed diagnosis
- Multiple, deep, or multiloculated lesions
- Coma
- Inappropriate antibiotics
- Large or metastatic abscesses
- Poor localization
- Ventricular rupture
- Fungal etiology
- Extremes of age

FIGURE 4-32 Factors associated with a poor prognosis. Several factors have been identified in a series of brain abscesses as being associated with a poor prognosis. With current management and recognition, the mortality of brain abscess has decreased to 0% to 24% in several recent studies.

Influence of preoperative mental status on mortality

Mental status	Patients, *n*	Mortality, %
Grade I (fully alert)	33	0
Grade II (drowsy)	55	4
Grade III (response to pain only)	61	59
Grade IV (coma, no pain response)	51	82

FIGURE 4-33 Influence of preoperative mental status on mortality. (*From* Wispelwey B, Scheld WM: Brain abscess. *In* Mandell GL, Douglas RG Jr, Bennett JE (eds.): *Principles and Practice of Infectious Diseases*, 3rd ed. New York: Churchill Livingstone; 1990:786; with permission.)

SELECTED BIBLIOGRAPHY

Chun CH, Johnson JD, Hofstetter M, Raff MJ: Brain abscess. *Medicine* 1986, 65:415–431.

Enzmann DR: Magnetic resonance imaging update on brain abscess and central nervous system aspergillosis. *Curr Clin Top Infect Dis* 1993, 13:269–292.

Rosenblum ML, Manpalam TJ, Pons VG: Controversies in the management of brain abscesses. *Clin Neurosurg* 1986, 33:603.

Wispelwey B, Dacey R, Scheld WM: Brain abscess. *In* Scheld WM, Durack D, Whitley R (eds.): *Infections of the Central Nervous System*. New York: Raven Press; 1991:457–486.

Wispelwey B, Scheld WM: Brain abscess. *In* Mandell GL, Bennett JE, Dolin C (eds.): *Principles and Practice of Infectious Diseases*, 4th ed. New York: Churchill Livingstone; 1994.

CHAPTER 5

Parasitic Diseases of the Nervous System

Joseph R. Berger

A. Parasitic infections of the nervous system: protozoa

Disease/parasite	Geographic distribution	Risk factors	Neurologic disease
Malaria			
Plasmodium falciparum	Tropics and subtropics	Mosquitoes	Acute encephalopathy
Trypanosomiasis			
African			
Trypanosoma gambiense	Tropical West African forest	Tsetse flies	Chronic encephalitis
T. rhodesiense	East equatorial Africa		Subacute meningoencephalitis
South American			
T. cruzi	Mexico to South America	Reduviid bugs	Acute meningoencephalitis (rare) Chronic parasympathetic denervation of GI tract
Amebiasis			
Entamoeba histolytica	Worldwide	Poor water and sewage, institutionalized persons, homosexuals	Brain abscess (rare)
Naegleria	Worldwide	Freshwater sports	Acute meningoencephalitis
Acanthamoeba	Worldwide	Immunosuppression	Subacute or chronic meningoencephalitis
Toxoplasmosis			
Toxoplasma gondii	Worldwide	Perinatal infection, immunosuppression	Diffuse, focal, or multifocal encephalitis, chorioretinitis

B. Parasitic infections of the nervous system: nematodes (roundworms)

Disease/parasite	Geographic distribution	Risk factors	Neurologic disease
Trichinella spiralis	Worldwide	Eating rare pork or bear meat	Acute meningoencephalitis, myositis
Angiostrongylus cantonensis	Southeast Asia, Oceania	Eating freshwater snails, crabs, and raw vegetables	Acute eosinophilic meningitis
Gnathostoma	Japan, Thailand, Philippines, Taiwan	Eating raw fish or meat	Hemorrhages, infarcts (rare)
Strongyloides	Tropics	Penetration of skin or gut by filariform; dissemination with immunosuppression	Meningitis (rare), paralytic ileus due to autonomic involvement
Toxocara	Worldwide	Children with pica, contamination with dog or cat feces	Small granulomas (rare), ocular granuloma
Filaria loa loa	Tropical Africa	Bites by deer flies, horseflies	Acute cerebral edema, subacute encephalitis (rare)
Onchocerca volvulus	Equatorial Africa, Latin America	Black flies	Chorioretinal lesions

FIGURE 5-1 Parasitic infections of the nervous system: geographic distribution and risk factors. **A**, Protozoa. **B**, Nematodes (roundworms). (*continued*)

C. Parasitic infections of the nervous system: trematodes (flukes)

Disease/parasite	Geographic distribution	Risk factors	Neurologic disease
Schistosomiasis			
Schistosoma japonicum	Far East	Walking or swimming in infested waters (snails)	Cerebral granulomas
S. mansoni	South America, Caribbean, Africa		Myelitis (rare)
S. hematobium	Africa, Middle East		Myelitis (rare)
Paragonimus sp.	Asia, Central Africa, Central and South America	Eating infected freshwater crabs and crayfish	Cerebral granulomas

D. Parasitic infections of the nervous system: cestodes (tapeworms)

Disease/parasite	Geographic distribution	Risk factors	Neurologic disease
Cysticercosis			
Taenia solium	Central and South America, Asia, Africa, East Europe	Ingestion of eggs in human fecal contamination	Small cysts or basilar arachnoiditis with hydrocephalus; ocular lesions
Hydatid disease			
Echinococcus granulosus	Worldwide	Ingestion of eggs in canine fecal contamination (sheep raising)	Large cysts
Coenurosi			
Multiceps multiceps	Europe, Americas	Ingestion of eggs in carnivore fecal contamination	Budding cysts (rare)

FIGURE 5-1 *(continued)* **C**, Trematodes (flukes). **D**, Cestodes (tapeworms). (*Adapted from* Johnson RT, Warren KS: Parasitic infections. *In* Asbury AK, McKhann GM, McDonald WI (eds.): *Diseases of the Nervous System: Clinical Neurobiology*, 2nd ed. Philadelphia: W.B. Saunders; 1992:1351; with permission.)

Major protozoan and helminthic infections of the central nervous system

Protozoan
- Cerebral malaria
- Trypanosomiasis
- *Entamoeba histolytica* cerebral abscess
- Toxoplasmosis
- Free-living ameba meningoencephaltis

Nematodes
- Eosinophilic meningoencephalitis
  - *Angiostrongylus cantonensis*
  - *Gnathostoma spinigerum*
- Toxocariasis (visceral larva migrans)
- *Trichinella spiralis*

Human filariases
- *Loa loa*
- *Dracunculus medinensis*
- *Onchocerca volvulus*
- *Strongyloides stercoralis*

Trematodes
- Schistosomiasis
- Paragonimiasis

Cestodes
- Neurocysticercosis
- Hydatid disease

FIGURE 5-2 Major protozoan and helminthic infections of the central nervous system. Worldwide, *Plasmodium falciparum* malaria is the most important protozoan infection and neurocysticercosis is probably the most important helminthic infection to cause severe cerebral disease. (*Adapted from* Cook GC: Protozoan and helminthic infections. *In* Lambert HP (ed.): *Infections of the Central Nervous System*. Philadelphia: B.C. Decker; 1991:265; with permission.)

PROTOZOA

Cerebral Malaria

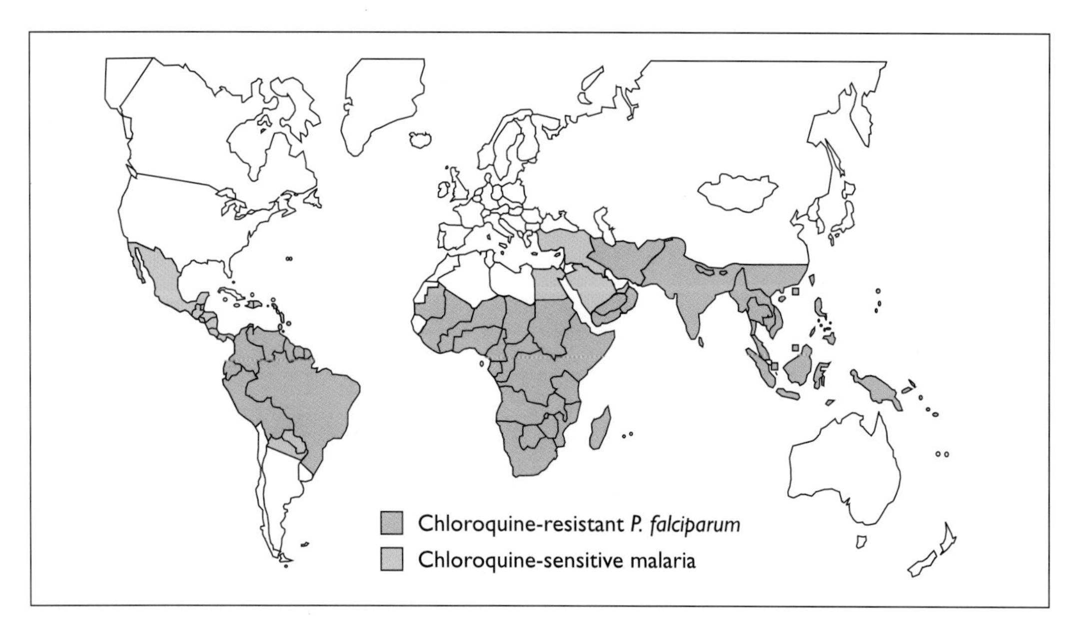

FIGURE 5-3 Geographic distribution of malaria, 1993. Malaria is the most important parasitic disease in humans, causing 1 to 2 million deaths per year. Although endemic malaria has been eradicated from North America, Europe, and Russia, a resurgence of disease has occurred in many parts of the tropics, with chloroquine-resistant strains posing increasing problems. Of the four species causing malaria, only *Plasmodium falciparum* causes cerebral malaria, and it accounts for almost all deaths. (*Adapted from* White NJ, Breman JG: Malaria and babesiosis. *In* Isselbacher KJ, *et al.* (eds.): *Harrison's Principles of Internal Medicine*, 13th ed. New York: McGraw-Hill; 1994:892; with permission.)

Clinical signs and symptoms of cerebral malaria	
Common	Possible systemic manifestations
Headache, meningismus, photophobia	Hyperpyrexia
Seizures	Anemia
Behavioral and cognitive changes	Hepatosplenomegaly
Delirium	Hypoglycemia
Coma	Disseminated intravascular coagulation
	Pulmonary edema
Less common	Shock
Monoparesis and hemiparesis	
Aphasia	
Hemianopia	
Ataxia, tremor, myoclonus	
Cranial nerve palsies	
Papilledema	
Blindness	
Deafness	

FIGURE 5-4 Clinical signs and symptoms of cerebral malaria. In falciparum malaria, high fever or severe headache, drowsiness, delirium, confusion, or parasitemia > 100,000 organisms/μL may predict impending cerebral malaria. It occurs most commonly in infants and young children, pregnant women, and nonimmune travelers to endemic areas. Coma is a characteristic and ominous finding, being associated with a mortality rate of 15% to 20%.

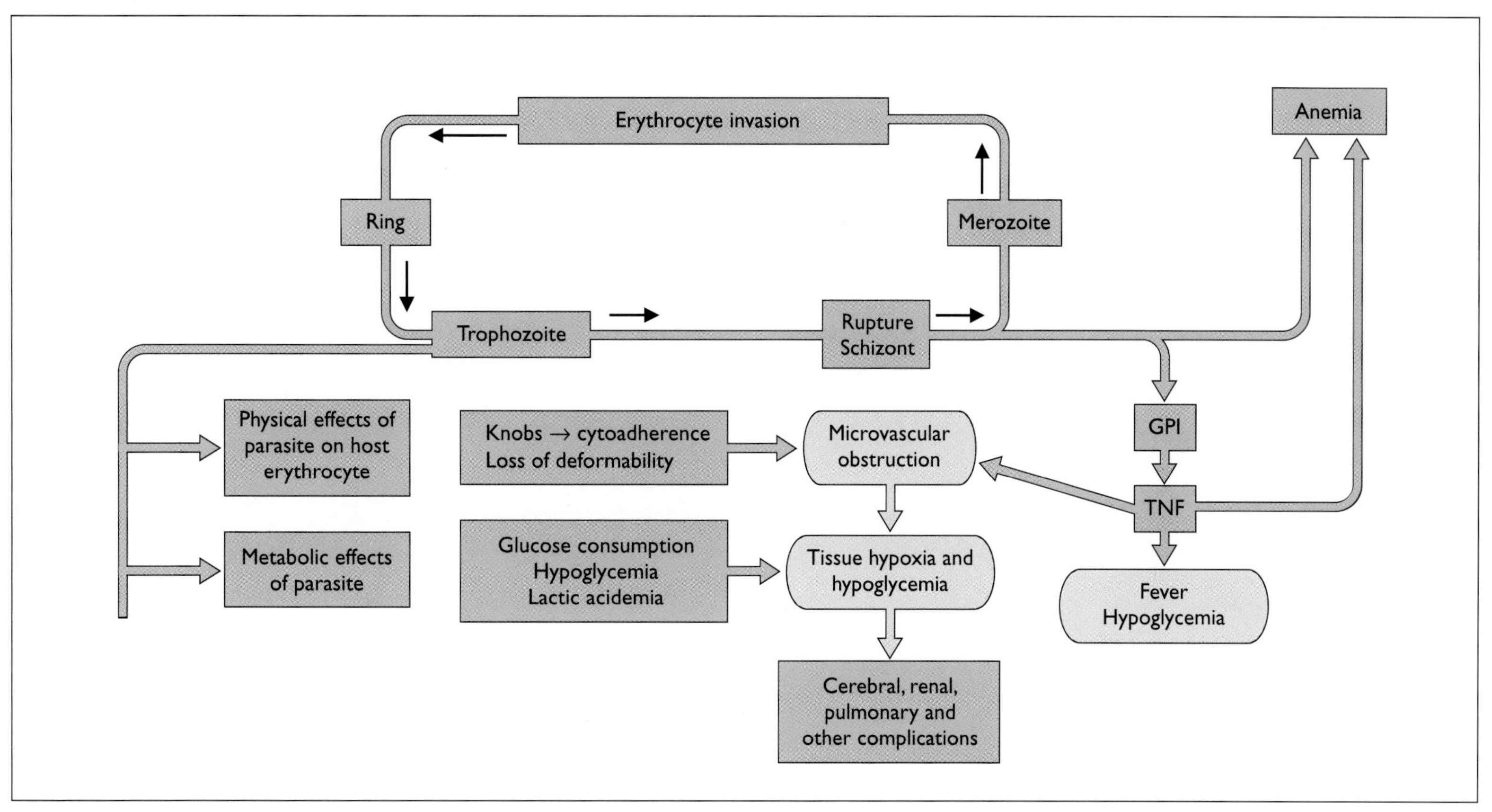

FIGURE 5-5 Pathogenesis of cerebral malaria. *Plasmodium falciparum* malaria is a microvascular disease with a strong metabolic component. Cytoadherence of *P. falciparum*–infected erythrocytes to endothelial cells in capillaries and postcapillary venules, plus the nondeformable nature of those cells, produces functional microvascular obstruction. Cytokines such as tumor necrosis factor (TNF)-α contribute to the process of enhancing expression of receptor molecules on the endothelial cell surface and thus further increase cytoadherence and obstruction to flow. It is a metabolic disease because consumption of glucose and production of lactate by the parasite plus the hypoglycemic effects of TNF-α (and possibly interleukin-1 and TNF-β) and treatment with quinine (or quinidine) all contribute to glucose deprivation, lactate excess, and acidemia at the tissue level. Anemia results acutely from erythrocyte lysis as schizont-stage parasites mature, and chronically from the effects of TNF-α. Rupture of schizont-stage parasites exposes glycosylphosphatidylinositol (GPI) anchors on the parasite and erythrocyte surface that elicit TNF-α and thus explains why the asexual erythrocytic cycle stimulates the release of TNF-α in the absence of the gram-negative endototoxin previously associated with the release of TNF-α from macrophages. (*Adapted from* Krogstad DJ: *Plasmodium* species (malaria). *In* Mandell GL, *et al.* (eds.): *Principles and Practice of Infectious Diseases*, 4th ed. New York: Churchill Livingstone; 1995:2419; with permission.)

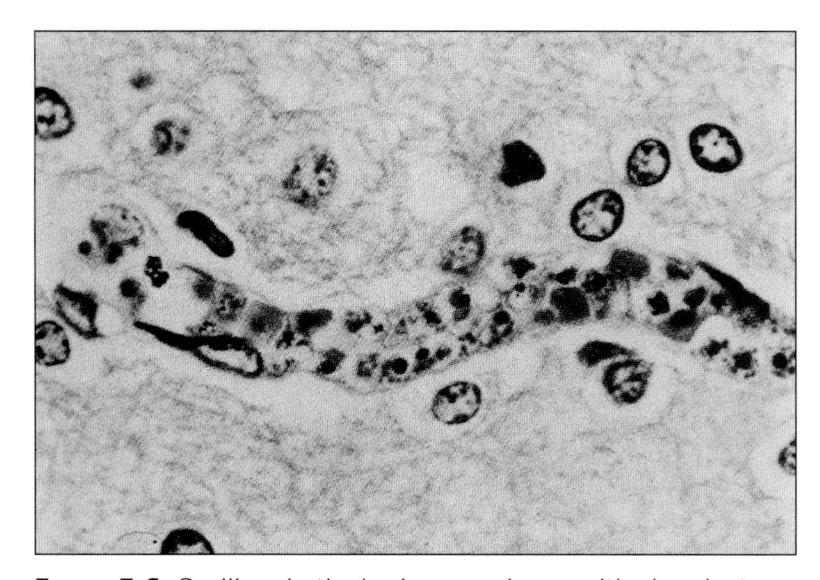

FIGURE 5-6 Capillary in the brain parenchyma with abundant parasitized erythrocytes. Parasitized erythrocytes are less deformable than normal parasites and are more adhesive to vascular endothelium. These alterations in the erythrocyte result in vascular occlusion chiefly affecting small cerebral vessels. (*From* Oo MM, Aikawa M, Than T, *et al.*: Human cerebral malaria: A pathological study. *J Neuropathol Exp Neurol* 1987, 46:223–231; with permission.)

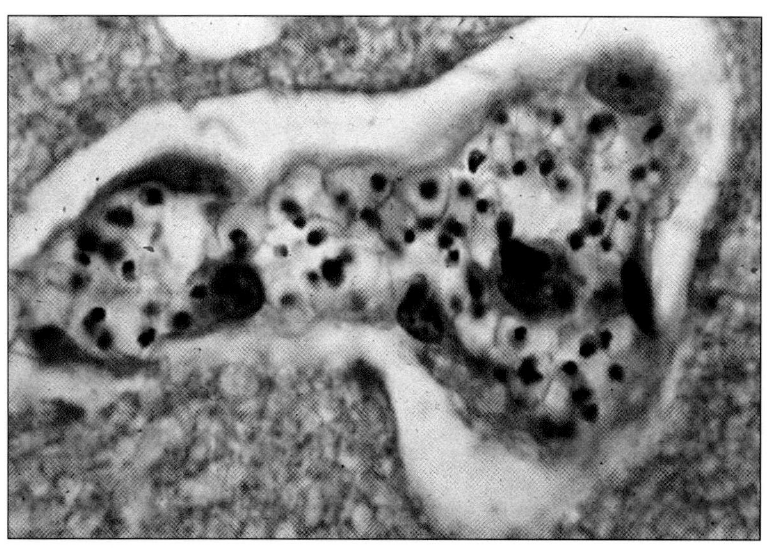

FIGURE 5-7 Darkly staining malarial parasites in erythrocytes distending a brain capillary. This distending process leads to ischemia and microhemorrhages in the surrounding tissue that is associated with altered mental status, focal neurologic findings, seizures, and death. (*From* Kepes JJ: *Pathology of Inflammatory Diseases*. New York: Medcom Inc.; 1971; with permission.)

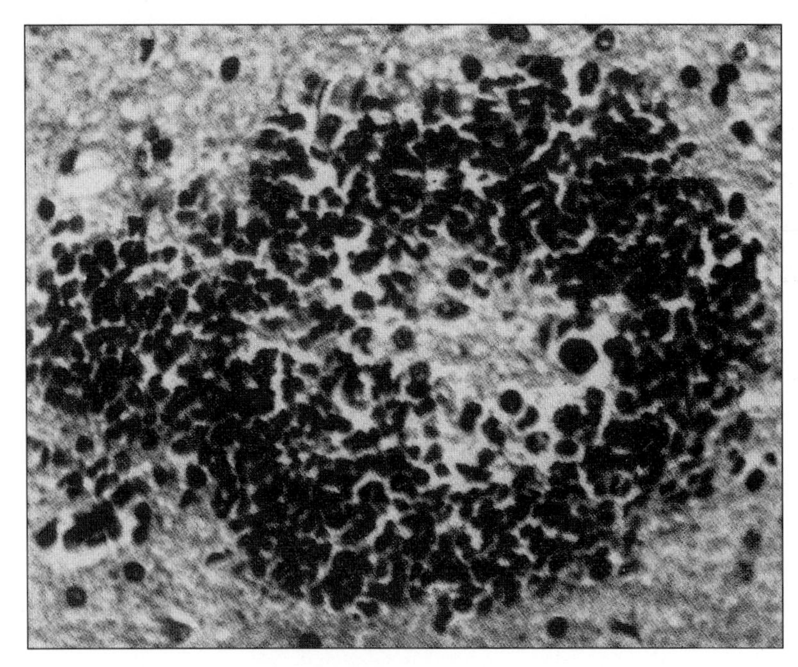

FIGURE 5-8 Ring hemorrhage in the brain with cerebral malaria. (*From* Thomas JD: Clinical and histopathological correlation of cerebral malaria. *Trop Geogr Med* 1971, 23:232–238; with permission.)

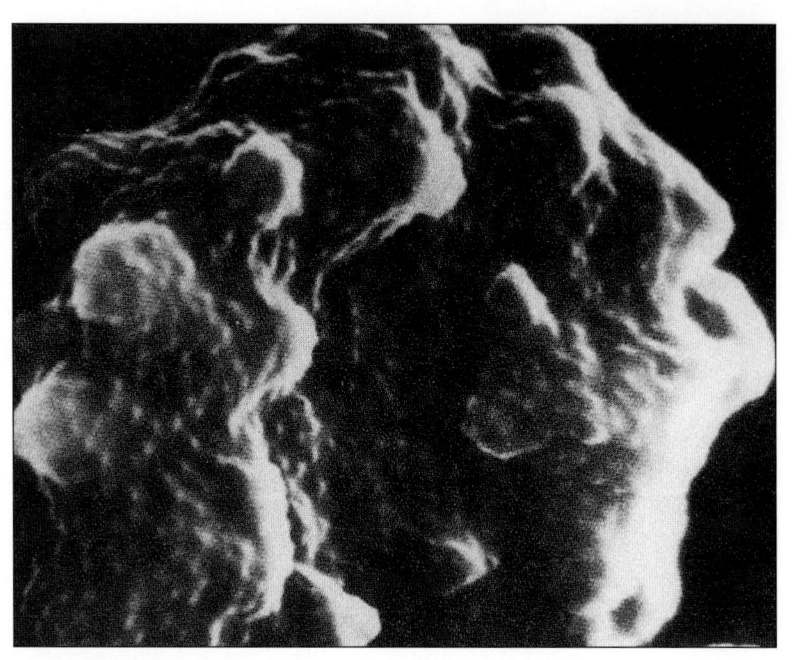

FIGURE 5-9 Scanning electron micrograph of an erythrocyte parasitized in malaria. Numerous knobs on its surface are important in mediating erythrocyte attachment to receptors on capillary endothelium, causing cytoadherence and occlusion (× 16,000.) (*From* Aikawa M: Fine structure of malaria parasites in the various stages of development. *In* Wernsdorfer WH, MCGregor I (eds.): *Malaria: Principles and Practice of Malariology.* Edinburgh: Churchill Livingstone; 1988:97–129; with permission.)

Treatment of cerebral malaria
Chloroquine-sensitive strains
Chloroquine base, 0.83 mg/kg body weight, by continuous iv infusion over 30 hrs
Chloroquine base, 3.5 mg/kg body weight iv or sc q6h, to a total dose of 25 mg/kg
Chloroquine syrup by NG tube: initial dose of 10 mg base/kg, followed by 5 mg/kg 6, 24, and 48 hrs later
Chloroquine-resistant strains
Quinine dihydrochloride, 10 mg base/kg body weight diluted in 10-mL of isotonic saline/kg, given by iv infusion over 4 hrs, every 8 hrs
May switch to oral quinine, 600 mg q8h, on return to consciousness

FIGURE 5-10 Treatment of cerebral malaria. Management can be summarized as including immediate administration of an effective schizonticidal agent, intensive care of the unconscious patient, and avoidance or early detection of complications. Treatment with an antimalarial agent must be started without delay because rapid clinical deterioration can occur. Selection of a drug and route should be based on the prevailing sensitivity of *Plasmodium falciparum* in the area and the patient's condition. NG—nasogastric tube. (*Adapted from* White NJ, Miller KD, Churchill FC, *et al.*: Chloroquine treatment of severe malaria in children: Pharmacokinetics, toxicity, and new dosage recommendations. *N Engl J Med* 1988, 319:1493–1500; with permission.)

Trypanosomiasis

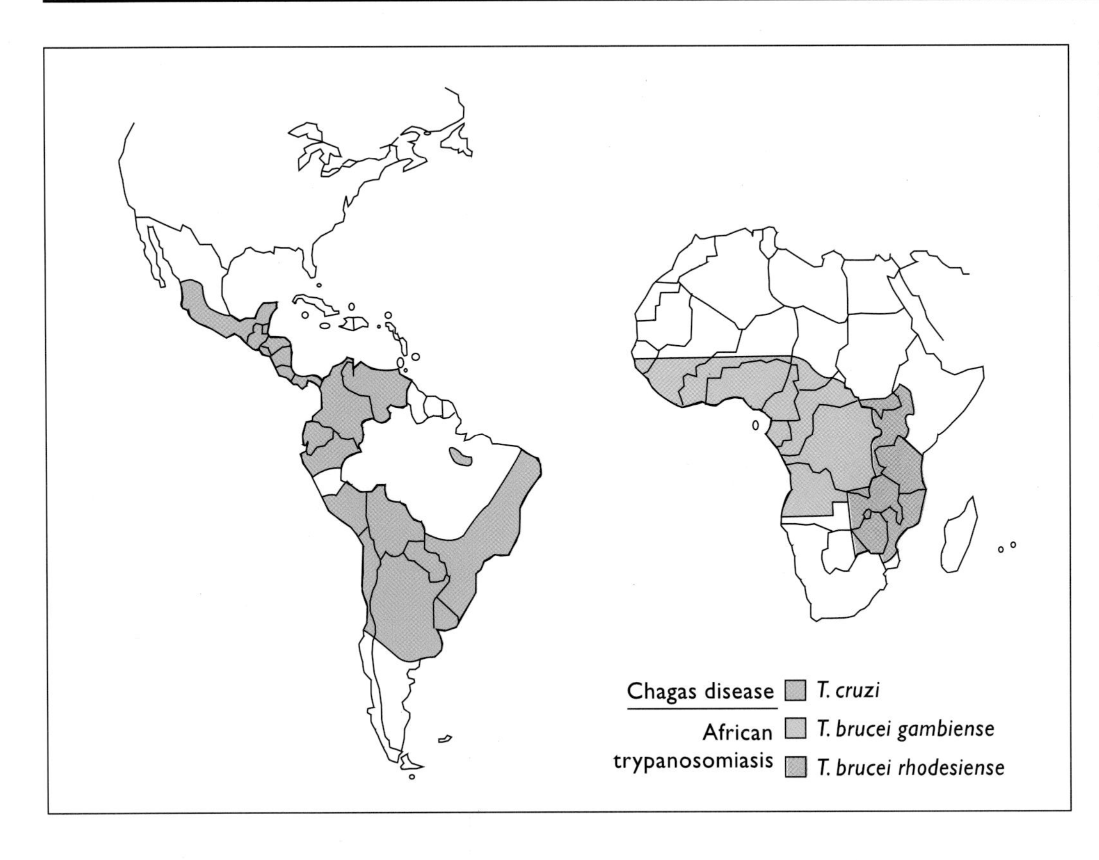

FIGURE 5-11 Geographic distribution of human trypanosomiasis. African trypanosomiasis, caused by *Trypanosoma brucei ssp. gambiense* or *rhodesiense*, and American trypanosomiasis (Chagas disease), caused by *T. cruzi*, have distinctly separate endemic areas. The two diseases differ significantly in transmission, pathogenesis, and clinical course and have little in common except morphologic similarities of the causative agents. (*Adapted from* Kirchhoff LV: *Trypanosoma* species (American trypanosomiasis, Chagas disease): Biology of trypanosomes. *In* Mandell GL, *et al.* (eds.): *Principles and Practice of Infectious Diseases*, 4th ed. New York: Churchill Livingstone; 1995:2443; with permission.)

Treatment of human trypanosomiasis

African trypanosomiasis
- Hemolymphatic (stage I)
  - Suramin, 100–200 mg test dose iv, *then* 1 g iv on days 1, 3, 7, 14, 21
  - *or*
  - Eflornithine, 100 mg/kg qid x 14 days, *then* 300 mg/kg/d po × 3–4 wks
- CNS involvement (stage II)
  - Eflornithine, 100 mg/kg qid × 14 days, *then* 300 mg/kg/d po × 3–4 wks
  - *or*
  - Melarsoprol, 2–3.6 mg/kg/d iv in 3 doses × 3 days, *then,* after 1 wk, 3.6 mg/kg/d iv in 3 doses × 3 days
  - Repeat latter course after 10–21 days

American trypanosomiasis
- Nifurtimox, 8–10 mg/kg/d po in 4 doses × 90–120 days

FIGURE 5-12 Treatment of human trypanosomiasis. For African trypanosomiasis, pentamidine isethionate may be an alternative for stage I disease. For stage II disease, eflornithine is the preferred treatment in West African trypanosomiasis, with pentamidine serving as an alternative; for stage II East African disease, melarsoprol should be used, with tryparsamide and suramin as alternatives. In Chagas disease, therapy is unsatisfactory. Nifurtimox markedly reduces the duration of symptoms and parasitemia and decreases mortality, but eradication of parasites is limited. Benznidazole and allopurinol may be alternatives. CNS—central nervous system. (Kirchhoff LV: Agents of African trypanosomiasis (sleeping sickness). *In* Mandell GL, *et al.* (eds.): *Principles and Practice of Infectious Diseases*, 4th ed. New York: Churchill Livingstone; 1995:2450–2454; with permission.)

African Trypanosomiasis (Sleeping Sickness)

Signs and symptoms of West African trypanosomiasis

Stage I (hemolymphatic)
- Spiking fever with afebrile periods
- Lymphadenopathy (Winterbottom's sign)
- Transient edema of face and hands
- Pruritus, circinate rash

Stage II (meningoencephalitis)
- Irritability
- Personality changes
- Loss of concentration
- Daytime somnolence
- Restlessness, insomnia at night
- Listless gaze
- Loss of spontaneity
- Indistinct speech
- Extrapyramidal signs
- Ataxia, parkinsonian symptoms

FIGURE 5-13 Signs and symptoms of West African trypanosomiasis. In West African trypanosomiasis (*Trypanosoma brucei gambiense*), additional signs and symptoms in stage I disease may include malaise, headache, vision abnormalities, weight loss, arthralgias, tachycardia, and hepatosplenomegaly. Stage II disease, marked by the onset of neurologic manifestations, progresses to coma and death months to years later. East African trypanosomiasis (*T. b. rhodesiense*) differs from the West African disease chiefly in its more acute course. (Kirchhoff LV: Agents of African trypanosomiasis (sleeping sickness). *In* Mandell GL, *et al.* (eds.): *Principles and Practice of Infectious Diseases*, 4th ed. New York: Churchill Livingstone; 1995:2450–2454; with permission.)

Comparison of West African and East African trypanosomiasis

	West African	East African
Organism	*T. b. gambiense*	*T. b. rhodesiense*
Vectors	Tsetse flies (*palpalis* group)	Tsetse flies (*morsitans* group)
Primary reservoir	Humans	Antelope and cattle
Human illness	Chronic (late CNS disease)	Acute (early CNS disease)
Duration of illness	Months to years	< 9 mos
Lymphadenopathy	Prominent	Minimal
Parasitemia	Low	High
Diagnosis by rodent inoculation	No	Yes
Epidemiology	Rural populations	Tourists in game parks Workers in wild areas Rural populations

FIGURE 5-14 Comparison of West African and East African trypanosomiasis. West African trypanosomiasis differs from East African trypanosomiasis chiefly in that the East African disease has a more acute course, leading to death within weeks to months. In East African trypanosomiasis, the lymphadenopathy also is not as striking, persistent tachycardia unrelated to fever is observed, and cardiac disease may result in death early, before the appearance of CNS manifestations. (*From* Kirchhoff LV: Agents of African trypanosomiasis (sleeping sickness). *In* Mandell GL, *et al.* (eds.): *Principles and Practice of Infectious Diseases*, 4th ed. New York: Churchill Livingstone; 1995:2452; with permission.)

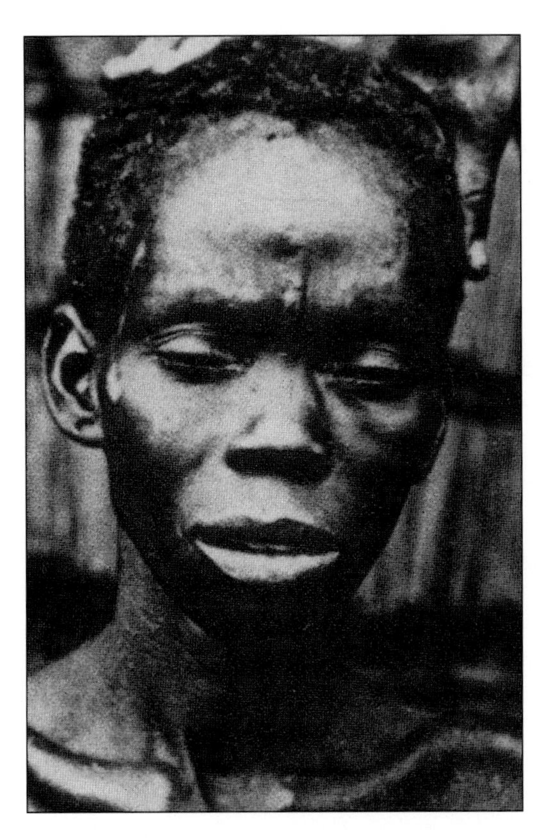

Figure 5-15 Characteristic facies of African trypanosomiasis. A stereotypic facial expression, characterized by somnolence and wasting, is seen with African trypanosomiasis in its advanced stages, which suggests the name sleeping sickness. (*From* Hutt MRS, Wilks NE: African trypanosomiasis (sleeping sickness). *In* Marcial-Rojas RA (ed.): *Pathology of Protozoal and Helminthic Diseases*. Huntington, NY: Robert E. Kreiger; 1975:57–68; with permission.)

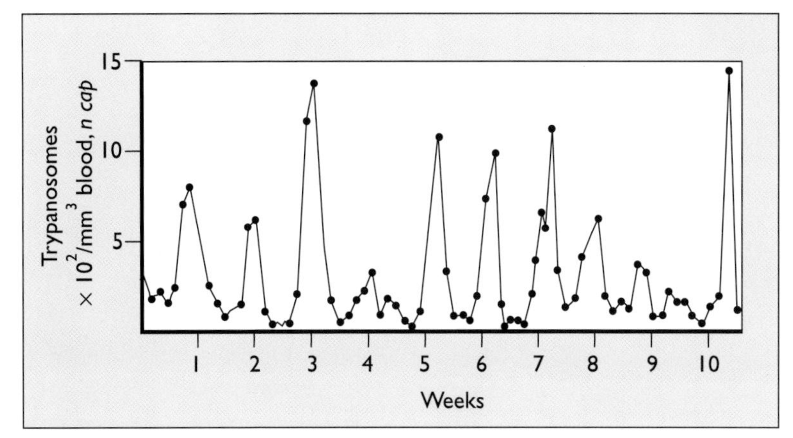

Figure 5-16 Cycles of parasitemia in African trypanosomiasis. Cycles of parasitemia, showing wide fluctuating in the number of parasites, correlate with the appearance of fever and constitutional features of the illness. The cycles are the result of the trypanosome's ability to change its surface glycoprotein. After the clearance of organisms with a particular surface antigen, the host needs to mount a second immune response when new surface glycoprotein is expressed. (*From* Vickerman K: Antigenic variation in African trypanosomes. *In* Porter P, Knight J (eds.): *Parasites in the Immunized Host: Mechanisms of Survival*. Ciba Foundation Symposium 25 (New Series). Amsterdam: Associated Scientific Publishers; 1974:53–80; with permission.)

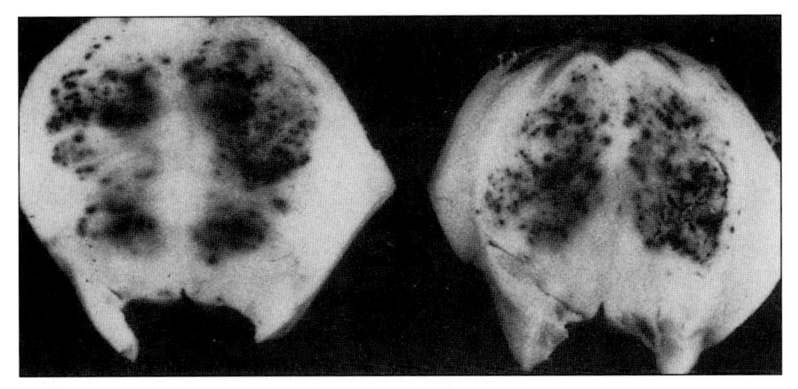

Figure 5-17 Sections of the pons in sleeping sickness showing acute hemorrhagic leukoencephalopathy with numerous discrete and confluent hemorrhages following treatment with an arsenical. (*From* Adams JH, Haller L, Boa FY, *et al.*: Human African trypanosomiasis (*T. b. gambiense*): A study of 16 fatal cases of sleeping sickness with some observations on acute reactive arsenical encephalopathy. *Neuropathol Appl Neurobiol* 1986; 12:81–94; with permission.)

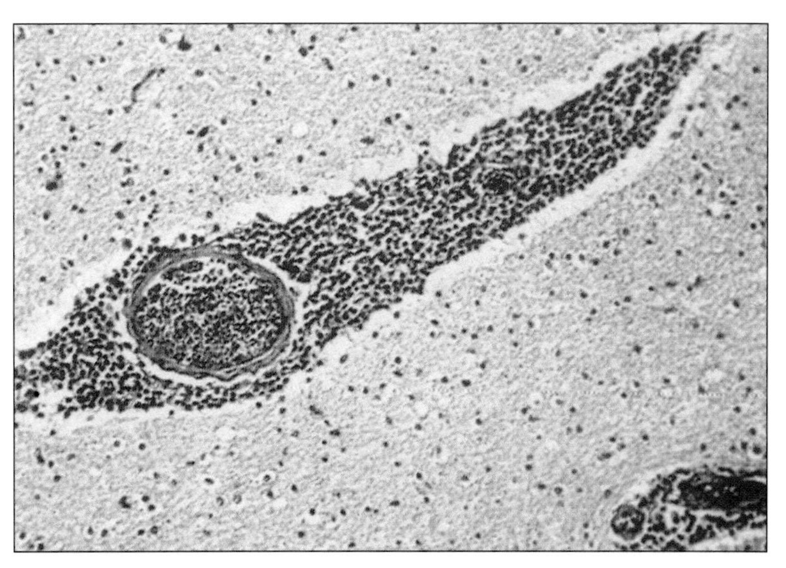

Figure 5-18 Perivascular infiltrates of *Trypanosoma brucei gambiense* in the temporal cortex associated with gliosis and inflammatory infiltrates. (*From* Vickerman K: Antigenic variation in African trypanosomes. *In* Porter P, Knight J (eds.): *Parasites in the Immunized Host: Mechanisms of Survival*. Ciba Foundation Symposium 25 (New Series). Amsterdam: Associated Scientific Publishers; 1974:53–80; with permission.)

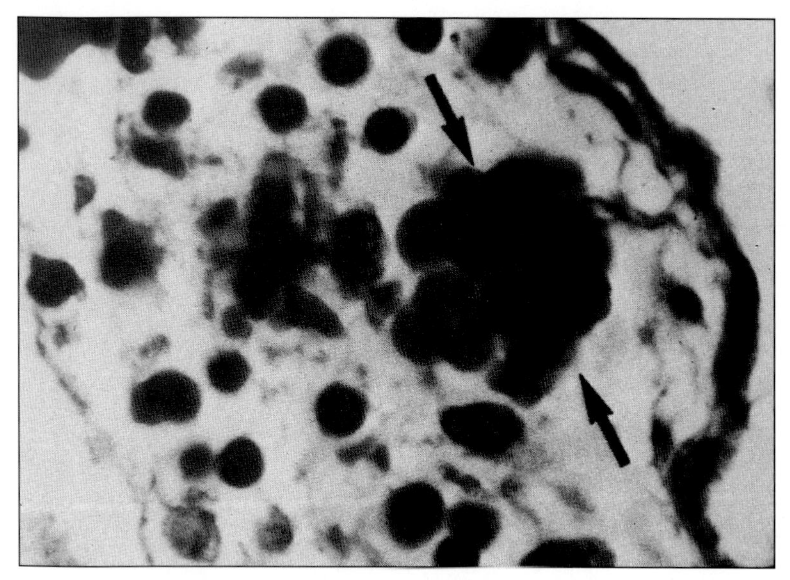

FIGURE 5-19 Morular cells in the meninges in African trypanosomiasis. Morular cells (between *arrows*), characteristic of sleeping sickness, are plasma cells with vacuoles containing immunoglobulin. Numerous lymphocytes and plasma cells are also observed. (*From* Vickerman K: Antigenic variation in African trypanosomes. *In* Porter P, Knight J (eds.): *Parasites in the Immunized Host: Mechanisms of Survival.* Ciba Foundation Symposium 25 (New Series). Amsterdam: Associated Scientific Publishers; 1974:53–80; with permission.

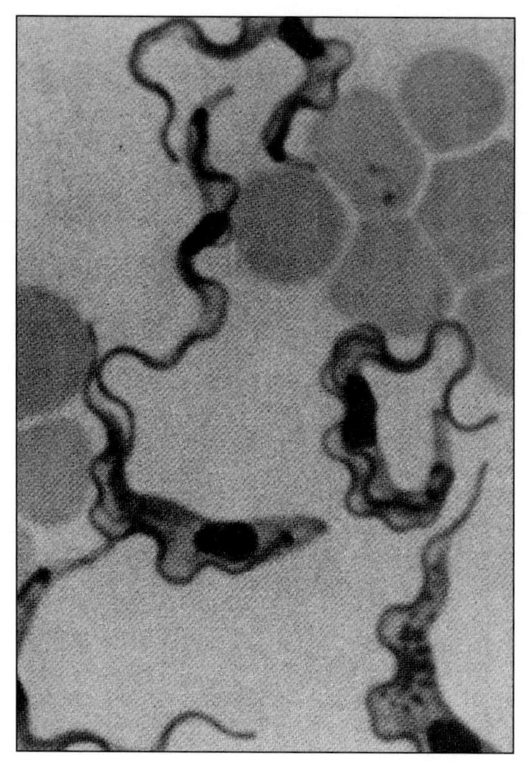

FIGURE 5-20 Trypomastigote form of *Trypanosoma brucei rhodesiense* is seen in a blood film. (*From* Hutt MRS, Wilks NE: African trypanosomiases (sleeping sickness). *In* Marcial-Rojas RA (ed.): *Pathology of Protozoal and Helminthic Diseases.* Huntington, NY: Robert E. Kreiger; 1975:57–68; with permission.)

American Trypanosomiasis (Chagas Disease)

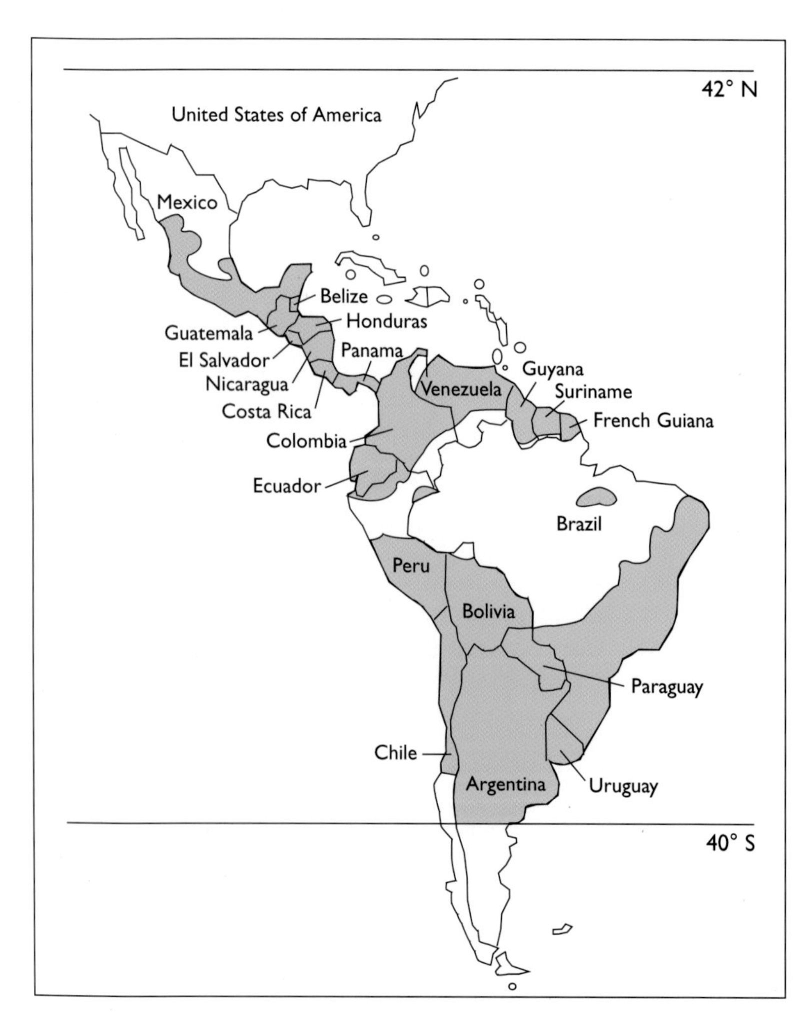

FIGURE 5-21 Geographic distribution of American trypanosomiasis. Chagas disease, caused by *Trypanosoma cruzi*, is endemic in Central and South America, where it is estimated to affect 16 million people. Most new infections occur in children living in rural areas. The disease is transmitted by the reduviid bug, which lives in the walls of the primitive houses in much of Latin America. (*Adapted from* Moncayo A: Chagas disease: Epidemiology and prospects for interruption of transmission in the Americas. *World Health Stat Q* 1992, 45:276; with permission.)

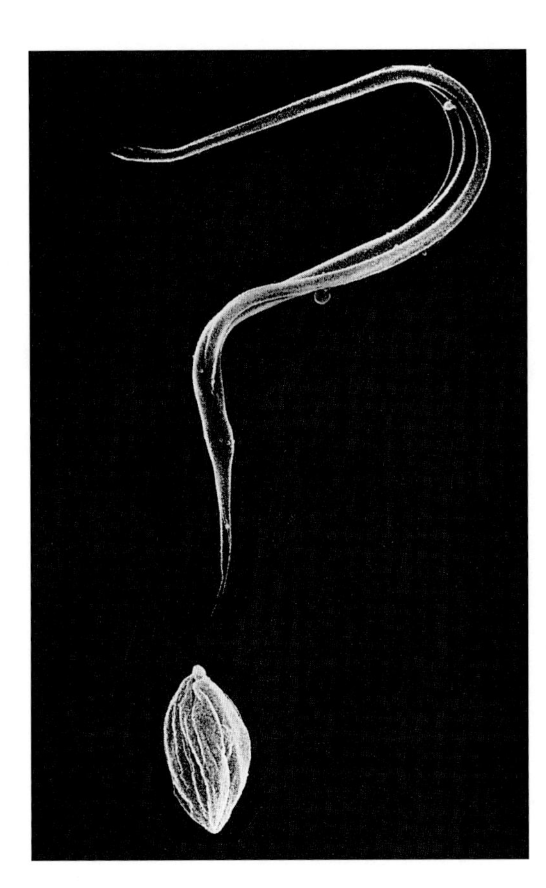

FIGURE 5-22 A composite scanning electron micrograph of two life-cycle stages of *Trypanosoma cruzi*, the agent of Chagas disease. The parasites were derived from infected cultured mammalian cells. The upper, elongated trypomastigote form is normally the bloodborne, infective stage, and the lower, rounded amastigote is the replicative, intracellular stage. (From research done in collaboration with Drs. Norma Andrews, Victoria Ley, and Victor Nussenzweig). (*Courtesy of* Dr. Edith S. Robbins.)

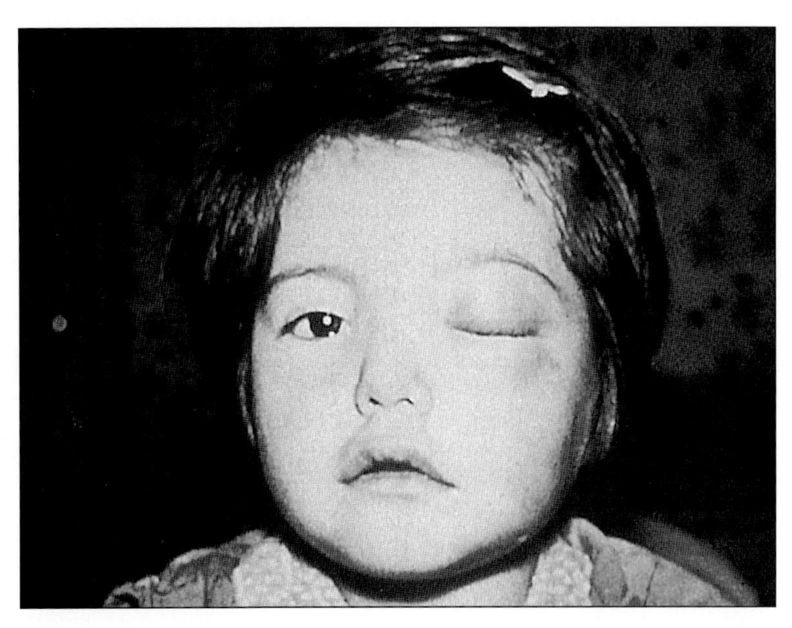

FIGURE 5-23 Romañna's sign in Chagas disease. Romañna's sign is a classic finding in acute Chagas disease and consists of unilateral painless edema of the palpebrae and periocular tissues that occurs when the conjunctiva is the portal of entry of the trypanosome. Malaise, fever, edema of face and lower extremities, generalized lymphadenopathy, and cardiac and gastrointestinal disorders subsequently appear. Meningoencephalitis is a rare complication. (*From* Moncayo A: Chagas disease. In *Tropical Disease Research: Progress 1991–1992 [11th Programme Report of the UNDP/World Bank/WHO Special Programme for Research and Training in Tropical Diseases]*. Geneva: World Health Organization; 1993:67; with permission.)

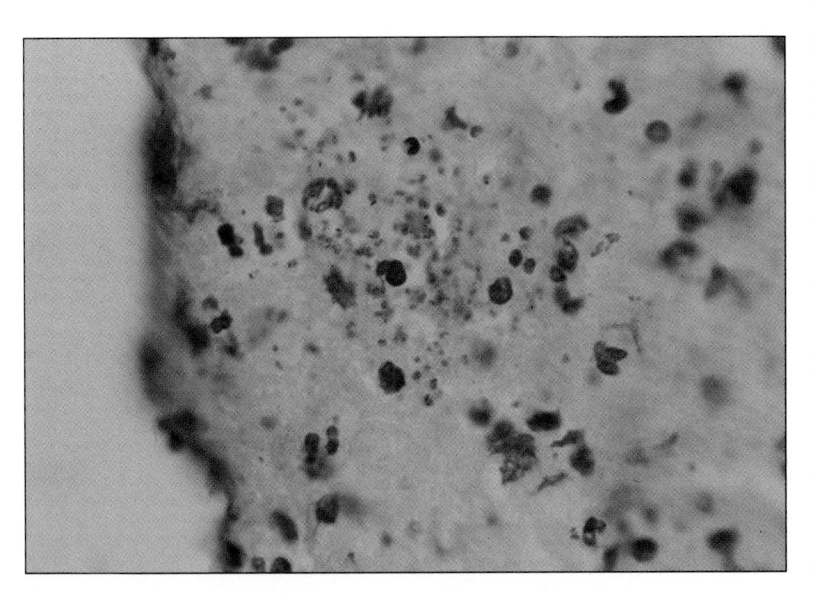

FIGURE 5-24 Active trypanosomiasis (Chagas disease) with numerous parasites within neurons, macrophages, and astrocytes. (*Courtesy of* Dr. Ramon Leigurda, Buenos Aires, Argentina.)

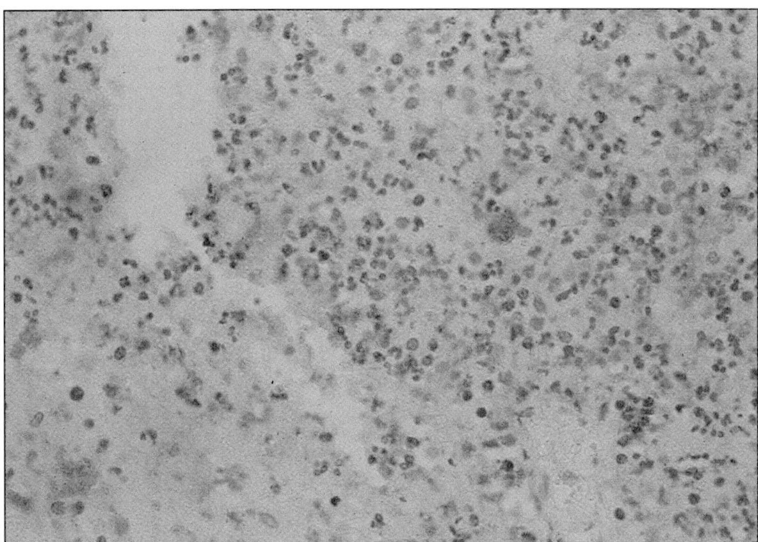

FIGURE 5-25 Positive immunostaining of brain tissues with antitrypanosomal polyclonal antibody and stretavidin-peroxidase. (*Courtesy of* Dr. Ramon Leigurda, Buenos Aires, Argentina.)

Infections with Free-Living Amebae

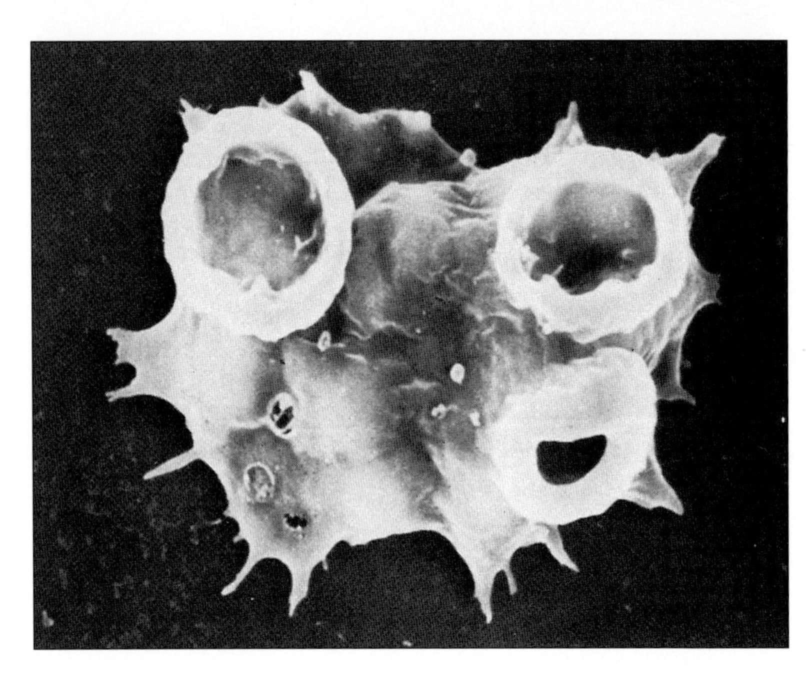

FIGURE 5-26 *Naegleria fowleri* ameba. Free-living ameboflagellates of the genus *Naegleria* are the most common cause of acute, rapidly fatal meningoencephalitis. *Acanthamoeba* more often causes a subacute or chronic meningoencephalitis typically observed in immunosuppressed patients. The frontal lobes and cerebellum are the regions chiefly affected. Invasion of the nasal mucosa typically occurs after swimming in freshwater that contains the ameba. Rare instances of survival have been documented; all survivors had received amphotericin B.

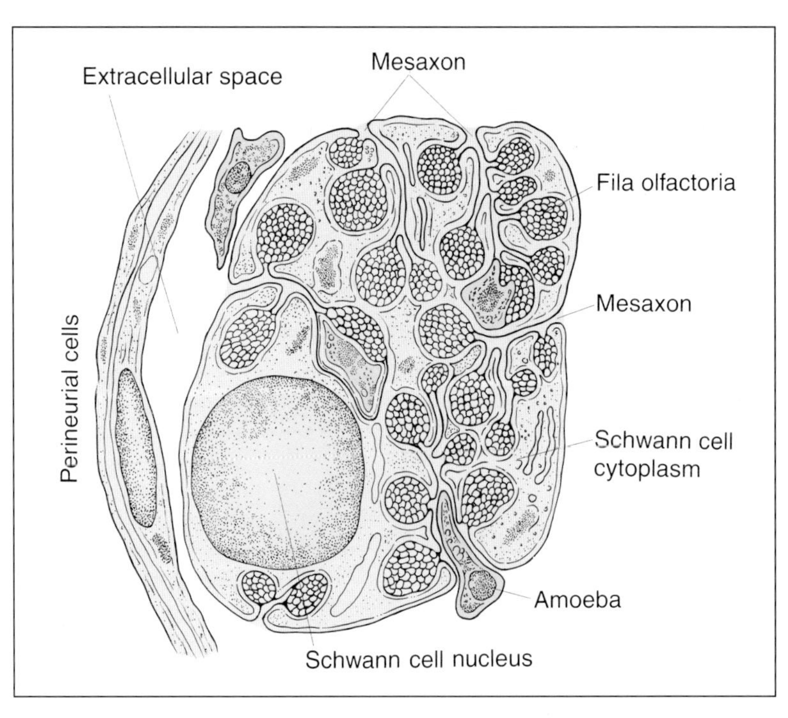

FIGURE 5-27 Diagram of the olfactory submucosal nerve plexus showing olfactory filia and invasion of several ameba into the mesaxon and extracellular spaces. (*From* Martinez AJ, Duma RJ, Nelson EC, Moretta FL: Experimental *Naegleria* meningoencephalitis in mice: Penetration of the olfactory mucosal epithelium by *Naegleria* and pathologic changes produced: A light and electron microscope study. *Lab Invest* 1973, 29:121–133; with permission.)

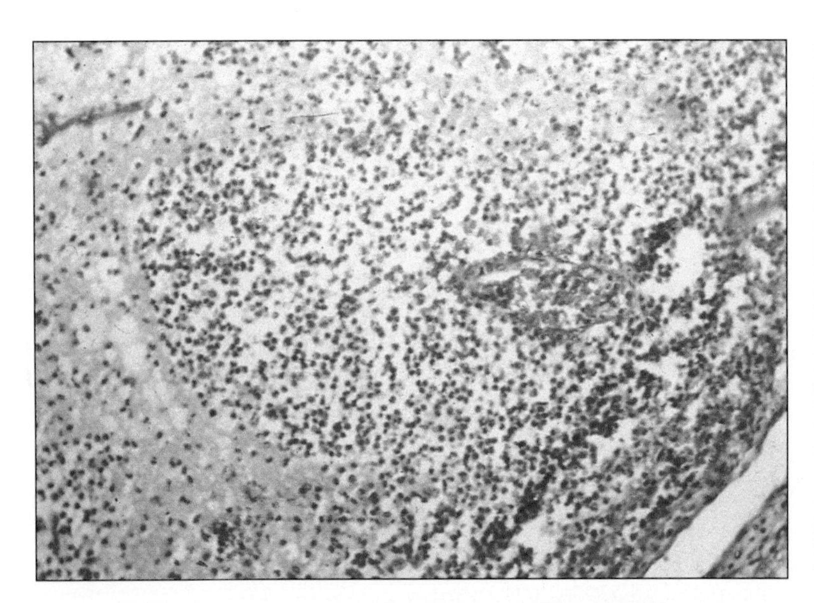

FIGURE 5-28 Severe amebic meningoencephalitis with massive purulent exudate covering the meninges and invading the underlying cortex. (*From* Kepes JJ: *Pathology of Inflammatory Diseases.* New York: Medcom Inc.; 1972; with permission.)

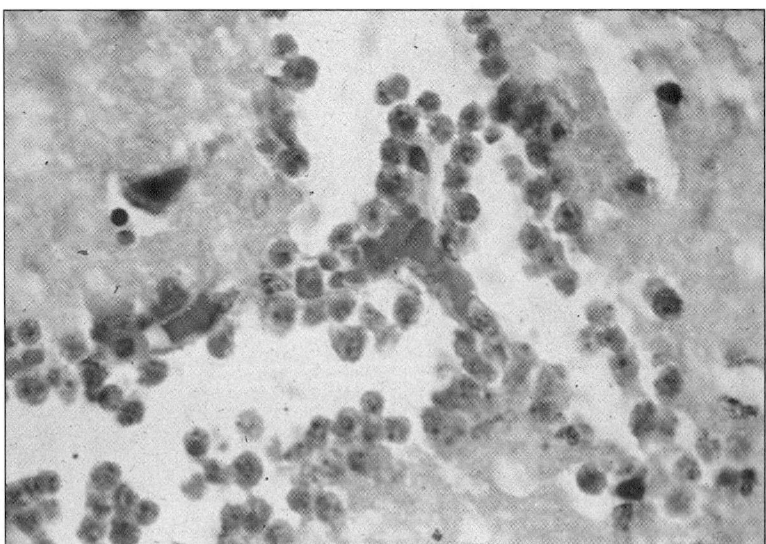

FIGURE 5-29 Masses of amebae surrounding the small blood vessels in a patient with amebic meningoencephalitis. The amebae can be distinguished from the host's macrophages by the purple (rather than blue) staining of their nuclei. (*From* Kepes JJ: *Pathology of Inflammatory Diseases.* New York: Medcom Inc.; 1972; with permission.)

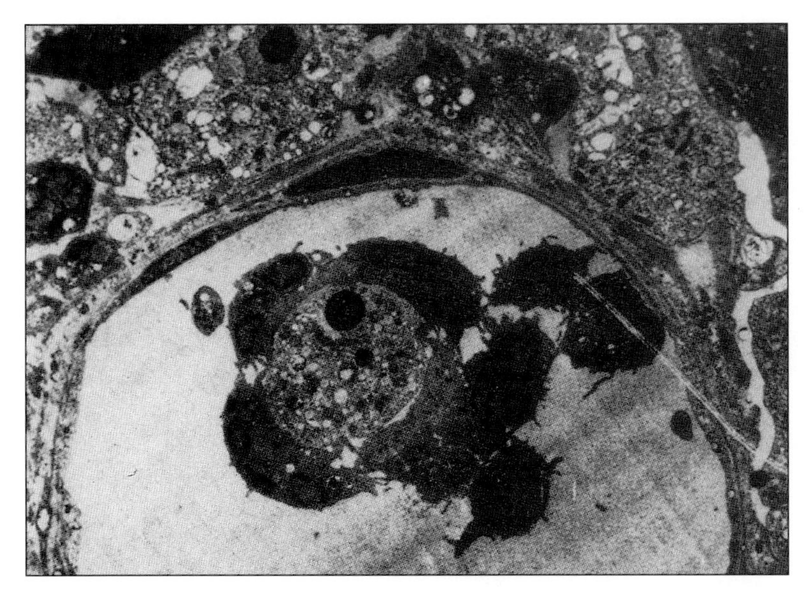

Figure 5-30 Electron micrograph showing a trophozoite of *Naegleria fowleri*, surrounded by neutrophils, in a blood vessel lumen in the olfactory mucosa of a mouse. The blood vessel is surrounded by amebae, some containing erythrocytes. (*From* Martinez AJ, Duma RJ, Nelson EC, Moretta FL: Experimental *Naegleria* meningoencephalitis in mice: Penetration of the olfactory mucosal epithelium by *Naegleria* and pathologic changes produced: A light and electron microscope study. *Lab Invest* 1993, 29:121–133; with permission.)

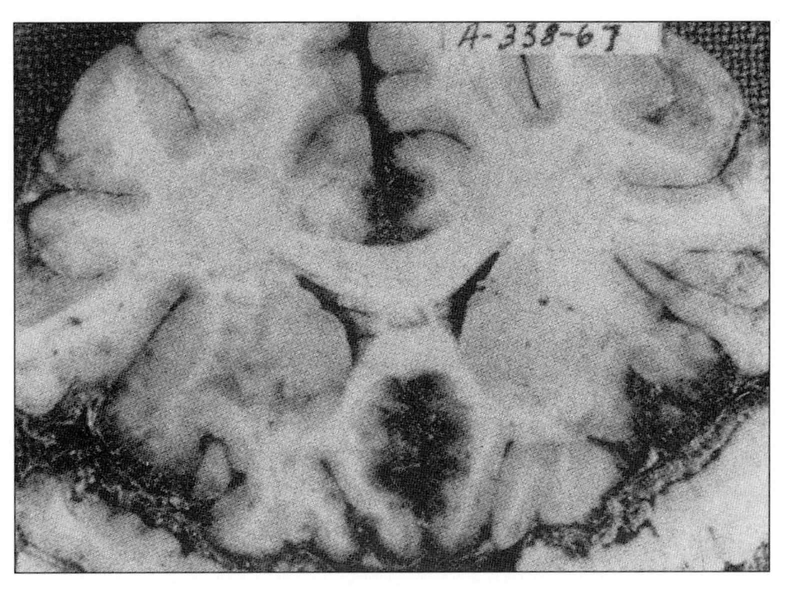

Figure 5-31 Gross photograph showing severe inflammation of the basal meninges and cortex with associated hemorrhage in acute primary amebic meningoencephalitis due to *Naegleria fowleri*. (*From* Martinez AJ: *Free-Living Amebas: Natural History, Prevention, Diagnosis, Pathology, and Treatment of Disease*. Boca Raton, FL: CRC Press; 1985; with permission.)

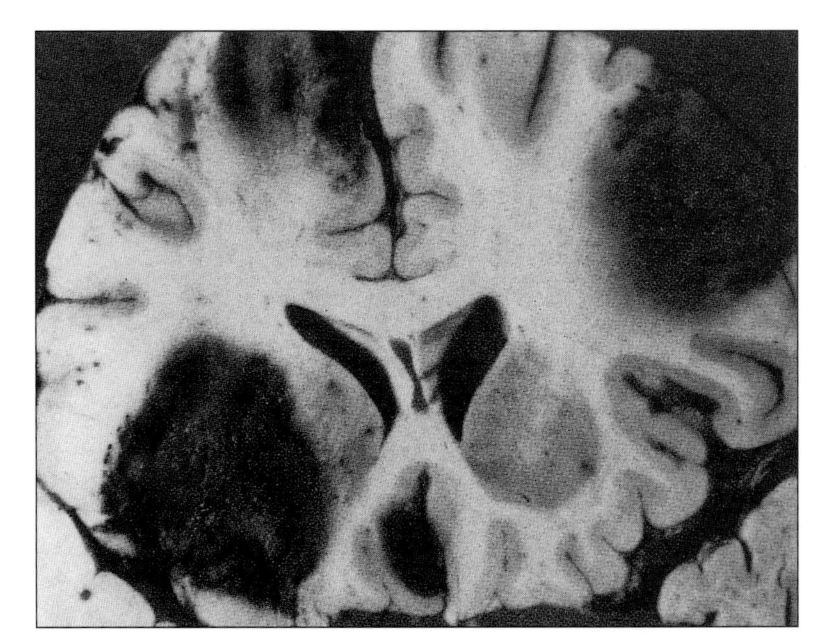

Figure 5-32 Gross photograph showing multifocal areas of encephalomalacia in the cerebral cortex, subcortical white matter, and basal ganglia in granulomatous amebic encephalitis. Granulomatous disease appears to result only from *Acanthamoeba* infection, whereas acute amebic meningoencephalitis most frequently is caused by *Naegleria fowleri*. (*From* Martinez AJ: *Free-Living Amebas: National History, Prevention, Diagnosis, Pathology, and Treatment of Disease*. Boca Raton, FL: CRC Press; 1985; with permission.)

Toxoplasmosis

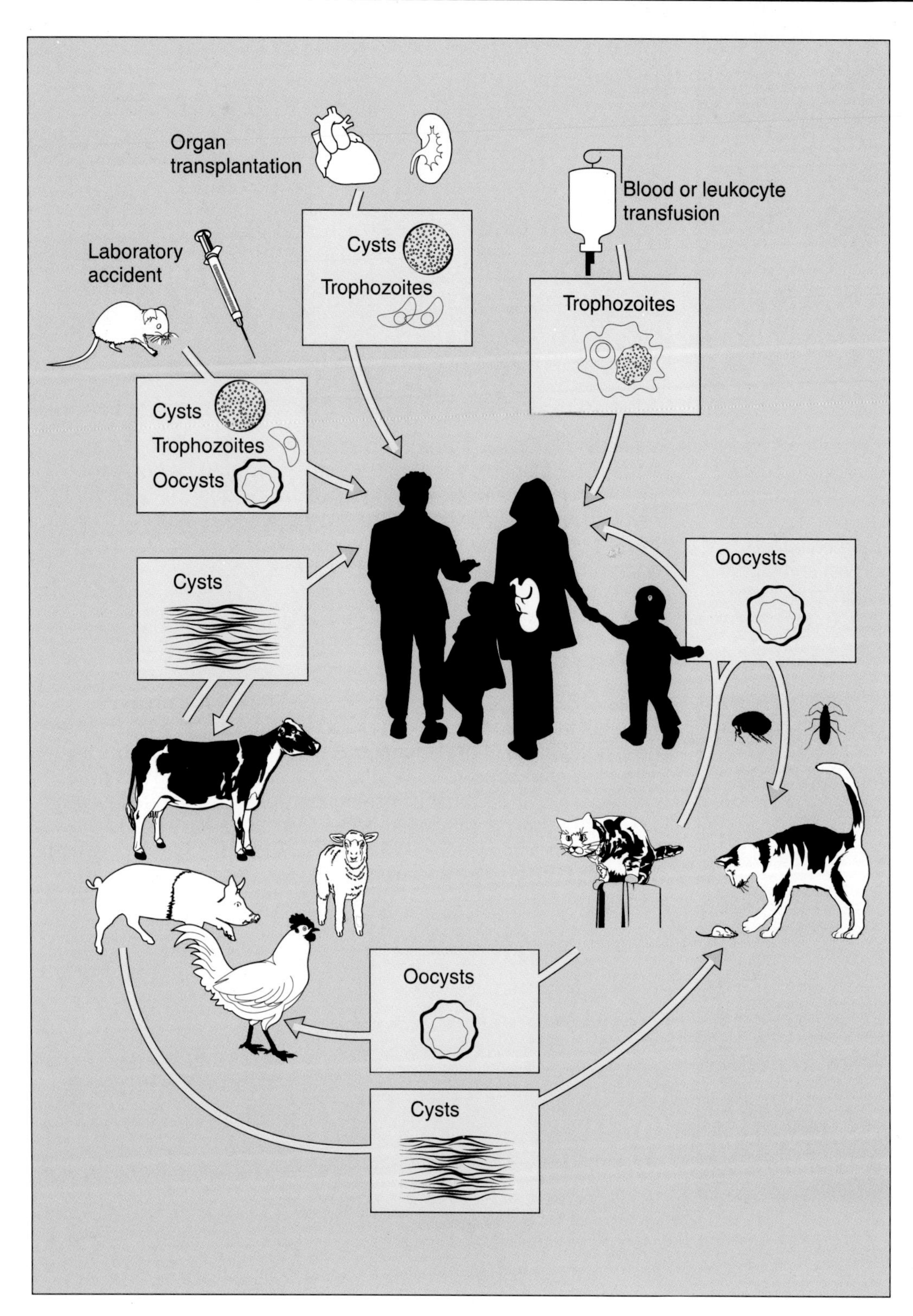

FIGURE 5-33 Modes of transmission of toxoplasmosis. Most commonly, *Toxoplasma gondii* infection of humans follows the ingestion of undercooked meat or foods contaminated by cat feces containing oocysts. The regional variations in the seropositivity of toxoplasmosis have correlated with a warm humid climate, poor sanitation, cat exposure, and consumption of undercooked meat.

Signs and symptoms of toxoplasmosis

Congenital disease		Immunocompromised host	
Retinochoroiditis	87%	Altered mental status	75%
Abnormal CSF	55%	Fever	10%–72%
Anemia	51%	Seizures	33%
Convulsions	50%	Headache	56%
Intracranial calcifications	50%	Focal neurologic signs	60%
Jaundice	29%	Motor deficits	
Fever	25%	Cranial nerve palsies	
Splenomegaly	21%	Movement disorders	
Hepatomegaly	17%	Dysmetria	
		Visual field loss	
		Aphasia	

FIGURE 5-34 Signs and symptoms of toxoplasmosis: congenital vs AIDS-related. Congenital toxoplasmosis is a systemic illness associated with meningoencephalitis and retinochoroiditis in the newborn. AIDS-related toxoplasmosis is seen in the adult and is usually a reactivation of latent infection. Radiographic imaging in AIDS patients shows focal mass lesions. CSF—cerebrospinal fluid. (Luft BJ, Remington JS: Toxoplasmosis of the central nervous system. *In* Remington SJ, Swartz MN (eds.): *Current Topics in Infectious Diseases*, vol 6. New York: McGraw-Hill; 1985:315–358.)

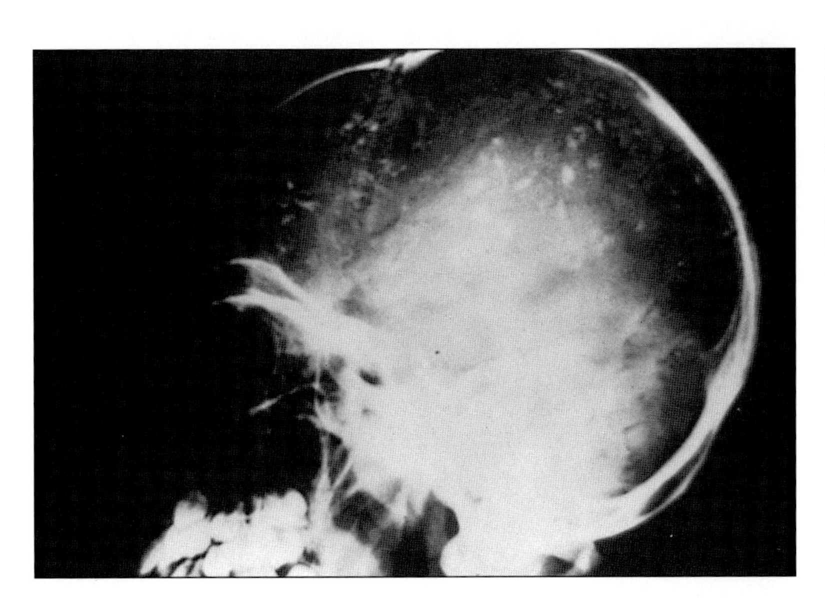

FIGURE 5-35 Intracerebral calcifications in congenital toxoplasmosis. Scattered calcifications of the brain are seen on a skull radiograph in an 8-year-old child with congenital toxoplasmosis. Calcifications are frequently periventricular but may be scattered. Hydrocephalus frequently is a coexistent finding. Congenital toxoplasmosis is asymptomatic in approximately two-thirds of individuals. (*From* Kepes JJ: *Pathology of Inflammatory Diseases*. New York: Medcom Inc.; 1972; with permission.)

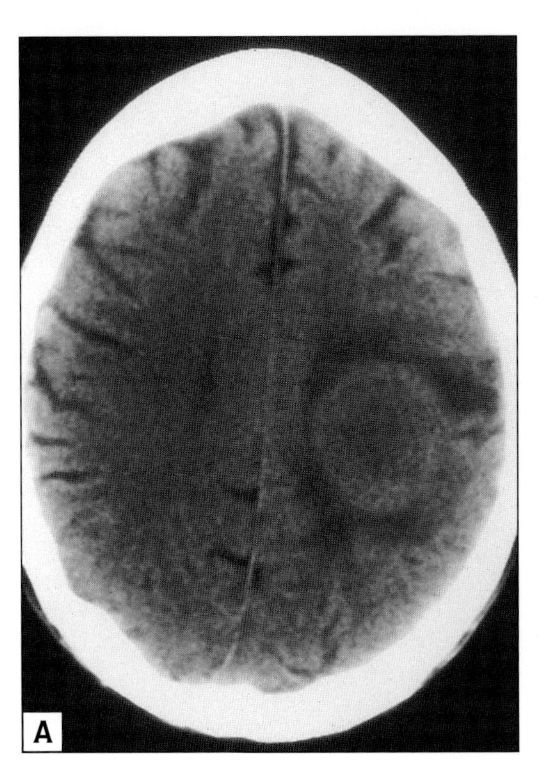

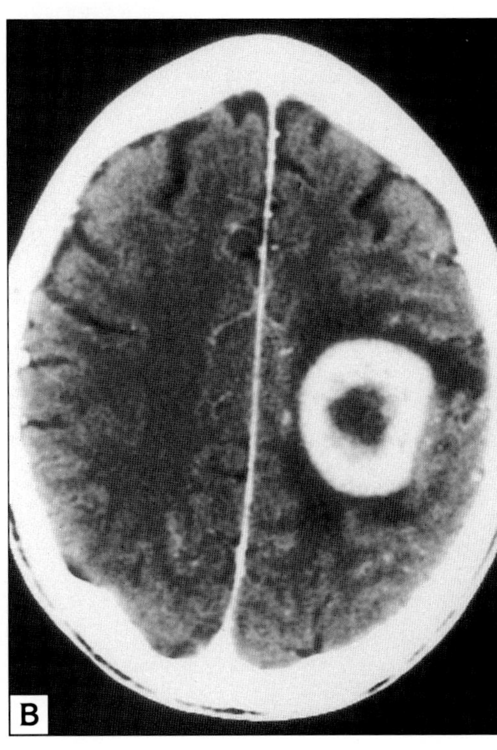

FIGURE 5-36 Computed tomographic (CT) scan of the brain in AIDS-related toxoplasmosis. **A**, CT scan without contrast reveals a large subcortical lesion of the left frontoparietal lobe in a patient with advanced AIDS who presented with right hemiparesis and a seizure disorder. Perilesional edema is evident. **B**, CT scan with contrast shows the typical ring-enhancing lesion of toxoplasmosis. This ring enhancement, however, is not diagnostic and may be seen with tumors, abscesses, and vascular lesions.

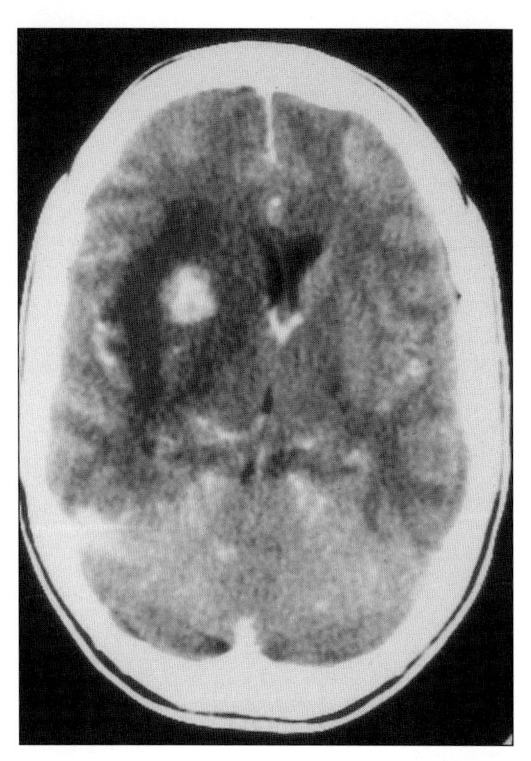

FIGURE 5-37
Nodular enhancing lesion of toxoplasmosis in the basal ganglia. A CT scan of the brain in a patient with AIDS and left hemiparesis reveals a homogeneously enhancing nodular lesion of the basal ganglia. There is significant edema and some mass effect on the frontal horn of the lateral ventricle. Toxoplasmosis appears to have a predilection for the basal ganglia.

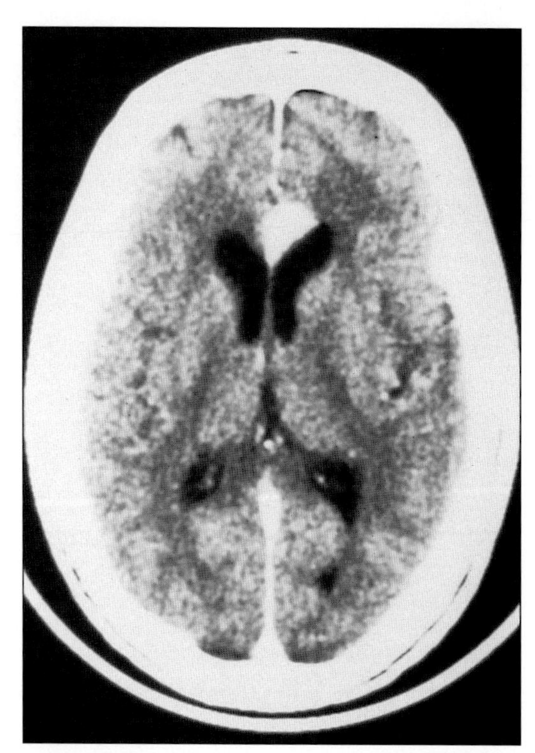

FIGURE 5-38
Nodular enhancing lesion of toxoplasmosis in the corpus callosum. Although the location of this lesion is suggestive of another etiology, such as cerebral lymphoma, biopsy established the diagnosis of toxoplasmosis in this patient.

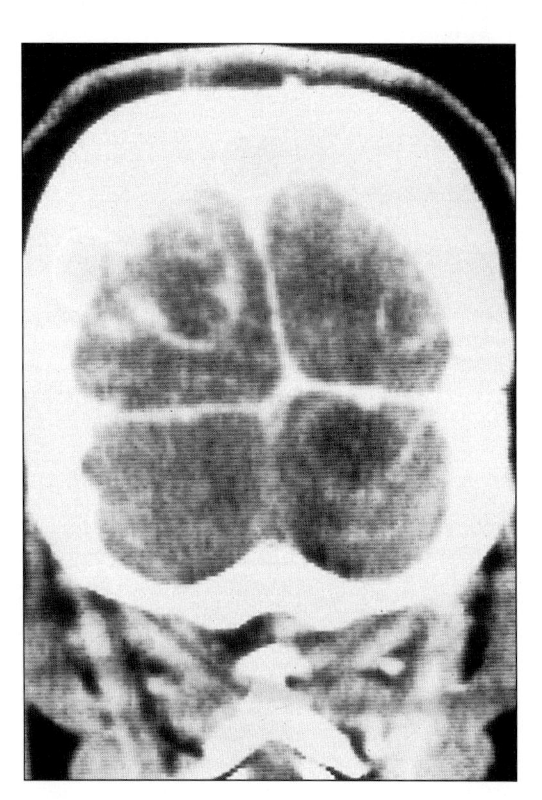

FIGURE 5-39
Multiple ring-enhancing lesions in cerebral toxoplasmosis. These lesions are located both supratentorially and infratentorially. Multiple lesions are a characteristic finding in cerebral toxoplasmosis.

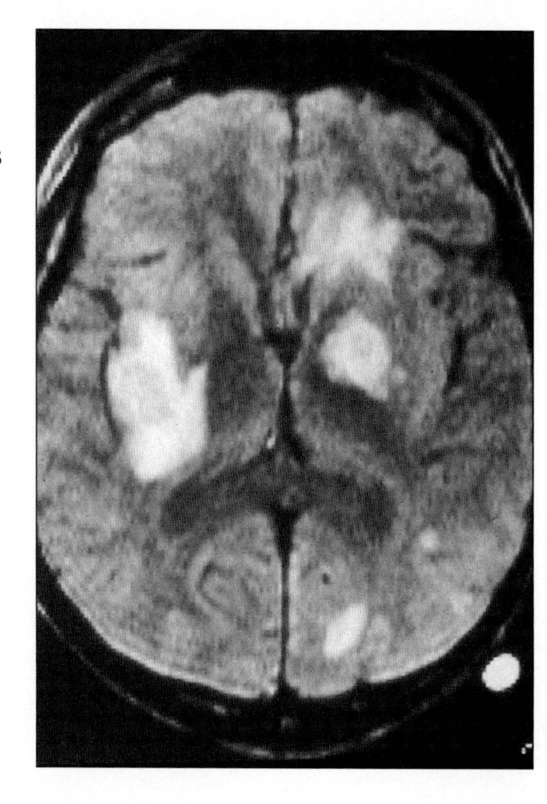

FIGURE 5-40
Cranial magnetic resonance image (MRI) reveals multiple T2 hyperintensities present subcortically and in the basal ganglia of a patient with toxoplasmosis.

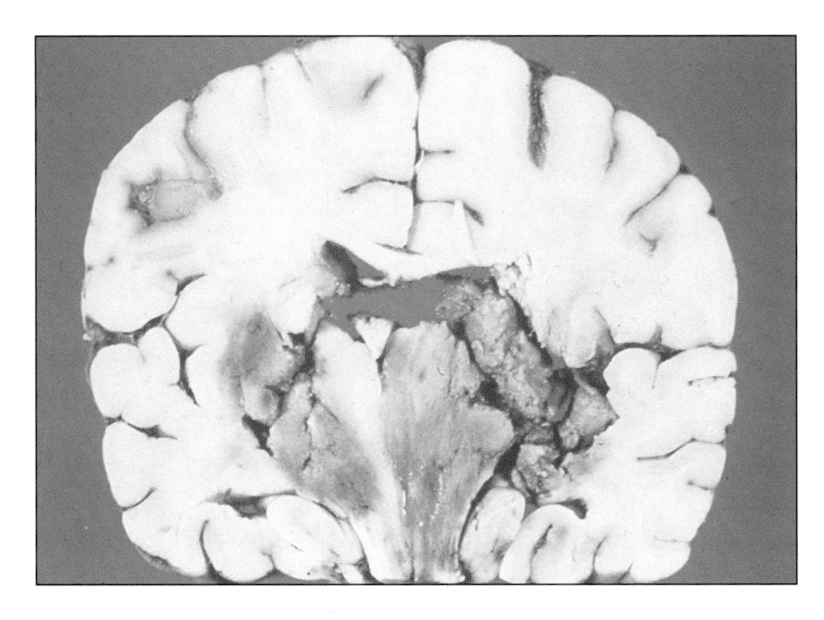

FIGURE 5-41 Gross brain specimen showing necrotic lesions of toxoplasma encephalitis. Lesions are present bilaterally in the basal ganglia and subcortically in the right frontal cortex.

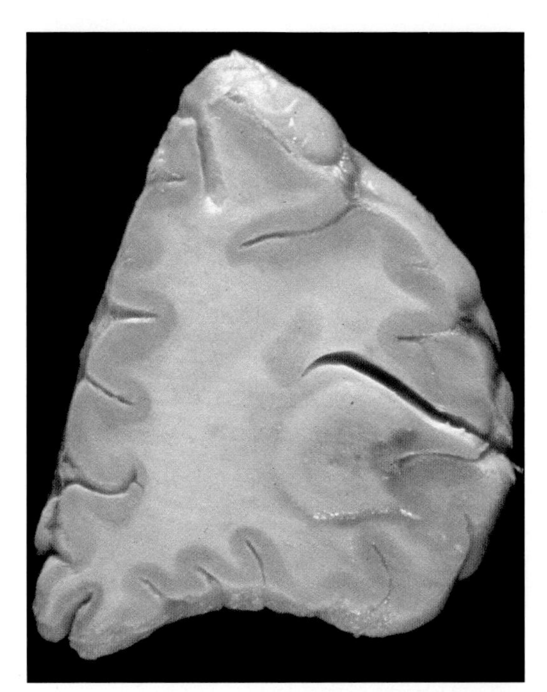

FIGURE 5-42 Gross brain specimen showing a subcortical lesion in toxoplasmosis.

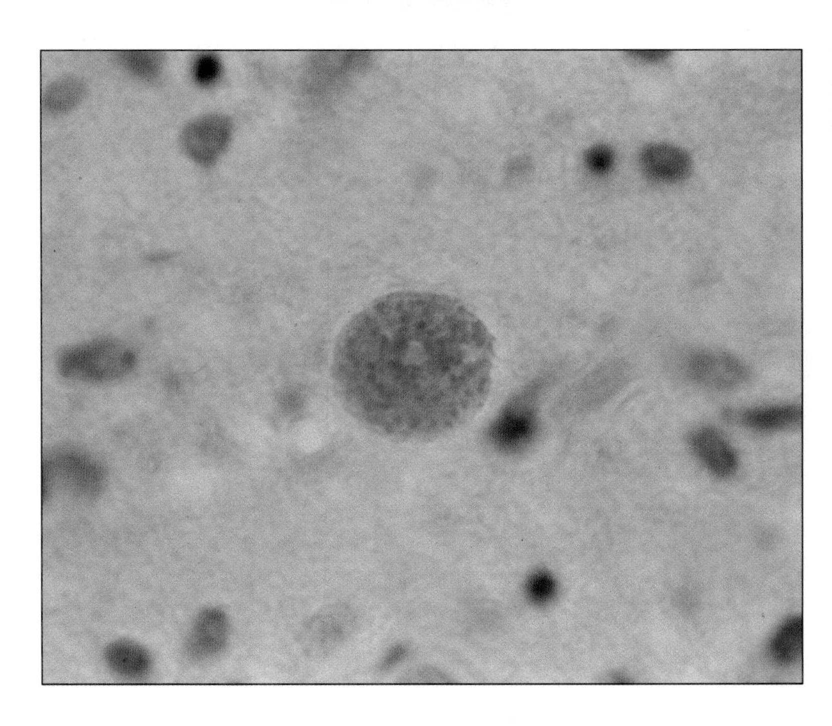

FIGURE 5-43 Tissue cyst of *Toxoplasma gondii* in the brain containing many bradyzoites. There is a relative absence of inflammation around the cyst.

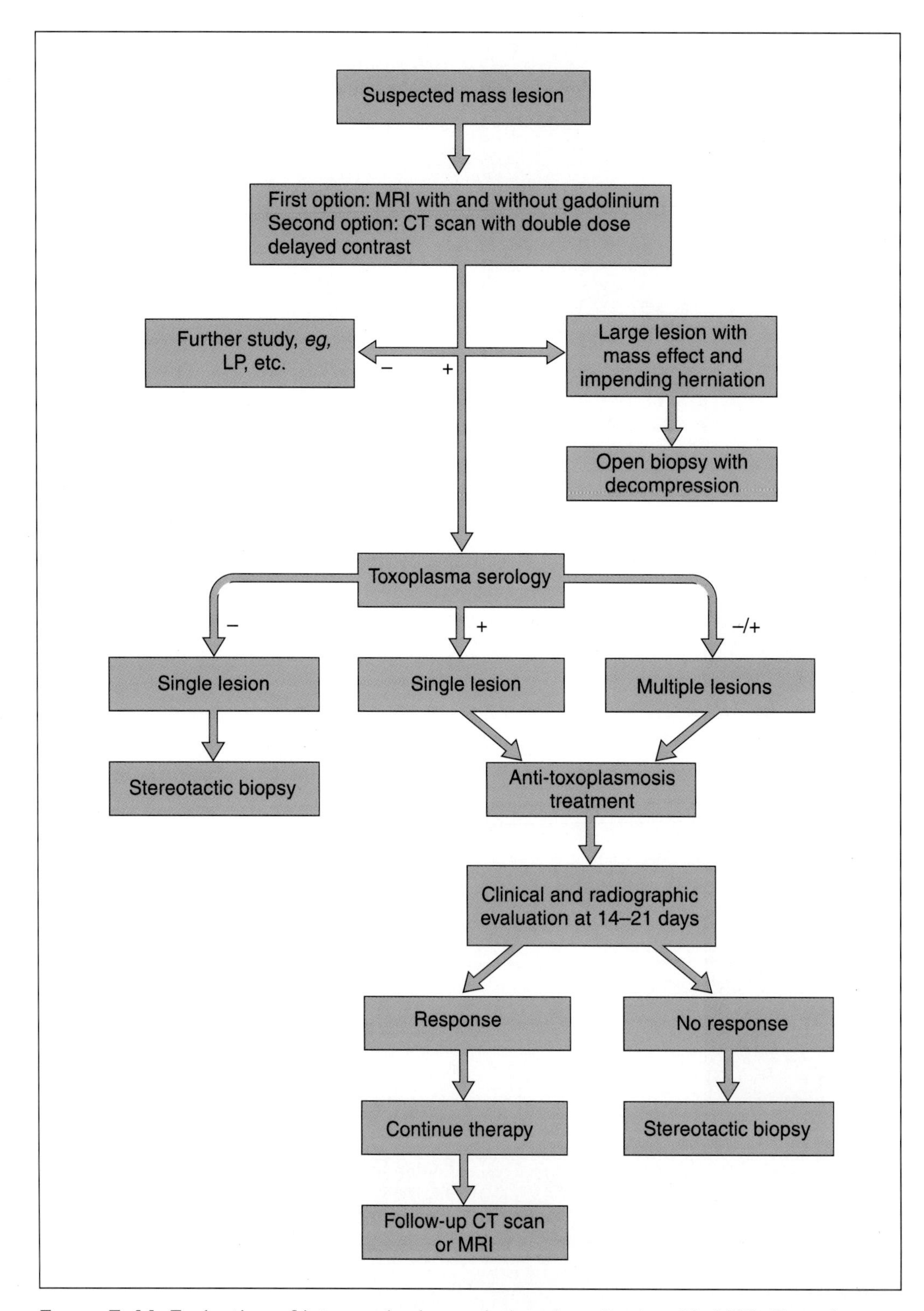

FIGURE 5-44 Evaluation of intracerebral mass lesions in patients with AIDS. Toxoplasmosis is the most common etiology of these mass lesions. Other possible diagnoses in AIDS patients include primary CNS lymphoma and abscess. LP—lumbar puncture. (*From* Berger JR: The neurological complications of human immunodeficiency virus infection. *In* Aminoff M (ed.): *Neurology and General Medicine*, 2nd ed. New York: Churchill Livingstone; 1994; with permission.)

Recommended treatment of toxoplasma encephalitis in AIDS	
Standard regimens	
Pyrimethamine	Oral 200-mg loading dose, then 50–75 mg daily
Folinic acid (leucovorin)	Oral, iv, or im 10–20 mg daily (up to 50 mg daily)
plus	
Sulfadiazine	Oral 1–1.5 g q6h
or	
Clindamycin	Oral or iv 600 mg q6h (up to iv 1200 mg q6h)
Alternative regimens	
Trimethoprim/sulfamethoxazole	Oral or iv 5 mg (TMP)/kg q6h
Pyrimethamine and folinic acid	As in standard regimens plus one of the following:
Clarithromycin	Oral 1 g q12h
Azithromycin	Oral 1200–1500 mg daily
Atovaquone	Oral 750 mg q6h
Dapsone	Oral 100 mg daily

FIGURE 5-45 Recommended treatment of toxoplasma encephalitis in AIDS. A high rate of side effects, chiefly skin rash, is observed with the use of sulfadiazine in AIDS patients, often necessitating the use of desensitization or other forms of therapy. The high rates of recurrent disease in AIDS patients mandate the use of secondary prophylaxis. The most effective regimen appears to be pyrimethamine, 25 mg/day, and sulfadiazine, 500 mg four times daily. However, other regimens, including trimethoprim (TMP)/sulfamethoxazole, have proven effective. (Luft BJ, Hafner R, Korzun AH, *et al.*: Toxoplasmic encephalitis in patients with the acquired immunodeficiency syndrome. *N Engl J Med* 1993, 329:995–1000. *From* Beaman MH, McCabe RE, Wong S-Y, Remington JS: *Toxoplasma gondii*. *In* Mandell GL, *et al.* (eds.): *Principles and Practice of Infectious Diseases*, 4th ed. New York: Churchill Livingstone; 1995:2467; with permission.)

TREMATODES (FLUKES)

Schistosomiasis

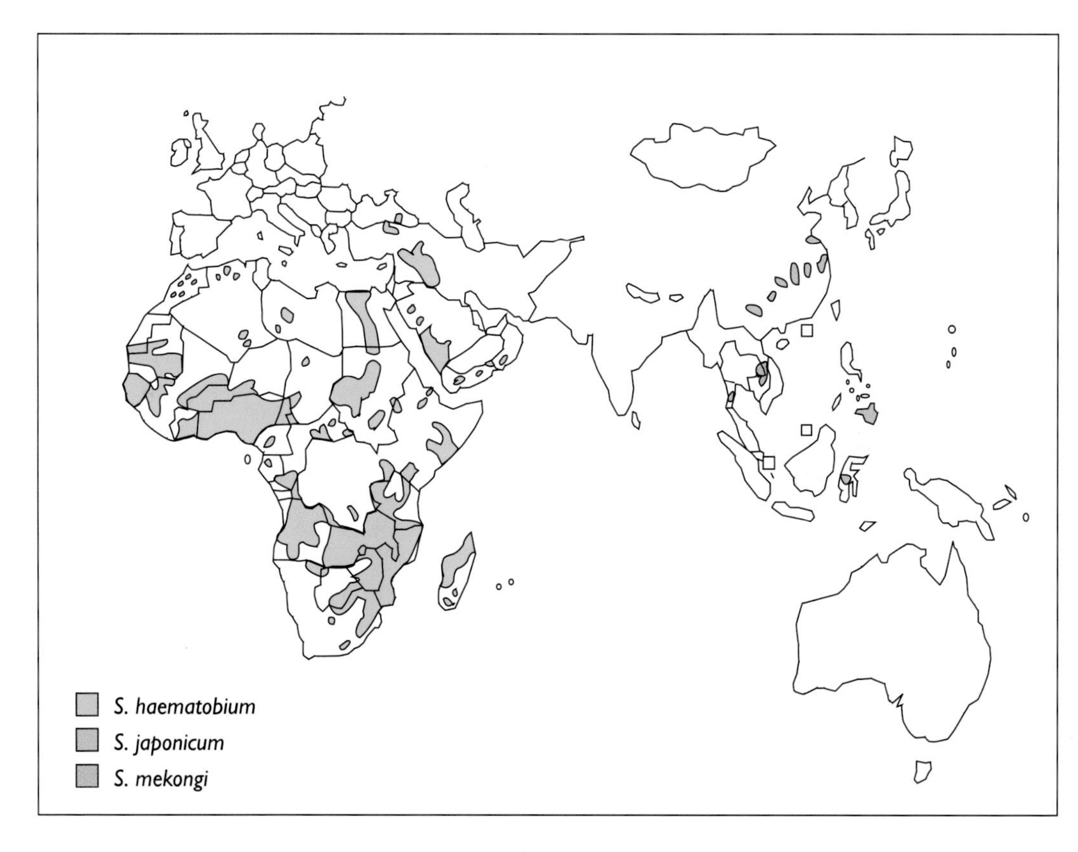

FIGURE 5-46 Global distribution of schistosomiasis. Schistosomiasis results from infection with one of three organisms: *Schistosoma mansoni*, *S. japonicum*, or *S. haematobium*. CNS disease is rare and is chiefly the result of deposition of eggs and the accompanying inflammatory response. On rare occasions, the adult worm may localize in the vasculature of the spinal cord or brain. The deposition of eggs is dependent on their size. The small eggs of *S. japonicum* frequently reach the brain, whereas the larger eggs of the other organisms most commonly affect the spinal cord. (Scrimegeour EM, Gajdusek DC: Involvement of the central nervous system in *Schistosoma mansoni* and *S. haëmatobium* infection. *Brain* 1985, 108:1023–1038.)

Cestodes (Tapeworms)

Cysticercosis

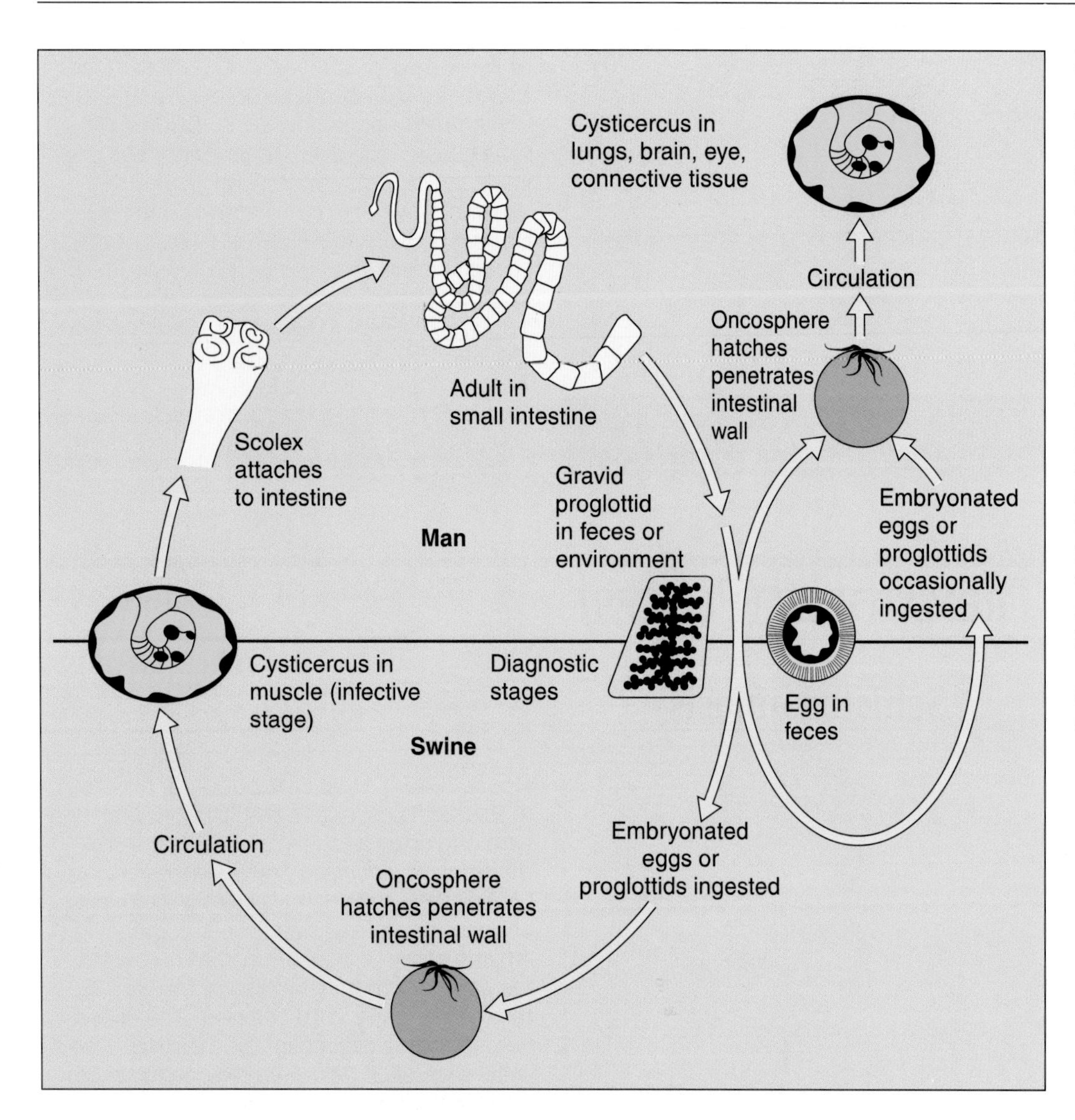

Figure 5-47 Life cycle of the cestode, *Taenia solium*. This common intestinal tapeworm is broadly distributed around the world, with particularly high incidences in Mexico, Central and South America, Africa, India, and China. The ingestion of pork infested with cysticerci, the tissue larval stage, results in infestation of the human small intestine (definitive host) by the adult tapeworm. The terminal gravid proglottids of the adult tapeworm that develop in the intestine are excreted in the feces. The eggs released from these proglottids contaminate the environment and can be ingested by pigs or man. The eggs mature into true larvae in the small intestine and migrate through the intestinal mucosa into blood vessels, migrating to various tissues including muscle (intermediate host). (*From* Melvin DM, Brooke MM, Sadun EH: *Common Intestinal Helminths of Man*. (DHEW publication no. [CDC] 72-8286.) Atlanta: Centers for Disease Control; 1964.)

Signs and symptoms of neurocysticercosis

Symptoms	Percent
Headache	23–98
Meningismus	29–33
Papilledema	48–84
Seizures	37–92
Abnormal mental status	74–80
Focal deficits (motor and/or sensory)	3–36
Ataxia	5–24
Myelopathy	<1
Cranial nerve palsies	1–36
Visual impairment	5–34

Figure 5-48 Signs and symptoms of neurocysticercosis. Symptoms and signs are highly dependent on the nature and location of the lesions in the brain. The forms of neurocysticercosis can be classified as asymptomatic, parenchymal, subarachnoid, intraventricular, spinal, and ocular. These forms of neurocysticercosis are not necessarily mutually exclusive. The frequencies of the initial symptoms and signs of neurocysticercosis are indicated. (*Adapted from* Cameron ML, Durack DT: Helminthic infections of the central nervous system. *In* Scheld WM, Whitley RJ, Durack DT (eds.): *Infections of the Central Nervous System*. New York: Raven Press; 1991:825–860; with permission.)

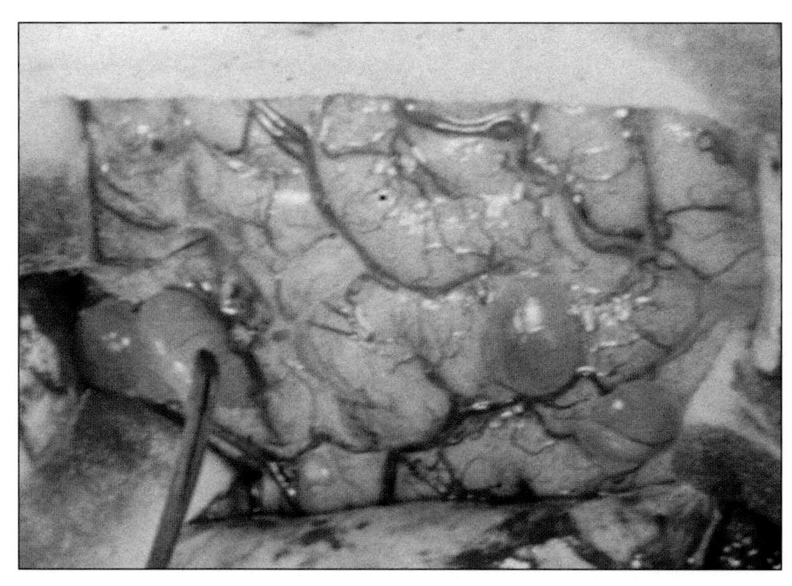

FIGURE 5-49 Surgical removal of superficial cortical cysts in neurocysticercosis. (*Courtesy of* Dr. Aldo Berti, Miami, FL.)

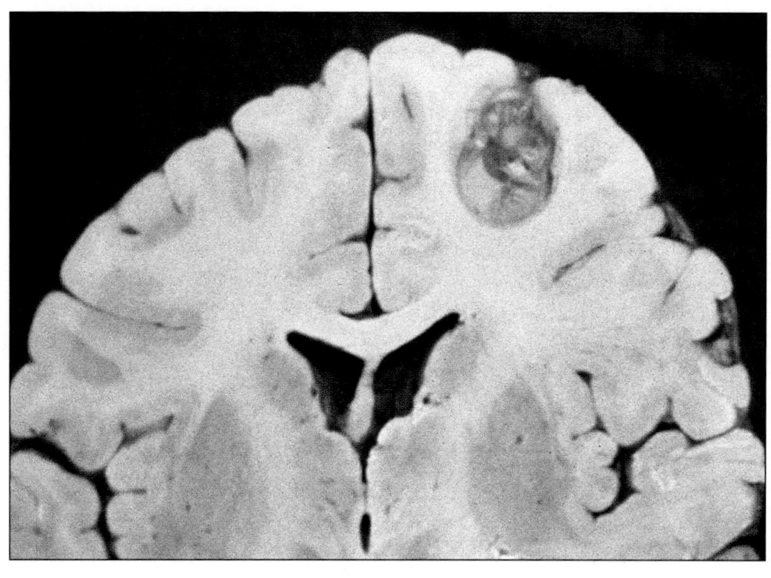

FIGURE 5-50 Parenchymal neurocysticercosis in a gross brain specimen. The cysts of parenchymal neurocysticercosis are typically observed at the gray-white junction. The most common manifestation is focal seizures. (*Courtesy of* Dr. Aldo Berti, Miami, FL.)

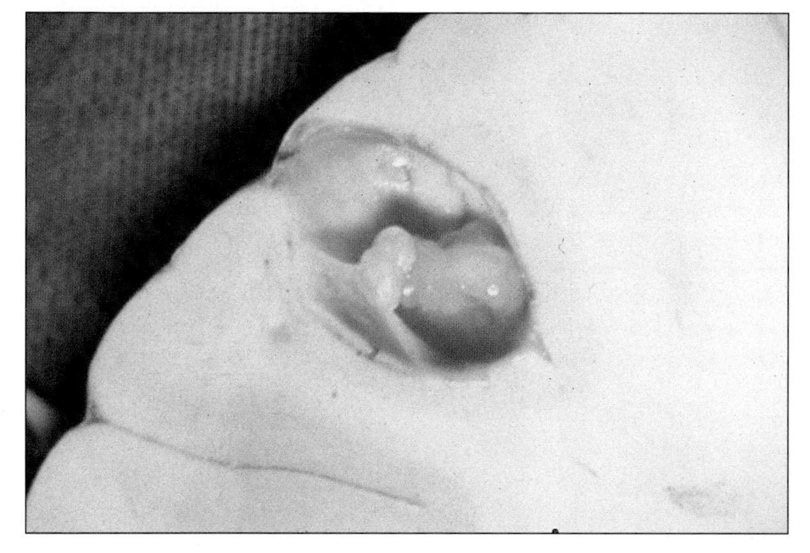

FIGURE 5-51 Higher magnification of a parenchymal cyst in neurocysticercosis. Death of the cysticerci, frequently precipitated by effective therapy, results in release of larval antigens which may stimulate an inflammatory host response and exacerbate symptoms. (*Courtesy of* Dr. Aldo Berti, Miami, FL.)

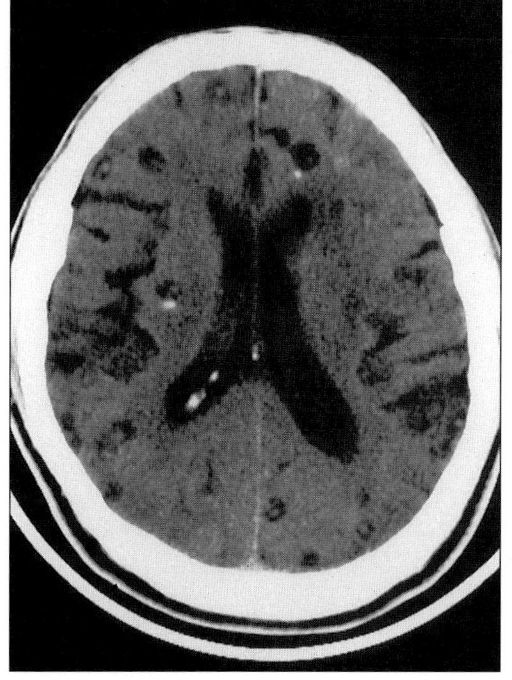

FIGURE 5-52 CT scan of the brain revealing multiple cysts within the parenchyma. The scolex of the cysticercus may be identified within many of these cysts, and calcification is observed as well. More than 50% of cases of neurocysticercosis are associated with calcification.

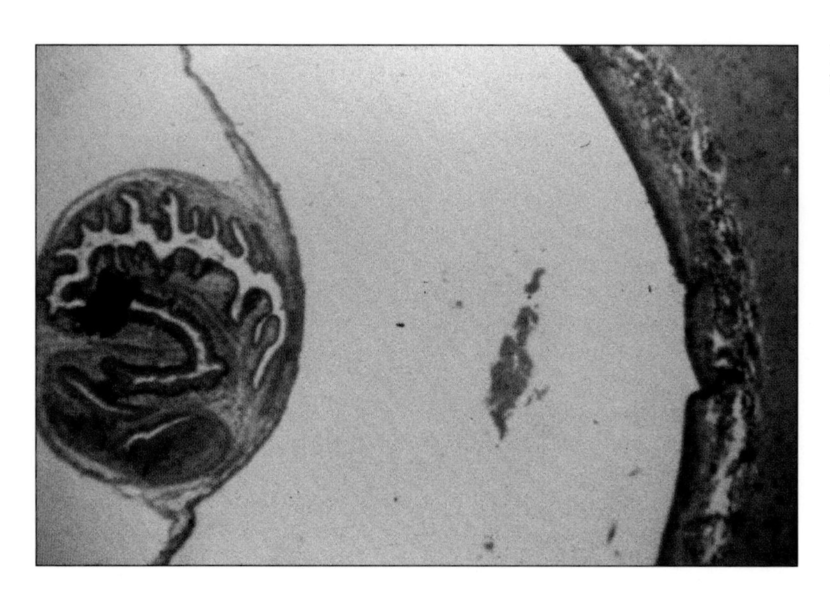

FIGURE 5-53 Photomicrograph of a neurocysticercosis cyst in the brain parenchyma. (*Courtesy of* Dr. Aldo Berti, Miami, FL.)

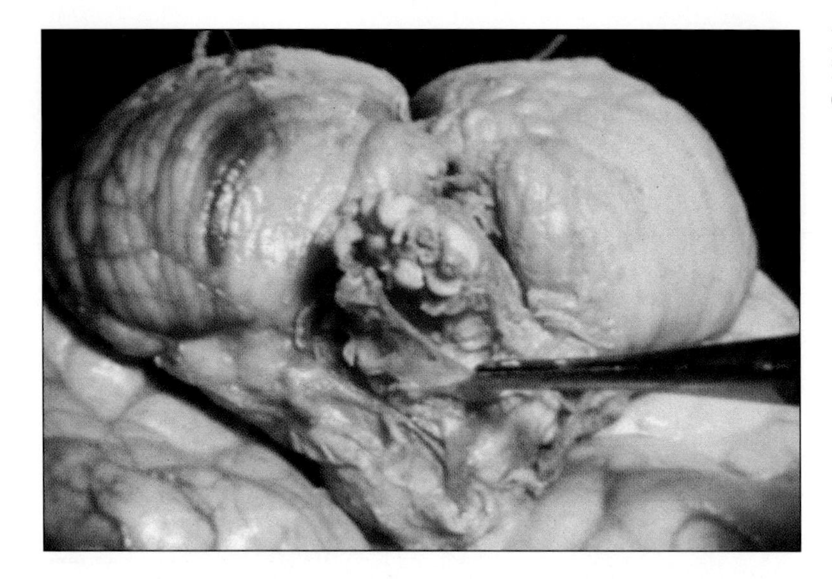

Figure 5-54 Racemose cysticercosis at the base of the brain resulting in dense fibrosis. Hydrocephalus frequently complicates this form of neurocysticercosis. (*Courtesy of* Dr. Aldo Berti, Miami, FL.)

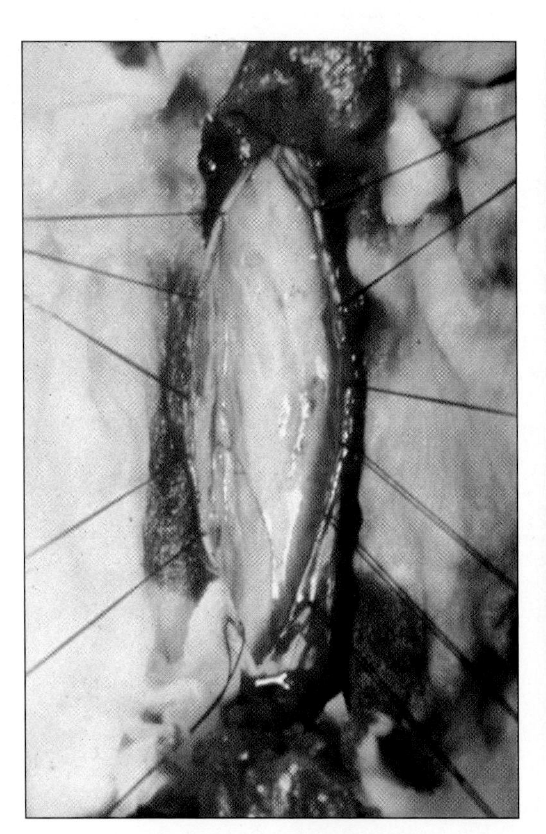

Figure 5-55 Spinal neurocysticercosis. Intense inflammation and fibrosis accompany extramedullary racemose lesions. Intramedullary cysts are occasionally observed in the spinal cord as well. (*Courtesy of* Dr. Aldo Berti, Miami, FL.)

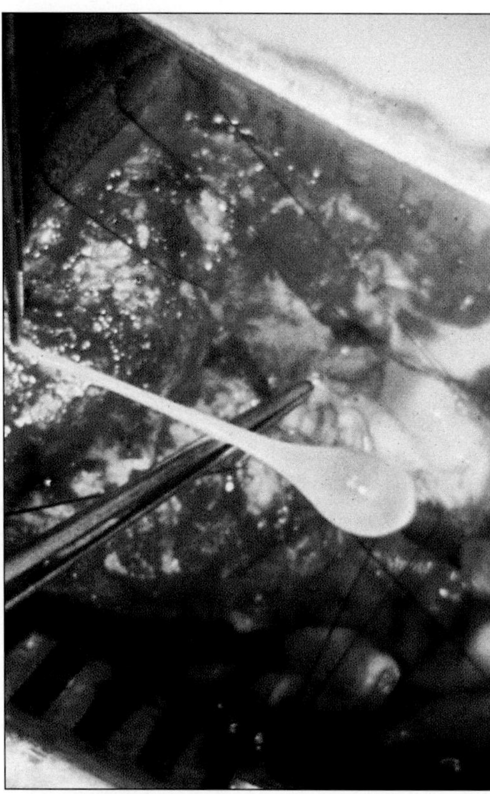

Figure 5-56 Careful surgical removal of an intact cyst in neurocysticercosis. (*Courtesy of* Dr. Aldo Berti, Miami, FL.)

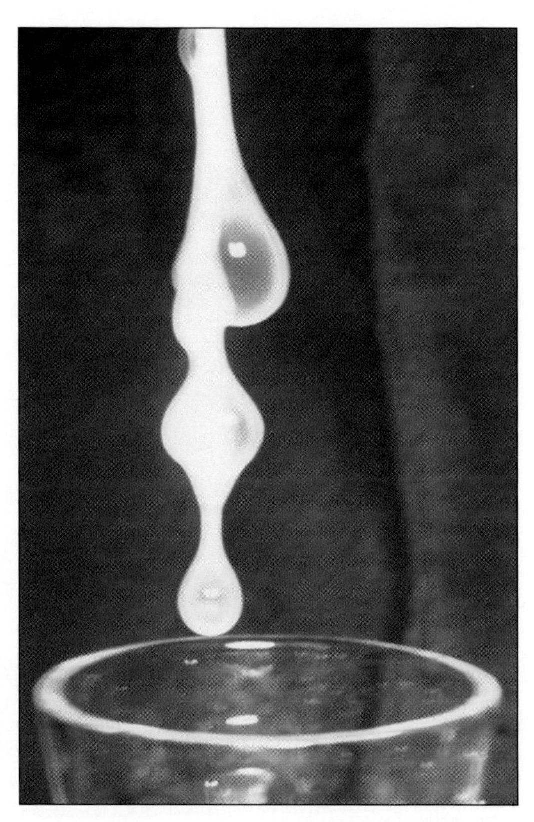

Figure 5-57 Multiple cysts of racemose neurocysticercosis following their removal from the subarachnoid space. (*Courtesy of* Dr. Aldo Berti, Miami, FL.)

Treatment of neurocysticercosis	
Medical therapy	
Praziquantel	50 mg/kg/d in 3 doses x 15 days
Albendazole	15 mg/kg/d in 3 doses x 8 days
Plus adjunctive corticosteroids	
or	
Surgical excision	

FIGURE 5-58 Treatment of neurocysticercosis. In symptomatic patients, both praziquantel and albendazole are effective. Because dying cysticerci provoke an inflammatory response, patients should be hospitalized and given high-dose glucocorticoids. Ocular, spinal, and ventricular lesions are best managed by surgical resection. (MaQuire JH, Spielman A: Ectoparasite infestations. *In* Isselbacher KJ, *et al.* (eds.): *Harrison's Principles of Internal Medicine*, 13th ed. New York: McGraw-Hill; 1992:931–934.)

Echinococcosis (Hydatid Disease)

Clinical manifestations of CNS echinococcosis
Headache
Nausea and vomiting
Papilledema
Seizures
Focal motor and sensory findings
Cranial nerve palsies
Disturbances of speech and language

FIGURE 5-59 Clinical manifestations of CNS echinococcosis. *Echinococcus* is a common tapeworm of dogs and sheep in some parts of the world. Four species have been described that affect humans: *E. chinococcus granulosus*, the most common in humans, *E. multilocularis*, *E. vogeli*, and *E. oligarthrus*. In the CNS, the manifestations of echinococcosis are chiefly those of slowly expanding mass lesions. (Aydin Y, Barlas O, Yolas C, *et al.*: Alveolar hydatid disease of the brain: report of four cases. *J Neurosurg* 1986, 65:115–119.)

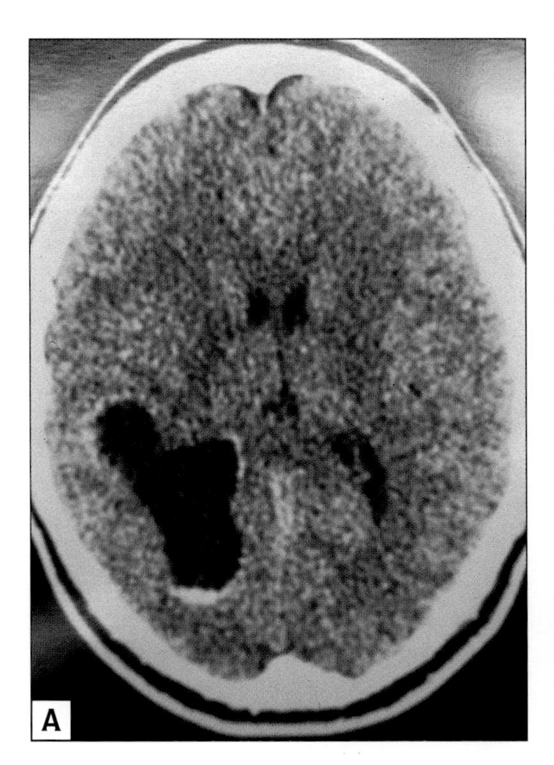

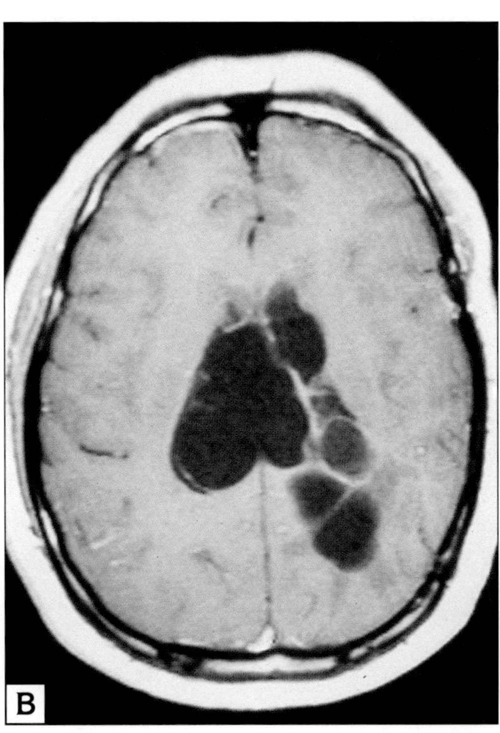

FIGURE 5-60 Intracranial hydatid cyst of echinococcosis. **A**, A CT scan of the brain shows a large cystic mass of the left temporoparietal region in a 40-year-old man from Honduras who presented with headache. At surgery, the cyst was inadvertently ruptured. Pathologic examination revealed hydatid disease. **B**, An MRI scan 31 months later shows multiple cystic lesions indicative of secondary hydatidosis. These lesions resulted from spillage of the contents of the initial hydatid cyst. (*Courtesy of* Dr. Sara G. Austin, Houston, TX.)

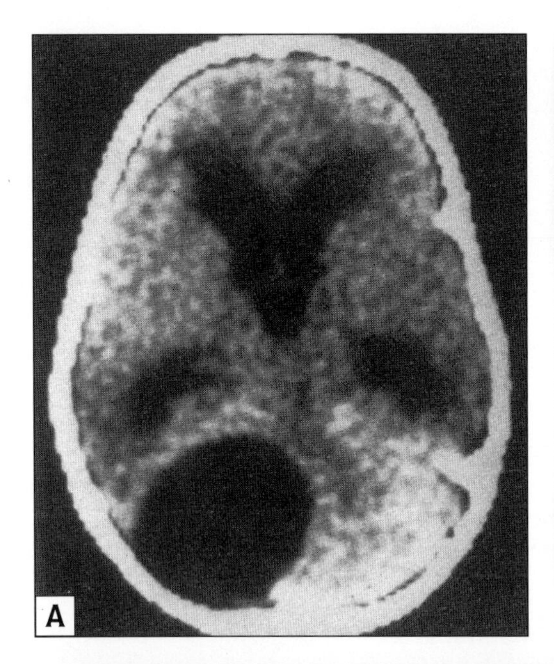

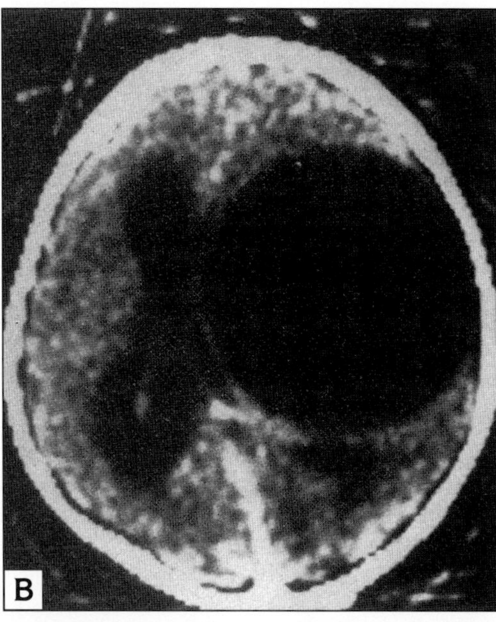

FIGURE 5-61 **A** and **B**, CT scans from two patients showing hydatid cysts in the brain. Characteristic findings include the spherical appearance, lack of enhancement, and absence of associated edema. (*From* Abbassioun K, Rahmat H, Ameli NO, Tafazoli M: Computerized tomography in hydatid cyst of the brain. *J Neurosurg* 1978, 49:408–411; with permission.)

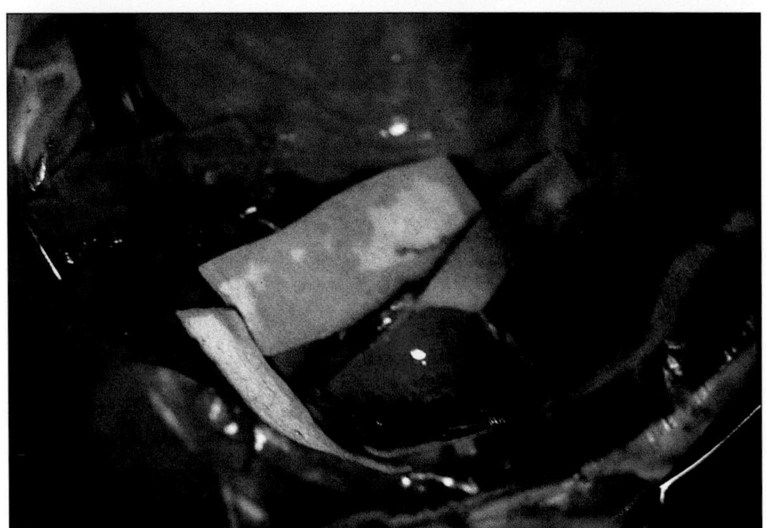

FIGURE 5-62 Removal of an intracerebral hydatid cyst. Care must be exercised to avoid spilling the contents of the cyst. (*Courtesy of* Dr. Ramon Leigurda, Buenos Aires, Argentina.)

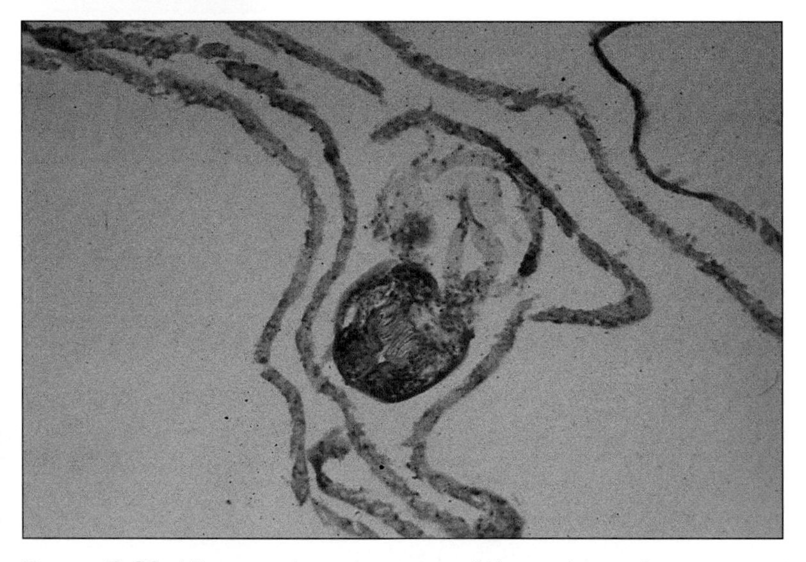

FIGURE 5-63 Microscopic appearance of the scolex and membranes of a hydatid cyst. (*Courtesy of* Dr. Ramon Leigurda, Buenos Aires, Argentina.)

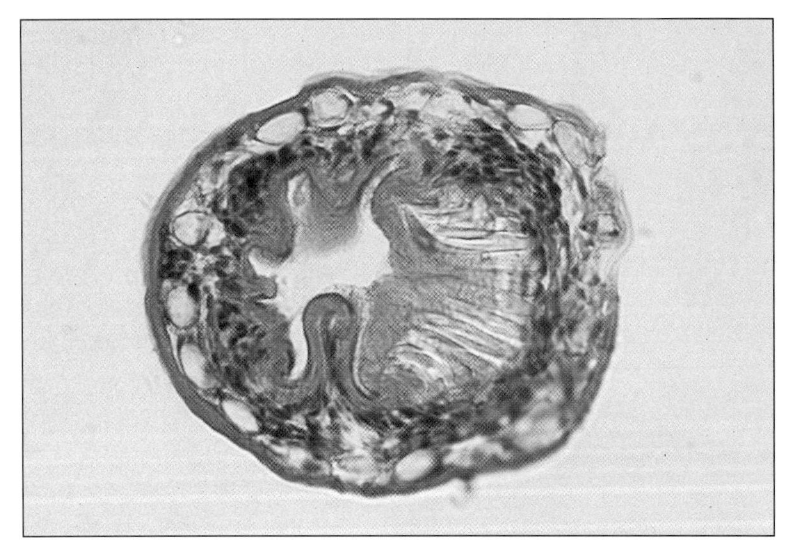

FIGURE 5-64 Histopathology of the scolex of a hydatid cyst. (*Courtesy of* Dr. Sara G. Austin, Houston, TX.)

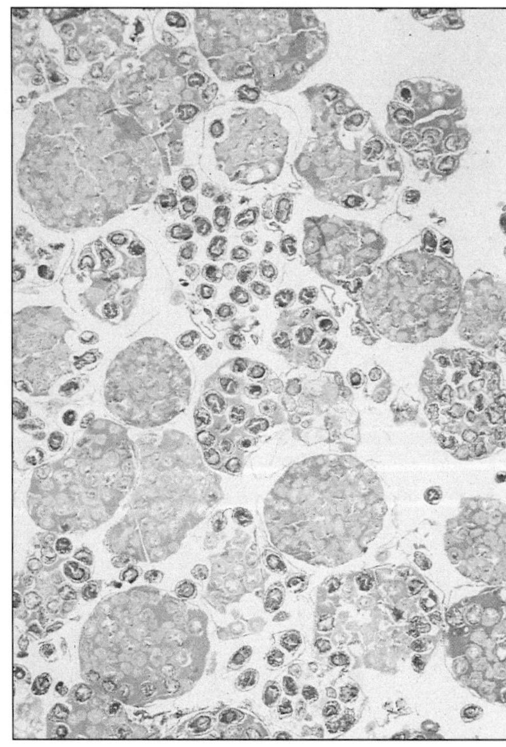

FIGURE 5-65 Histopathology of protoscoleces. (*Courtesy of* Dr. Sara G. Austin, Houston, TX.)

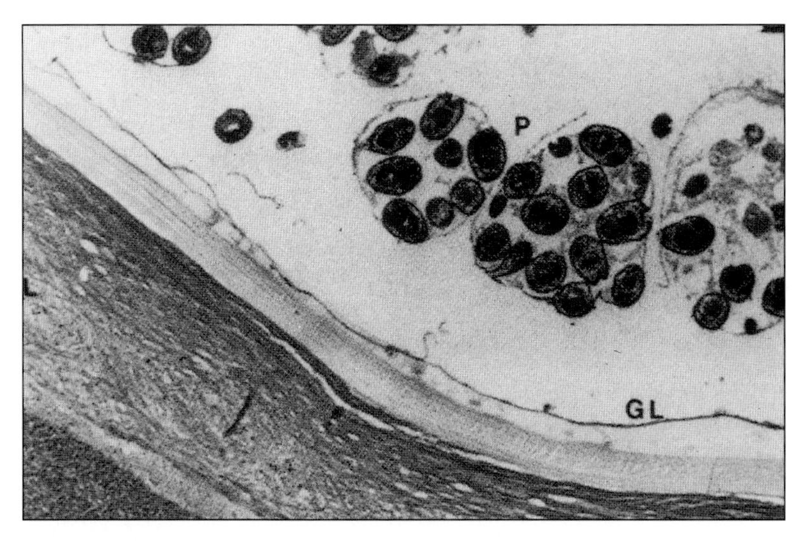

FIGURE 5-66 Cross-section of a hydatid cyst. Section of a hydatid cyst shows protoscoleces (*P*) in brood capsules within an echinococcal cyst. The cyst wall consists of the germinative layer (*GL*), laminated membrane, and adventitial layer. (*From* Schantz PM, Okelo GBA: Echinococcosis (hydatidosis). *In* Warren KS, Mahmoud AAF (eds.): *Tropical and Geographic Medicine*, 2nd ed. New York: McGraw-Hill; 1990:505–518; with permission.)

Treatment of echinococcosis
Surgical excision ± albendazole preoperatively *or* Albendazole, 400 mg bid x 28 days, repeated as needed 1–8 times every 2–3 wks

FIGURE 5-67 Treatment of echinococcosis. Surgery, when feasible, is the definitive treatment for removing cysts or resecting tissue that contains cysts. Chemotherapy with albendazole, combined with percutaneous drainage, may be effective for hepatic and pulmonary lesions.

NEMATODES (ROUNDWORMS)

Onchocerciasis

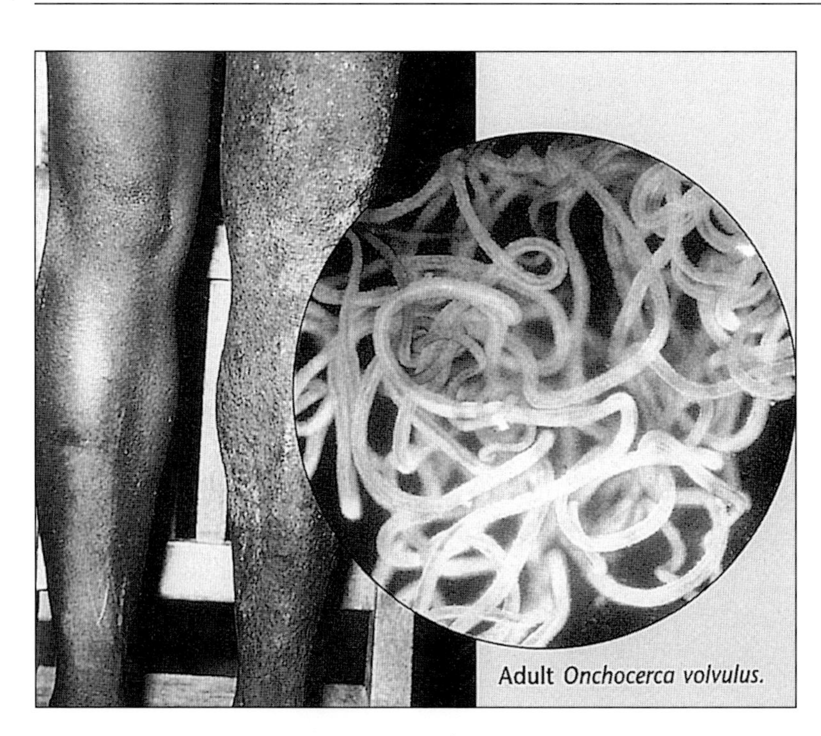

FIGURE 5-68 Onchocerciasis, or river blindness, is the result of infestation with the threadworm, *Onchocerca volvulus*, and is one of the leading causes of blindness in the developing world. After the entry of microfilaria into the skin via the bite of the simulium fly (black fly), subcutaneous nodules and an intense pruritic rash may develop. The adult worm lives in cutaneous fibrous tissues and discharges large numbers of microfilaria. (*From* Ramachandran CP: Lymphatic filariasis and onchocerciasis. In *Tropical Disease Research: Progress 1991–1992 [11th Programme Report of the UNDP/World Bank/WHO Special Programme for Research and Training in Tropical Diseases]*. Geneva: World Health Organization; 1993:37; with permission.)

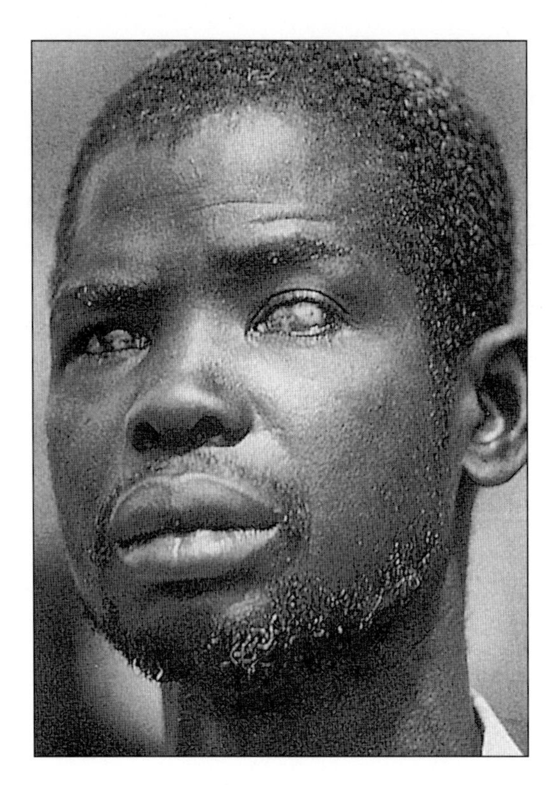

FIGURE 5-69 Blindness due to onchocerciasis. Microfilaria migrate into the conjunctiva and cornea, resulting in blindness. (*From* Ramachandran CP: Lymphatic filariasis and onchocerciasis. In *Tropical Disease Research: Progress 1991–1992 [11th Programme Report of the UNDP/World Bank/WHO Special Programme for Research and Training in Tropical Diseases]*. Geneva: World Health Organization; 1993:37; with permission.)

SELECTED BIBLIOGRAPHY

Cameron ML, Durack DT: Helminthic infections of the central nervous system. *In* Scheld WM, Whitley RJ, Durack DT (eds.): *Infections of the Central Nervous System*. New York: Raven Press; 1991:825–860.

Cegielski JP, Durack DT: Protozoal infections of the central nervous system. *In* Scheld WM, Whitley RJ, Durack DT (eds.): *Infections of the Central Nervous System*. New York: Raven Press; 1991:767–800.

Del Brutto OH, Sotelo J: Neurocysticercosis: an update. *Rev Infect Dis* 1988, 10:1075–1087.

Marsden PD, Bruce-Chwatt LJ: Cerebral malaria. *Contemp Neurol Ser* 1975, 12:29–44.

Porter SB, Sande MA: Toxoplasmosis of the central nervous system in the acquired immunodeficiency syndrome. *N Engl J Med* 1992, 327:1643–1648.

CHAPTER 6

Epidural Abscess and Subdural Empyema

David G. Brock

INTRACRANIAL SUBDURAL EMPYEMA AND EPIDURAL ABSCESS

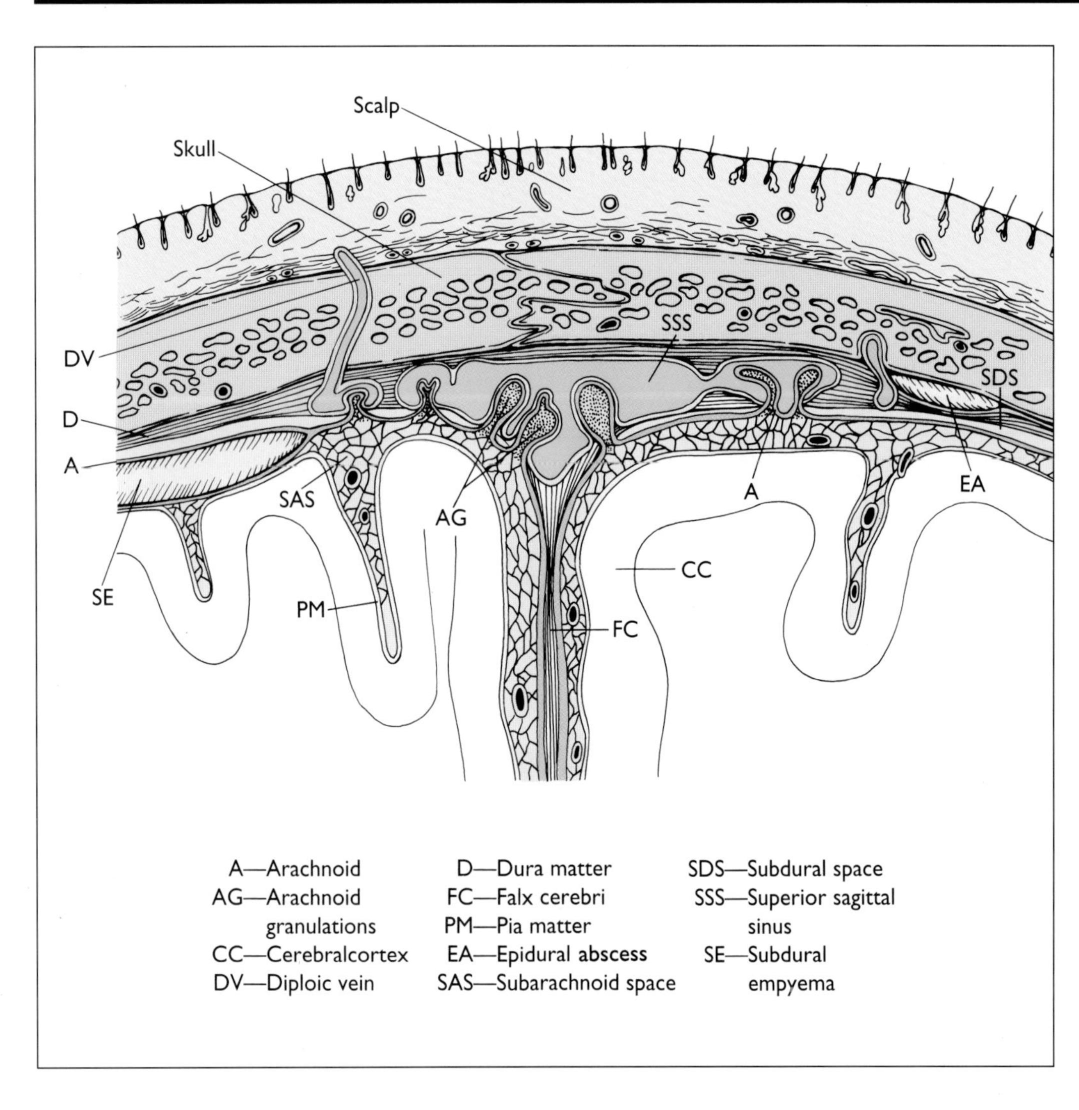

FIGURE 6-1 Anatomy of the intracranial dural spaces. Intracranial subdural empyema and epidural abscess are suppurative infections of the cerebral dural spaces and constitute neurologic emergencies. Intracranial subdural empyema may represent up to 23% of all intracranial infections, with intracranial epidural abscess being about half as common. A subdural empyema develops in the existing space between the dura and arachnoid, whereas cranial epidural abscess forms in the potential space between the dura and skull. The anatomy of the dural spaces helps explain the characteristic distribution of these infections. Intracranial epidural abscesses tend to be localized, limited by the dural attachment to the skull. Intracranial subdural empyemas are usually diffuse and occur most commonly over the cerebral hemispheres, where the subdural space is largest. Parafalcine, subtentorial, and multiple empyemas may be present in up to 20% of cases. (Small M, Dale BA: Intracranial suppuration 1968–1982—A 15-year review. *Clin Otolaryngol* 1984, 9:315–321.)

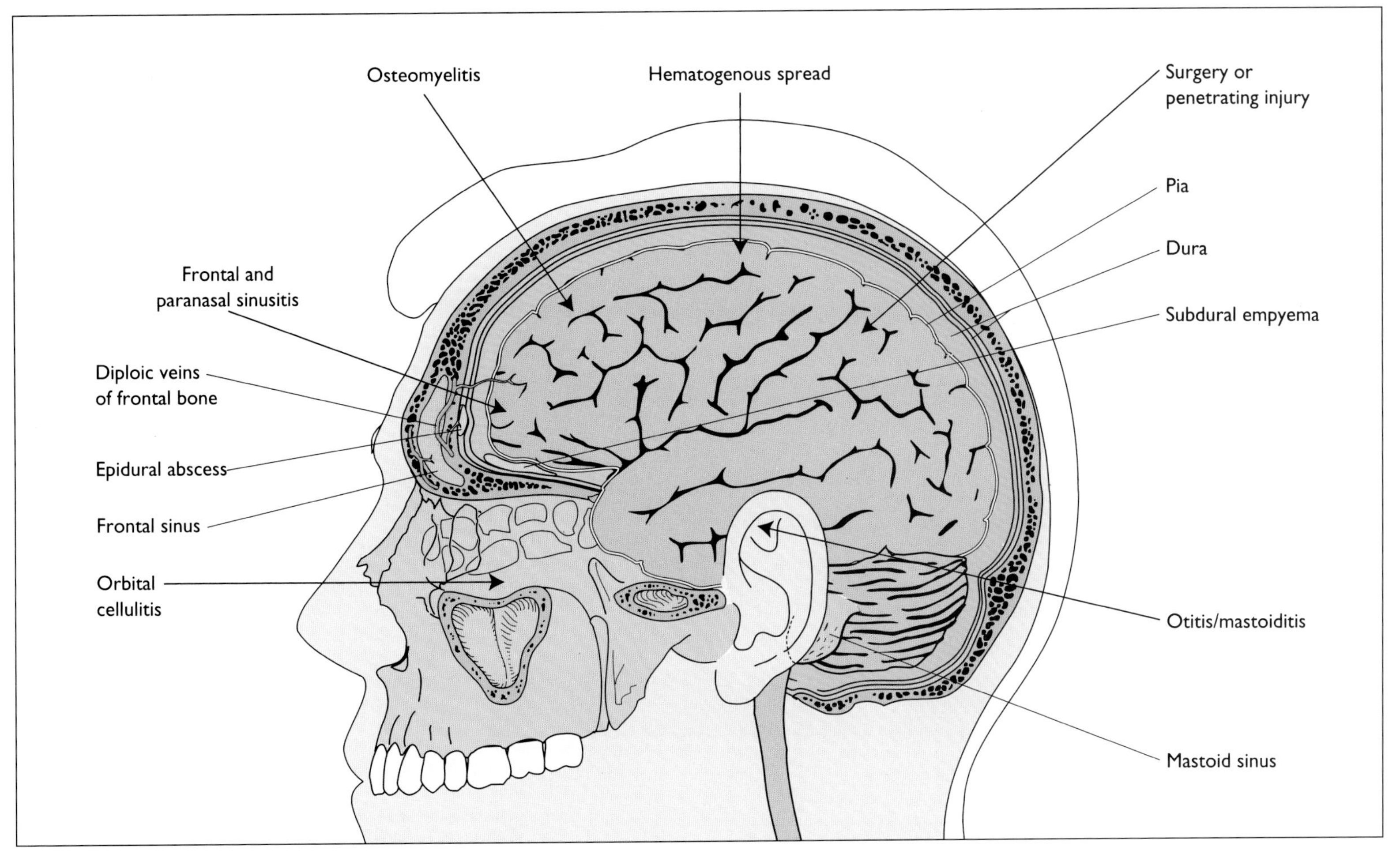

FIGURE 6-2 Pathogenesis of intracranial epidural abscess and subdural empyema. The most frequent sites of primary infection leading to cranial subdural empyema or epidural abscess are the paranasal sinuses. Cranial bones, dura, and galea have an interconnected blood supply with diploic (valveless) veins. These veins can allow sinus or superficial skin infections access to the dural spaces via hematogenous spread. Cranial epidural abscess usually arises by contiguous spread of infection from the sinuses or adjacent osteomyelitis but may even develop as a complication of cranial subdural empyema. Organisms commonly causing intracranial epidural abscess and subdural empyema are related to the primary source of infection. Aerobic and anaerobic streptococci are most common with sinus sources, and staphylococci are more often seen with facial infections, penetrating injuries, or cranial surgery. (Mauser HW, Tulleken CA: Subdural empyema: a review of 48 patients. *Clin Neurol Neurosurg* 1984, 86:255–263.)

Organisms causing intracranial parameningeal infections	
Staphylococci	
Staphylococcus aureus	16%
Coagulase-negative staphylococci	2%
Streptococci	
Streptococcus pneumoniae	3%
Other streptococci	27%
Aerobic bacilli	
Enterobacteriaceae	12%
Other aerobes	12%
Anaerobic bacilli	10%
Culture negative	28%
Mixed infection	9%

FIGURE 6-3 Organisms causing intracranial parameningeal infections. Exact incidence data are unknown but can be estimated from case reports. The data in this table are compiled from three recent case series totaling over 150 patients. There is a high proportion of *Streptococcus milleri* found among the other streptococcal infections. In the anaerobic group, *Bacteroides fragilis* is the most common organism isolated. Aerobic bacilli include a wide variety of pathogens, including *Haemophilus influenzae, Pseudomonas aeruginosa*, and other gram-negative rods. In contrast, a review by Helfgott *et al.* of over 200 case reports prior to 1989 showed streptococci to be the predominant organism (48% of the total). Coagulase-positive staphylococci were present in 11%, coagulase-negative staphylococci in 5%, and a variety of gram-negative and anaerobic bacilli in 13%. No organisms were identified in 34% of the cases. (Hlavin ML, Kaminiski HJ, Fenstermaker RA, White RJ: Intracranial suppuration: a modern decade of postoperative subdural empyema and epidural abscess. *Neurosurgery* 1994, 34:974–981. Pathak A, Sharma BS, Mathuriya SN, *et al.*: Controversies in the management of subdural empyema. *Acta Neurochir* 1990, 102:25–32. Bok APL, Peter JC: Subdural empyema: burr holes or craniotomy. *J Neurosurg* 1993, 78:574–578. Helfgott DC, Weingarten K, Hartman BJ: Subdural empyema. *In* Scheld WM, *et al.* (eds.): *Infections of the Central Nervous System.* New York: Raven Press; 1991:487–498.)

Primary source infections causing cranial subdural empyema

	Study, *n*			
	Zimmerman	Bannister	Pathak	Bok
Sinus	41	68	0	59
Otic	2	23	37	21
Trauma or neurosurgery	33	8	32	9
Hematogenous	2	3	0	0
Meningitis	14	0	5	0
Other	0	0	2	0
Unknown	8	0	24	11

FIGURE 6-4 Primary source infections causing cranial subdural empyema. By far, the most common cause of intracranial subdural empyema is paranasal sinusitis, accounting for approximately 50% of cases in most series. Cranial epidural abscess arises most often by contiguous spread of infection. A recent series of 27 patients with postoperative parameningeal infections found 14 epidural abscesses, four subdural empyemas, and nine patients with both infections simultaneously. (Hlavin ML, Kaminiski HJ, Fenstermaker RA, White RJ: Intracranial suppuration: a modern decade of postoperative subdural empyema and epidural abscess. *Neurosurgery* 1994, 34:974–981. Zimmerman RD, Leeds NE, Danzinger A: Subdural empyema: CT findings. *Radiology* 1984, 150:417–422. Bannister G, Williams B, Smith S: Treatment of subdural empyema. *J Neurosurg* 1981, 55:82–88. Pathak A, Sharma BS, Mathuriya SN, *et al.*: Controversies in the management of subdural empyema. *Acta Neurochir* 1990, 102:25–32. Bok APL, Peter JC: Subdural empyema: burr holes or craniotomy. *J Neurosurg* 1993, 78:574–578.

Presenting signs and symptoms of intracranial subdural empyema and epidural abscess

Cranial subdural empyema	Cranial epidural abscess
Patient usually acutely ill at presentation:	Infection often an indolent course:
Fever	Headache
Headache	Fever
Depressed consciousness	Seizures
Hemiparesis	Focal neurologic signs
Seizures	Altered mental status
Malaise	
Gaze palsies/ataxia	
Nuchal rigidity	

Figure 6-5 Presenting signs and symptoms of intracranial subdural empyema and epidural abscess. Cranial subdural empyema and epidural abscess should be included in the differential diagnosis of any patient presenting with fever and focal neurologic deficits. Routine serologic testing rarely helps in diagnosing these disorders. Patients usually have a mild leukocytosis, but in some cases the total leukocyte count may be normal. Cerebrospinal fluid (CSF) may demonstrate signs of inflammation, including polymorphonuclear cells and elevated protein level. Particularly in cases of cranial epidural abscess, however, the CSF results may be normal. Blood and CSF cultures can assist in identifying the causative organism.

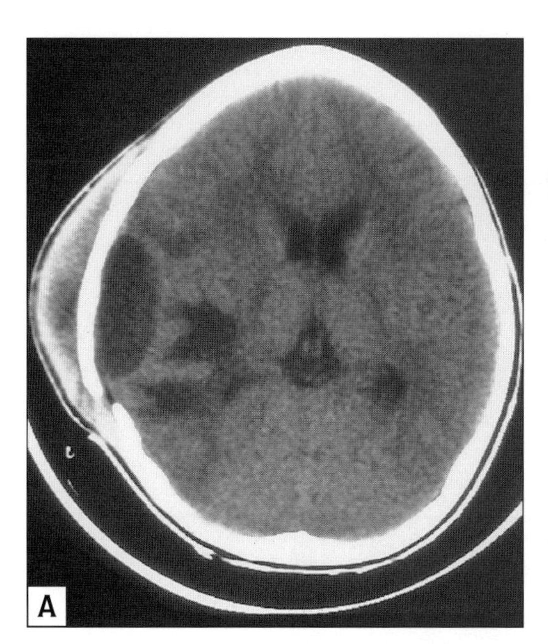

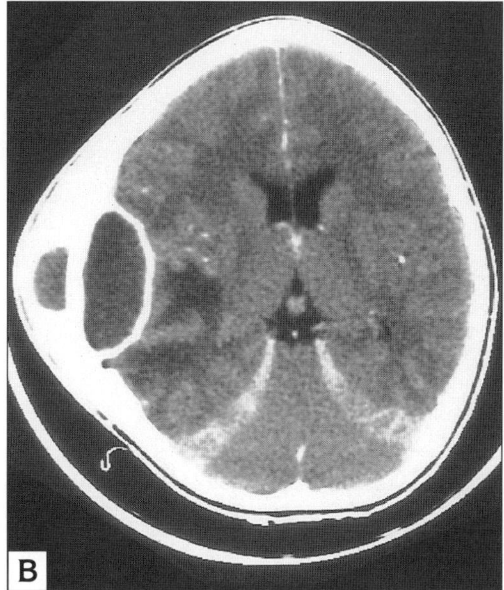

Figure 6-6 Typical computed tomographic (CT) appearance of an intracranial epidural abscess. This patient had an infected subgaleal hematoma which caused the epidural abscess. **A**, An uncontrasted CT scan shows a large, low-density mass with well-defined margins where the dura is being pulled away from the skull. There is prominent edema of the underlying cerebral hemisphere. **B**, The second CT with contrast demonstrates very intense contrast enhancement of the abscess rim. Note that the subgaleal abscess also enhances. Although CT scanning is usually adequate to diagnose an intracranial epidural abscess, some infections may be missed so magnetic resonance (MR) imaging should be considered if CT scanning is not diagnostic.

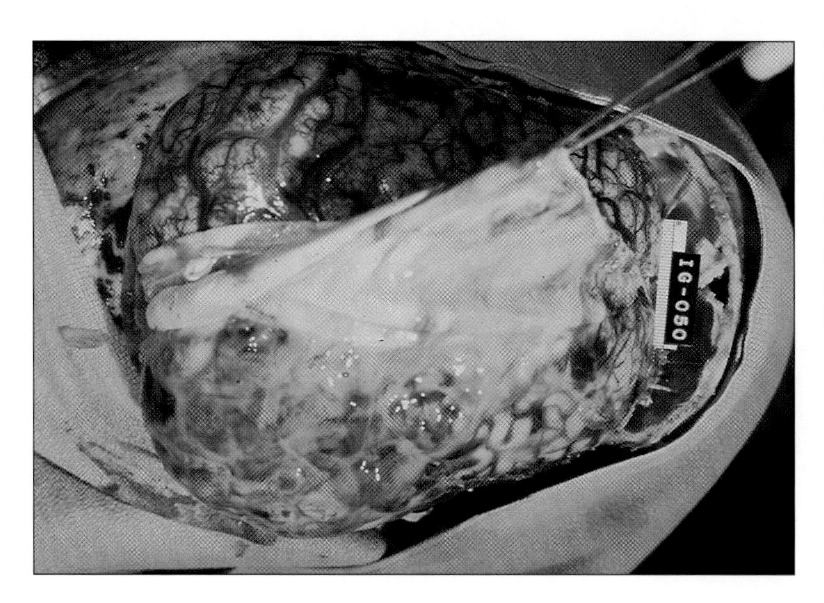

Figure 6-7 An autopsy specimen showing a cranial subdural empyema. Note the thick purulent material coating the surface of the brain and dura. The left hemisphere, seen in the upper portion of the picture, is not involved. In comparison, meningitis, an infection in the subarachnoid space, usually affects the entire surface of the brain. This photograph clearly demonstrates pus between the arachnoid membrane and dura. Although cranial subdural empyema is often associated with brain abscess or cranial epidural abscess, it is rarely a complication of bacterial meningitis, except in children. (*Courtesy of* Dr. R. Scott Vandenberg.)

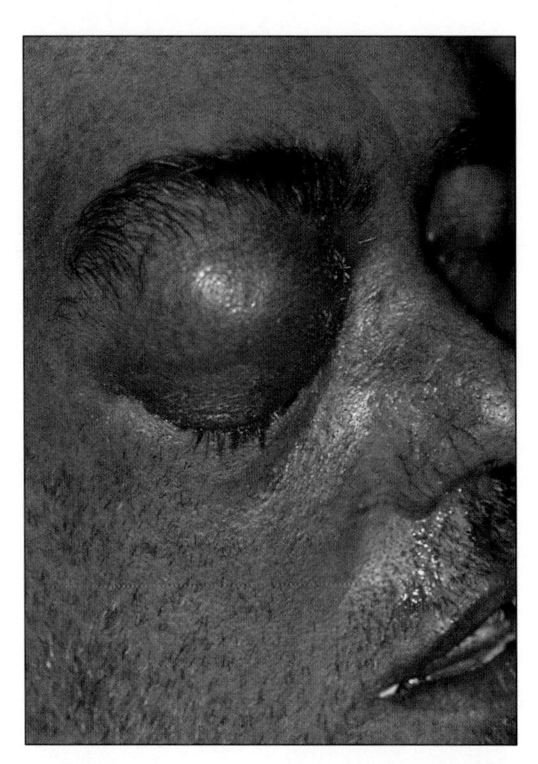

Figure 6-8 Clinical presentation of intracranial subdural empyema. Severe proptosis and orbital cellulitis are evident in a patient with known sinus disease. At presentation, he had a decreased level of consciousness, fever, and leukocytosis. Diagnosis of intracranial subdural empyema requires a high index of clinical suspicion because it can mimic other intracranial processes including meningitis, venous sinus thrombosis, and brain abscess. This patient's clinical presentation could be consistent with any of these diagnoses. (*Courtesy of* Dr. Stephen Park.)

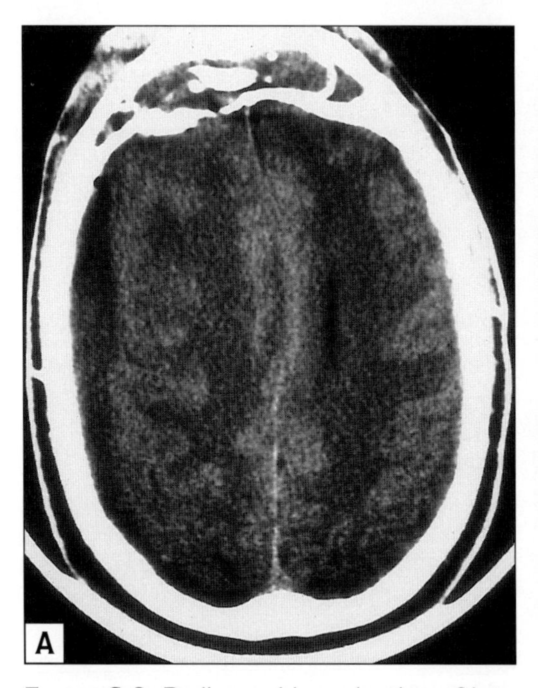

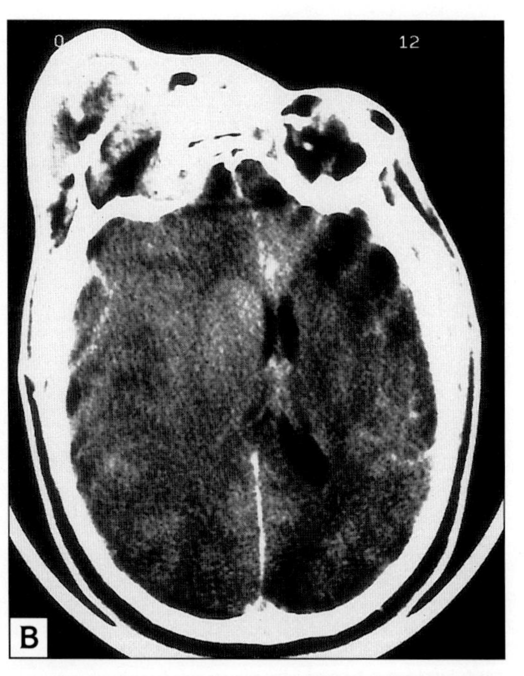

Figure 6-9 Radiographic evaluation of intracranial subdural empyema. **A**, An uncontrasted CT scan of the patient seen in Figure 6-8 shows the classic appearance of a subdural fluid collection. The fluid has a lentiform shape with a radiographic density similar to that of CSF and there is a mass effect on the underlying cortex. As opposed to a cranial epidural abscess, subdural empyema is more diffuse, with less distinct margins. **B**, CT image after intravenous contrast administration in the same patient again shows the prominent proptosis and mass effect with midline shift. There is only mild contrast enhancement of the empyema, in contrast to the dense enhancement seen with an intracranial epidural abscess. CT scanning is adequate in most cases of cranial subdural empyema, although a small or immature empyema might be missed. A subdural empyema might be mistaken for a chronic subdural hematoma if contrast is not given. If there is clinical suspicion of empyema and CT scanning is not diagnostic, then MR imaging is warranted.

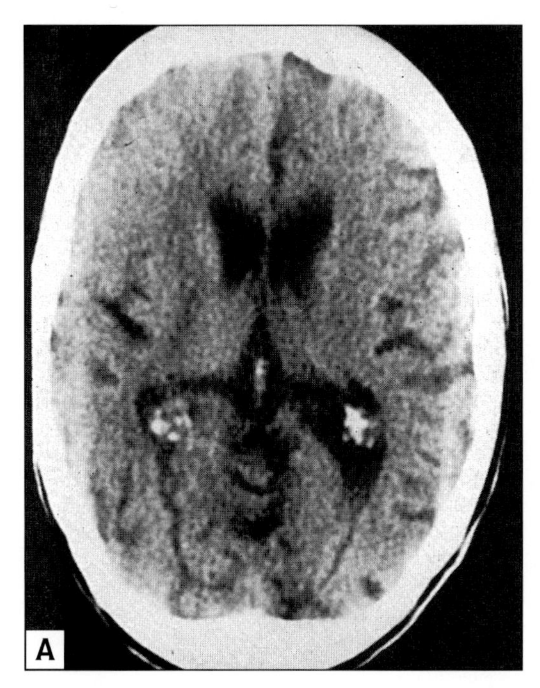

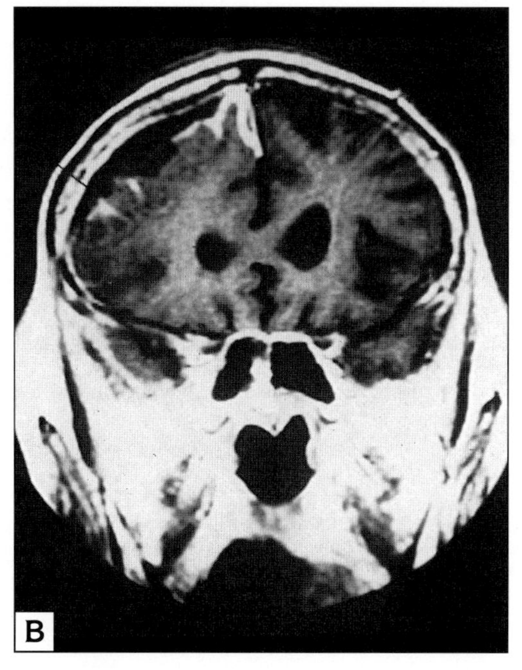

FIGURE 6-10 CT scan (**A**) and gadolinium-enhanced MR image (**B**) in cranial subdural empyema. Although adequate in most cases, a contrast-enhanced CT scan may miss some cases of cranial subdural empyema. The advantages of CT scanning are its speed and the relative ease of obtaining a quality image, as well as its availability in most hospitals. In one community hospital-based study five of six cranial subdural empyemas and two of two cranial epidural abscesses were correctly identified by CT scanning. (Harris LF, Haws FP, Triplett JN Jr, Maccubin DA: Subdural empyema and epidural abscess. *South Med J* 1987, 80:1254–1258.) The utility of CT scanning may be diminished in postneurosurgical patients. In a recent study of 27 patients with postsurgical abscesses, the CT scan was misread as showing no infection in eight cases (30%). (Hlavin ML, Kaminiski HJ, Fenstermaker RA, White RJ: Intracranial suppuration: a modern decade of postoperative subdural empyema and epidural abscess. *Neurosurgery* 1994, 34:974–981.) MRI is not only better able to detect and appropriately identify parameningeal infections but it more definitively demonstrates the extent and complexity (*ie*, loculations) of the infection. (Weingarten K, Zimmerman RD, Becker RD, *et al.*: Subdural and epidural empyemas: MR imaging. *AJR* 1989, 152:615–621. The CT scan (*panel A*) shows effacement of the sulci over the right hemisphere, without obvious fluid collection or evidence of empyema. Gadolinium-enhanced coronal MR image (*panel B*) obtained shortly after the CT scan shows a large subdural empyema. (*Courtesy of* Dr. Rick Harnsberger. *From* Greenlee JE: Subdural empyema. *In* Mandell GL, *et al.* (eds.): *Principles and Practice of Infectious Diseases*, 4th ed. New York: Churchill Livingstone; 1995:901; with permission.)

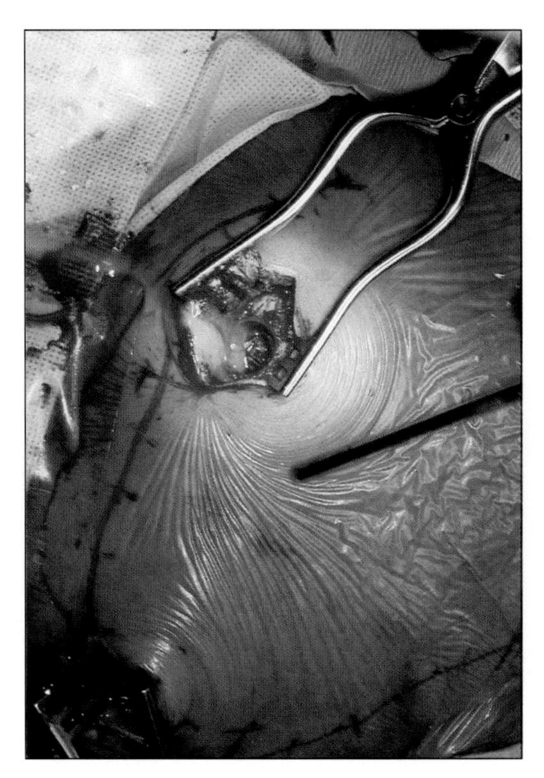

FIGURE 6-11 Burr hole drainage of intracranial subdural empyema. Extensive purulent material is evident at the burr hole site in the patient seen in Figure 6-8. The subdural space was irrigated and material sent for culture, which grew *Streptococcus intermedius.* Controversy abounds about whether burr holes are sufficient for drainage or whether craniotomy is needed. Two studies comparing outcomes in patients treated with burr holes versus craniotomy found a clear benefit for craniotomy. It may be that the wider opening allows for more complete draining of pus as well as helps to find hidden loculated areas. (Wackym PA, Canalis RF, Feuerman T: Subdural empyema of otorhinological origin. *J Laryngol Otol* 1990, 104:118–122.) Another study, however, demonstrated excellent results with burr hole drainage. (Bok APL, Peter JC: Subdural empyema: Burr holes or craniotomy? *J Neurosurg* 1993, 78:574–578.) Craniotomy is a more extensive surgical procedure, with a greater risk of complication. These authors attributed their good outcome to use of CT scanning to localize collections of pus. (*Courtesy of* Dr. Stephen Park.)

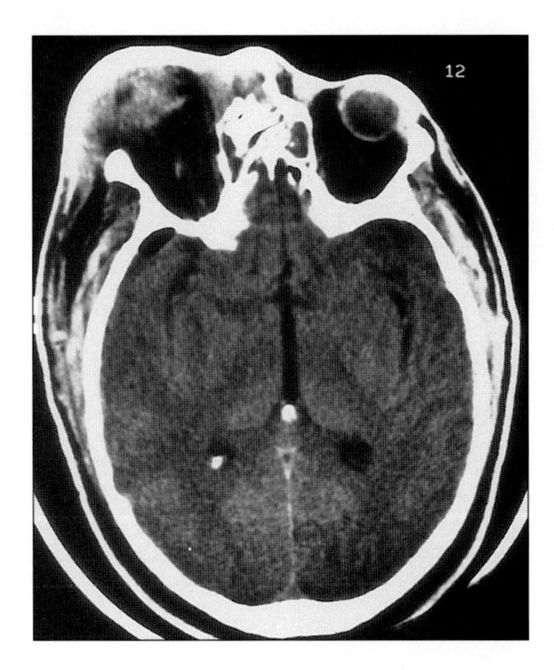

Figure 6-12 Postdrainage CT scan in intracranial subdural empyema. A CT scan the day after drainage of the cranial subdural empyema shows complete resolution of the empyema, edema, and mass effect. Outcome in cases of intracranial subdural empyema is largely related to the patient's level of responsiveness on presentation; in general, a lower level of consciousness is associated with a poorer outcome. Patients who are initially unresponsive have a greater than 50% mortality. Neurologic sequelae in survivors include seizures (up to 40% of cases), hemiparesis, and cognitive dysfunction.

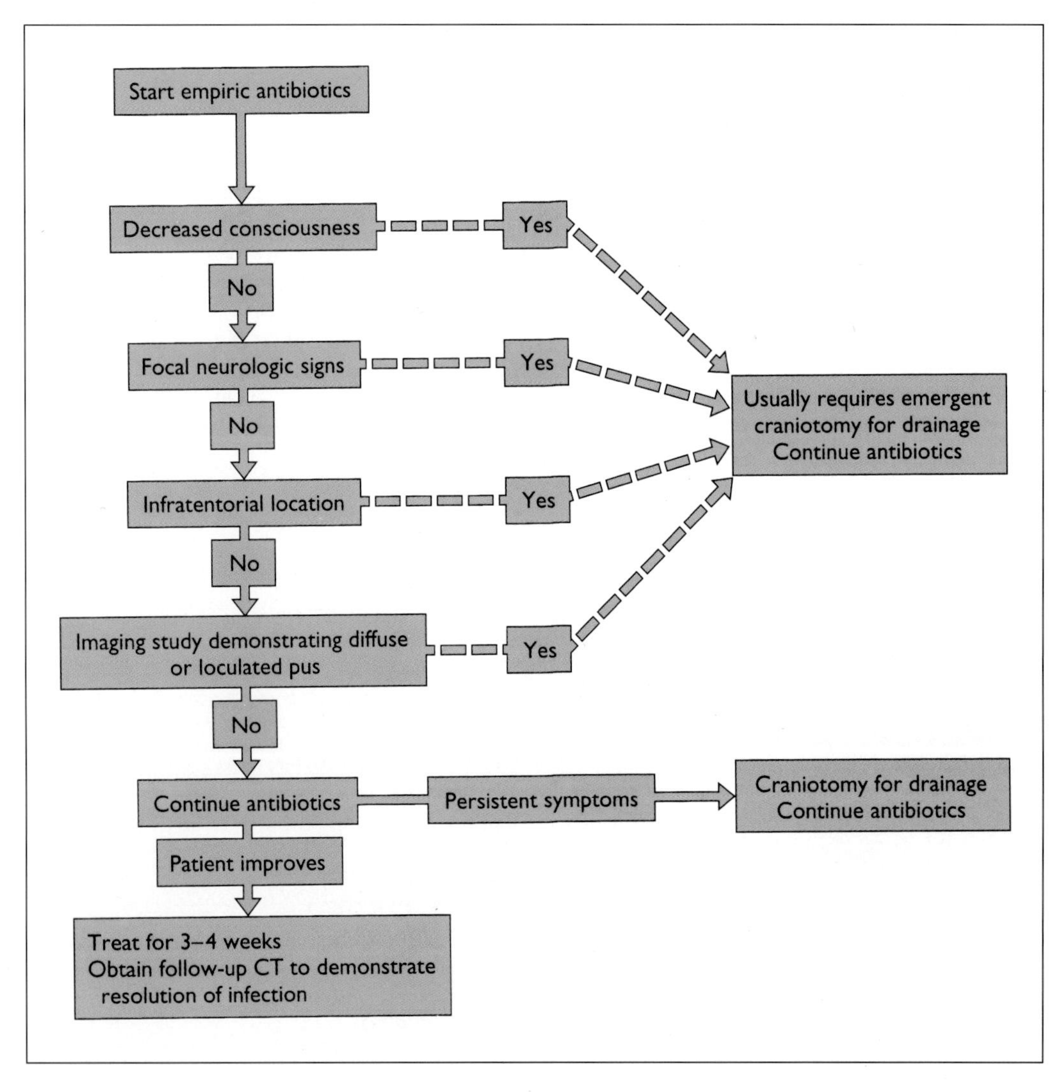

Figure 6-13 Decision tree for treatment of cranial epidural abscess and subdural empyema. The key to a good outcome in cranial subdural empyema or epidural abscess is rapid diagnosis. The clinician must not delay in initiating antibiotic therapy (*see* Figure 6-14). Lumbar puncture is not routinely indicated, as the findings are frequently nonspecific, the procedure consumes valuable time, and there is the risk of cerebral herniation. Conservative treatment of cranial infections demands continuous neurologic monitoring for clinical deterioration. Any worsening in the patient's status requires prompt imaging and possible surgical intervention.

Empiric antibiotic therapy for cranial or spinal infections

Presumed etiology	Likely pathogens	Empiric antibiotics
Hematogenous spread or unknown source	*Staphylococcus aureus* Streptococci including *viridans* Gram-negative organisms	Penicillinase-resistant penicillin *plus* 3rd generation cephalosporin
Postsurgical or penetrating injury	*Staphylococcus aureus* Gram-negative organisms *Staphylococcus epidermidis* (rarely)	Penicillinase-resistant penicillin *plus* 3rd-generation cephalosporin Vancomycin *plus* 3rd-generation cephalosporin
Contiguous spread	*Staphylococcus aureus* Gram-negative organisms Anaerobes	Penicillinase-resistant penicillin *plus* 3rd-generation cephalosporin *plus* metronidazole

FIGURE 6-14 Empirical antibiotic therapy for cranial or spinal infections. Empirical treatment for infections of the dural spaces is based upon the presumed mechanism of infection. The considerations are the same for intracranial and intraspinal infections. Antibiotic therapy can be adjusted accordingly when culture and sensitivity data become available; however, in a significant proportion of these infections, no organisms can be cultured, due to prior antibiotic treatment or poor specimen handling. If *Pseudomonas aeruginosa* is a suspected pathogen, an antipseudomonal cephalosporin (ceftazidime) and an aminoglycoside should be used. Multiple organisms can often be cultured from a single abscess or empyema, and these and anaerobic infections frequently may be missed by inadequate specimen handling.

SPINAL EPIDURAL ABSCESS AND SUBDURAL EMPYEMA

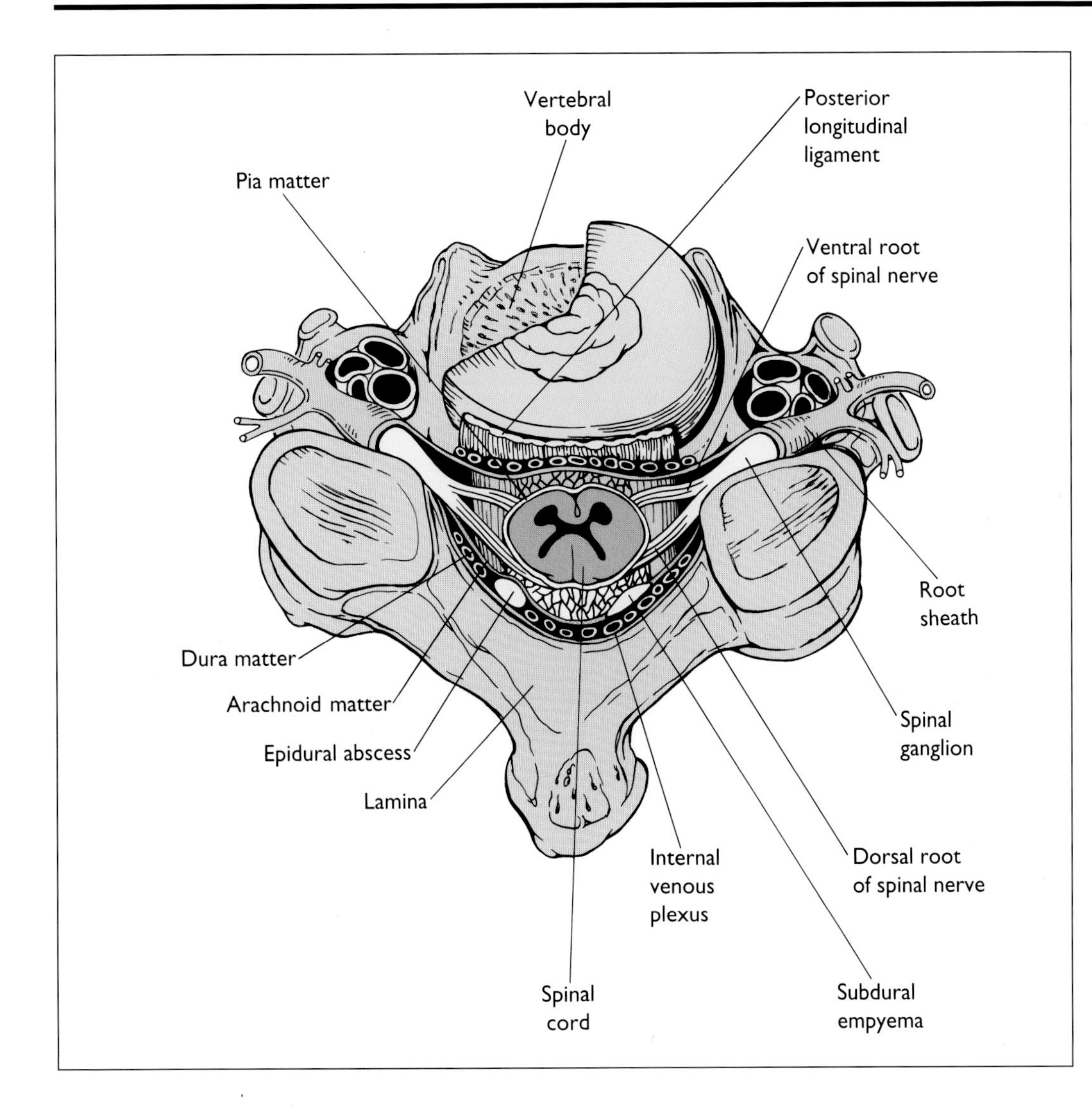

FIGURE 6-15 Anatomy of the spinal column. The arachnoid and dura are closely approximated, so the spinal subdural space is only a potential space. Infection of this space, spinal subdural empyema, is quite rare; no more than 50 cases are reported in the literature. Spinal epidural abscess, however, is quite common, with an incidence that may approach 2/10,000 hospital admissions. The epidural space is a true space, containing fat and the internal venous plexus, making it an ideal site for seeding from blood-borne infections. (Hlavin ML, Kaminski HJ, Ross JS, Ganz E: Spinal epidural abscess: a ten year perspective. *Neurosurgery* 1990, 27:177–184.)

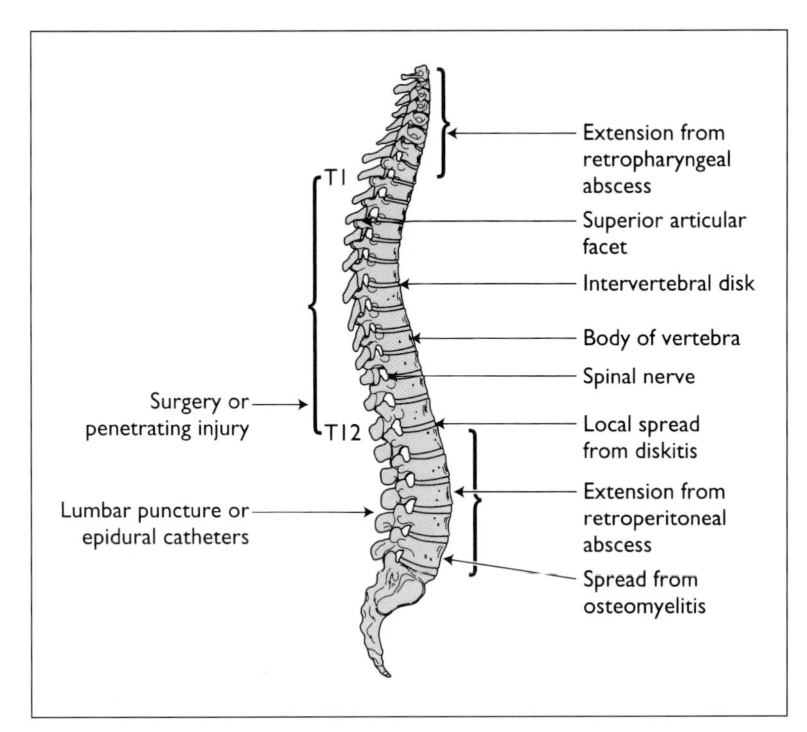

FIGURE 6-16 Pathogenesis of spinal epidural abscess. Hematogenous spread is most often the cause of spinal epidural abscess, although up to 50% of cases may have no primary source identified. Primary sources include infections of the soft tissue, skin, urinary tract, upper respiratory tract, abdomen, and heart (endocarditis). Intravenous drug abuse is also implicated. Direct extension from vertebral osteomyelitis or diskitis or iatrogenic (*ie*, epidural catheters) is also common. Spinal epidural abscess can occur anywhere along the spinal cord, but there is a predilection for the lumbar (40%–50%) and thoracic (30%–40%) regions, with the cervical region less frequently involved (10%–20%). The lower portion of the spinal canal is wider and contains more epidural fat, which is thought to favor the formation of infection in these segments. Infections may be localized, often involving only one spinal segment, but usually several segments are affected. Occasionally, spinal epidural abscesses can be extensive and involve most of the length of the cord. (Hlavin ML, Kaminski HJ, Ross JS, Ganz E: Spinal epidural abscess: a ten year perspective. *Neurosurgery* 1990, 27:177–184.)

Microbiology of spinal epidural abscess

	Study, *n*			
	Darouiche (n = 43)	Hlavin (n = 40)	Nussbaum (n = 40)	Curling (n = 29)
Coagulase-negative staphylococci	4	2	2	1
Staphylococcus aureus	28	24	27	13
Streptococci	4	4	3	5
Pseudomonas aeruginosa	2	0	3	2
Escherichia coli	3	1	4	2
Other gram-negative bacilli	2	2	1	1
Anaerobes	1	1	0	1
Other	0	3	0	4
None isolated	1	0	3	0

FIGURE 6-17 Microbiology of spinal epidural abscess. The microbiology of spinal epidural abscess has changed dramatically from early reports when 95% of cases were caused by *Staphylococcus aureus*. Although *S. aureus* remains the predominant pathogen, infections due to streptococci, gram-negative bacilli, and multiple pathogens are increasing in numbers. Conversely, *Mycobacterium tuberculosis* is now isolated uncommonly. (Darouiche RO, Hamill RJ, Greenberg SB, *et al.*: Bacterial spinal epidural abscess: review of 43 cases and literature survey. *Medicine* 1992, 71:369–385. Hlavin ML, Kaminski HJ, Ross JS, Ganz E: Spinal epidural abscess: a ten year prospective. *Neurosurgery* 1990, 27:177–184. Nussbaum ES, Rigamonti D, Standiford H, *et al.*: Spinal epidural abscess: a report of 40 cases and review. *Surg Neurol* 1992, 38:225–231. Curling OD, Gower DJ, McWhorter JM: Changing concepts in spinal epidural abscess: a report of 29 cases. *Neurosurgery* 1990, 27:185–192.)

Clinical stages of spinal epidural abscess	
Stage I	Spinal ache usually at level of infection Possibly local edema, erythema, or percussion tenderness May last for weeks to months
Stage II	Radicular pain and paresthesias Progression over several days or < 1 day Headache, fever, and meningismus possible
Stage III	Impaired spinal cord function Urinary retention with progressive anesthesia and weakness May occur rapidly or over several days
Stage IV	Complete paralysis and anesthesia below the level of the abscess May develop within hours of the onset of Stage III

Figure 6-18 Clinical stages of spinal epidural abscess. The clinical features of spinal epidural abscess were first described in 1948 by Heusner and are still valid today. The rate of progression from stage I to stage IV varies dramatically between patients, and acute decompensation may occur over hours. (Heusner AP: Nontuberculous spinal epidural infections. *N Engl J Med* 1948, 239:845–854.)

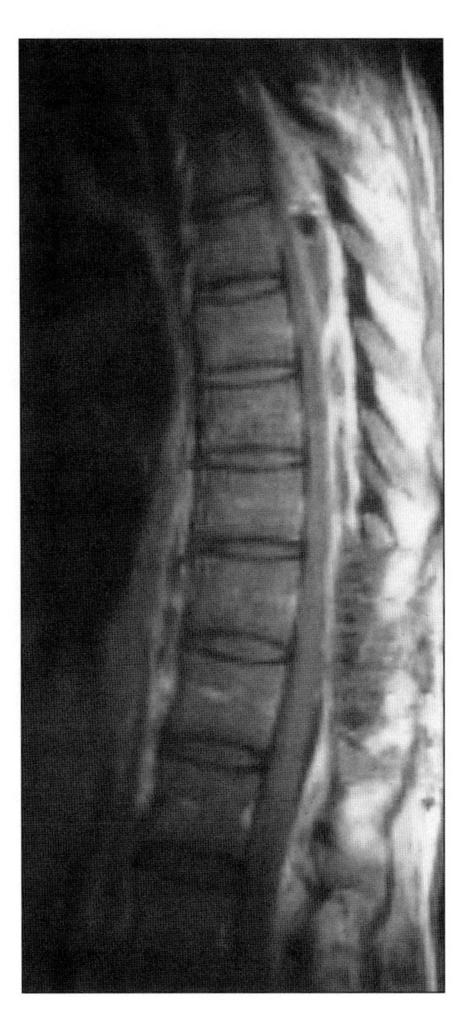

Figure 6-19 MR evaluation of spinal epidural abscess. A sagittal T1-weighted MR image after gadolinium-DTPA contrast administration demonstrates a large spinal epidural abscess in a patient who developed fever and back pain after a motor vehicle accident. There is an irregular enhancing septate lesion extending the length of the epidural space. The patient has already had a partial decompressive laminectomy from T9–11. MRI is becoming the preferred imaging study for spinal infections because of its high resolution, ability to image the entire length of the cord, ability to both localize infection and identify contiguous infections, and noninvasiveness. (Post MJD, Sze G, Quencer RM, *et al.*: Gadolinium-enhanced MR in spinal infection. *J Comput Assist Tomogr* 1990, 14:721–725.)

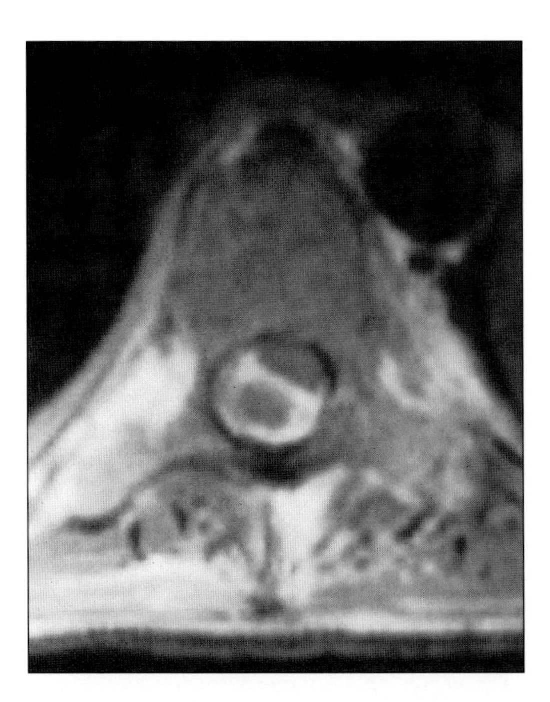

Figure 6-20 Prelaminectomy transverse MR image at T8 in the patient shown in Figure 6-19. An MR scan demonstrates a rim-enhancing extradural lesion that is clearly compressing and displacing the spinal cord. A history of antecedent back trauma is reported in as many as 35% of patients with spinal epidural abscess. The injury often occurs several days to weeks before the onset of symptoms and may be only a minor sprain or contusion. It is speculated that the injury causes a small hematoma in the epidural space, which acts as nidus for infection.

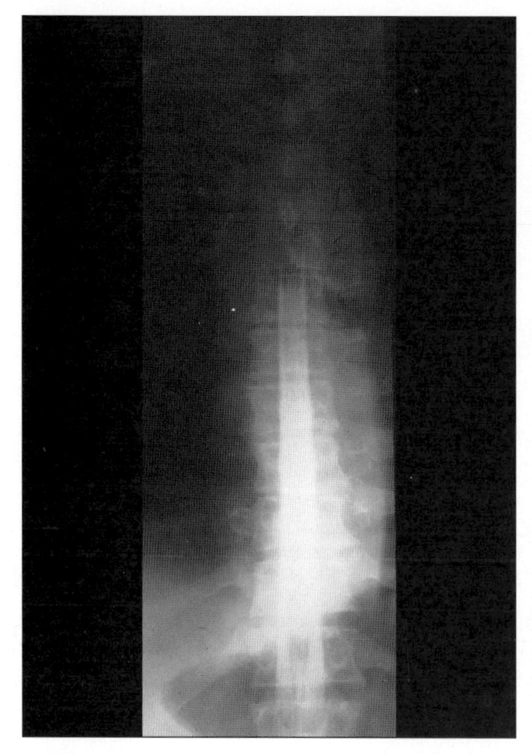

Figure 6-21 Lumbar myelogram revealing a complete spinal block in the thoracic region. The "feathered" appearance of the dye column at the level of the block is a typical sign of an epidural mass. Although myelography had been the study of choice for identifying spinal epidural abscess, MRI is now preferred. A lumbar myelogram can localize only the lower level of a spinal block and gives no information about the extent of the process. Any epidural lesion that compresses the thecal sac can cause a spinal block, so the finding is not specific for abscess.

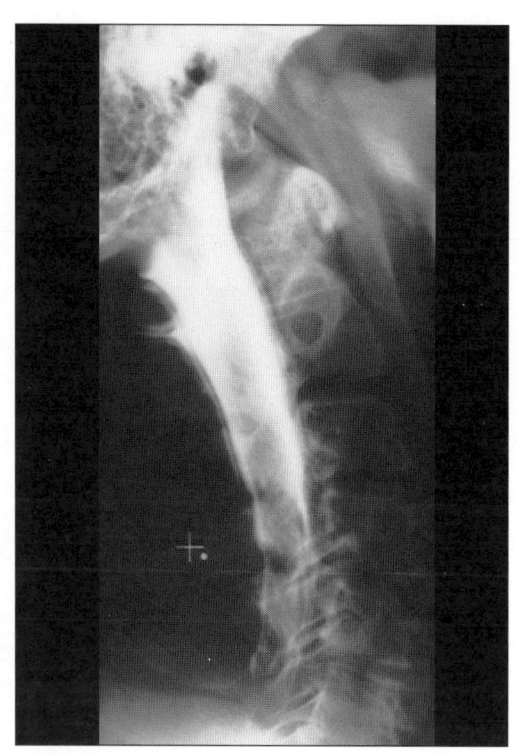

Figure 6-22 Cervical myelogram demonstrating a complete spinal block in the cervical region. To localize a spinal epidural abscess completely, myelograms must be performed from both above and below the abscess. A myelogram may fail to identify a spinal epidural abscess if it only displaces epidural fat without compressing the thecal sac.

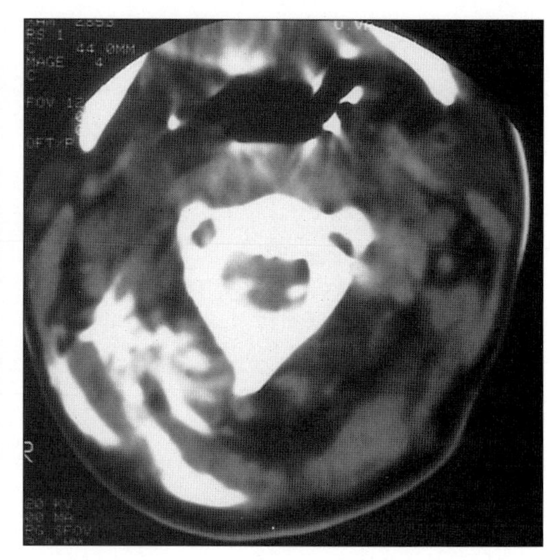

Figure 6-23 CT-myelography of a cervical epidural abscess. This CT-myelogram shows a contrast-enhancing rim around the cervical spinal cord that is being compressed by an epidural mass. CT scanning after myelography can offer more information about an epidural abscess than either study alone. In one study of 11 patients who had both CT-myelograms and MRI, the MRI was found superior in four cases, the CT scan better in three cases, and the studies of equal value in four cases. MRI has the overall advantage in that it avoids the additional complications and morbidity associated with an invasive procedure.

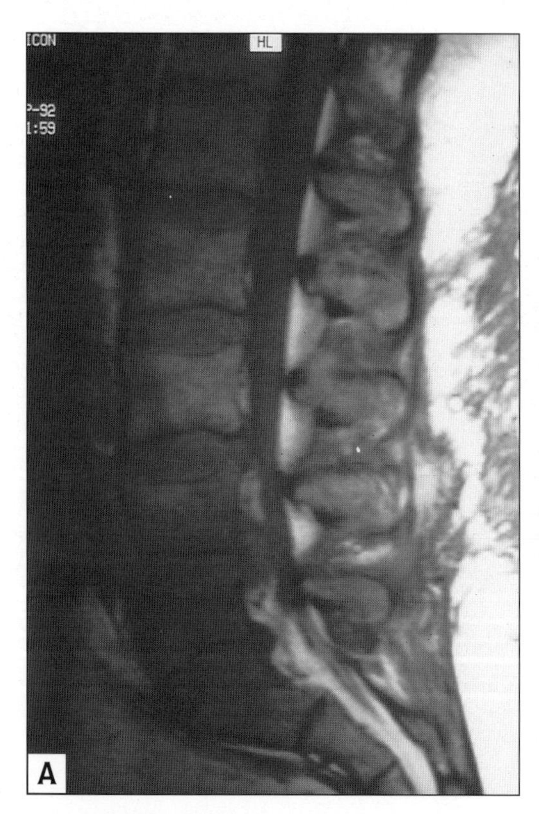

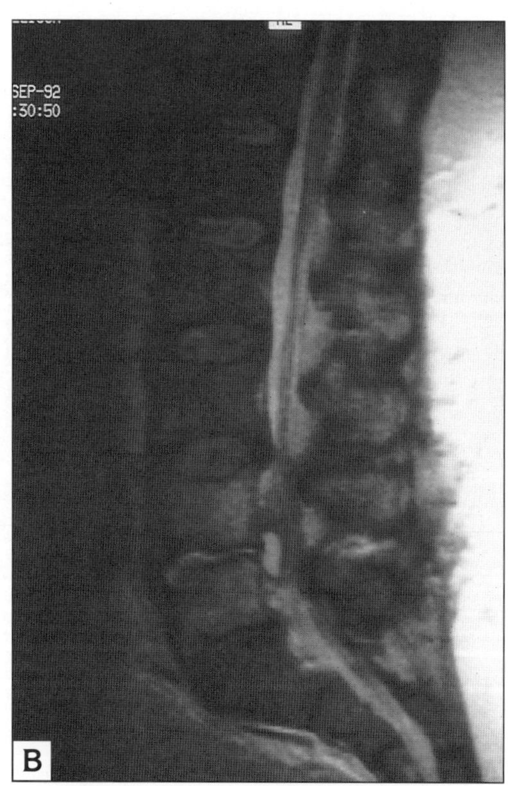

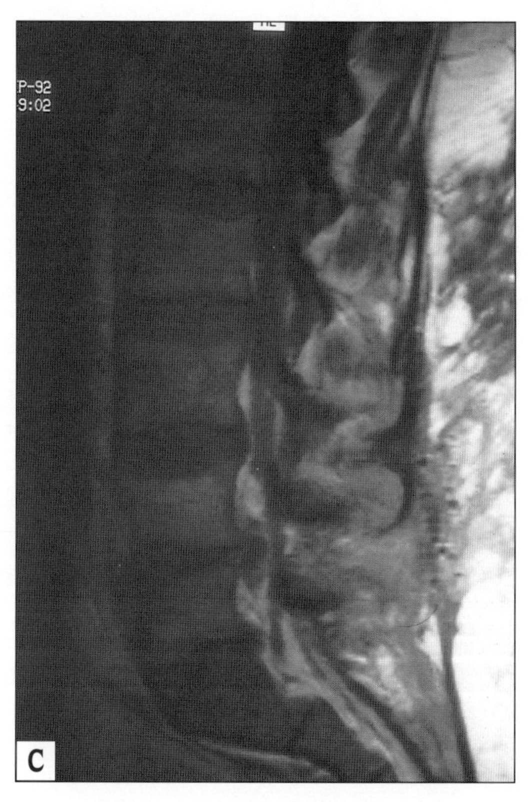

Figure 6-24 Classic appearance of a spinal epidural abscess in a standard MRI sequence. A 37-year-old woman had a 1-week history of back pain. No primary source of infection was identified. **A**, The T1-weighted image shows a low-density mass posterior to the L4–5 vertebral bodies. **B**, On T2 weighting, the abscess appears as a hyperintense lesion compressing the thecal sac. Note the different appearance of the mild disk herniation at L3–4. **C**, Intravenous gadolinium-DTPA produces a mild rim enhancement of the abscess.

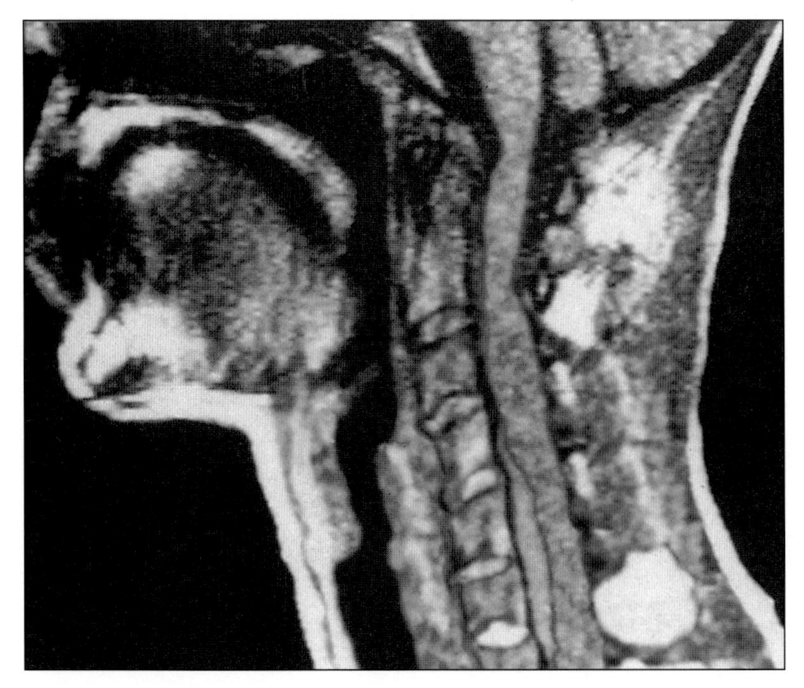

FIGURE 6-25 T1-weighted MR scan of a cervical spinal subdural empyema. The presentation of spinal subdural empyema is similar to that of spinal epidural abscess, with fever, back pain, and radiculopathy being most common. Mild symptoms may be present for several weeks, but then patients may rapidly develop para- or quadraparesis over a few hours. MR scanning will reveal an extra-axial inflammatory mass, often displacing the spinal cord. MR imaging cannot, however, differentiate spinal epidural abscess from subdural empyema. The diagnosis can only be confirmed surgically by opening the dura and demonstrating a subdural location for the infection. In this image, increased signal intensity is apparent anterior to the cord at C4–6 (*arrow*). There is reversal of the normal lordotic curve and spinal stenosis with cord compression. (Levy ML, Wieder BH, Schneider J, *et al.*: Subdural empyema of the cervical spine: clinicopathological correlates and magnetic resonance imaging. *J Neurosurg* 1993, 79:929–935; with permission.)

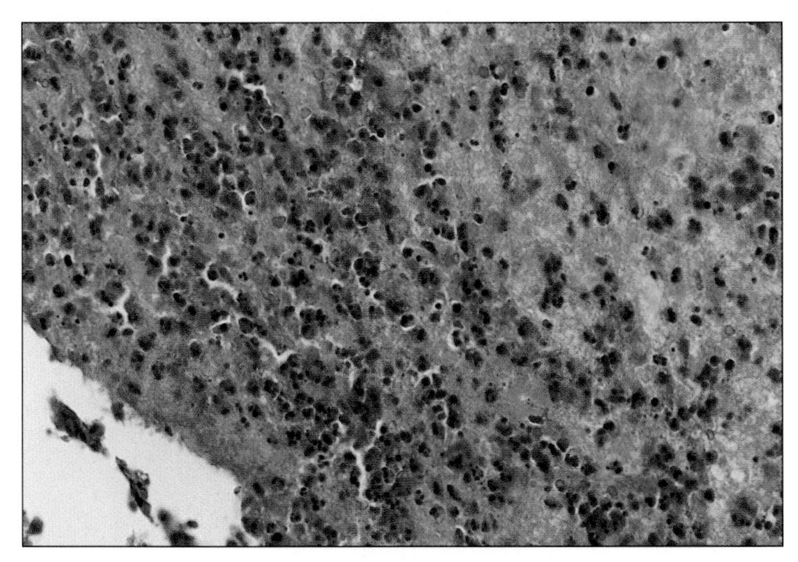

FIGURE 6-26 Histopathologic examination revealing pus in material obtained from the site of a spinal epidural abscess. The patient had fever, back pain, and radicular symptoms after lumbar laminectomy. The histopathologic findings are typical for an acute suppurative infection (pus), consisting of prominent inflammatory cells on an amorphous background of protein and cellular debris. No bacteria are seen in this specimen. Greater than 90% of patients will have an infectious agent identified, either from the operative site or by blood culture. Inability to culture organisms may be caused by antibiotic treatment prior to debridement or by inadequate specimen handling. (Hematoxylin-eosin stain.) (*Courtesy of* Dr. David Eberhard.)

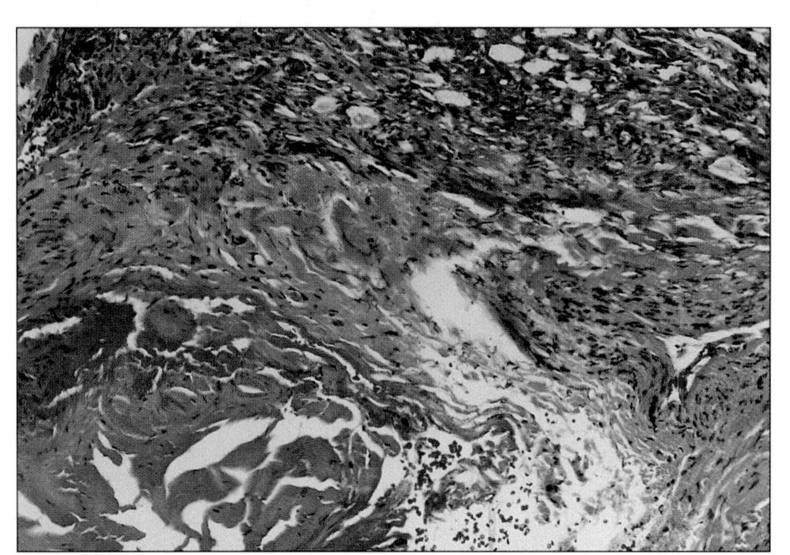

FIGURE 6-27 Histopathologic examination revealing granulation tissue in material obtained from the site of a spinal epidural abscess. This patient had back pain, fever, and a history of osteomyelitis. The upper portion of the field demonstrates an area of organizing inflammatory tissue (granulation tissue). There is a dense mononuclear infiltrate and formation of neovascular channels. The inflammatory mass is tightly adherent to underlying fibrous tissue, the dura. Spinal epidural abscesses have classically been divided into two types: an acute group with rapid progression of neurologic deficits over hours to days, and a chronic group with an indolent or fluctuating course over weeks to years. This distinction, however, does not appear to have any bearing on overall outcome, nor does it relate to the pathologic findings of pus or granulation tissue. (Hematoxylin-eosin stain.) (Del Curling O Jr, Gower DJ, McWhorter JM: Changing concepts in spinal epidural abscess: a report of 29 cases. *Neurosurgery* 1990, 27:185–192.)

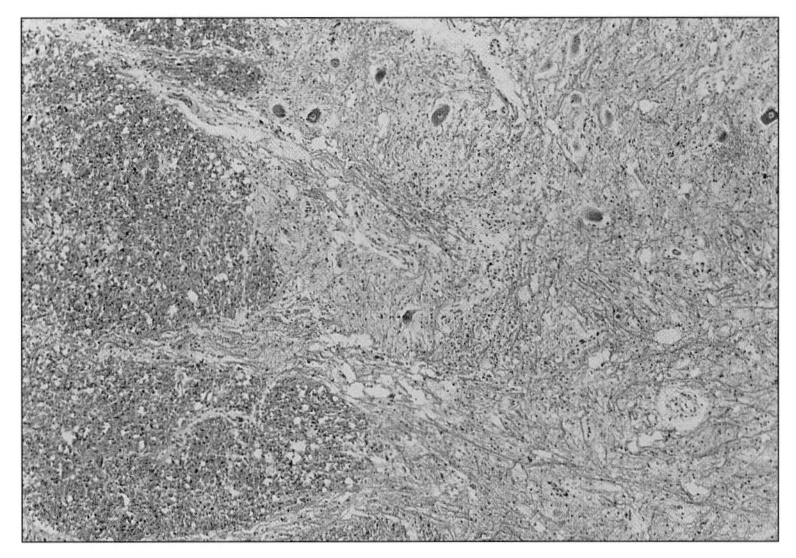

FIGURE 6-28 Photomicrograph of spinal cord underlying an epidural abscess. A specimen obtained at autopsy shows features of subacute to chronic injury to the spinal cord, with edema, neuronal loss, and inflammatory infiltrate. The exact mechanism by which a spinal epidural abscess can cause acute cord injury is debated. Some authors favor a vascular mechanism, involving either arterial infarction, venous congestion leading to edema and ischemia, or venous thrombophlebitis. Others believe that mechanical compression is the primary insult. Regardless of the mechanism, patients who appear stable can progress rapidly from no neurologic deficit to paraplegia in a few hours. (Luxol fast blue stain). (Baker AS, Ojemann RG, Swartz MN, *et al.*: Spinal epidural abscess. *N Engl J Med* 1975, 293:463–468. Lasker BR, Harter DH: Cervical epidural abscess. *Neurology* 1987, 37:1747–1753.)

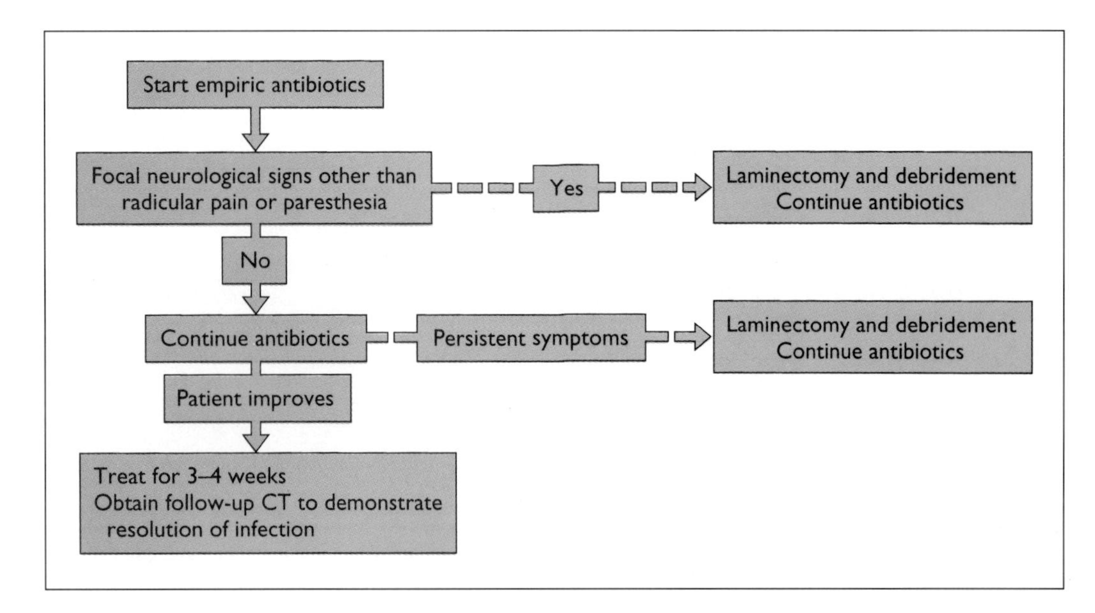

FIGURE 6-29 Decision tree for treatment of spinal epidural abscess. The key to a good outcome in treatment of spinal epidural abscess is prompt treatment. The diagnosis of spinal epidural abscess may be difficult, as the presenting symptoms are often mild. The diagnosis needs to be considered in any patient with fever and back pain or radicular symptoms. Conservative treatment of spinal infections demands continuous neurologic monitoring for clinical deterioration. Any worsening in the patient's status requires prompt imaging and possible surgical intervention. If there is an associated osteomyelitis, at least 4 weeks of therapy is required, and a longer duration may be needed if chronic osteomyelitis is suspected. There is limited information about ideal therapy for spinal subdural empyema because the condition is rare. Most authors recommend immediate laminectomy, drainage, and irrigation in addition to antibiotic therapy. (*See* Fig. 6-14).

SELECTED BIBLIOGRAPHY

Brock DG, Bleck TP: Extra-axial suppurations of the central nervous system. *Semin Neurol* 1992, 12:263–272.

Gellin BG, Weingarten K, Gamache FW Jr, Hartman BJ: Epidural abscess. *In* Scheld WM, Whitley RJ, Durack DT (eds.): *Infections of the Central Nervous System*. New York: Raven Press; 1991:499–514.

Harris LF, Haws FP, Triplett JN Jr, Maccubbin DA: Subdural empyema and epidural abscess. *South Med J* 1987, 80:1254–1258.

Helfgott DC, Weingarten K, Hartman BJ: Subdural empyema. *In* Scheld WM, Whitley RJ, Durack DT (eds.): *Infections of the Central Nervous System*. New York: Raven Press; 1991:487–498.

CHAPTER 7

Venous Sinus Infections

Oren Sagher

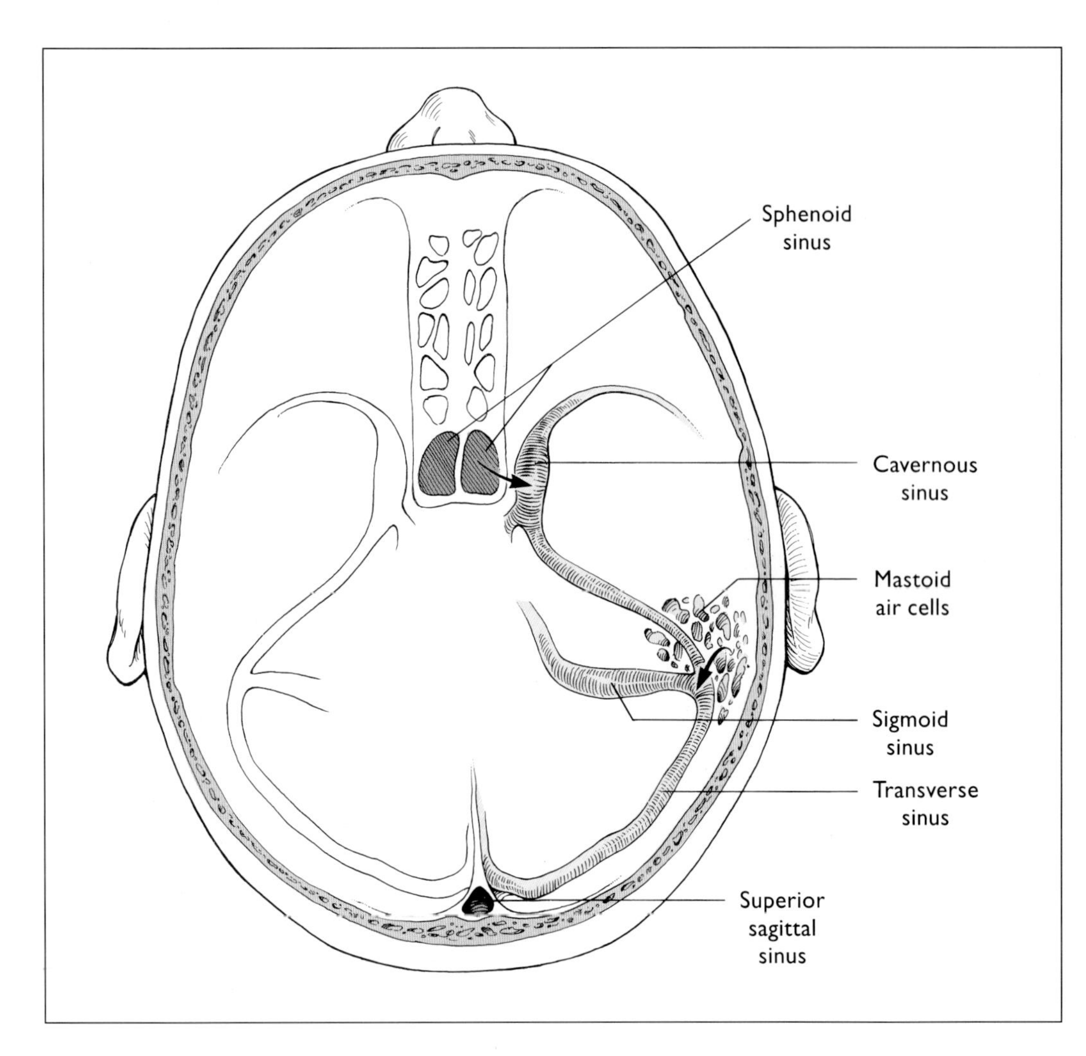

FIGURE 7-1 Dural venous sinuses. Septic thrombophlebitis may occur in any of the sinuses, but it is characteristically encountered in regions where the venous sinuses are in close proximity to air sinuses. Infectious processes within the air sinuses may extend to adjacent venous sinuses, either from direct involvement of the dura or by spread along emissary veins. As illustrated here, the cavernous sinus and sigmoid sinus are at risk for this type of direct extension.

Typical CSF findings in venous sinus infections

Opening pressure	↑
WBCs	10–300/mm^3, neutrophilic predominance
Glucose	Normal
Protein	50–200 mg/dL
Organisms	Only if accompanied by meningitis or abscess

FIGURE 7-2 Typical cerebrospinal fluid (CSF) findings in venous sinus infections. Analysis of CSF in venous sinus infection often reveals increased intracranial pressure but is otherwise nonspecific. Lumbar puncture therefore is not of significant diagnostic value unless there is clinical suspicion of coexisting meningitis.

Microbial etiology in venous sinus infections

Site of primary infection	Possible organisms
Paranasal sinuses	Aerobic and anaerobic streptococci Other anaerobes *Staphylococcus aureus* Facultative gram-negative bacilli (rare) Fungi (rare)
Otitis media or mastoiditis	*S. aureus* Aerobic and anaerobic streptococci Other anaerobes Facultative gram-negative bacilli

FIGURE 7-3 Microbial etiology in venous sinus infections. Organisms that colonize the paranasal sinuses are most commonly responsible for infection of the venous sinuses. Consequently streptococci and *Staphylococcus aureus* account for the majority of venous sinus infections. Fungal venous sinus infections may occur in immunocompromised or diabetic patients, but this is rather uncommon.

Initial antibiotic therapy for venous sinus infections	
Suggested initial therapy	**Alternative in penicillin allergy**
Nafcillin, 1.5 g iv q4h, *plus either* metronidazole *or* chloramphenicol	Vancomycin, 500 mg iv q6h, *plus either* metronidazole *or* chloramphenicol

Figure 7-4 Initial antibiotic therapy in venous sinus infections. After obtaining a culture of the infected air sinus, initial therapy empirically targets streptococci and *Staphylococcus aureus*. Treatment for fungal venous sinus infection (*eg*, with amphotericin) should only be instituted if a fungus has been identified on histologic analysis or culture of an adjacent infected air sinus.

Sigmoid Sinus Infection

Sigmoid sinus septic thrombosis: diagnosis	
Risk factors Otitis media Mastoiditis Symptoms Headache Ear pain Ear drainage Nausea/vomiting Fever Lethargy	Signs Infected middle ear Postauricular swelling, tenderness Obtundation ± Cranial nerve VI palsy Papilledema Hemiparesis (rare)

Figure 7-5 Sigmoid sinus septic thrombosis: diagnosis. Patients with sigmoid sinus septic thrombosis typically present with a history of partially treated ear infection and progressive headache, fever, and vomiting. Patients may be lethargic or obtunded due to elevated intracranial pressure. Focal neurologic findings (*eg*, hemiparesis) may also be present but raise the suspicion of a mass lesion, such as a brain abscess.

Sigmoid sinus septic thrombosis: differential diagnosis
Intracranial abscess
Meningitis
Subdural empyema
Intracranial tumor
Cerebral ischemia or infarction

Figure 7-6 Sigmoid sinus septic thrombosis: differential diagnosis. Central nervous system (CNS) extension of air sinus infection may include meningitis, abscess, and subdural empyema, as well as venous sinus thrombosis. These conditions may have a similar history and findings and must always be considered in the differential diagnosis. Vascular events and brain neoplasms must also be considered, as many of the signs and symptoms of venous sinus infection are nonspecific.

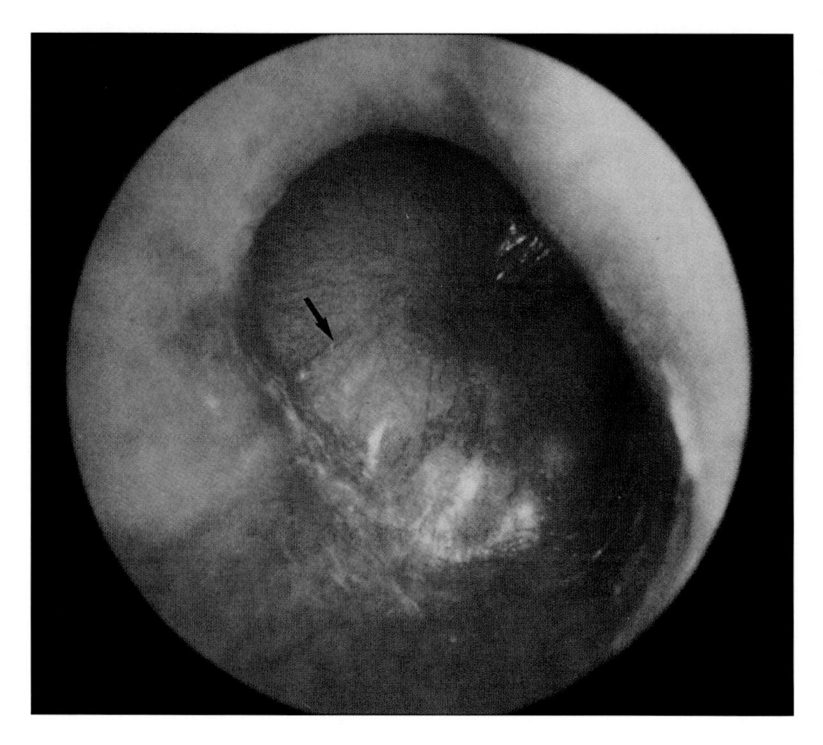

Figure 7-7 Acute otitis media with the characteristic bulging, red tympanic membrane (*arrow*). Such infections may progress to mastoiditis, and sigmoid sinus septic thrombophlebitis may ensue. (*Courtesy of* Dr. H. Alex Arts.)

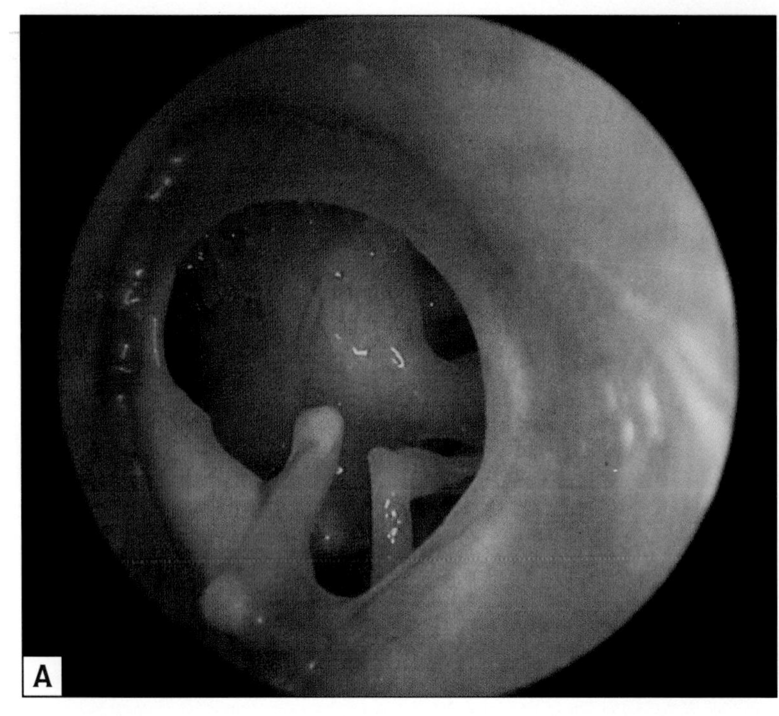

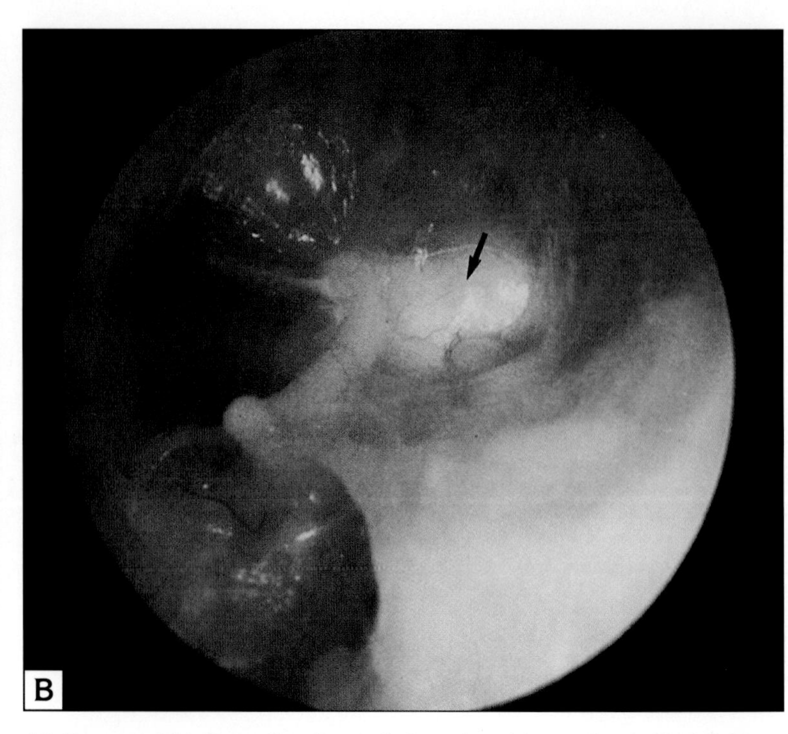

FIGURE 7-8 Chronic otitis media. **A**, Chronic otitis media with a large perforation in the tympanic membrane. Extension of the inflammatory process in chronic otitis media to the mastoid may result in sigmoid sinus occlusion. Typically, cultures reveal multiple pathogens, including *Proteus* spp., *Staphylococcus aureus*, *Bacteroides* spp., *Escherichia coli*, as well as aerobic and anaerobic streptococci. (Harris JP, Darrow DH: Complications of chronic otitis media. *In* Nadol JB Jr (ed.): *Surgery of the Ear and Temporal Bone*. New York: Raven Press; 1993:171–191.) **B**, The formation of a cholesteatoma (*arrow*) may also occur in the setting of chronic otitis media. Cholesteatomas may extend intracranially, causing distortion of the brain, brain stem, or cranial nerves. (*Courtesy of* Dr. H. Alex Arts.)

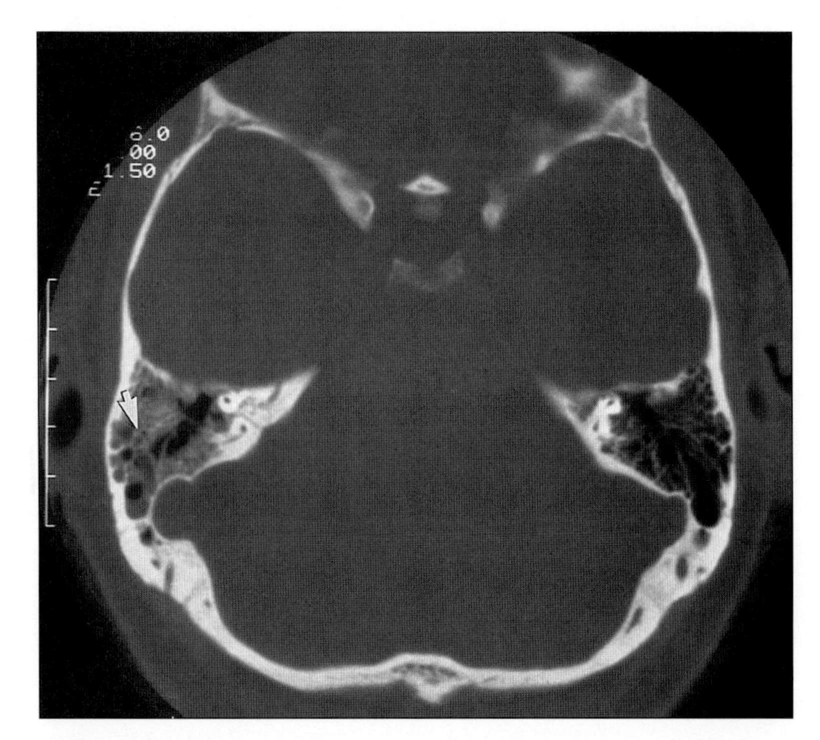

FIGURE 7-9 Mastoiditis. Computed tomographic (CT) scan of the head shows the presence of fluid and granulation tissue within an infected mastoid (*arrow*). This is the typical radiologic appearance of mastoiditis. In long-standing infections, the mastoid air cells may become completely obliterated. In cases of severe acute mastoiditis, necrosis of the air cell walls may develop, eventually perforating the mastoid cortex. This patient had a chronic otitis media, which resulted in mastoiditis and thrombophlebitis of the adjacent sigmoid sinus.

Sigmoid sinus septic thrombosis: radiologic findings
CT of the head
Fluid in mastoid
"Delta sign" in transverse and/or sigmoid sinus
Brain swelling
Midline shift
Hemorrhagic infarction
MRI of the head
As for CT, also:
Soft tissue in major dural venous sinuses
Dural enhancement around sinuses
Absence of signal in occluded venous sinus (MRA)
Angiography
Absence of flow in lateral or sigmoid sinus
Venous "blush" in collateral veins

FIGURE 7-10 Sigmoid sinus septic thrombosis: radiologic findings. The diagnosis of venous sinus occlusion is best confirmed with radiologic studies that delineate blood flow. Consequently, cerebral angiography has been the most sensitive examination used for this purpose. More recently, however, magnetic resonance imaging (MRI) sequences capable of delineating blood flow have been developed (magnetic resonance angiography, MRA). MRI/MRA is now used with increased frequency to visualize sinus occlusion.

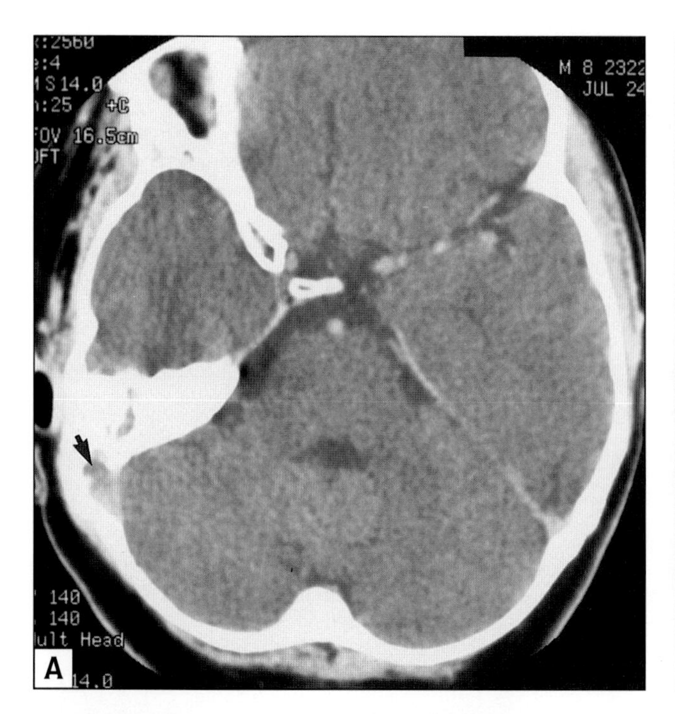

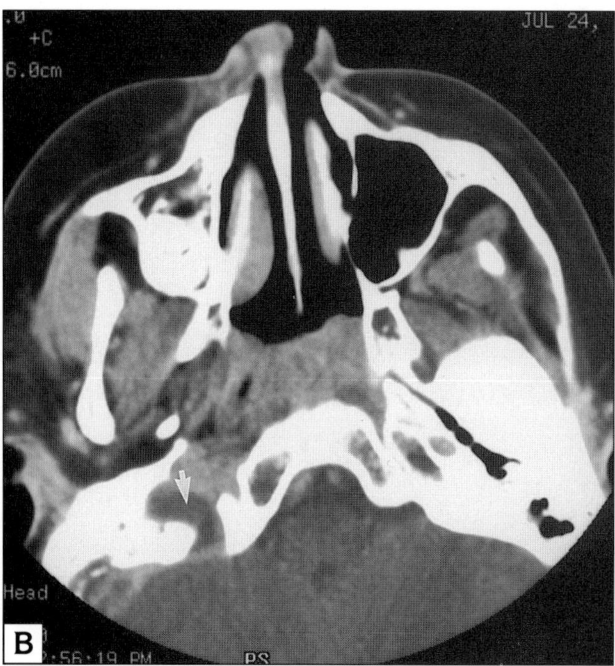

Figure 7-11 Sigmoid sinus septic thrombophlebitis complicating a case of chronic mastoiditis. **A**, A CT scan of the head following the administration of contrast shows the filling defect within the sigmoid sinus (*arrow*). **B**, The filling defect is seen on a lower scan to extend into the jugular bulb (*arrow*). The filling defect within a thrombosed sinus is known as a *delta sign*.

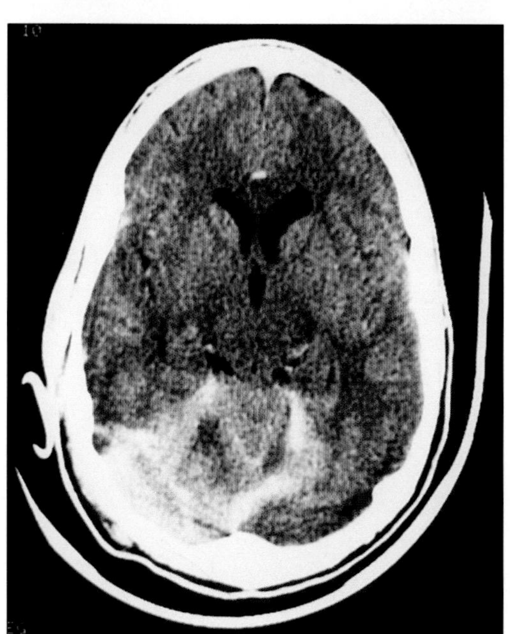

Figure 7-12 CT scan of the head (with contrast) shows increased vascularity in the tentorium adjacent to an occluded sigmoid sinus. This represents increased collateral venous drainage caused by the occlusion of primary drainage pathways. (*Courtesy of* Dr. Steve Telian.)

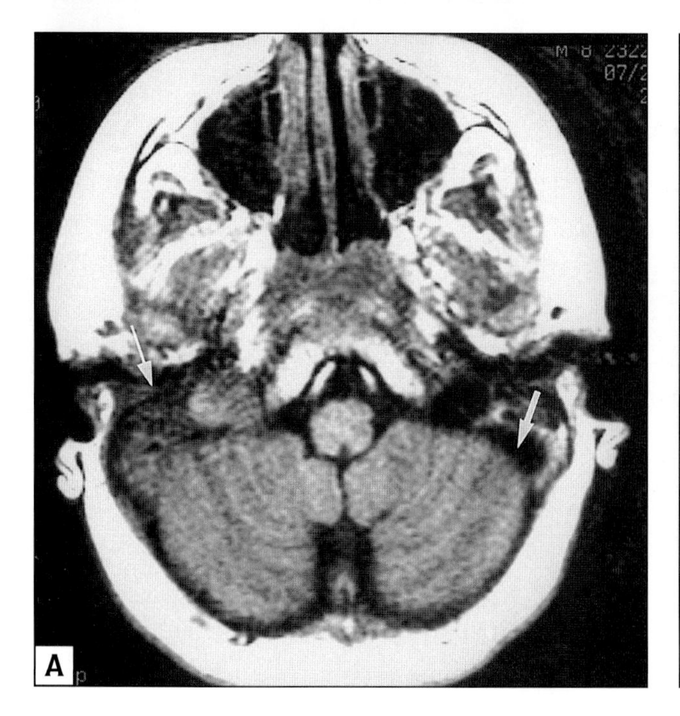

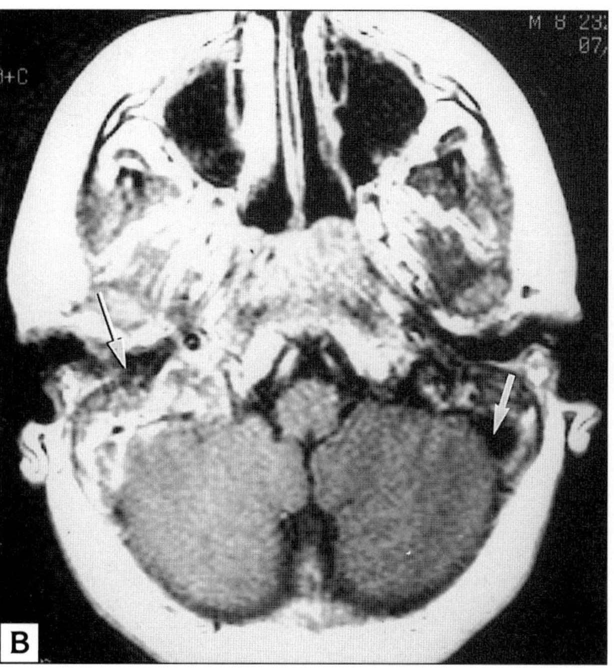

Figure 7-13 Mastoiditis and sigmoid sinus thrombosis in an 8-year-old boy with chronic otitis media. **A** and **B**, MRIs of the head before (*panel A*) and after (*panel B*) the administration of contrast. The inflammatory tissue within the right mastoid enhances brightly (*thin arrow*). The adjacent sigmoid sinus is occluded with inflammatory tissue and does not demonstrate the normal low signal seen in the sigmoid sinus on the other side (compare *thick arrow*).

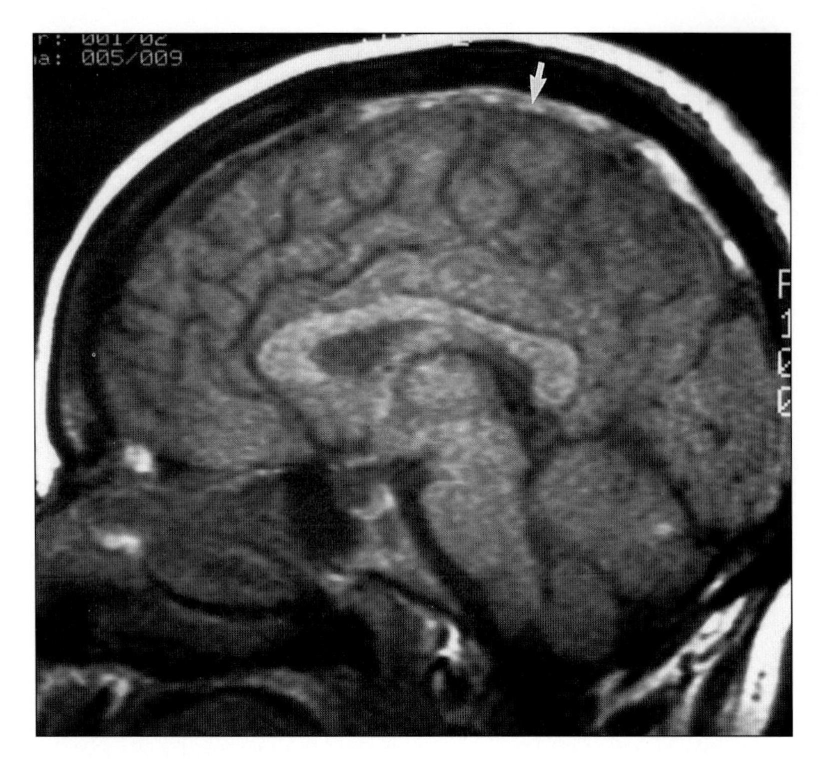

FIGURE 7-14 Frequently, the occlusion of a venous sinus results in retrograde thrombosis in proximal sinuses. In this patient, septic occlusion of the sigmoid sinus resulted in thrombosis of the transverse sinus and superior sagittal sinus. An MRI scan of the brain illustrates high signal within the posterior portion of the superior sagittal sinus (*arrow*), indicating the presence of thrombus within this sinus.

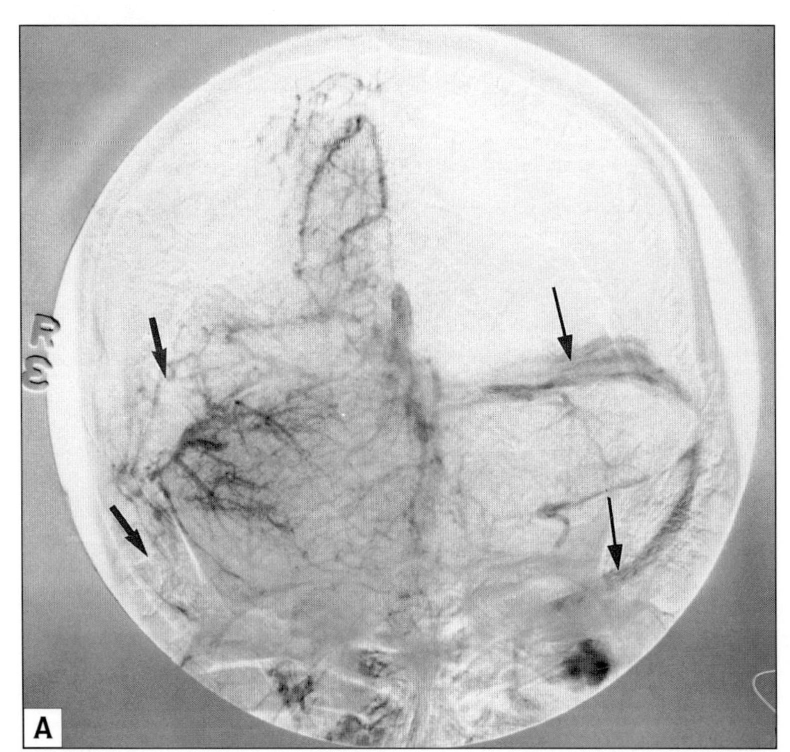

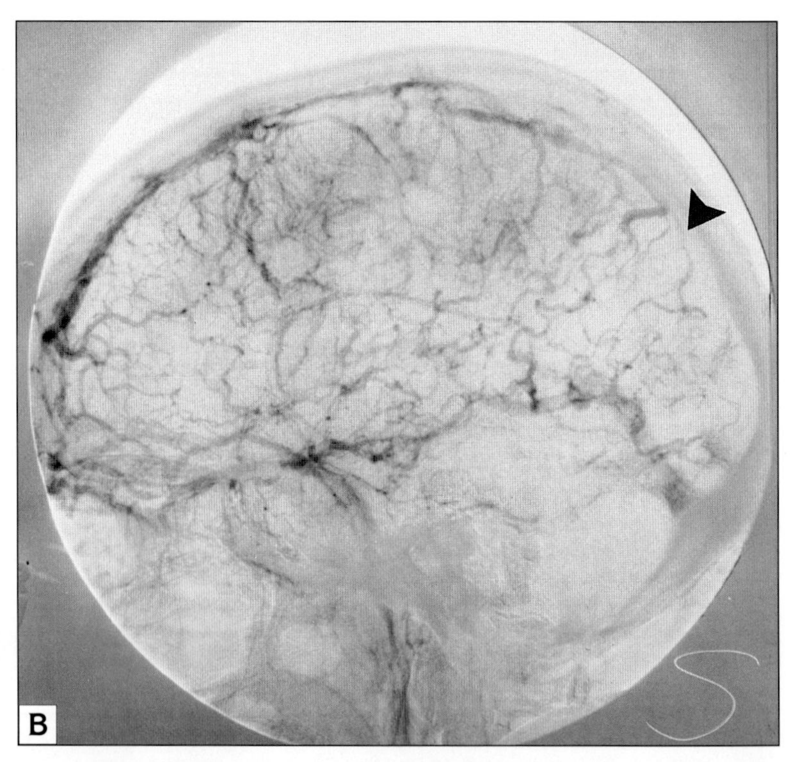

FIGURE 7-15 Cerebral angiogram (venous phase) of a patient with septic thrombophlebitis of the right sigmoid sinus. **A**, The left transverse and sigmoid sinuses fill normally (*thin arrows*), whereas the corresponding sinuses on the right do not (*thick arrows*), indicating that these sinuses have thrombosed. Stasis within the venous system and collateralized pial venous drainage on the right give rise to the vascular blush seen on the right. **B**, Lateral projection of the same study illustrates retrograde thrombosis of the posterior portion of the superior sagittal sinus (*arrowhead*).

Sigmoid sinus septic thrombosis: complications
Progression of thrombosis
Hemorrhagic infarction
Meningitis
Brain abscess
Brain herniation

FIGURE 7-16 Sigmoid sinus septic thrombosis: complications. Septic thrombophlebitis of the sigmoid sinus may cause complications related either to progression of the infectious process or to venous stasis and elevation of intracranial pressure.

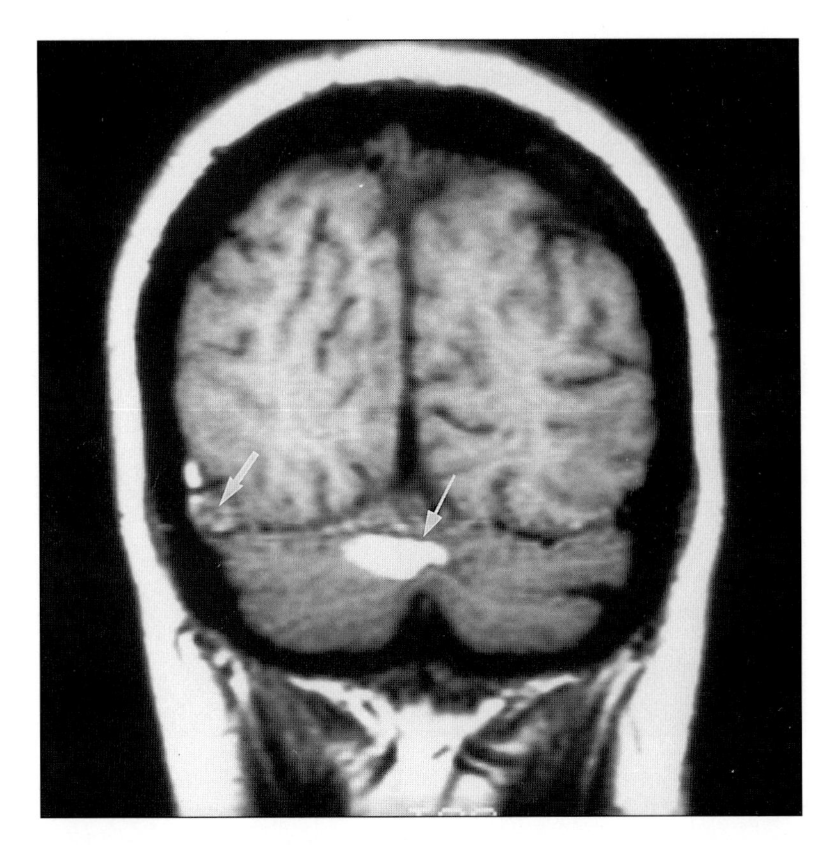

Figure 7-17 Cerebellar venous infarction. The occlusion of venous sinuses may result in stasis of venous drainage, causing edema and occasional venous infarctions. An MRI scan of the brain shows a cerebellar venous infarction. The high signal within the vermis of the cerebellum (*thin arrow*) indicates the presence of clotted blood, characteristic of a venous infarction. Also, note the presence of thrombus within the right transverse sinus (*thick arrow*).

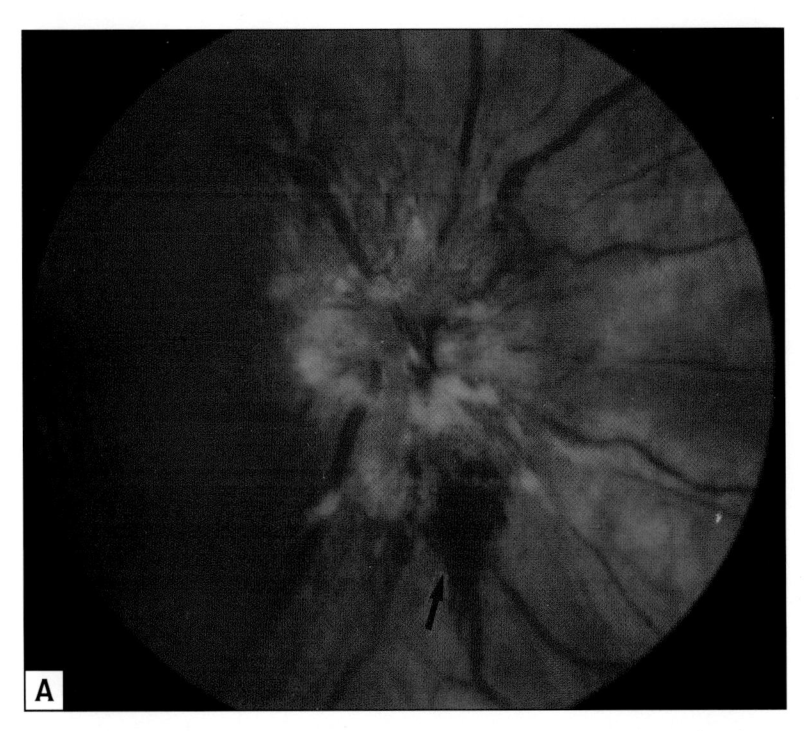

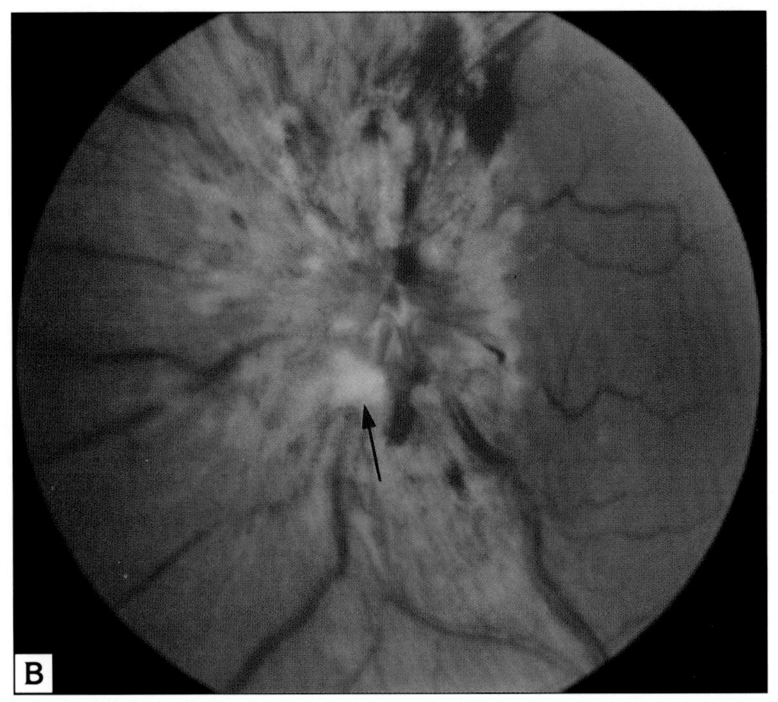

Figure 7-18 Thrombosis of the dural venous sinuses may lead to the development of increased intracranial pressure. Headache, nausea, and changes in the level of consciousness may result. **A** and **B**, Examination of the optic discs may reveal papilledema, as it has in this patient (*panel A*, right eye; *panel B*, left eye). Both optic discs are swollen, and numerous white exudates (*ie, thin arrow*) and flame-shaped hemorrhages (*ie, thick arrow*) are seen. (*Courtesy of* Dr. Wayne Cornblath.)

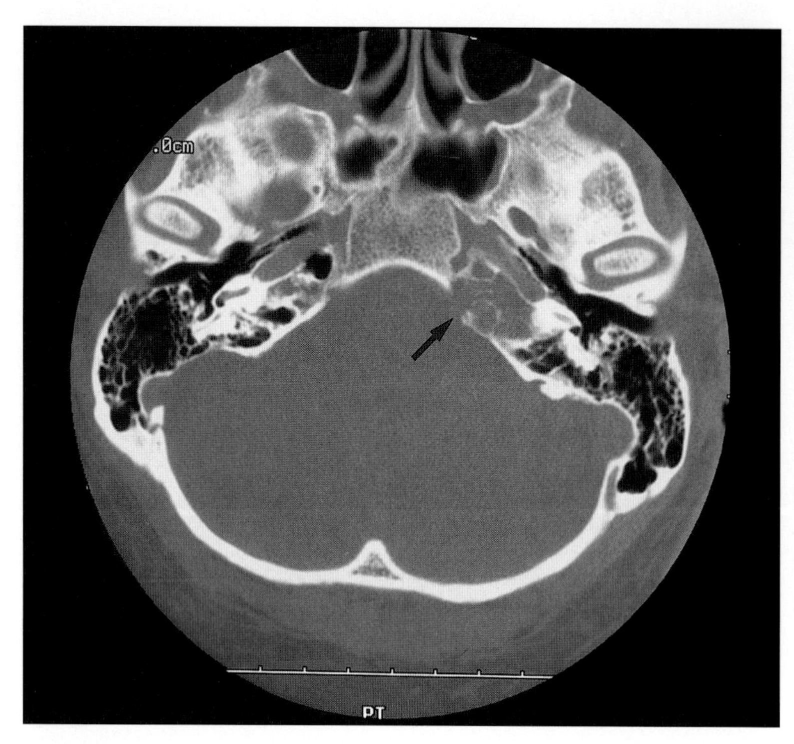

FIGURE 7-19 Petrous apex infection. CT scan of the head demonstrates an inflammatory process involving the air cells in the apex of the left petrous bone (*arrow*). Inflammation of the petrous apex may be complicated by septic thrombophlebitis of the nearby cavernous sinus or the sigmoid sinus (via spread through the superior petrosal sinus). Infection involving the petrous apex may present as a clinical syndrome consisting of retro-orbital pain, a draining ear, and diplopia caused by involvement of cranial nerve VI (Gradenigo's syndrome).

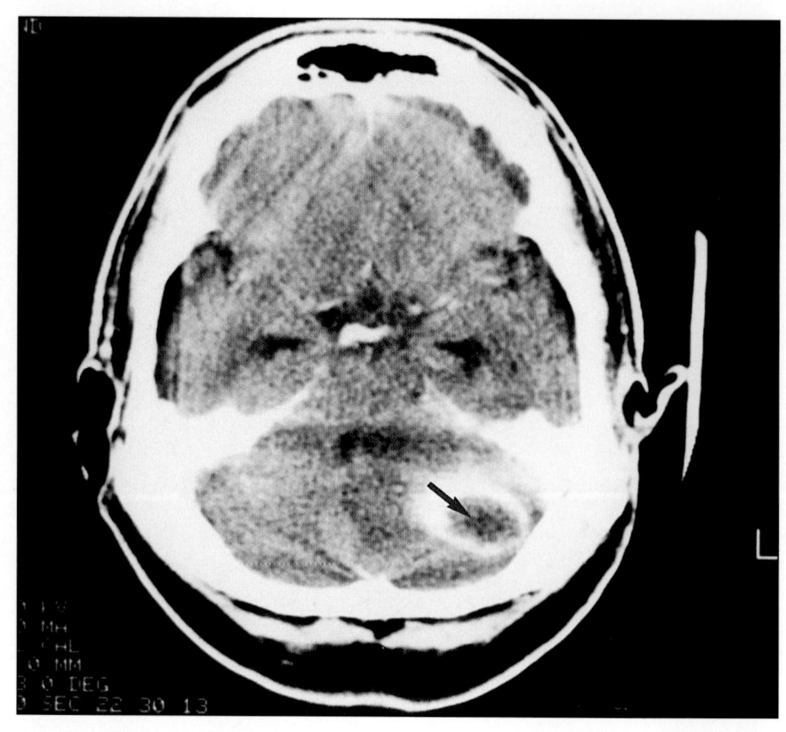

FIGURE 7-20 Cerebellar abscess. A CT scan of the head (with contrast) shows a cerebellar abscess (*arrow*) complicating a case of mastoiditis and sigmoid sinus septic thrombophlebitis. (*Courtesy of* Dr. Steve Telian.)

Sigmoid sinus septic thrombosis: interventions
Drainage and culture of infected middle ear
Vigorous antibiotic therapy
Mastoidectomy (occasional)
Supportive therapy for ↑ ICP
± Heparinization (if no evidence of hemorrhagic infarction)

FIGURE 7-21 Sigmoid sinus septic thrombosis: interventions. The treatment of sigmoid sinus infection should be rapid, targeting both the suppurative process and the increased intracranial pressure (ICP). Therapy should consist of culturing and draining the adjacent infected mastoid as well as instituting empirical antibiotics. In addition, the patient's head should be elevated, and respiratory compromise and fluid overload should be avoided. Aggressive reduction of ICP through osmotic agents and hyperventilation should be undertaken only after consultation with a neurosurgeon, as these may be complicated by extension of the venous occlusion and worsening cerebral ischemia. The use of heparinization to prevent extension of venous sinus occlusion is controversial and may be complicated by intracranial hemorrhage.

Cavernous Sinus Infection

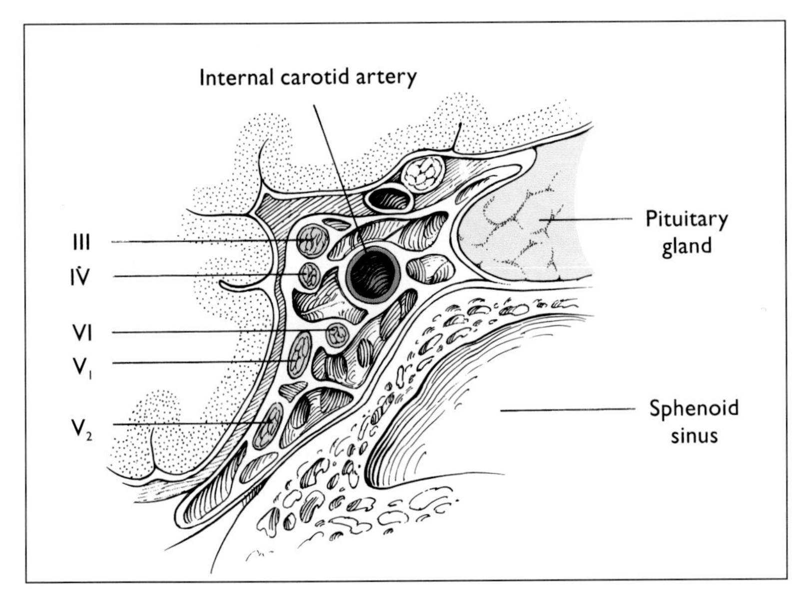

Figure 7-22 The cavernous sinus in cross-section. Infection and occlusion of this sinus may follow sphenoid sinusitis or septic thrombophlebitis of the orbital veins. The neurovascular structures within the cavernous sinus may be involved in the inflammatory process, resulting in a number of clinical signs and symptoms. Spread of the inflammation into the internal carotid artery may lead to narrowing or occlusion of the artery, an event which may result in a cerebral infarction. Cranial nerves III, IV, and VI are frequently involved in cavernous sinus thrombophlebitis, resulting in varying degrees of ocular motility deficits. Symptoms of involvement of cranial nerves V_1 and V_2 (*ie*, facial numbness or pain) are possible but are not frequently observed.

Cavernous sinus septic thrombosis: diagnosis

Risk factors	Signs
Paranasal sinusitis	Periorbital edema
Facial infection	Chemosis
Dental infection	Papillitis
Symptoms	Oculomotor palsies
Headache	Proptosis
Facial pain	± Facial sensory changes
Vision loss	
Fever	
Double vision	

Figure 7-23 Cavernous sinus septic thrombosis: diagnosis. Patients with cavernous sinus septic thrombosis typically present with headache, fever, and diplopia. A history of paranasal sinus infection may be obtained but is not necessary. Ophthalmoplegia and proptosis are often seen on examination.

Cavernous sinus septic thrombosis: differential diagnosis

- Orbital cellulitis or abscess
- Idiopathic granulomatous cavernous sinus thrombosis (Tolosa-Hunt Syndrome)
- Carotid-cavernous sinus fistula
- Intracavernous carotid artery aneurysm
- Cavernous sinus or orbital tumor
- Polyarteritis nodosa with cerebral venous thrombosis (Cogan's syndrome)

Figure 7-24 Cavernous sinus septic thrombosis: differential diagnosis. The differential diagnosis for cavernous sinus thrombophlebitis must include other conditions characterized by cavernous sinus compression or occlusion, such as intracavernous tumors or vascular lesions. Orbital processes such as infection and tumors must also be considered.

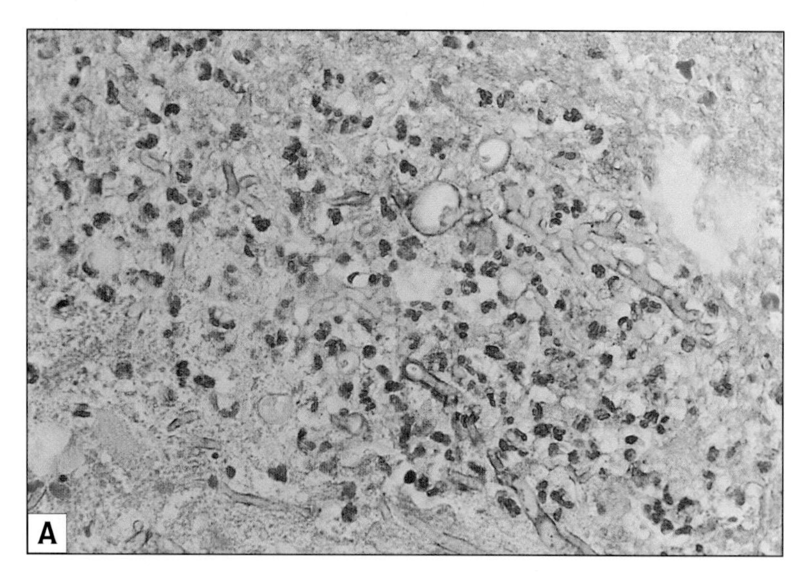

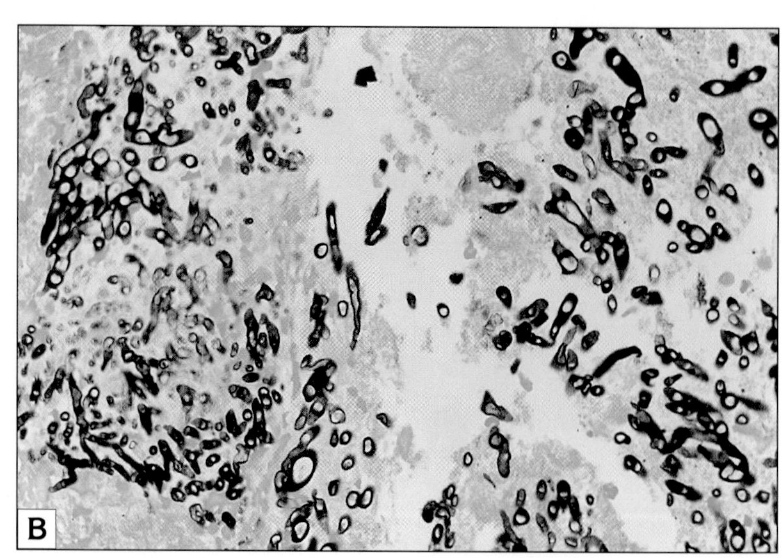

Figure 7-25 Histologic appearance of cavernous sinus infection caused by *Aspergillus*. **A**, Hematoxylin-eosin stain shows necrosis and infiltration with neutrophils. Fungal organisms, with characteristic branching hyphae, are seen throughout (*arrow*). **B**, Gomori's methenamine silver (GMS) stain for fungi shows outlining of the darkly staining *Aspergillus* organisms.

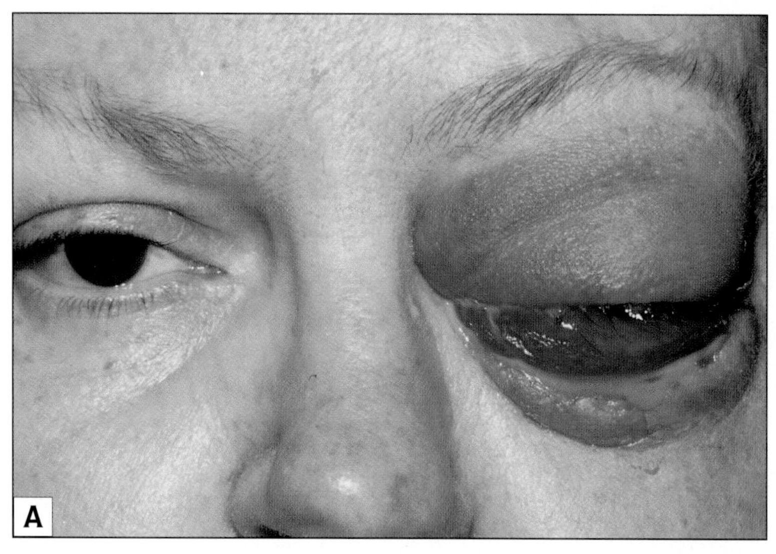

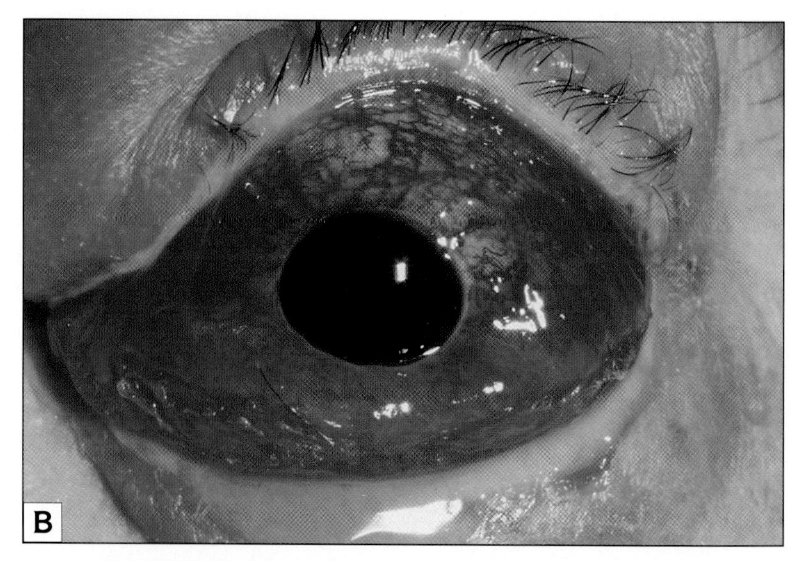

Figure 7-26 Proptosis, ptosis, and chemosis caused by impaired venous drainage from the orbit in a patient with occlusion of the cavernous sinus. **A**, With the patient in neutral gaze, complete ptosis and gross swelling of the orbit are apparent. **B**, On forced elevation of the upper lid, severe conjunctival swelling and hyperemia are seen. The pupil has been dilated pharmacologically in this patient. The pupil may also be dilated and unreactive if the oculomotor nerve (cranial nerve III) is involved within the infected cavernous sinus. (*Courtesy of* Dr. Wayne Cornblath.)

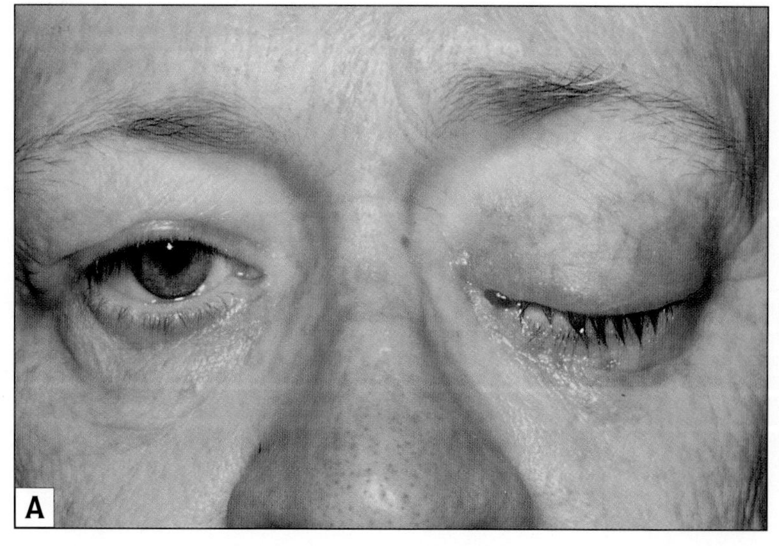

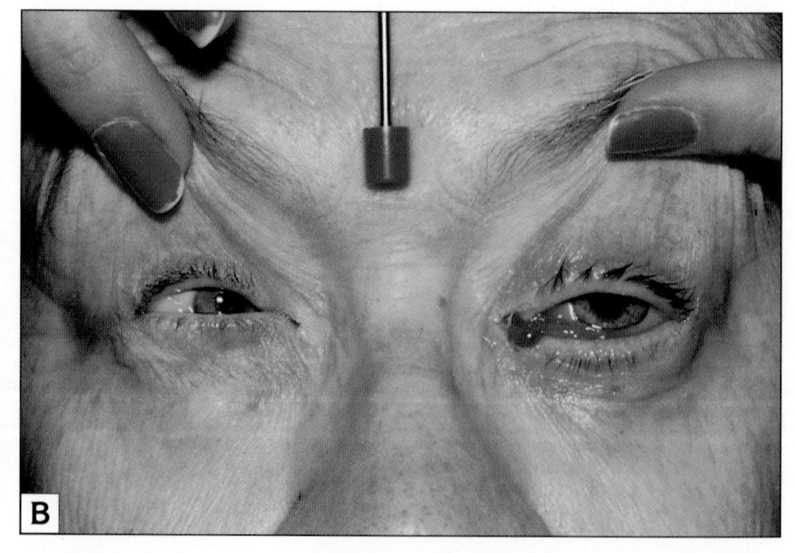

Figure 7-27 Ptosis and complete ophthalmoplegia of the left eye caused by involvement of cranial nerves III, IV, and VI within the thrombosed cavernous sinus. **A–F**, Sequential photographs document the inability of the left eye to move in any direction as the patient attempts to look at a red pin. (*Courtesy of* Dr. Wayne Cornblath.) (*continued*)

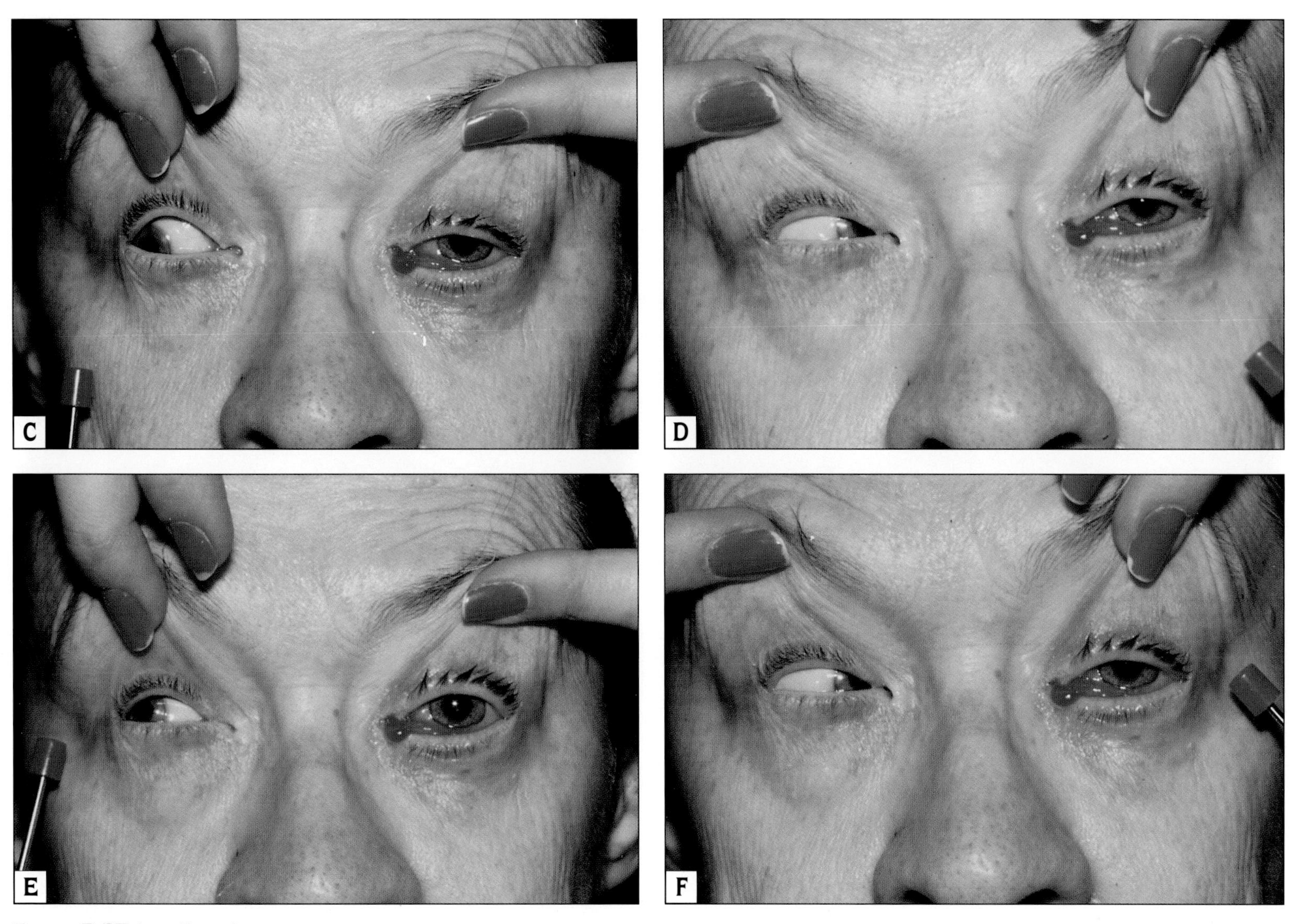

Figure 7-27 (*continued*)

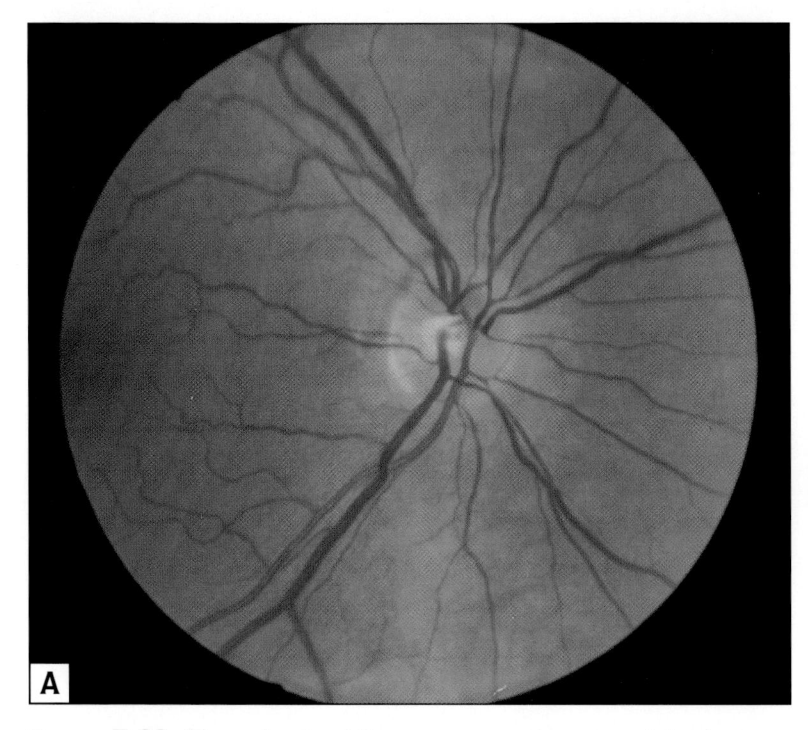

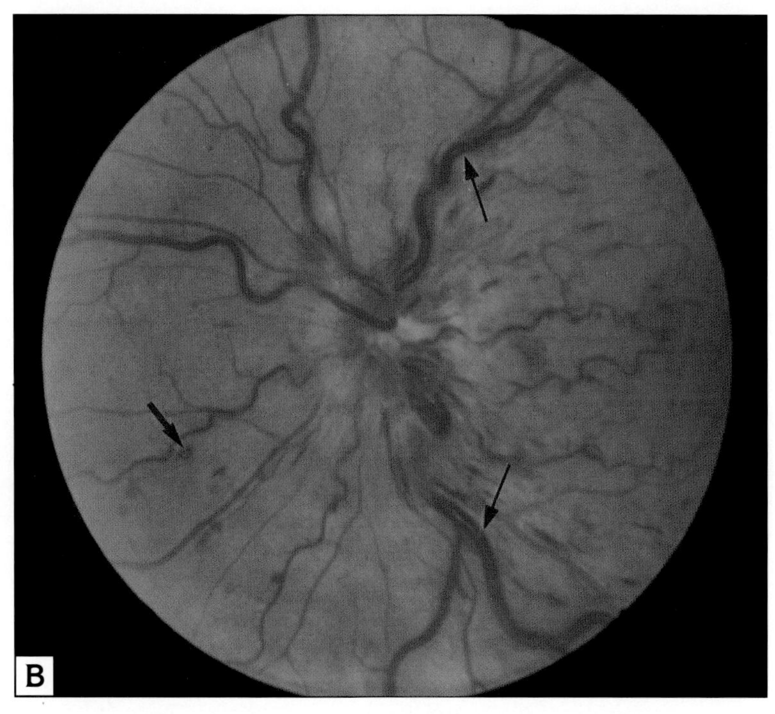

Figure 7-28 Thrombosis of the cavernous sinus may interfere with venous drainage from the eye. The venous obstruction may lead to retinal venous engorgement and impairment of visual acuity. **A**, The right eye (unaffected) shows a normal fundus. **B**, On the left eye (on the side of thrombosis), the retina shows abnormally engorged veins (*thin arrows*) and numerous flame-shaped hemorrhages (*ie*, *thick arrow*). (*Courtesy of* Dr. Wayne Cornblath.)

Cavernous sinus septic thrombosis: radiologic findings
CT and MRI Fullness in cavernous sinus region ± Paranasal sinus fluid
Angiography Absence of venous flow in cavernous sinus ± Narrowing of internal carotid artery

FIGURE 7-29 Cavernous sinus septic thrombosis: radiologic findings. As is the case with sigmoid sinus infections, the diagnosis of cavernous sinus thrombophlebitis is best confirmed with radiologic studies that delineate blood flow, such as cerebral angiography or MRI/MRA.

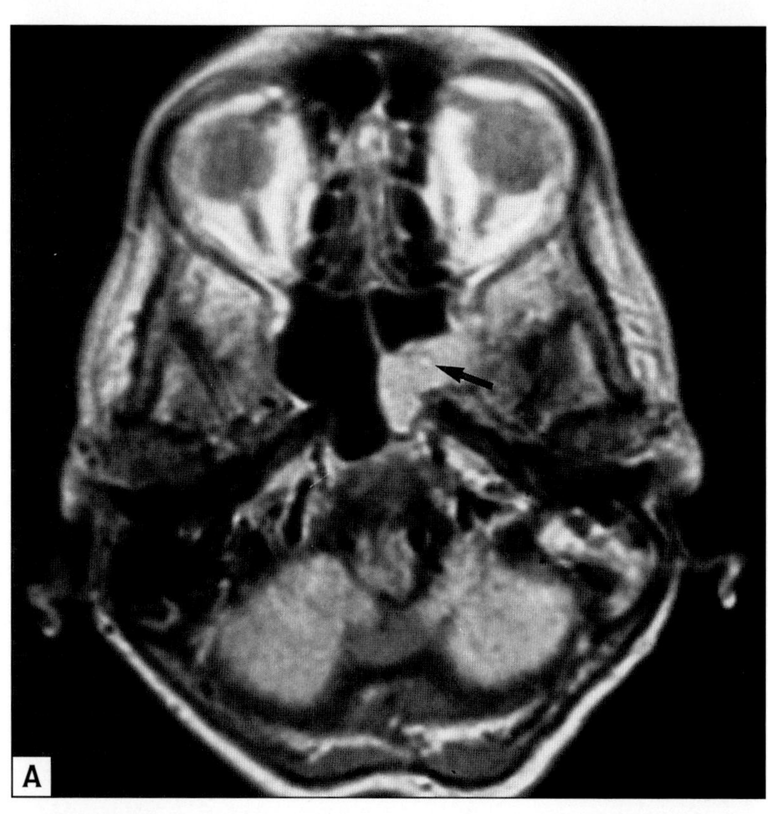

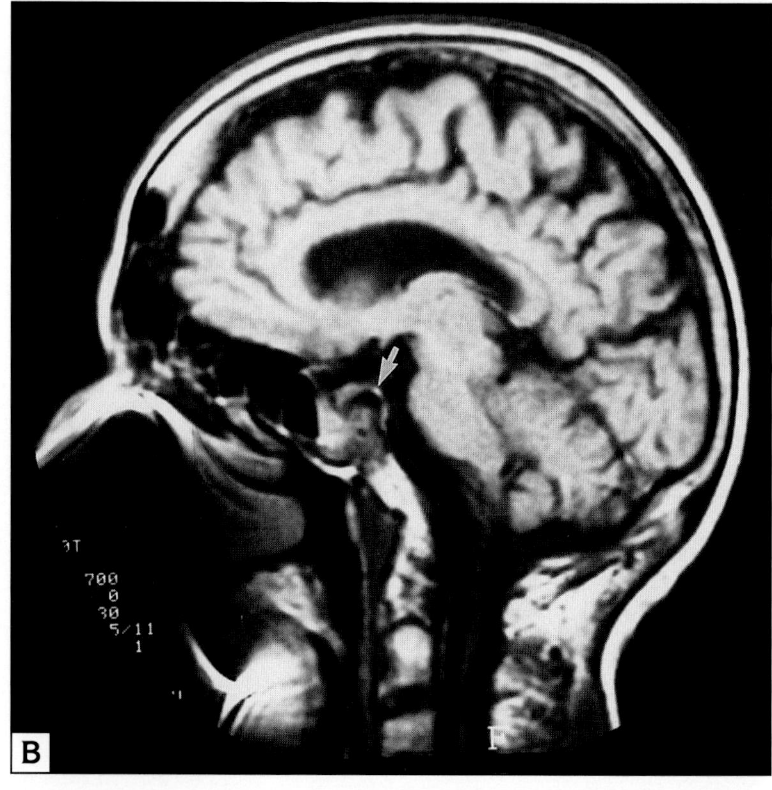

FIGURE 7-30 Sphenoid sinusitis with direct extension into the cavernous sinus. **A**, MRI scan of the head shows inflammation of the sphenoid sinus and adjacent cavernous sinus (*arrow*). **B**, Sagittal projection of the same study demonstrates the engulfment of the intracavernous internal carotid artery (*arrow*) in inflammatory tissue.

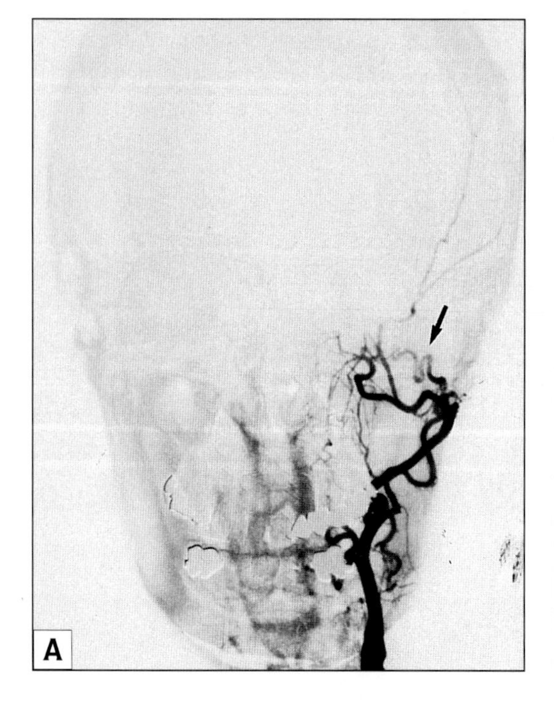

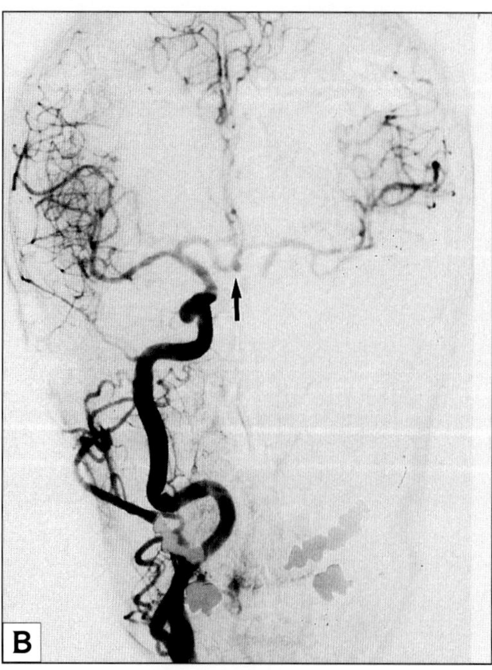

FIGURE 7-31 Thrombosis of the left internal carotid artery in an infected cavernous sinus. **A**, Cerebral angiogram with injection of the left common carotid artery. Note the absence of filling of intracranial vessels on the affected side. Only external carotid branches are filling in this study (*arrow*). **B**, Cerebral angiogram with injection of the right common carotid artery. The left intracranial circulation is supplied by the right internal carotid artery via a patent anterior communicating artery (*arrow*). Involvement of the internal carotid artery may result in embolic or ischemic infarction. In addition, intravascular dissemination of the infection may occur, resulting in miliary abscesses and mycotic aneurysms; this is a rare but potentially lethal complication.

CHAPTER 8

Infections of the Skull and Bony Sinuses

Hans-Walter Pfister
Eberhard Wilmes

Cranial Osteomyelitis

Causes of cranial osteomyelitis
Complication of craniotomy or cranioplasty
Contamination of open skull wound
Extension of infection from contiguous sites (*eg*, otitis media or chronic sinusitis, esp. frontal sinusitis)
Hematogenous seeding

Figure 8-1 Causes of cranial osteomyelitis. Cranial osteomyelitis is a rare infection that usually occurs as a complication of craniotomy/cranioplasty or frontal sinusitis. Hematogenous seeding is a rare cause of cranial osteomyelitis. The clinical hallmarks are local symptoms, including pain, swelling, and tenderness. (*Adapted from* Apuzzo MLJ (ed.): *Brain Surgery: Complication Avoidance and Management*, vol 2. New York: Churchill Livingstone; 1993; with permission.)

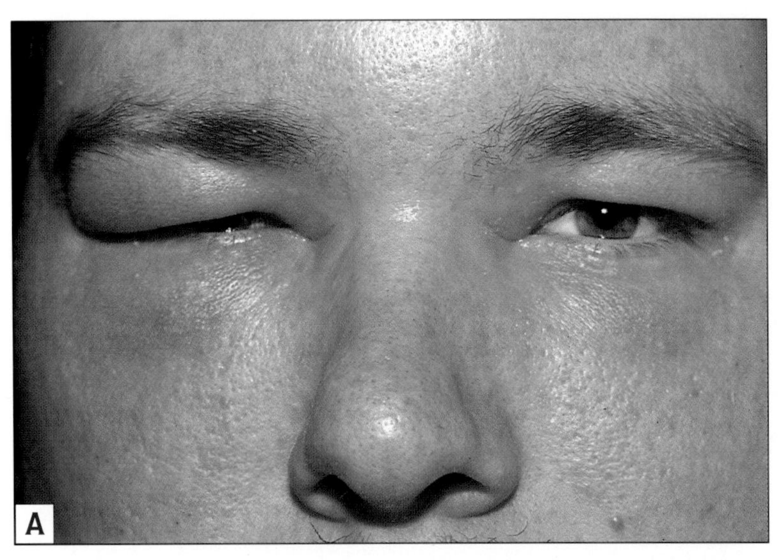

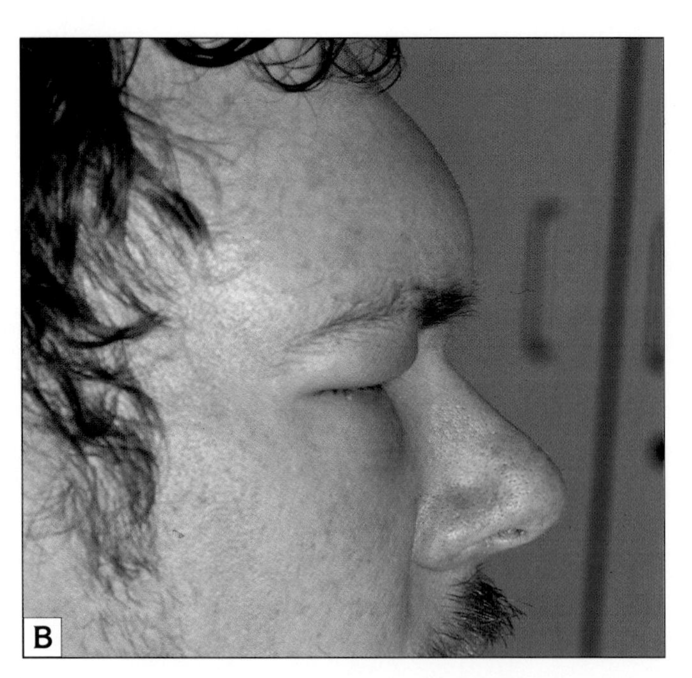

Figure 8-2 Osteomyelitis of the frontal bone. **A** and **B**, Frontal and side views of the patient show marked edema of the periorbita and doughy swelling of the forehead.

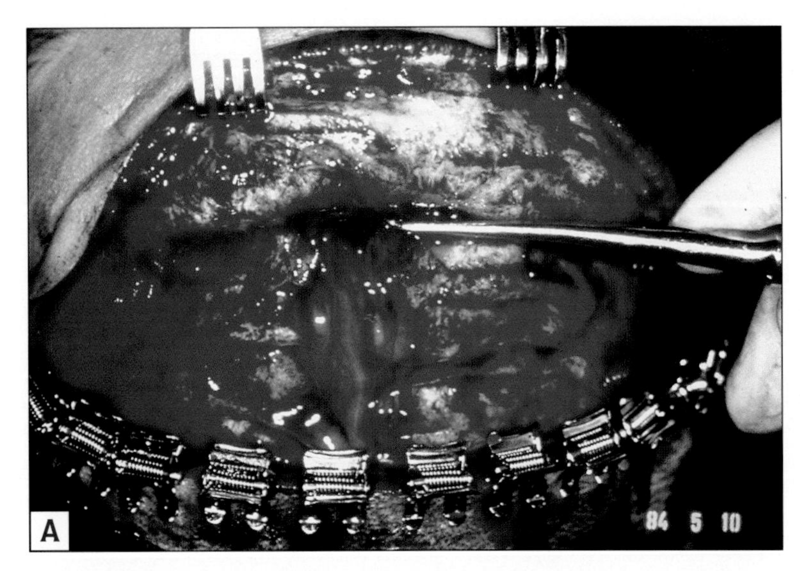

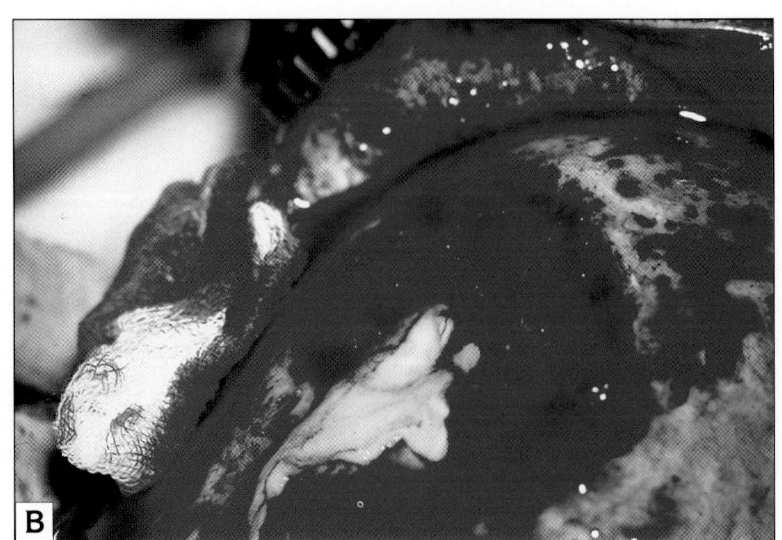

Figure 8-3 Cranial osteomyelitis of the frontal bone. **A** and **B**, Intraoperative views showing purulent discharge.

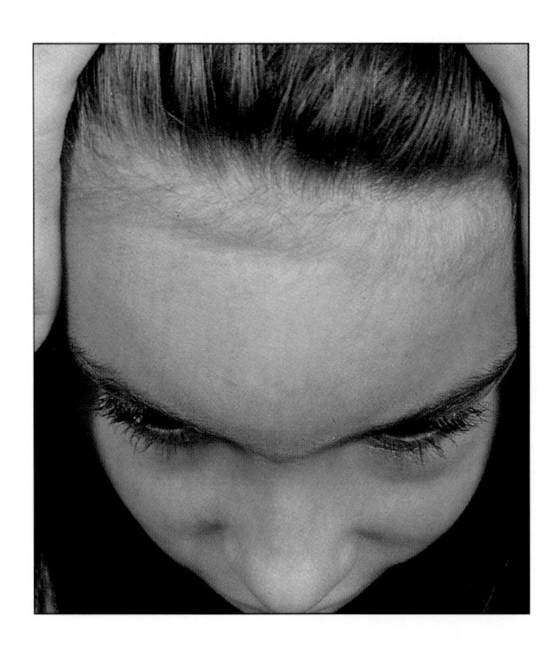

FIGURE 8-4 Osteomyelitis of the frontal bone. Doughy swelling of the forehead (Pott's puffy tumor).

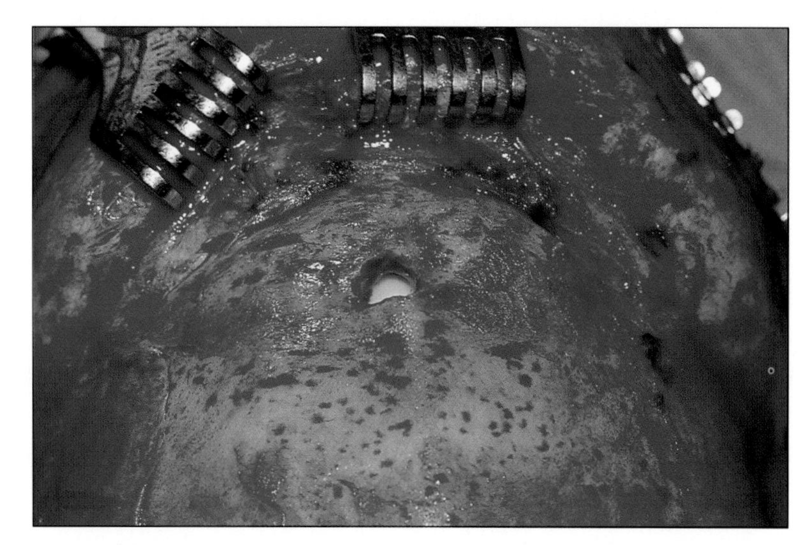

FIGURE 8-5 Cranial osteomyelitis. Intraoperative view revealing pus median in the frontal bone with osteodestruction.

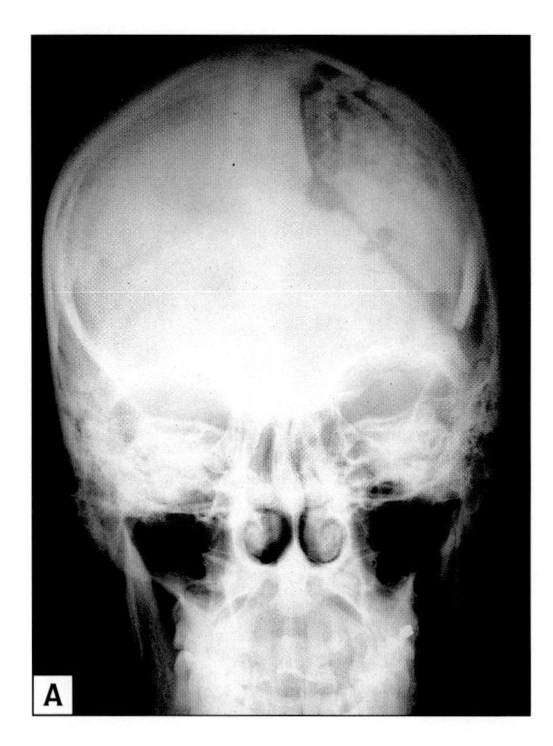

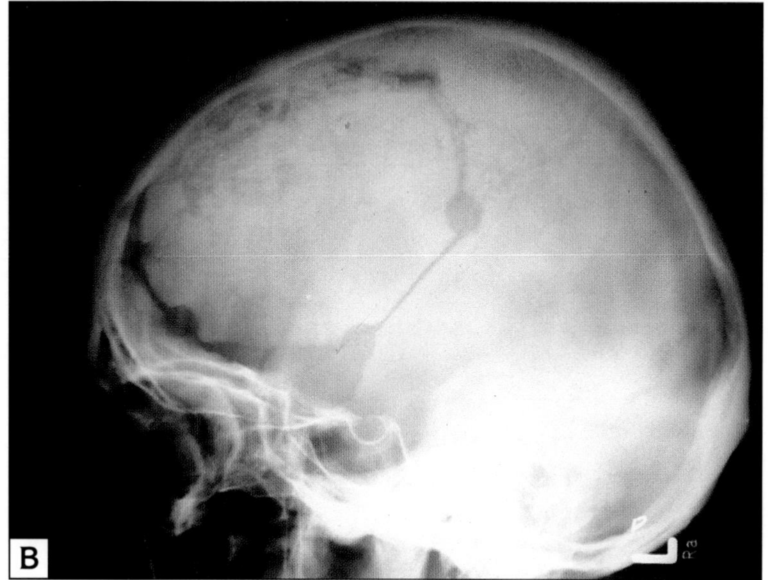

FIGURE 8-6 Osteomyelitis of a craniotomy bone flap. **A** and **B**, Anteroposterior and lateral radiographs reveal an irregular destructive process. (*Courtesy of* Dr. H. Steinhoff.)

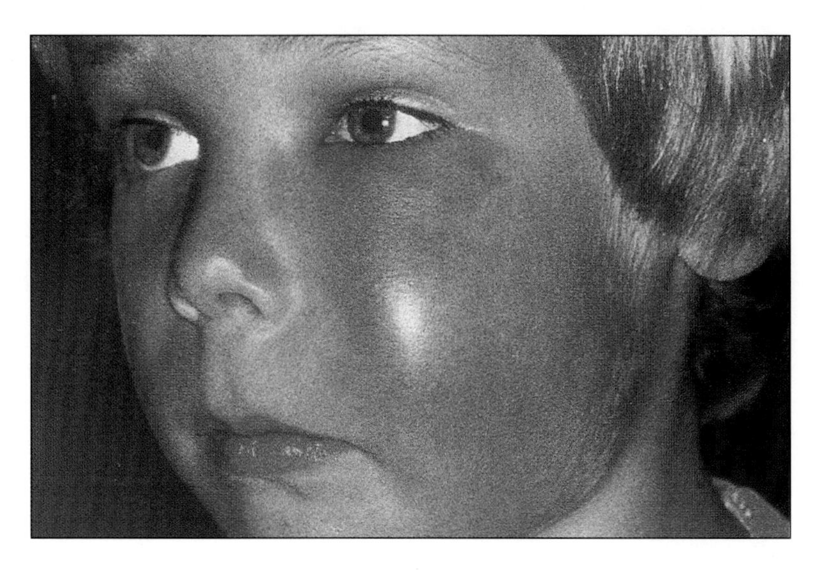

FIGURE 8-7 Acute antral sinusitis and osteomyelitis of the upper jaw in a 4-year-old boy. There is severe redness and swelling of the left cheek as well as edema of the eyelids. (*Adapted from* Thomae K (ed.): *Klinische Visite, Bildtafeln Thomae: Bakterielle Infektionen.* Biberach, Germany; 1984, 122:1–12; with permission.)

Management options for cranial osteomyelitis
Excision (debridement) of involved necrotic bone
Removal of alloplastic plate
Surgical drainage of involved area
Intravenous antibiotics

FIGURE 8-8 Management options for cranial osteomyelitis. Appropriate treatment of cranial osteomyelitis includes surgery and antibiotic therapy. Antibiotics are directed against the causative organisms identified by intraoperative cultures. *Staphylococcus aureus* is the most common pathogen, but gram-negative bacteria, nonenterococcal streptococci, and anaerobes may be involved in cases secondary to sinusitis and otitis. (*Adapted from* Apuzzo MLJ (ed.): *Brain Surgery: Complication Avoidance and Management*, vol 2. New York: Churchill Livingstone; 1993; with permission.)

Bacterial etiology of intracranial epidural abscess

Primary infection	Probable organism
Paranasal sinusitis	Aerobic or anaerobic streptococci Other anaerobes *Staphylococcus aureus*
Otitis media and mastoiditis	*S. aureus* Aerobic or anaerobic streptococci Other anaerobes Facultative gram-negative bacilli
Postsurgical infection	*S. aureus* Facultative gram-negative bacilli

FIGURE 8-9 Bacterial etiology of intracranial epidural abscess. Most cases of intracranial epidural abscess follow frontal sinusitis, craniotomy, or mastoiditis. Causative organisms can usually be predicted on the basis of the primary source of infection, directing the choice of initial empiric antimicrobial therapy. (*Adapted from* Greenlee SJ: Subdural empyema. *In* Mandell G, Douglas RG, Bennett JE (eds.): *Principles and Practice of Infectious Diseases*, 3rd ed. New York: Churchill Livingstone; 1990:790; with permission.)

INTRACRANIAL EPIDURAL ABSCESS

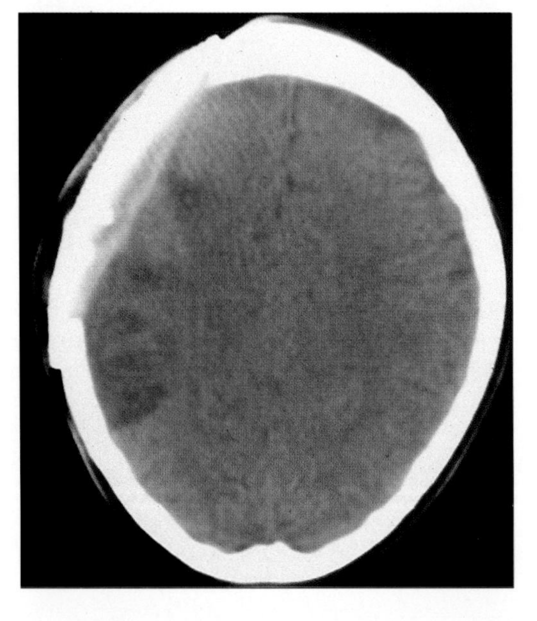

FIGURE 8-10 Cranial computed tomographic (CT) scan (axial section with bone window setting) revealing epidural empyema at the site of a previous cranioplasty with prosthetic material. Previous craniotomy was performed in this 23-year-old patient because of brain infarction with mass effect. (*Courtesy* of Dr. C. Hamburger.)

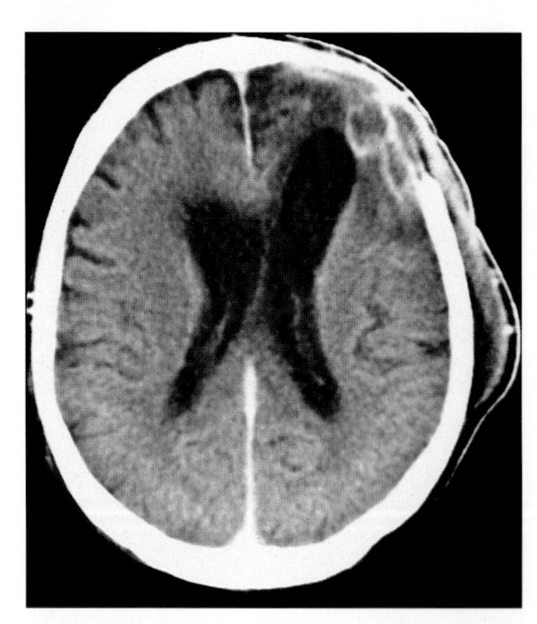

FIGURE 8-11 Cranial CT scan (axial section with bone window setting) revealing epidural empyema at the site of craniotomy. Previous craniotomy was performed in this 66-year-old patient because of severe intracerebral hemorrhage. The patient died of septic shock due to *Staphylococcus aureus*. (*Courtesy* of Dr. C. Hamburger.)

Treatment of intracranial epidural abscess
Consider as neurosurgical emergency
Drain by burr holes or craniotomy/craniectomy
Follow with antibiotic therapy
Initial: Nafcillin, 1.5 g iv q4h, with metronidazole or chloramphenicol, x 3–4 wks
In penicillin allergy: vancomycin, 500 mg iv q6h, with metronidazole or chloramphenicol
Final antibiotic selection guided by culture results
Follow with repeat CT or MRI scans for up to 1 y

FIGURE 8-12 Treatment of intracranial epidural abscess. Intracranial epidural abscesses generally require emergency surgical drainage to avoid the development of subdural empyema. Antibiotic therapy should be directed against aerobic and anaerobic streptococci and *Staphylococcus aureus* (dosages given are for adults with normal renal function). Concomitant surgery of infected sinuses or bone may be necessary. (Greenlee SJ: Epidural abscess. *In* Mandell G, Douglas RG, Bennett JE (eds.): *Principles and Practice of Infectious Diseases*, 3rd ed. New York: Churchill Livingstone; 1990:791–793.)

MUCOCELE/PYOCELE

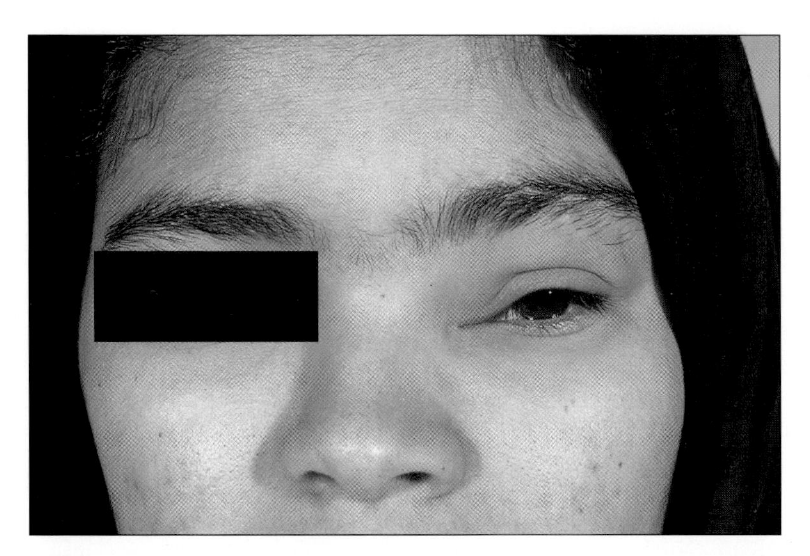

FIGURE 8-13 Mucocele of the frontal sinus with extension to the orbit. Swelling of the left upper eyelid is apparent.

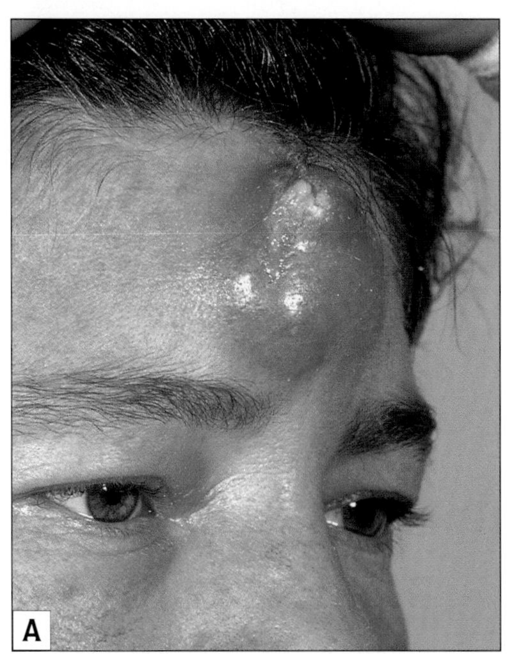

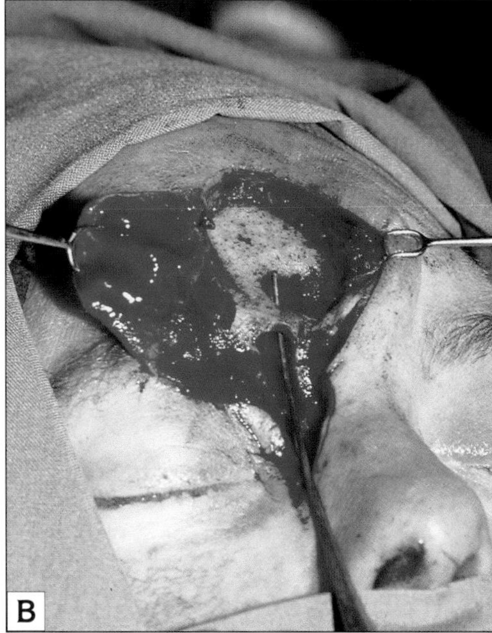

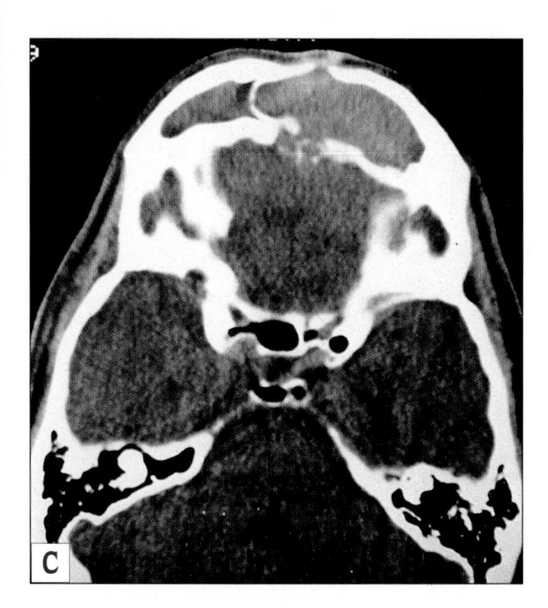

FIGURE 8-14 **A** and **B**, Mucopyocele of the frontal sinus with perforation. Preoperative (*panel A*) and operative (*panel B*) views. **C**, Axial cranial CT scan reveals mucopyocele of the frontal sinus with destruction of the anterior and posterior table of the frontal sinus.

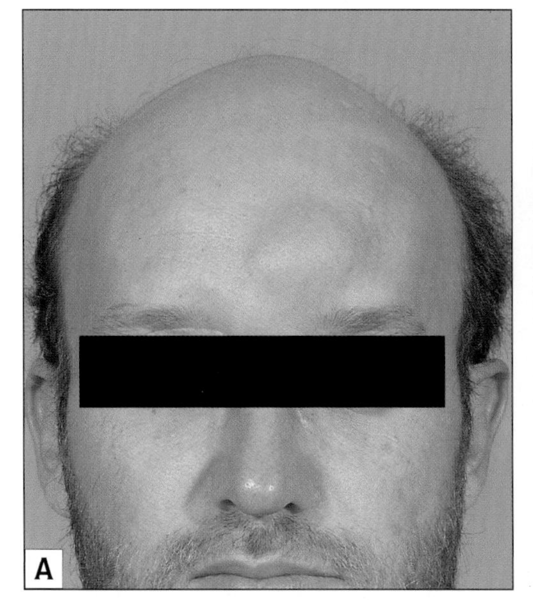

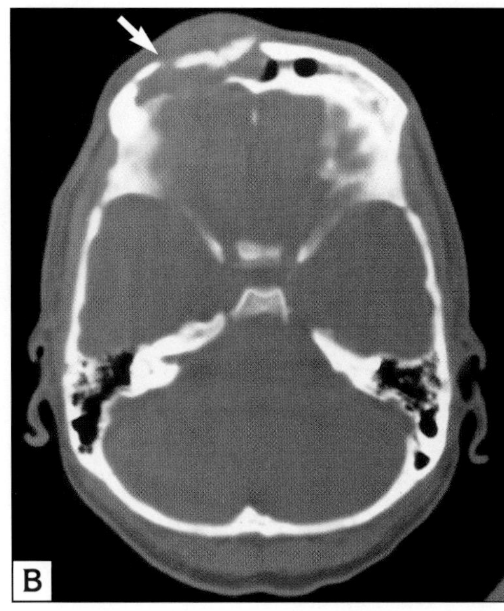

FIGURE 8-15 Pyocele of the frontal sinus in a patient who had previous surgery for a frontobasal fracture. **A**, Localized swelling at the forehead. **B**, A CT scan reveals a destructive process of the anterior (*arrow*) and posterior tables of the frontal sinus.

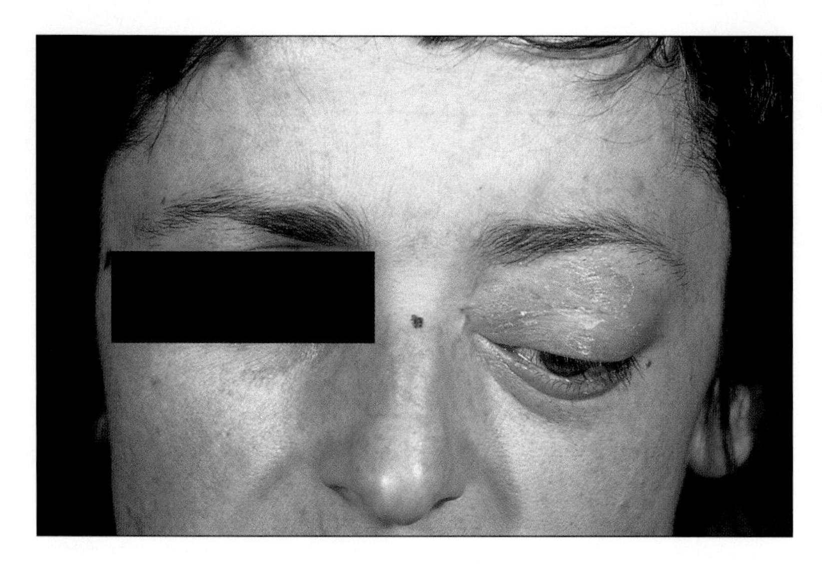

FIGURE 8-16 Pyocele of the frontal and ethmoid sinuses with extension into the orbit, resulting in swelling of the eyelids and downward displacement of the globe.

A. Characteristic findings in mucoceles: frontoethmoidal mucocele
Clinical findings
Frontal headache (deep nasal or periorbital pain)
Proptosis
Globe displacement downward and outward, resulting in diplopia
Nasal obstruction and rhinorrhea (rare)
Radiographic findings
Clouding of the sinus
Loss of typical scalloped outline of frontal sinus
Sclerosis of surrounding skull

B. Characteristic findings in mucoceles: sphenoethmoidal mucocele
Clinical findings
Headache with occipital, vertex, or deep nasal pain
Globe displacement, diplopia, visual field disturbances
Pituitary disturbances (rare)
Radiographic findings
Clouding of the sinus
Loss of typical scalloped outline of sinus
Sclerosis of surrounding skull

C. Characteristic findings in mucoceles: maxillary mucocele
Frequently an incidental finding on radiographs
Often clinically asymptomatic
Frequently spontaneous regression

FIGURE 8-17 Characteristic findings in mucoceles. A mucocele develops when accumulation and retention of mucoid material occurs within a sinus as a result of continuous or periodic obstruction of the ostium of the sinus. The frontal sinus is most commonly involved. The symptoms depend on the mucocele's location and the bony erosion. Frontoethmoidal and sphenoethmoidal mucoceles require surgical removal. A pyocele is the result of an infected mucocele; treatment includes surgery and antibiotics directed against *Staphylococcus aureus*, nonenterococcal streptococci, and oral anaerobes. **A**, Frontoethmoidal mucocele; **B**, sphenoethmoidal mucocele; **C**, maxillary mucocele. (*Adapted from* Johnson JT: Infections. *In* Cummings CW (ed.): *Otolaryngology—Head and Neck Surgery*, vol 1. St. Louis: Mosby Year Book; 1993:928–940.)

Sinusitis

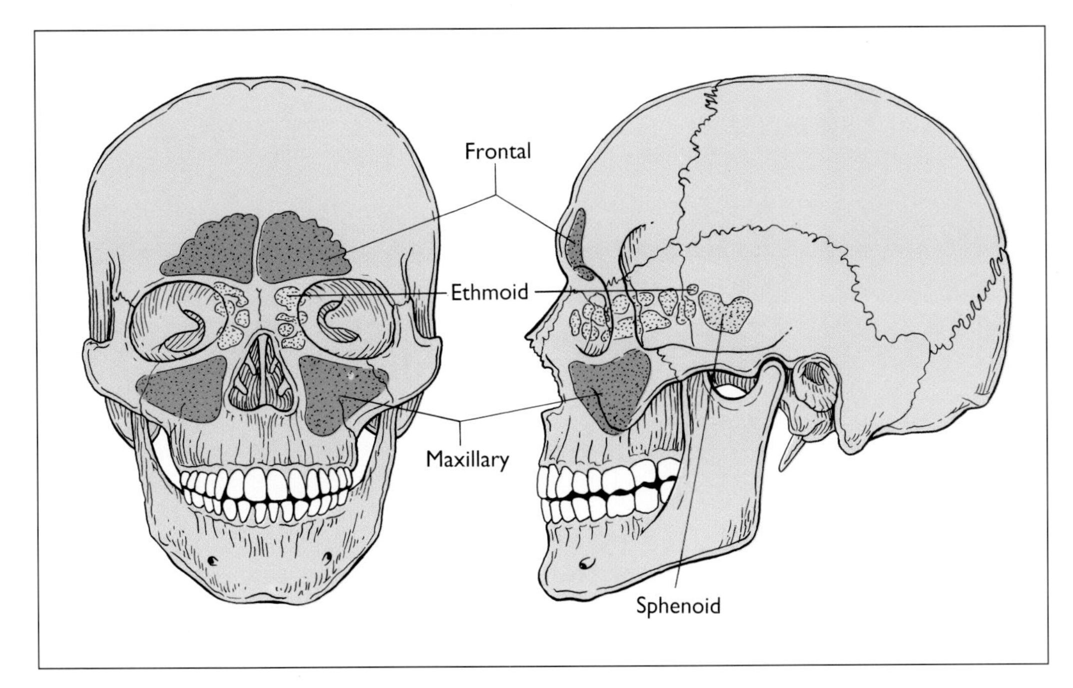

Figure 8-18 Anatomy of the paranasal sinuses. The frontal, anterior, ethmoidal, and maxillary sinuses drain into the middle meatus, whereas the posterior ethmoidal and sphenoidal sinuses open into the superior meatus. Note that the ostium of the maxillary sinus drains at an obtuse angle toward the roof. The floor of the maxillary sinus is close to the superior alveolar ridge. (*From* Vortel JJ, Chow AW: Infections of the sinuses and parameningeal structures. *In* Gorbach SL, Bartlett JG, Blacklow NR (eds.): *Infectious Diseases*. Philadelphia: W.B. Saunders; 1992:431; with permission.)

Symptoms and signs of acute sinusitis

- Facial pain
- Headache
- Purulent nasal discharge
- Nasal obstruction
- Disorders of smell
- Nasal quality to the voice
- Erythema, tenderness over involved sinus
- Fever
- Cough
- Fetid breath
- Eyelid edema, excessive tearing (ethmoid sinusitis)

Figure 8-19 Symptoms and signs of acute sinusitis. Typically, acute sinusitis develops during the course of a common cold or influenza, occurring more frequently in adults than children. Because its symptoms frequently overlap those of a prolonged cold, its diagnosis is often not possible from history and physical findings alone. Radiographic examination of the sinuses is the most sensitive test for diagnosis, with opacity, air-fluid levels, and mucosal thickening on films indicating active infection. CT and magnetic resonance imaging (MRI) are useful in evaluating the paranasal sinuses in cases with suspected complications.

Microbial etiology of acute sinusitis

	Frequency, %	
Agent	**Adults**	**Children**
Streptococcus pneumoniae	31	36
Haemophilus influenzae (unencapsulated)	21	23
Branhamella catarrhalis	2	19
Rhinovirus	15	—
Gram-negative bacteria	9	2
Anaerobic bacteria	6	—
Combined *S. pneumoniae* and *H. influenzae*	5	—
Influenza virus	5	—

Figure 8-20 Microbial etiology of acute sinusitis. *Streptococcus pneumoniae* and *Haemophilus influenzae* account for about one half of all cases in adults and children. Less-frequent causes (< 5% recovery rate each) include *Staphylococcus aureus*, *Streptococcus pyogenes*, and the parainfluenza and adenoviruses. (*Adapted from* Gwaltney JM Jr: Sinusitis. *In* Mandell GL, Douglas RG Jr, Bennett JE (eds.): *Principles and Practice of Infectious Diseases*, 3rd ed. New York: Churchill Livingstone; 1990:510–514; with permission.)

Diagnostic procedures in sinusitis

- Transillumination
- Radiography
- Ultrasonography
- CT/MRI
- Sinus aspiration
- Endoscopic sinoscopy

Figure 8-21 Diagnostic procedures in sinusitis. Because the signs and symptoms of sinusitis are often nonspecific, additional diagnostic procedures may be helpful. Transillumination is used to assess the maxillary and frontal sinuses for opacification, which indicates trapped fluid. Radiography is useful in confirming the clinical suspicion of acute sinusitis, with ultrasonography, CT, and MRI, reserved for patients with protracted symptoms or complications. Sinus aspiration is considered the gold standard of diagnostic measures, as it yields material for microbiologic culture. (Vortel JJ, Chow AW: Infections of the sinuses and parameningeal structures. *In* Gorbach SL, Bartlett JG, Blacklow NR (eds.): *Infectious Diseases*. Philadelphia: W.B. Saunders; 1992:431–448).

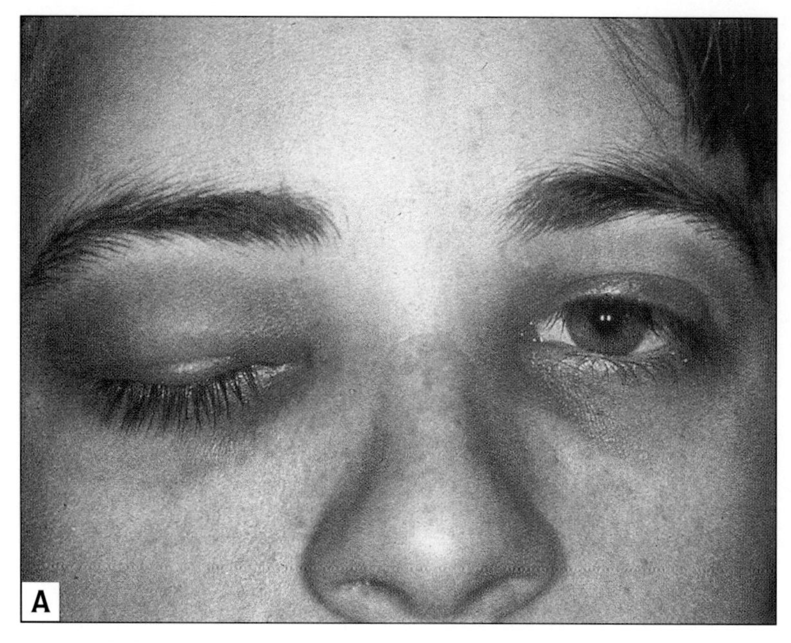

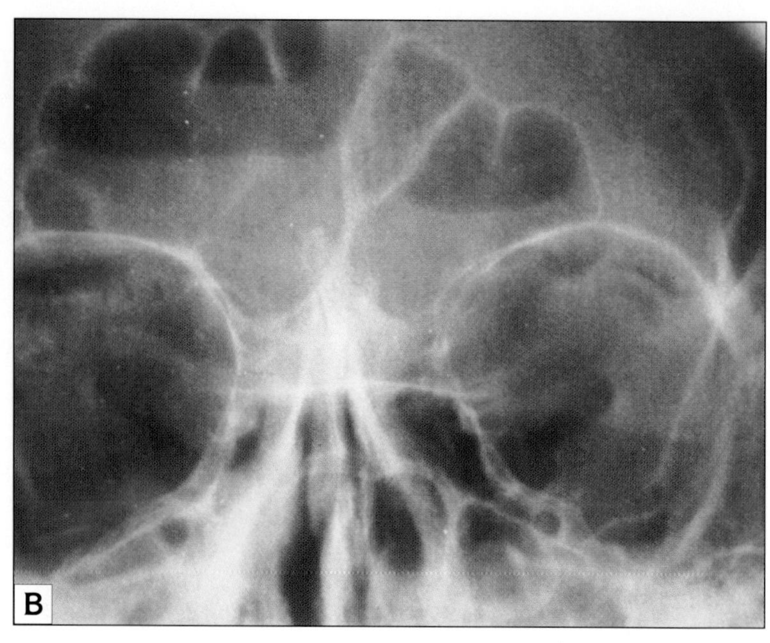

Figure 8-22 Acute bilateral frontal sinusitis. **A**, Acute bilateral frontal sinusitis (right > left) with bilateral periorbital erythema, edema of the right upper eyelid, and impaired ocular motility of 3 days' duration in a 17-year-old patient. **B**, Radiologic examination of the sinuses (occipitofrontal views) reveals an air-fluid level in both frontal sinuses (right > left). (*Adapted from* Thomae K (ed.): *Klinische Visite, Bildtafeln Thomae: Bakterielle Infektionen*. Biberach, Germany; 1984, 122:1–12; with permission.)

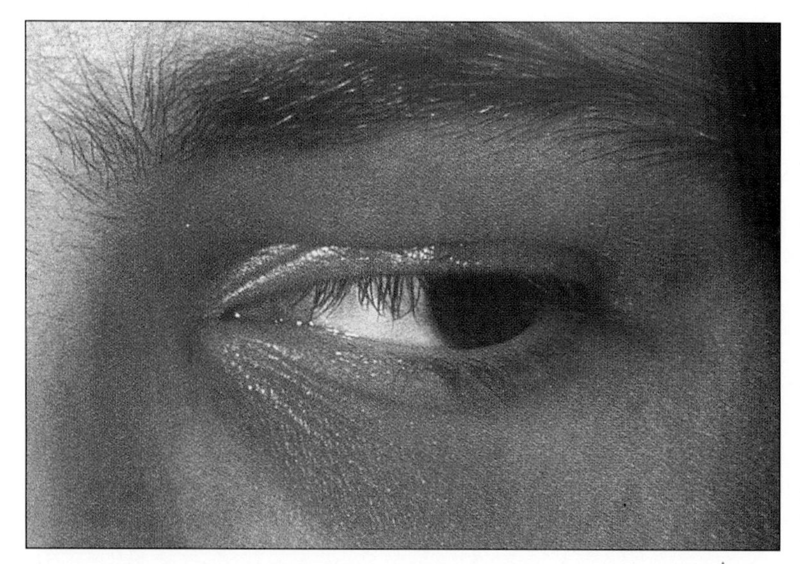

Figure 8-23 Supra- and infraorbital edema with redness in a 16-year-old patient with acute frontal and antral sinusitis. (*Adapted from* Thomae K (ed.): *Klinische Visite, Bildtafeln Thomae: Bakterielle Infektionen*. Biberach, Germany; 1984, 122:1–12; with permission.)

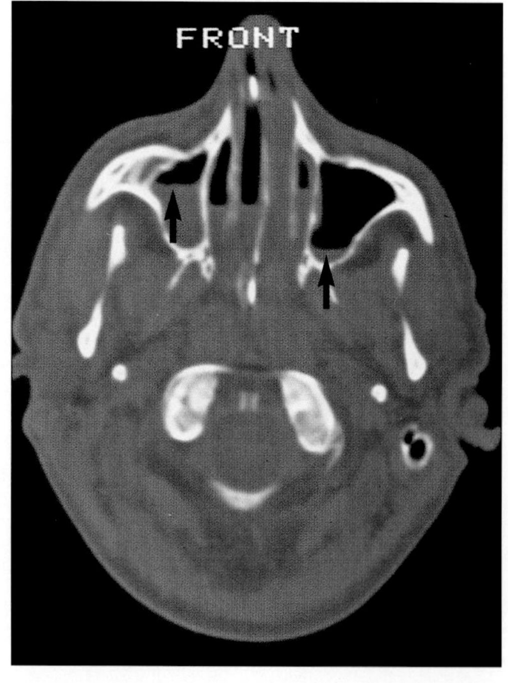

Figure 8-24 Bilateral antral sinusitis and ethmoid sinusitis. Cranial CT scanning (axial section with bone window setting) disclosed air-fluid levels in both antral sinuses (left > right) (*arrows*).

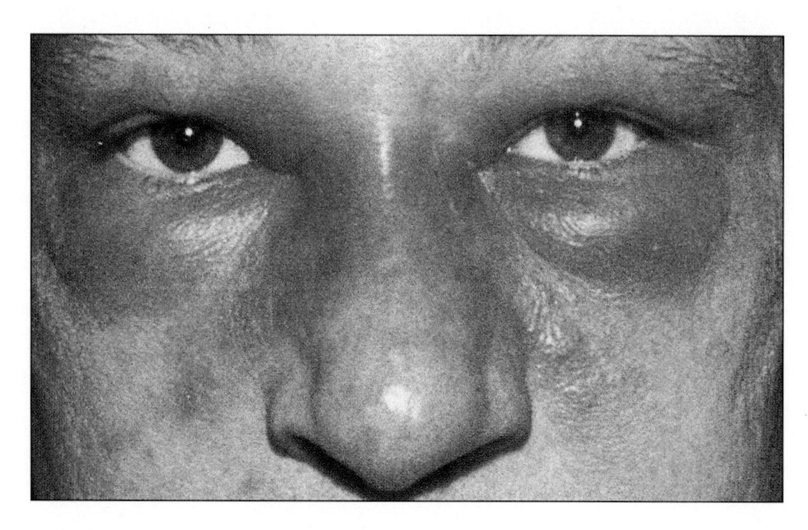

Figure 8-25 Erythema and edema of the eyelids and the dorsum of the nose secondary to acute ethmoid sinusitis of 10 days' duration in a 47-year-old patient. (*Adapted from* Thomae K (ed.): *Klinische Visite, Bildtafeln Thomae: Bakterielle Infektionen*. Biberach, Germany; 1984, 122:1–12; with permission.)

Management options in the treatment of sinusitis

Medical	Surgical
Topical nasal decongestants	Endoscopic opening of the ethmoid and maxillary infundibulum
Antimicrobials	Opening of the frontal recessus to the frontal sinus, drainage of the sphenoid sinus (if necessary)
Anti-inflammatory or antiallergic agents, analgesics (if necessary)	Correct intranasal abnormalities (*eg*, septal surgery, polypectomy) (if necessary)

FIGURE 8-26 Management options in the treatment of sinusitis. Nasal decongestant drops and sprays as well as oral antibiotics covering *Streptococcus pneumoniae* and *Haemophilus influenzae* are effective in most patients. Surgery is indicated for severe cases or those with intracranial or orbital complications, with corrective surgery reserved for cases of chronic sinusitis.

Antimicrobial regimens for acute sinusitis

Agent	Adults, *mg po*	Children, *mg/kg/d*
Ampicillin	500 qid	50–100
Amoxicillin	500 tid	40
Trimethoprim (80 mg)–sulfamethoxazole (40 mg)	160–800 bid	8–40
Erythromycin plus sulfisoxazole	500 qid 500 qid	50 150
Cefaclor	500 tid	40
Amoxicillin-potassium clavulanate	500 tid	40
Cefuroxime axetil	250 bid	45–60

FIGURE 8-27 Antimicrobial regimens for acute sinusitis. Antibiotics are the mainstay of treatment for acute sinusitis. A 10- to 14-day course of ampicillin or amoxicillin is used initially, with either trimethoprim-sulfamethoxazole or erythromycin-sulfisoxazole used for penicillin-allergic patients. (*From* Vortel JJ, Chow AW: Infections of the sinuses and parameningeal structures. *In* Gorbach SL, Bartlett JG, Blacklow NR (eds.): *Infectious Diseases*. Philadelphia: W.B. Saunders; 1992:436; with permission.)

Complications of sinusitis

Orbital complications	Intracranial complications
Eyelid edema (periorbital cellulitis, periostitis)	Meningitis
Orbital cellulitis (diffuse inflammation of the orbital contents)	Subdural empyema
Subperiosteal abscess	Epidural abscess
Orbital abscess (phlegmon)	Brain abscess
	Cavernous sinus thrombosis
	Osteomyelitis

FIGURE 8-28 Complications of sinusitis. Orbital complications of sinusitis result from extension of infections of the paranasal sinuses to the orbit (*eg*, direct extension through the paper-thin lamina papyracea, which divides the ethmoid from the orbit, or indirectly by retrograde thrombophlebitis). Despite a marked reduction in the frequency of intracranial complications through progress in antibiotic therapy, these complications are potentially life-threatening and require immediate therapy.

Orbital Complications of Sinusitis

Clinical signs of orbital complications of sinusitis

Eyelid edema
Chemosis
Proptosis
Displacement of the globe
Painful ocular movement
Impairment of ocular motility (ophthalmoplegia)
Decreased visual acuity
Funduscopic changes

Figure 8-29 Clinical signs of orbital complications of sinusitis. Orbital complications of sinusitis range from mild cellulitis to frank abscess. The majority of cases involve the eyelids, which become swollen without evidence of orbital infection.

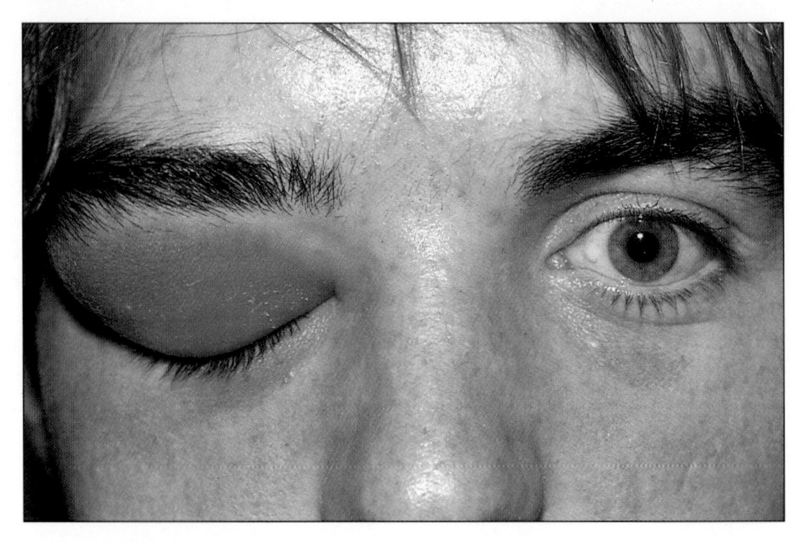

Figure 8-30 Orbital complication of ethmoid sinusitis. Marked swelling has completely closed the involved right eye.

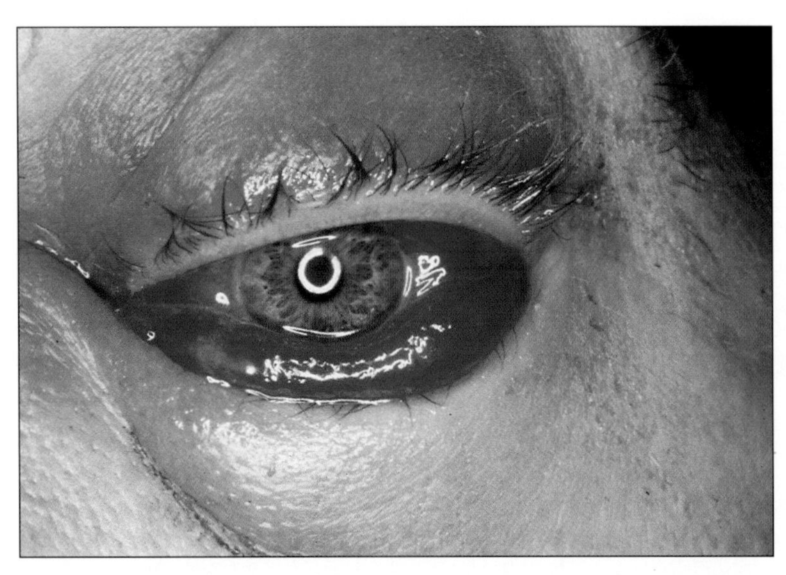

Figure 8-31 Subperiosteal abscess of the ethmoid sinus. Manual forced opening of the eye reveals intense congestion and swelling of the eyelids and conjunctiva (chemosis) with conjunctival bleeding.

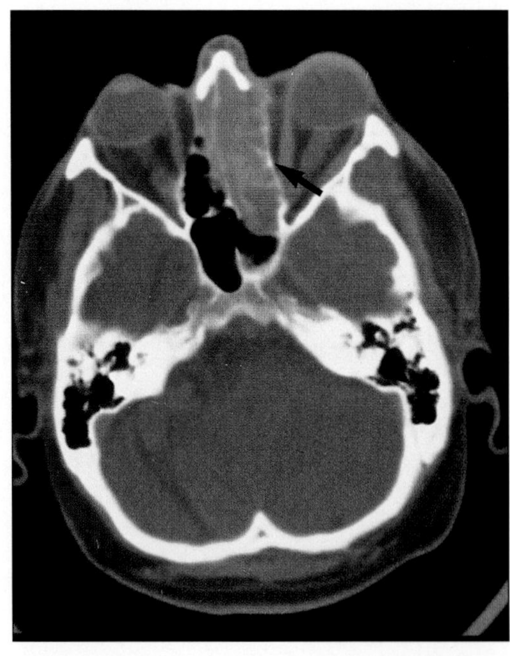

Figure 8-32 An axial cranial CT scan shows acute ethmoid sinusitis (*arrow*) with left proptosis.

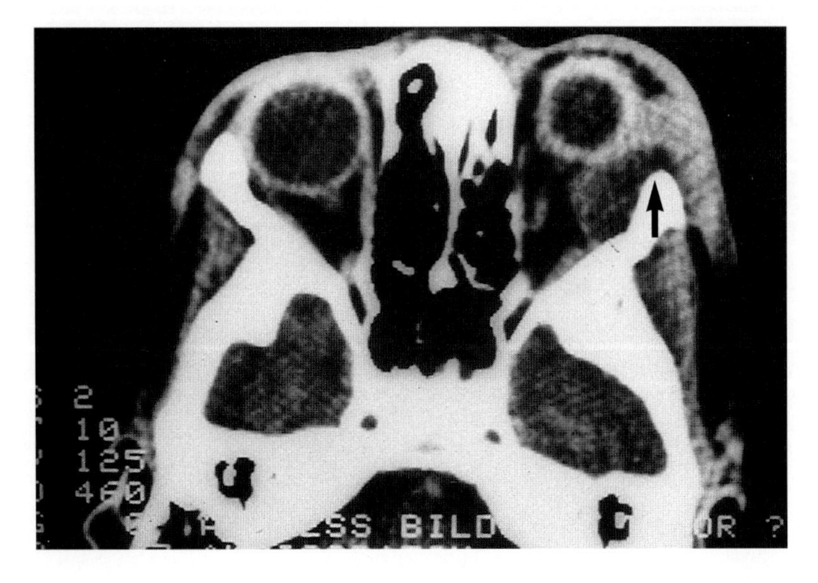

Figure 8-33 CT scan reveals the formation of an abscess in the lateral orbit (*arrow*), secondary to ethmoid sinusitis and causing exophthalmos.

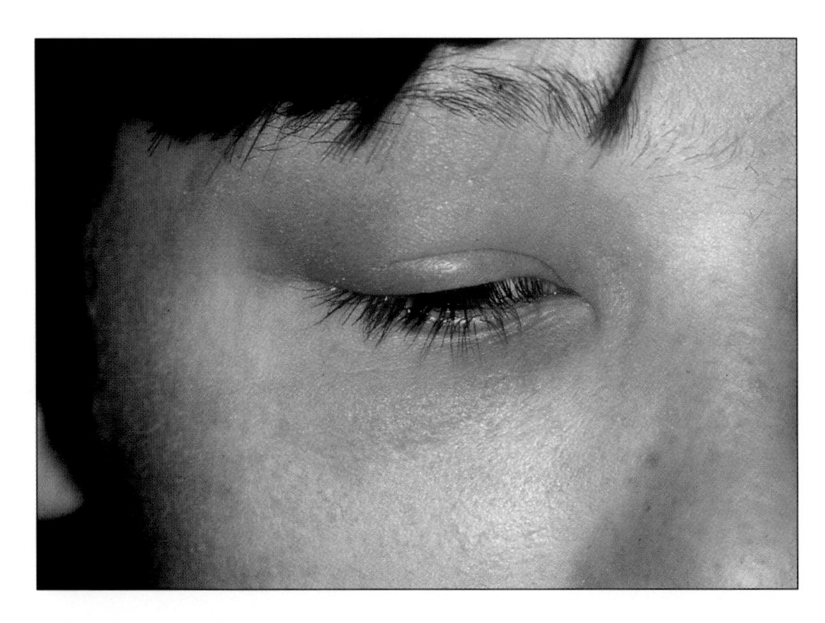

Figure 8-34 Early stage of orbital complication secondary to periostitis and ethmoiditis revealing periorbital redness and swelling of the upper eyelid.

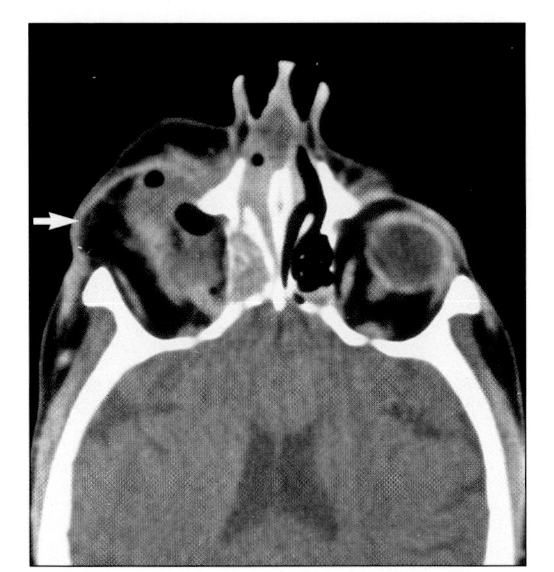

Figure 8-35 Cranial CT scan (axial section) discloses pyocele and orbit phlegmon (*arrow*) secondary to ethmoid infection in an immunosuppressed patient.

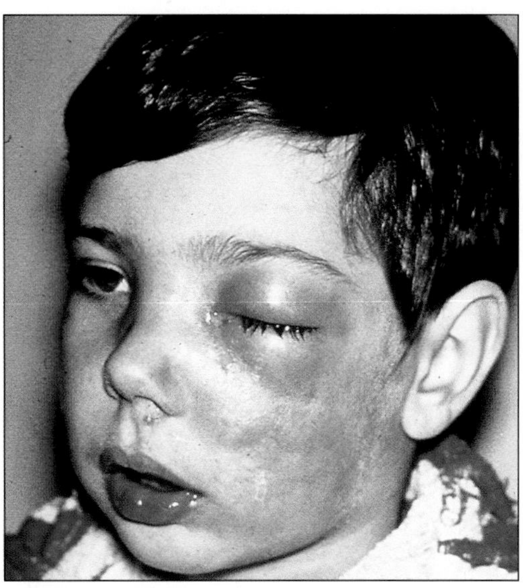

Figure 8-36 A boy with a phlegmon of the orbit, with redness and severe periorbital edema that completely closes the eye.

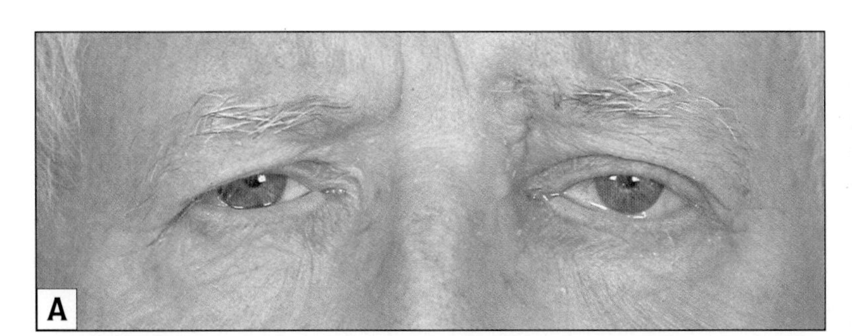

Figure 8-37 Retrobulbar abscess secondary to ethmoid sinusitis in a 71-year-old man who suffered from headache and diplopia. **A**, Slight left exophthalmos resulting in a difference of the palpebral fissures. **B**, The CT scan reveals a left retrobulbar abscess (*arrow*). The patient's clinical condition improved after surgery and intravenous antibiotic therapy.

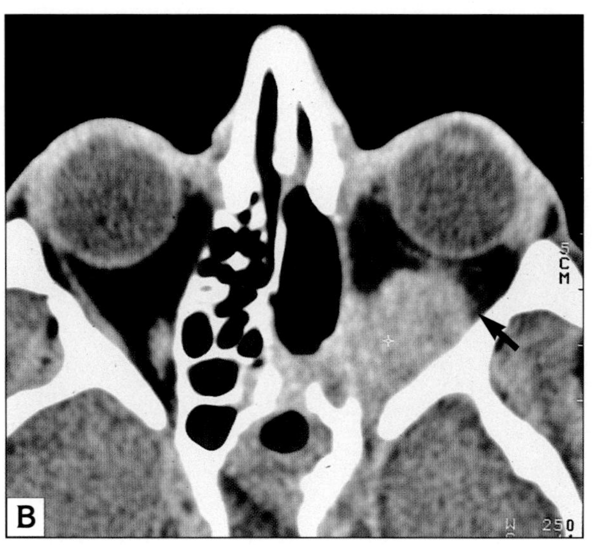

Intracranial Complications of Sinusitis

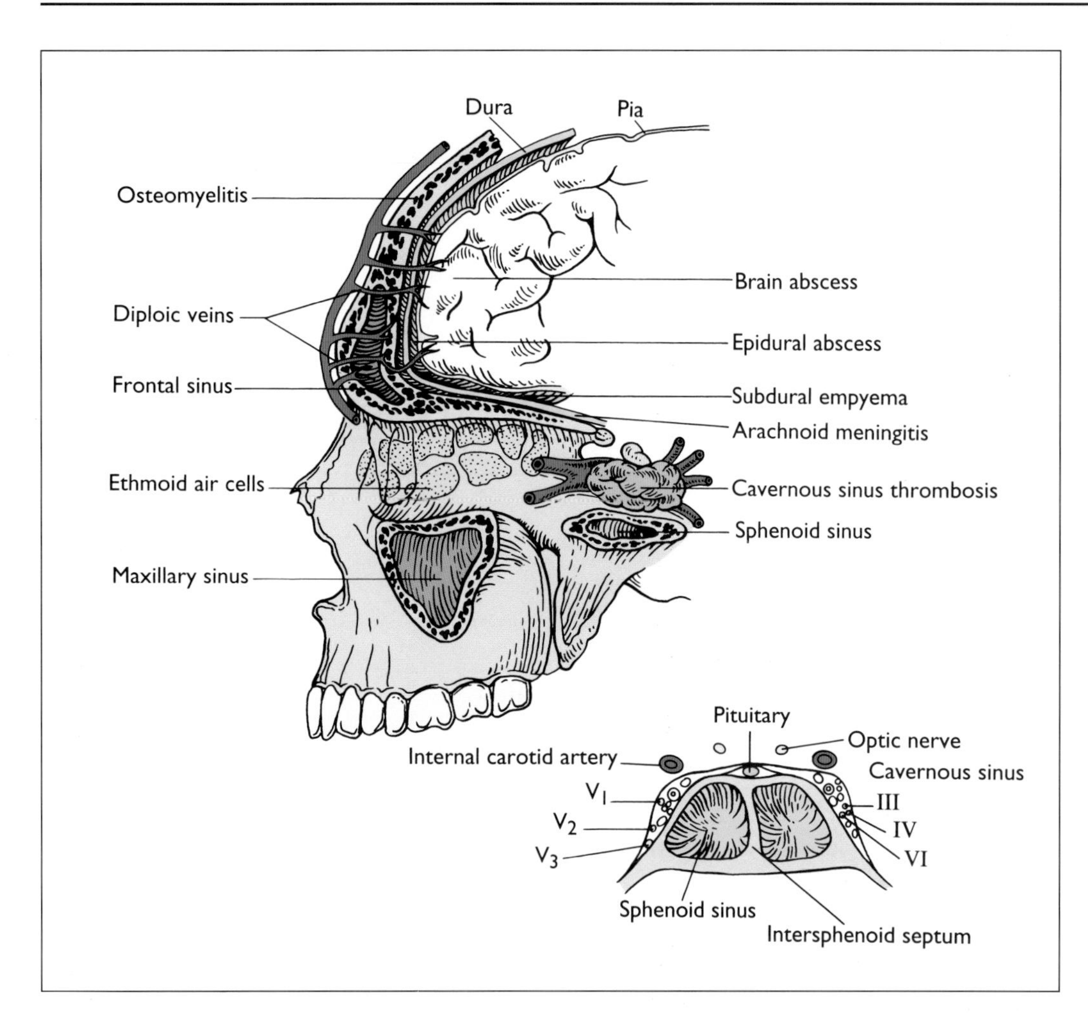

FIGURE 8-38 Intracranial complications of sinusitis. The sagittal section shows the major routes for intracranial extension of infection, either directly or via the vascular supply. Note the proximity of the diploic veins to the frontal sinus and of the cavernous sinuses to the sphenoid sinus. The coronal section (*inset*) demonstrates the structures adjoining the sphenoid sinus. (*From* Vortel JJ, Chow AW: Infections of the sinuses and parameningeal structures. *In* Gorbach SL, Bartlett JG, Blacklow NR (eds.): *Infectious Diseases*. Philadelphia: W.B. Saunders; 1992:432; with permission.)

Evaluation of intracranial complications of sinusitis

			CT	
Complication	**Clinical signs**	**CSF Findings**	**Plain**	**Contrast-enhanced**
Meningitis	Headache, fever, stiff neck, lethargy, rapid death	High PMN count and protein; low glucose	Normal	Diffusely enhanced
Osteomyelitis	Pott's puffy tumor	Normal	Bony defect	Bony defect
Epidural abscess or mucocele	Headache, fever	Normal	Lucent area	Biconvex capsule
Subdural empyema	Headache, convulsions, hemiplegia, rapid death	High PMN count and protein; normal glucose	Lucent area	Crescent-shaped enhancement
Cerebral abscess	Convulsions, headache, personality change	Lymphocytosis; normal glucose	Lucency with mass effect	Capsule
Venous sinus thrombosis (cavernous)	"Picket-fence" fever, rapid death (orbital edema, ocular palsies)	Normal or high PMN count	Nonspecific	Enhancing lesion

FIGURE 8-39 Evaluation of intracranial complications of sinusitis. The clinical spectrum of intracranial complications of sinusitis are quite varied. Management of these should be aggressive and include cerebrospinal fluid (CSF) evaluation and CT. Life-threatening and suppurative complications have become rare with antibiotic therapy. PMN—polymorphonuclear leukocytes. (*Adapted from* Vortel JJ, Chow AW: Infections of the sinuses and parameningeal structures. *In* Gorbach SL, Bartlett JG, Blacklow NR (eds.): *Infectious Diseases*. Philadelphia: W.B. Saunders; 1992:436; with permission.)

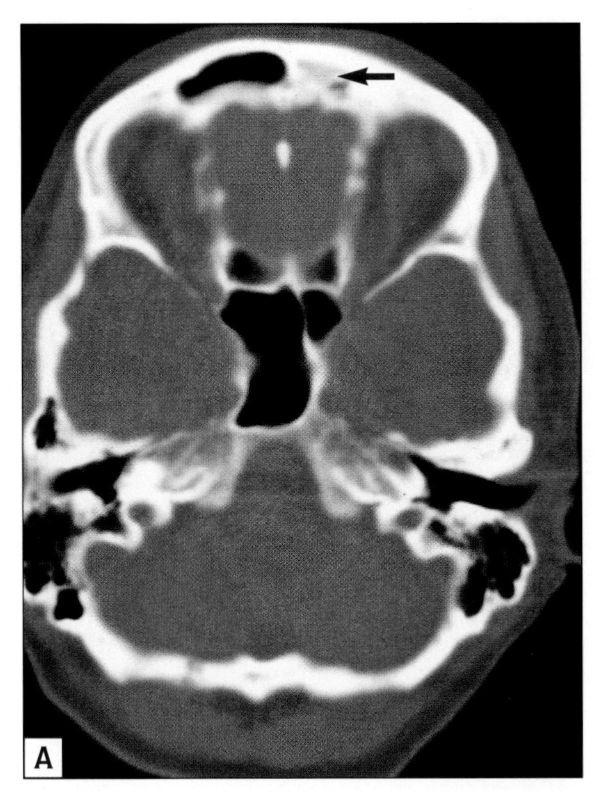

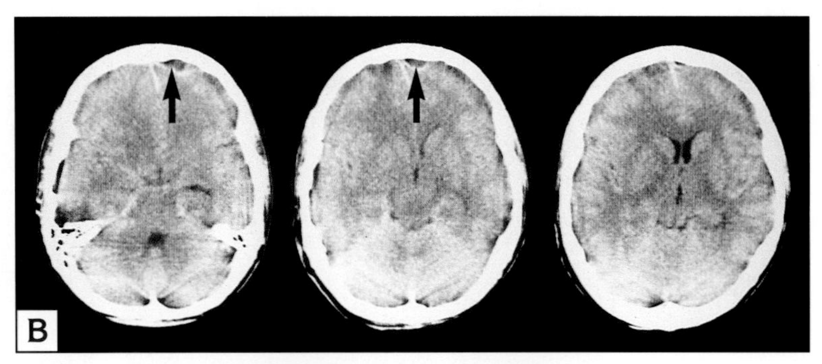

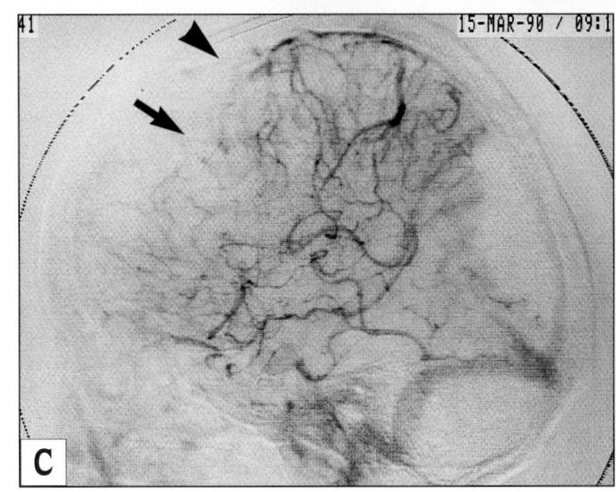

Figure 8-40 Frontal sinusitis complicated by purulent meningitis, subdural empyema, and septic sinus venous thrombosis in a 48-year-old patient. **A**, Cranial CT scan (axial section with bone window setting) discloses opacity of the frontal sinus (*arrow*). **B**, Another cranial CT scan shows subdural empyema in the right frontal region (*arrows*) and along the falx as well as swelling of the left hemisphere and a midline shift due to septic sinus venous thrombosis. **C**, Right carotid angiography (lateral subtraction view) reveals nonvisualization of parts of the superior sagittal sinus (*arrowhead*) and broken bridging veins (*arrow*). The patient had surgery of the frontal sinus and subdural empyema and associated intravenous antibiotic therapy. She survived with moderate disability (hemiparesis, psychosyndrome).

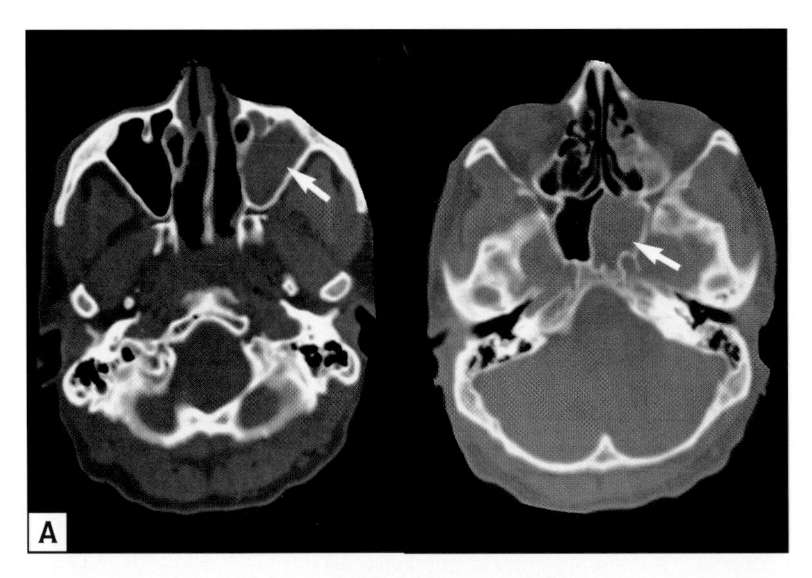

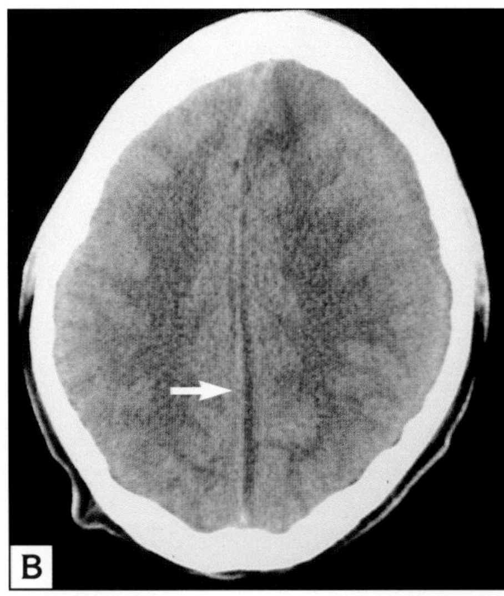

Figure 8-41 Right antral and sphenoid sinusitis complicated by subdural empyema. **A**, Cranial CT scan (axial section with bone window setting) discloses an opacity of the right antral sinus (*arrow, left panel*) and sphenoid sinus (*arrow, right panel*). **B**, Cranial CT scan with contrast enhancement reveals subdural empyema in the interhemispheric space (*arrow*).

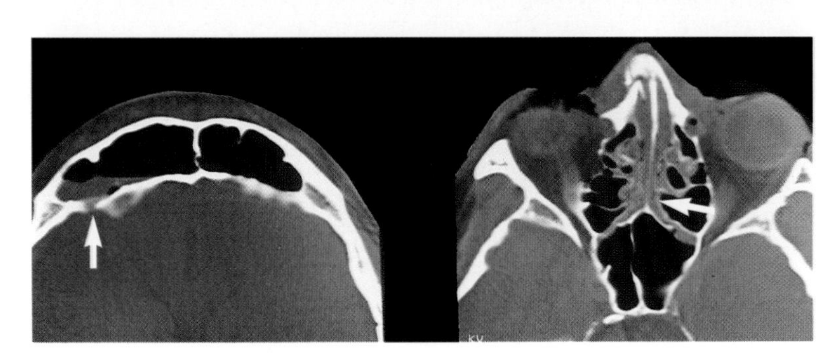

Figure 8-42 Cranial CT scan (axial section with bone window setting, *left panel*) reveals a defect of the posterior table of the frontal sinus (*arrow*) after a recent head trauma complicated by *Haemophilus influenzae* meningitis. The CT scan in the *right panel* shows ethmoid sinusitis (*arrow*).

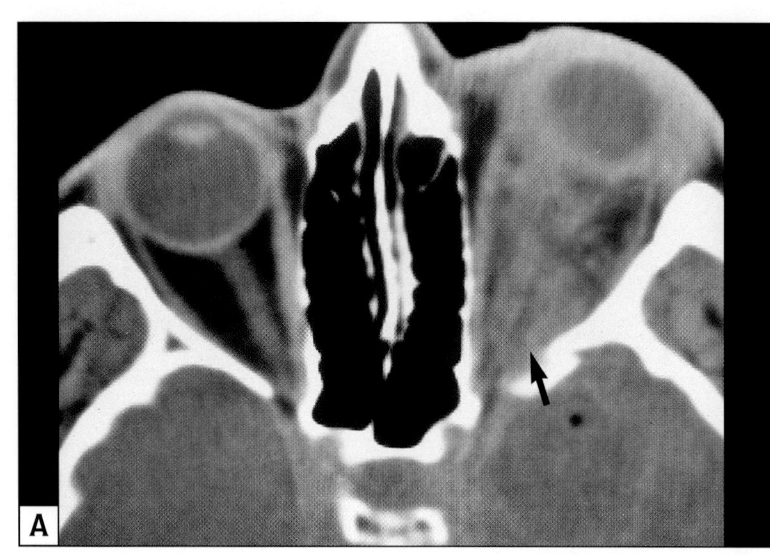

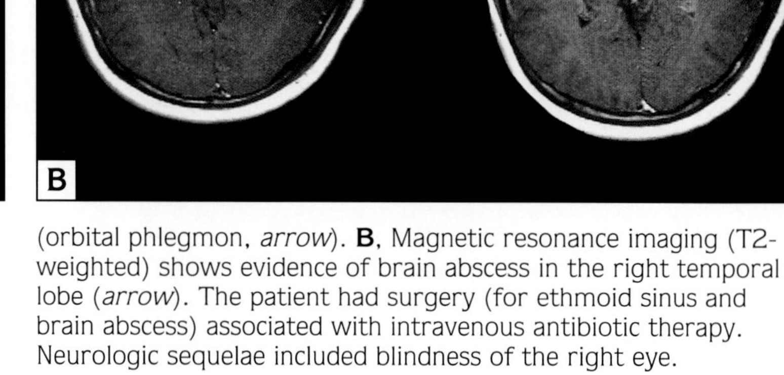

FIGURE 8-43 Right orbital phlegmon due to *S. aureus* complicated by purulent meningitis and brain abscess in the right temporal lobe developed after perforating orbital trauma in a 29-year-old patient. **A**, CT scan of the head (axial section with bone window setting) shows right proptosis and a mass in the right orbit (orbital phlegmon, *arrow*). **B**, Magnetic resonance imaging (T2-weighted) shows evidence of brain abscess in the right temporal lobe (*arrow*). The patient had surgery (for ethmoid sinus and brain abscess) associated with intravenous antibiotic therapy. Neurologic sequelae included blindness of the right eye.

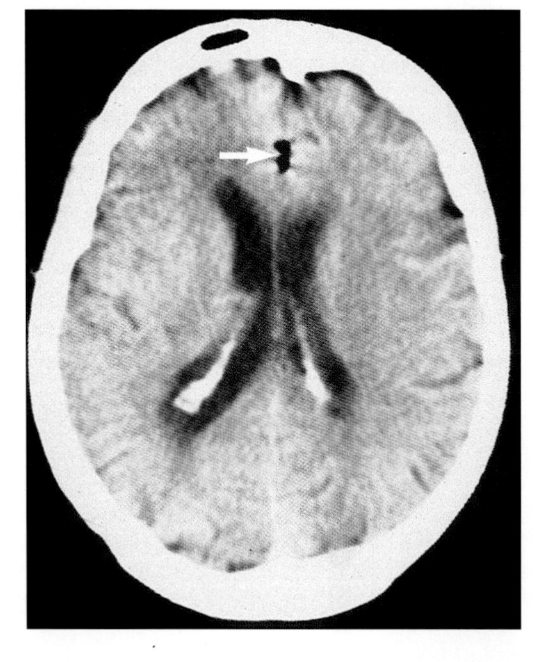

FIGURE 8-44 CT scan in a 67-year-old patient with sphenoid sinusitis and dural leak (after a previous neurosurgical procedure) complicated by pneumococcal meningitis. On admission, the patient was somnolent with a stiff neck and high fever; the CT scan disclosed intracranial free air (*arrow*).

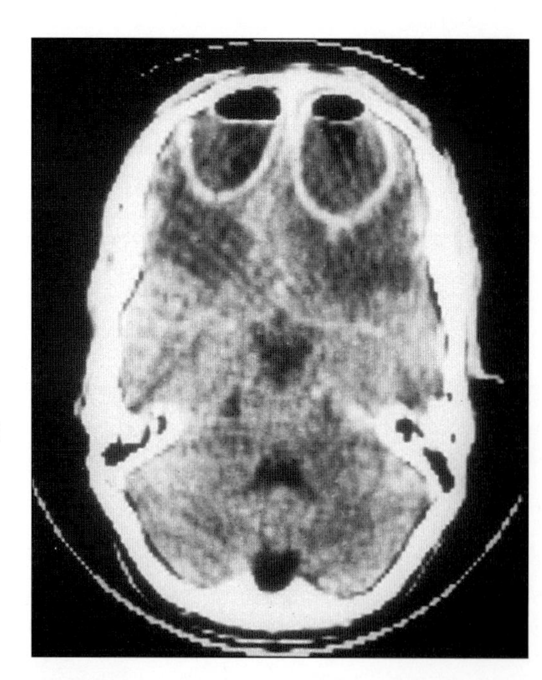

FIGURE 8-45 Sinusitis complicated by bilateral frontal lobe abscesses. A CT scan shows prominent ring-enhancement, air within the abscesses, and surrounding edema.

MASTOIDITIS

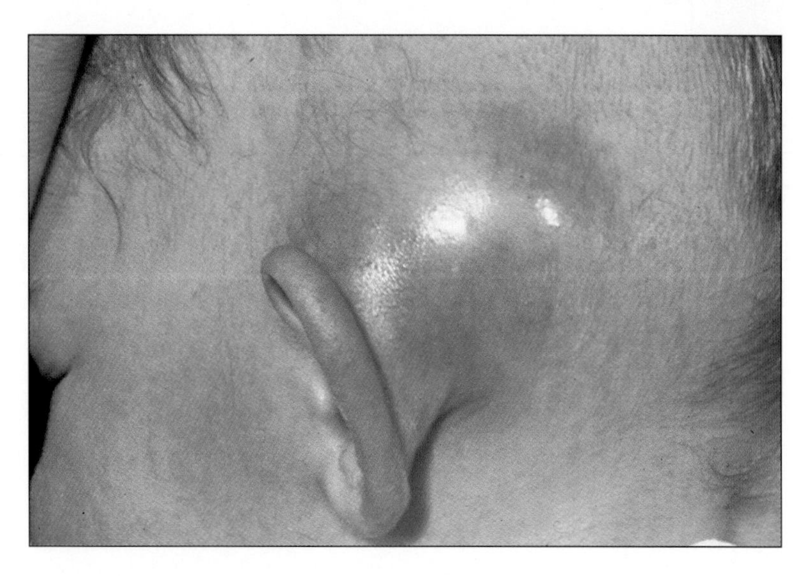

FIGURE 8-46 Acute mastoiditis. Physical findings include red swelling, pain, and tenderness over the mastoid process, with proptosis of the auricle. (*Adapted from* Thomae K (ed.): *Klinische Visite, Bildtafeln Thomae: Bakterielle Infektionen*. Biberach, Germany; 1984, 123:1–12; with permission.)

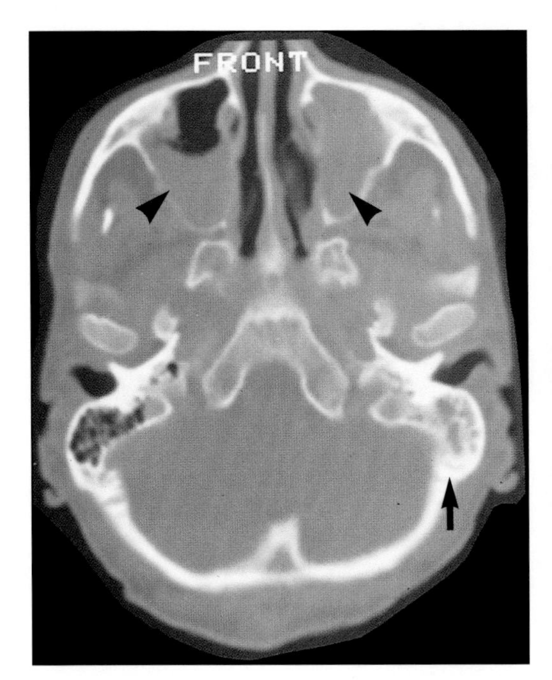

FIGURE 8-47 Right mastoiditis and bilateral antral sinusitis in a patient with *Streptococcus pyogenes* group A endocarditis. Cranial CT (bone window setting) reveals a homogeneous opacity of the right mastoid (*arrow*) and antral sinuses (*arrowheads*) (right > left).

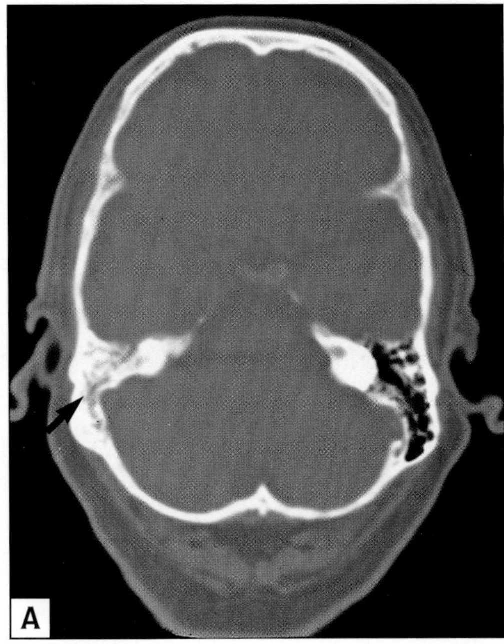

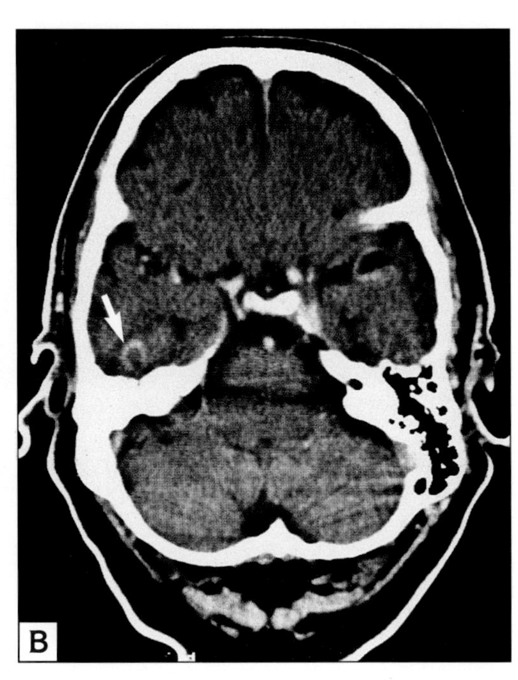

FIGURE 8-48 Left mastoiditis complicated by purulent meningitis and brain abscess due to *Streptococcus pneumoniae* in a 64-year-old patient. **A**, Cranial CT scan (axial section with bone window setting) reveals a homogenous opacity of the left mastoid (*arrow*). **B**, Axial cranial CT scan following contrast injection reveals ring enhancement of a brain abscess in the left temporal lobe (*arrow*). Following mastoidectomy and intravenous antibiotic therapy, the patient had complete recovery.

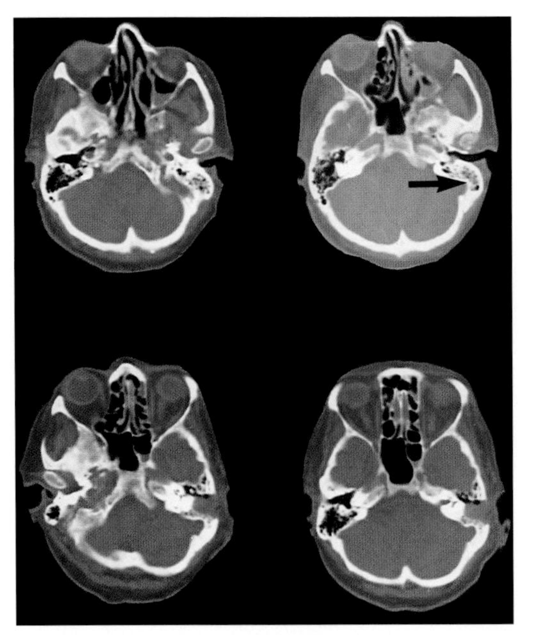

FIGURE 8-49 Right mastoiditis due to *Streptococcus pneumoniae* complicated by bacterial meningitis. *Upper row*, Cranial CT scans (axial section with bone window setting) reveal opacity of the right mastoid (*arrow*). *Lower row*, CT scans following mastoidectomy. Intraoperative cultures revealed *S. pneumoniae*, *Enterococcus* spp., and *Staphylococcus aureus*.

Complications of acute mastoiditis
Subperiosteal abscess
Facial paralysis
Suppurative labyrinthitis
Intracranial complications
Meningitis
Epidural abscess
Brain abscess
Lateral sinus thrombophlebitis

FIGURE 8-50 Complications of acute mastoiditis. Complications of acute mastoiditis are due to extension of infection beyond the mastoid air cells to contiguous areas, such as the labyrinth, sigmoid sinus, facial nerve, intracranial cavity, and/or soft tissues of the neck. Treatment of acute mastoiditis includes mastoidectomy and antibiotics (*eg*, a semisynthetic penicillin and chloramphenicol). (*Adapted from* McKenna MJ, Eavey RD: Acute mastoiditis. *In* Nadol JB Jr, Schuknecht HF (eds.): *Surgery of the Ear and Temporal Bone*. New York: Raven Press; 1993:145–154; with permission.)

Antimicrobial agents for common pathogens in acute otitis media and mastoiditis

Antimicrobial agent	*S. pneumoniae* (30%)	*H. influenzae* (20%)	*M. catarrhalis* (< 20%)	*S. pyogenes* (< 10%)	*S. aureus* (< 5%)
Ampicillin or amoxicillin	+	±	±	+	±
Amoxicillin-clavulanate	+	+	+	+	+
Penicillin	+	-	±	+	±
Clindamycin	+	-	+	+	+
Erythromycin	+	-	+	+	+
Sulfonamides	-	+	+	-	-
Erythromycin-sulfisoxazole	+	+	+	+	+
Trimethoprim-sulfamethoxazole	+	+	+	-	+
Cefaclor	+	+	±	+	+
Cefuroxime axetil	+	+	+	+	+
Cefixime	+	+	+	+	-

Figure 8-51 Antimicrobial agents for common pathogens in acute otitis media and mastoiditis. Amoxicillin (or ampicillin) is the drug currently preferred for initial empiric therapy of acute otitis media and mastoiditis, since it is active both in vitro and in vivo against *Streptococcus pneumoniae* and most strains of *Haemophilus influenzae* and it is relatively inexpensive. Amoxicillin is recommended since it can be given in three divided doses and produces fewer adverse reactions than ampicillin; 10 days' treatment is recommended. If the patient is allergic to penicillin, a combination of erythromycin and sulfisoxazole can be used. *S. pneumoniae* is pathogenic in approximately 30% of cases, *H. influenzae* in 20%, *Moraxella (Branhamella) catarrhalis* in < 20%, *Streptococcus pyogenes* in < 10%, and *Staphylococcus aureus* in < 5%. (+, effective; ±, effective for non–beta-lactamase-producing strains; –, not effective.) (*From* Vortel JJ, Chow AW: Infections of the sinuses and parameningeal structures. *In* Gorbach SL, Bartlett JG, Blacklow NR (eds.): *Infectious Diseases*. Philadelphia: W.B. Saunders; 1992:443; with permission.)

Fungal Infections

Fungi causing sinusitis

Phycomycetes (esp. *Mucor* spp.; also *Absidia, Rhizopus*)
Aspergillus (esp. *fumigatus*; also *niger, flavus, oryzae, nidulans*)
Histoplasma
Candida
Coccidioides
Alternaria

Figure 8-52 Fungi causing sinusitis. The most common fungal pathogens are of the class Phycomycetes and *Aspergillus* spp. All these fungi are saprophytic and ubiquitous in soil and can be found in the oral cavity. They may become pathogenic in individuals with altered immune functions. (*Adapted from* White JA: Paranasal sinus infections. *In* Ballenger JJ (ed.): *Diseases of the Nose, Throat, Ear, Head, and Neck*, 14th ed. Philadelphia: Lea & Febiger; 1991:184–202; with permission.)

Conditions predisposing to fungal infections of the sinuses

Prolonged steroid therapy (and other immunosuppressive drugs), broad-spectrum antibiotics
Organ transplant recipients
Malignancy, leukemia, lymphoma
Metabolic abnormalities (*eg*, diabetes mellitus, uremia)
AIDS

Figure 8-53 Conditions predisposing to fungal infections of the sinuses. Immunosuppressed patients are at highest risk to acquire fungal infections of the sinuses.

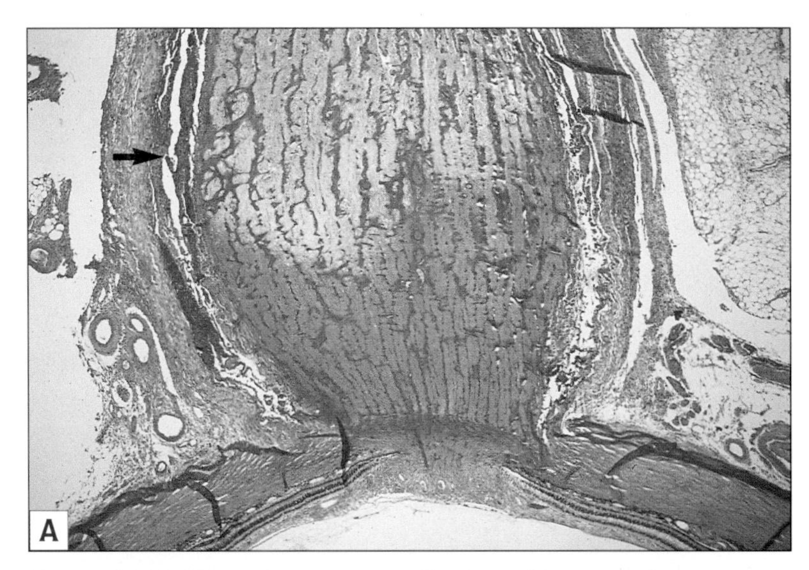

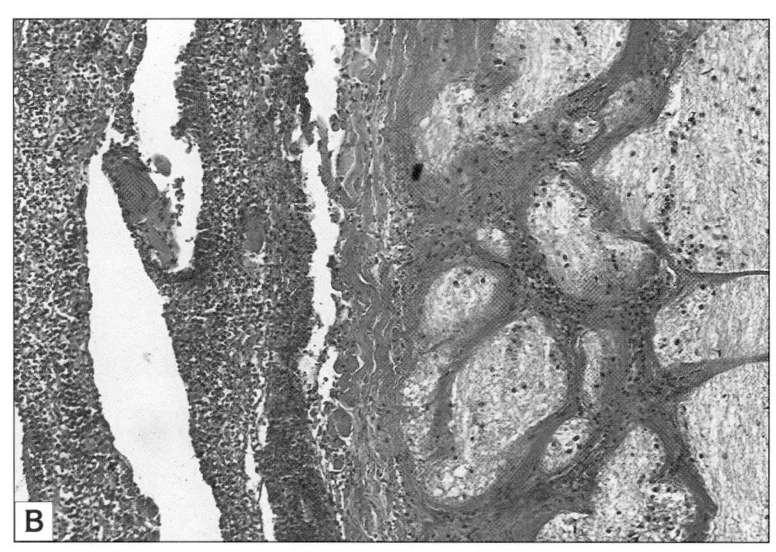

Figure 8-54 Disseminated aspergillosis. **A**, Hematoxylin-eosin staining reveals a granulocytic infiltrate of the meninges (*arrow*) surrounding the optic nerve in a patient with malignancy and diabetes mellitus. **B**, Higher magnification discloses marked granulocytic meningeal inflammation. (*Courtesy of* Dr. K. Bise.)

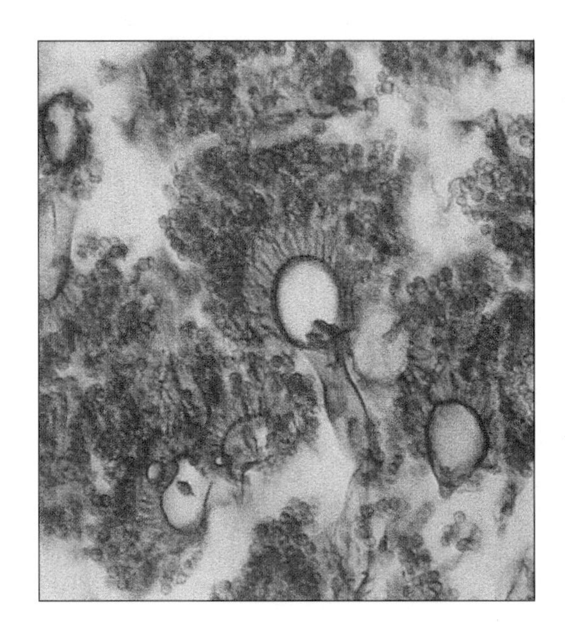

Figure 8-55 Microscopic view of the spore-bearing structures of *Aspergillus fumigatus*, demonstrating conidiophores of aspergillus (periodic acid–Schiff stain). (*Adapted from* Thomae K (ed.): *Klinische Visite, Bildtafeln Thomae: Bronchopulmonale Infektionen*. Biberach, Germany; 1984, 128:1–16; with permission.)

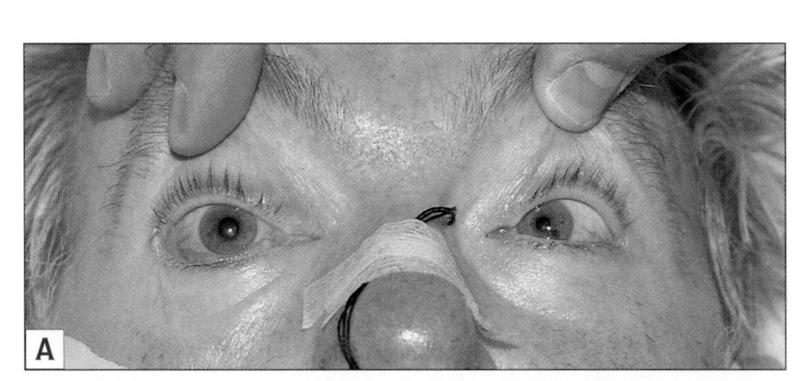

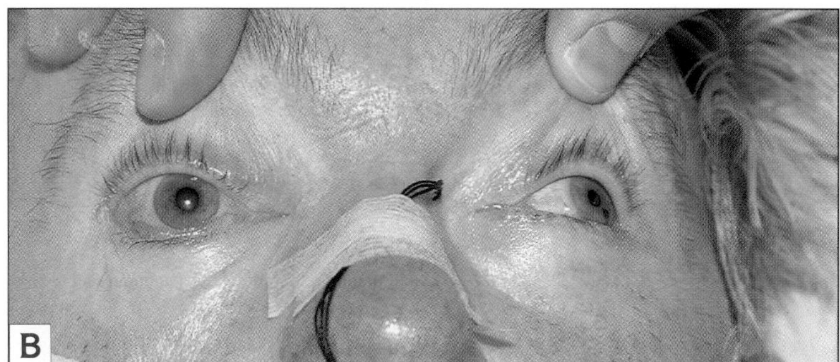

Figure 8-56 Fungal infection of the paranasal sinuses in a 75-year-old patient with diabetes complicated by septic cavernous sinus syndrome. The patient had right ophthalmoplegia associated with visual loss, chemosis, slight proptosis, conjunctival injection, and a sensibility disorder in the trigeminal distribution of the right ophthalmic division. **A**, A lack of abduction of the right eye in left-gaze. **B**, A lack of adduction of the right eye in right-gaze. (*continued*)

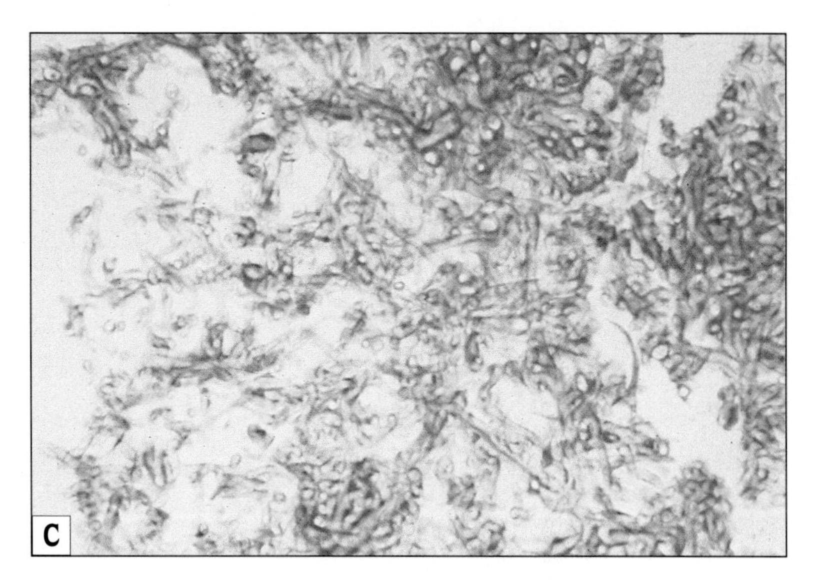

FIGURE 8-56 (*continued*) **C**, Periodic acid–Schiff stain of material obtained from the right maxillary sinus shows septate hyphae and dichotomous branching which is characteristic of *Aspergillus* spp. Despite surgical therapy for sinusitis and intravenous antibiotic and antimycotic therapy, the patient died of septic shock. (*Courtesy of* Dr. H. Arnholdt.)

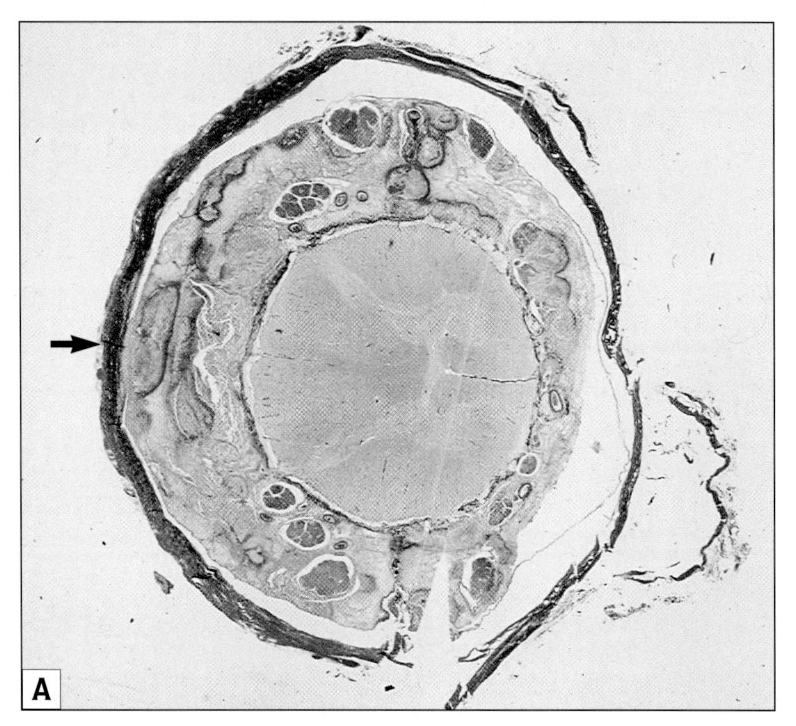

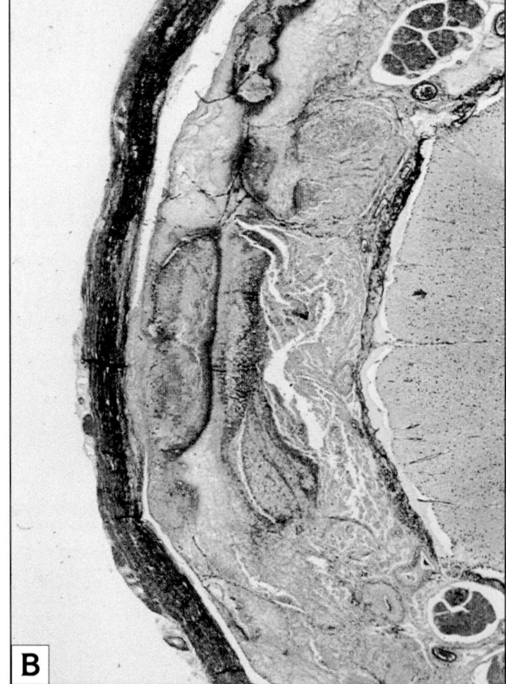

FIGURE 8-57 Mucormycosis. **A** and **B**, Mucormycosis in a 32-year-old patient with pineoblastoma who developed granulocytic meningitis of the cerebral and spinal meninges. Marked granulocytic infiltrates of the spinal meninges are shown (*arrow*, Grocott stain). (*Courtesy of* Dr. K. Bise.)

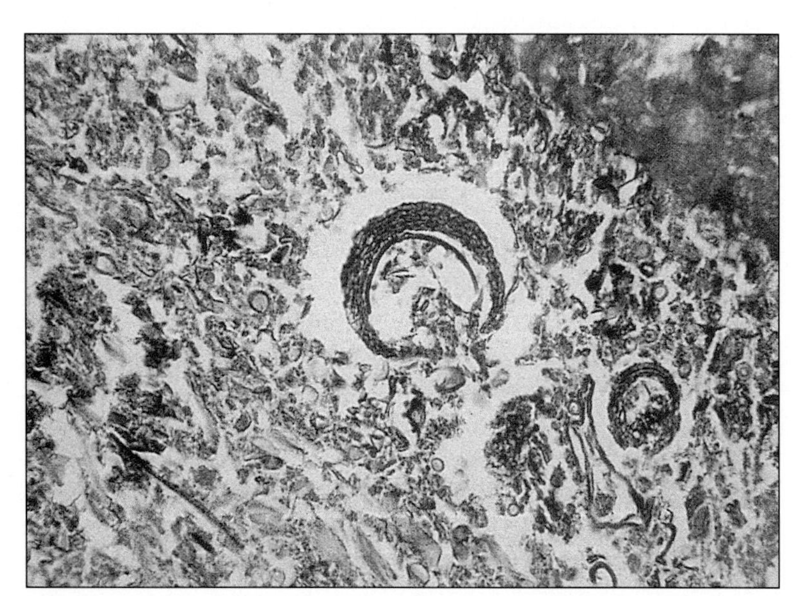

FIGURE 8-58 Sporangium in mucormycosis (*Rhizopus oryzae*) in necrosis of the nose cartilage in a young patient with diabetes mellitus (periodic acid–Schiff stain). (*Adapted from* Thomae H (ed.): *Klinische Visite, Bildtafeln Thomae: Bronchopulmonale Infektionen*. Biberach, Germany; 1987, 128:1–16; with permission.)

Clinical presentation of craniofacial mucormycosis
Ketoacidosis, neutropenia
Bloody nasal discharge
Ulcerations or crusting on the palate or nasal cavity (classical finding: black, encrusted middle turbinate)
Chemosis, proptosis, periorbital edema, obtundation, ophthalmoplegia, trigeminal anesthesia, facial palsy
Headache, facial swelling
Hemiplegia (with extension of the fungal infection to the internal carotid artery)

FIGURE 8-59 Clinical presentation of craniofacial mucormycosis. Ethmoid sinuses are most often affected, followed by the sphenoid and maxillary sinuses. Invasion of the ophthalmic and carotid arteries may occur.

Management of craniofacial mucormycosis
Aggressive debridement of all necrotic tissue (orbital exenteration may be necessary in orbital involvement) Correct underlying diabetic ketoacidosis Intravenous amphotericin B (*eg*, 0.5–0.7 mg/kg/d × 8–10 wks)

FIGURE 8-60 Management of craniofacial mucormycosis. Fungal infection in an immunocompromised patient is a medical emergency. If untreated, severe complications (*eg*, blindness, cranial nerve deficits, hemiplegia) or death may occur within 2 to 5 days. Appropriate treatment can result in survival of 60%–85% of patients with craniofacial mucormycosis. (*Adapted from* Kwon-Chung KJ, Bennett JE (eds.): *Medical Mycology*. Philadelphia: Lea & Febiger; 1992:524–559; with permission.)

SELECTED BIBLIOGRAPHY

Chow AW, Vortel J: Infections of the sinuses and parameningeal structures. *In* Gorbach SL, Bartlett JG, Blacklow NR (eds.): *Infectious Diseases*. Philadelphia: W.B. Saunders Co.; 1992:431–448.

Gwaltney JM Jr: Sinusitis. *In* Mandell GL, Douglas RG Jr, Bennett JE (eds.): *Principles and Practice of Infectious Diseases*, 3rd ed. New York: Churchill Livingstone; 1990:510–514.

Lawson W: Orbital complications of sinusitis. *In* Blitzer A, Lawson W, Friedman WH (eds.): *Surgery of the Paranasal Sinuses*, 2nd ed. Philadelphia: W.B. Saunders Co.; 1991:457–470.

Neu HC: Infectious diseases of the sinuses. *In* Blitzer A, Lawson W, Friedman WH (eds.): *Surgery of the Paranasal Sinuses*, 2nd ed. Philadelphia: W.B. Saunders Co.; 1991:161–167.

Stankiewicz JA, Nevell DJ, Park AH: Complications of inflammatory diseases of the sinuses. *Otolaryngol Clin North Am* 1993, 26:639–655.

Waith JA: Paranasal sinus infections. *In* Ballenger JJ, (ed.): *Diseases of the Nose, Throat, Ear, Head, and Neck*, 14th ed. Philadelphia: Lea & Febiger; 1991:184–202.

CHAPTER 9

The Nervous System in Sepsis and Endocarditis

David A. Ramsay
G. Bryan Young

Neurologic Complications of Sepsis

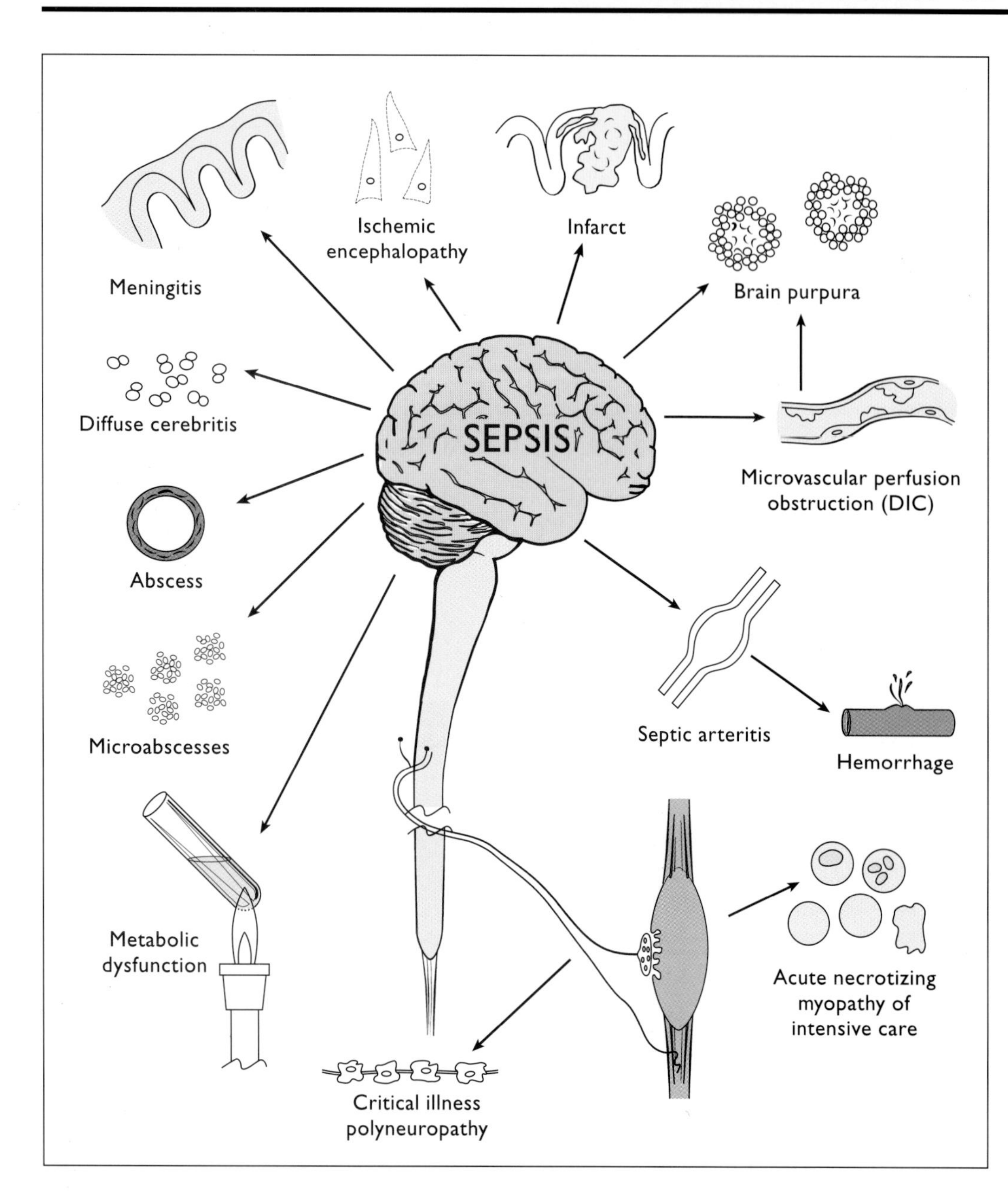

Figure 9-1 The effects of sepsis on the nervous system. *Sepsis* is a term that implies the presence of microorganisms or their toxins in the blood or tissues of the body *and* a systemic response or effect on at least one organ system. It must be emphasized that the otherwise helpful localizing signs and symptoms that characterize some of these disorders are masked in critically ill, often comatose, septic patients, who are, owing to their attachment to ventilators, monitors, and various lines, difficult to assess neurologically. Accordingly, extensive investigation, including electroencephalography, neuroimaging, and cerebrospinal fluid and blood analysis, is usually necessary to identify which of these often diffuse or multifocal complications of sepsis are present. DIC—disseminated intravascular coagulation. (Barton R, Cerra FB: The hypermetabolism–multiple organ failure syndrome. *Chest* 1989, 115:136–140. Bone RC: Sepsis syndrome: New insights into its pathogenesis and treatment. *Intensive Care World* 1992, 4:50–59. Nava E, Palmer RMF, Moncada S: Inhibition of nitric oxide synthesis in septic shock: How much is beneficial? *Lancet* 1991, 338:1557–1558. Sprung C, Cerra FB, Freund HR, *et al.*: Plasma amino acids as predictors of the severity and outcome of sepsis. *Crit Care Med* 1991, 19:753–757.)

Classification of the effects of sepsis on the nervous system	
Direct effects	Microabscesses Acute pyogenic encephalitis Vasculitis Acute and chronic meningitis Meningoencephalitis
Indirect complications	Cerebrovascular complications Visible metabolic defects Sepsis-associated encephalopathy Neuromuscular complications

Figure 9-2 Classification of the effect of sepsis on the nervous system. Sepsis can affect the nervous system directly (*eg*, diffuse "cerebritis," abscess formation, microabscesses, meningitis, septic arteritis) or indirectly (by the effects of circulating microperfusion modifiers, including cytokines, nitric oxide and altered regulation of leukocyte cell adhesion molecules, or the metabolic and hypotensive effects of failure of other organs).

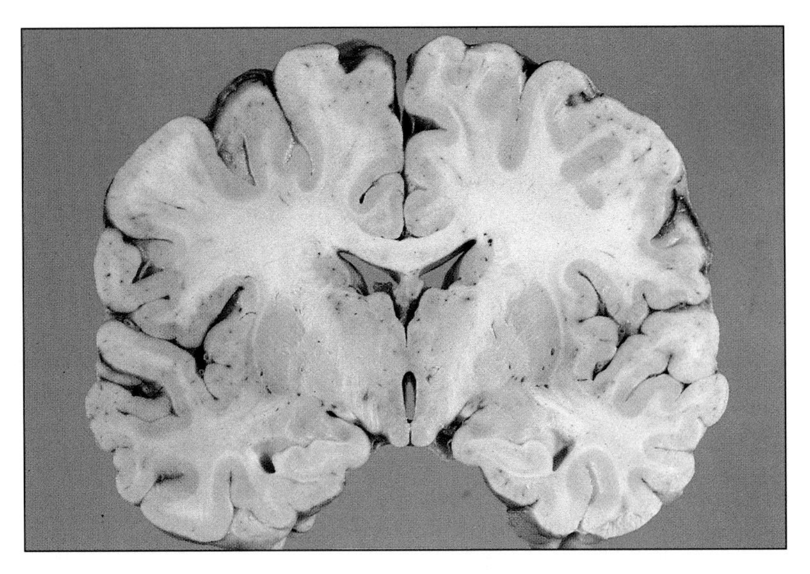

Figure 9-3 Normal brain. A coronal slice through a grossly normal brain serves as a reminder that, in many cases of sepsis and unequivocal sepsis-associated encephalopathy, the central nervous system (CNS) is grossly and microscopically unremarkable or significant structural abnormalities may not be noticed until microscopic examination of the tissue is performed. This is of particular relevance to the interpretation of neuroimaging studies, which may be reported as normal in a neurologically severely disabled patient. (Young GB, Bolton CF, Austin TW, *et al.*: The encephalopathy associated with septic illness. *Clin Invest Med* 1990, 13:297–304.)

Direct Neurologic Infection in Sepsis

Microabscesses

Microbiology of sepsis-associated brain microabscesses

Organism	Percent
Staphylococcus aureus	29
Candida albicans	24
Mixed flora	21
Escherichia coli	6
Klebsiella pneumoniae	6
Pseudomonas aeruginosa	4
Other organisms	6
Unknown	4

Figure 9-4 Microbiology of sepsis-associated brain microabscesses. Although the clinical suspicion of their existence may be well founded, the diagnosis of cerebral microabscesses in life is practically impossible. Accordingly, in most cases, this condition receives "bystander" treatment when antibiotics are administered to counter organisms isolated from sites other than the brain. (Jackson AC, Gilbert JJ, Young GB, Bolton CF: The encephalopathy of sepsis. *Can J Neurol Sci* 1985, 12:303–307. Pendlebury WW, Perl DP, Munoz DG: Multiple microabscesses in the central nervous system: A clinicopathological study. *J Neuropathol Exp Neurol* 1989, 48:290–300.)

Extraneural sources of infection in sepsis-associated brain microabscesses

Source	Percent
Lungs	32
Abdomen (perforated viscus, cholecystitis)	21
Heart valves	15
Unknown	13
Other (genitourinary system, intravenous line, joint, vascular graft, wound)	19

Figure 9-5 Extraneural sources of infection in sepsis-associated brain microabscesses. The most likely sources of extraneural infection associated with brain microabscesses are the lungs and abdominal cavity. (Jackson AC, Gilbert JJ, Young GB, Bolton CF: The encephalopathy of sepsis. *Can J Neurol Sci* 1985, 12:303–307. Pendlebury WW, Perl DP, Munoz DG: Multiple microabscesses in the central nervous system: a clinicopathological study. *J Neuropathol Exp Neurol* 1989, 48:290–300.)

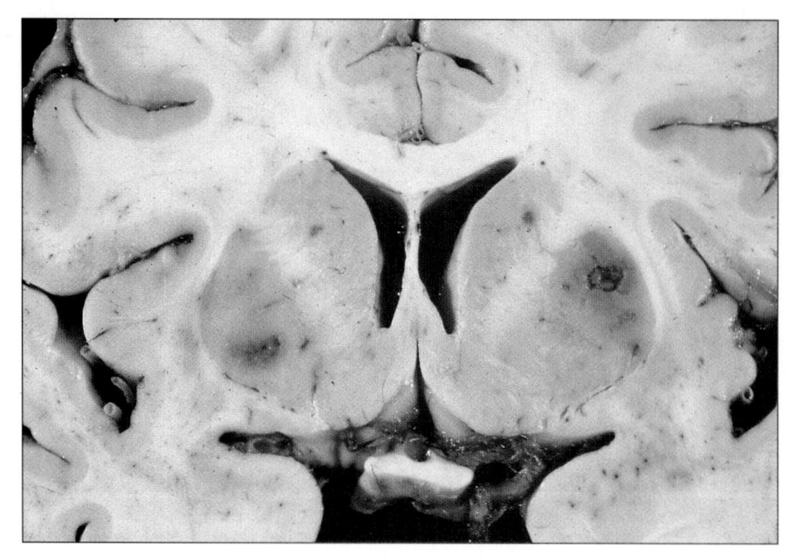

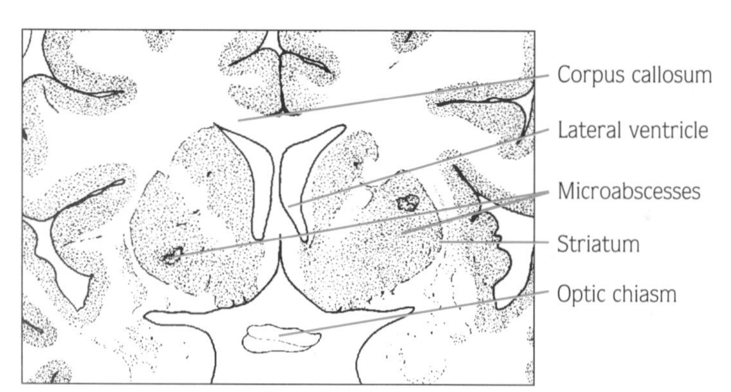

FIGURE 9-6 Microabscesses, gross appearance. The most commonly encountered structural abnormalities of the CNS in sepsis are microabscesses. Although fundoscopic examination may reveal retinal microabscesses, which suggest the presence of brain microabscesses, these inflammatory collections are usually not identified unless the brain is examined at autopsy. This coronal slice through the rostral basal ganglia contains bilateral punctate areas of hemorrhagic softening in the putamen, which are rare, gross examples of microabscesses. (Jackson AC, Gilbert JJ, Young GB, Bolton CF: The encephalopathy of sepsis. *Can J Neurol Sci* 1985, 12:303–307. Pendlebury WW, Perl DP, Munoz DG: Multiple microabscesses in the central nervous system: A clinicopathological study. *J Neuropathol Exp Neurol* 1989, 48:290–300.)

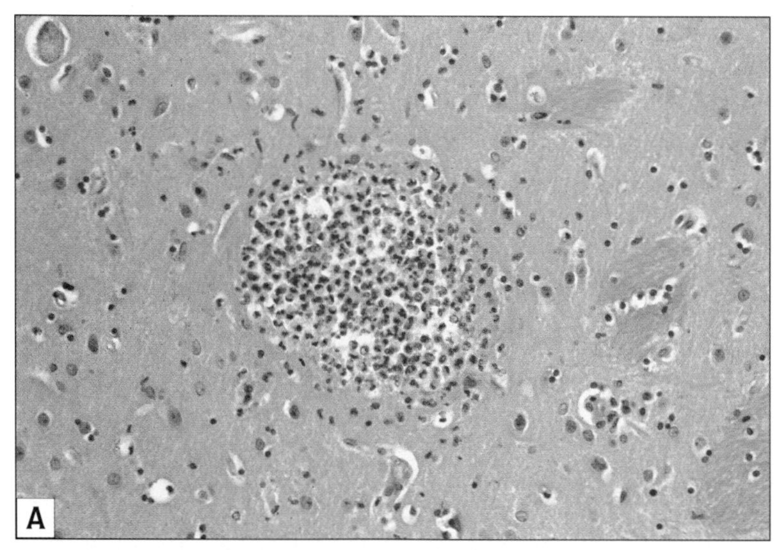

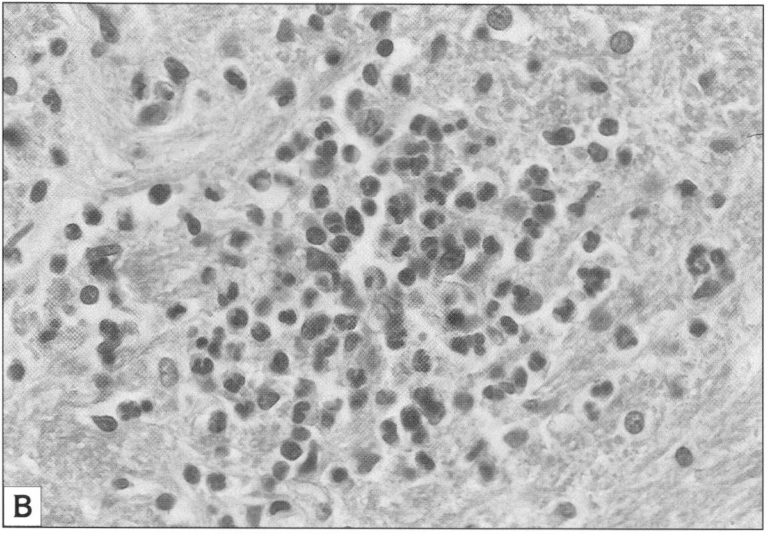

FIGURE 9-7 Microabscesses, histologic appearances. Microabscesses may not be discovered until the brain is examined microscopically. They are found throughout the CNS (including the spinal cord), most commonly in the cortex and deep gray matter. **A**, At low power, they appear as more or less well-circumscribed, nodular collections of inflammatory cells, sometimes around a capillary and associated with a variable degree of neuroparenchymal necrosis. (Hematoxylin and eosin, × 45.) **B**, At higher magnification, the acute microabscesses contain numerous polymorphonuclear leukocytes. (Hematoxylin, eosin, and solochrome, × 155.)

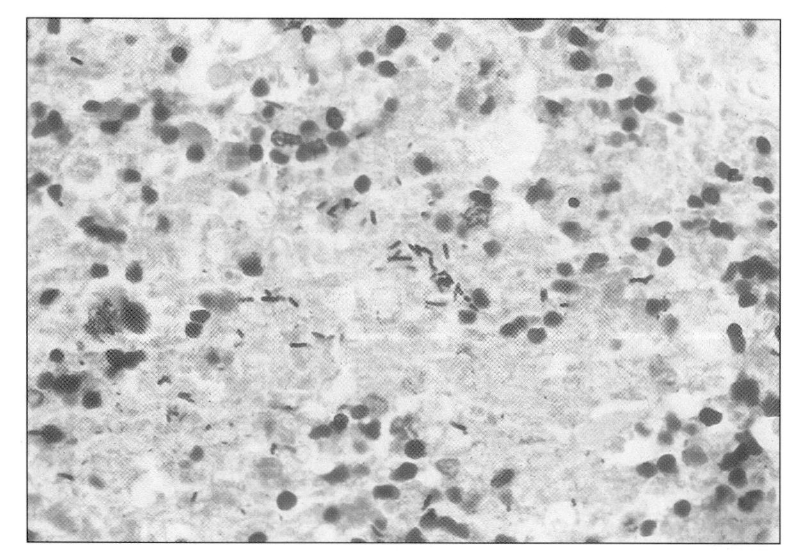

FIGURE 9-8 Bacterial microabscesses. The bacterial species most commonly implicated in the formation of brain microabscesses is *Staphylococcus aureus*. However, in many cases, the organisms cannot be identified in histologic sections, probably because they have been "cleared" by antecedent antibiotic treatment. The bacterial basis of the microabscesses is, therefore, inferred from antemortem investigation, which usually provides evidence of an infection, often a septicemia. In the case illustrated here, however, gram-variable bacilli are demonstrated and there was a history consistent with a *Haemophilus influenzae* pneumonia (Gram, × 155).

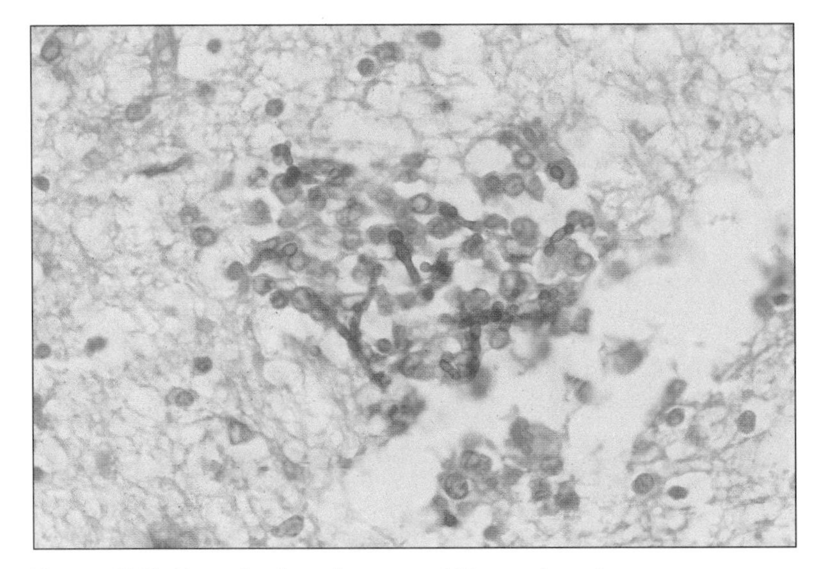

FIGURE 9-9 Fungal microabscesses. When microabscesses are associated with fungal sepsis, it is easier than in cases of bacterial origin to demonstrate the organism in tissue sections; the commonest agent is *Candida albicans*. This photomicrograph shows a small microabscess that contains budding spores and pseudohyphae, which are characteristic of candidal species. (Periodic acid–Schiff, × 155.)

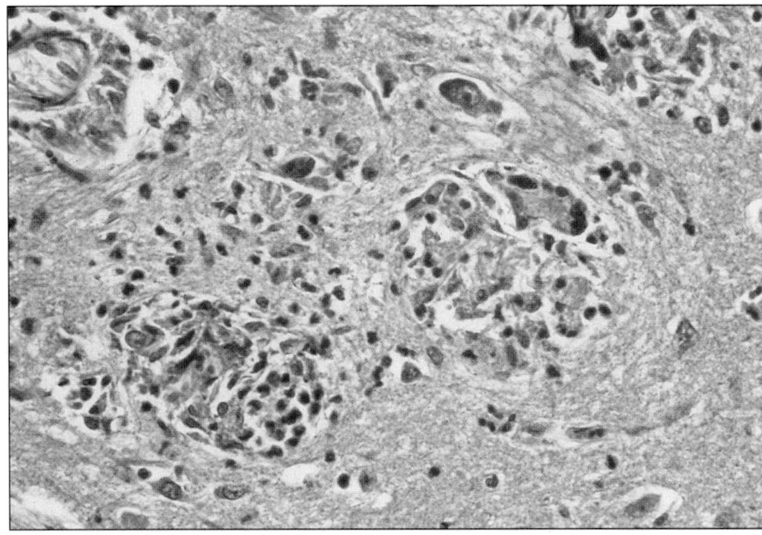

FIGURE 9-10 Chronic microabscesses. An abscess is a discrete, usually walled-off collection of acute polymorphonuclear leukocytes. The term *microabscess* is therefore something of a misnomer since the acute inflammatory cells are never enclosed by granulation tissue. Moreover, microabscess formation is dynamic, and the cytologic constituents change with time. At first, the inflammatory cells are polymorphonuclear leukocytes, but, with control of the infection, the granulocytes may be replaced by chronic inflammatory cells, including macrophages and lymphocytes, and the adjacent microglia are "activated." In cases of fungal infections, characteristic multinucleated macrophages (giant cells) appear, as shown in this photomicrograph. (Hematoxylin and eosin, × 80.)

Acute Pyogenic CNS Infections

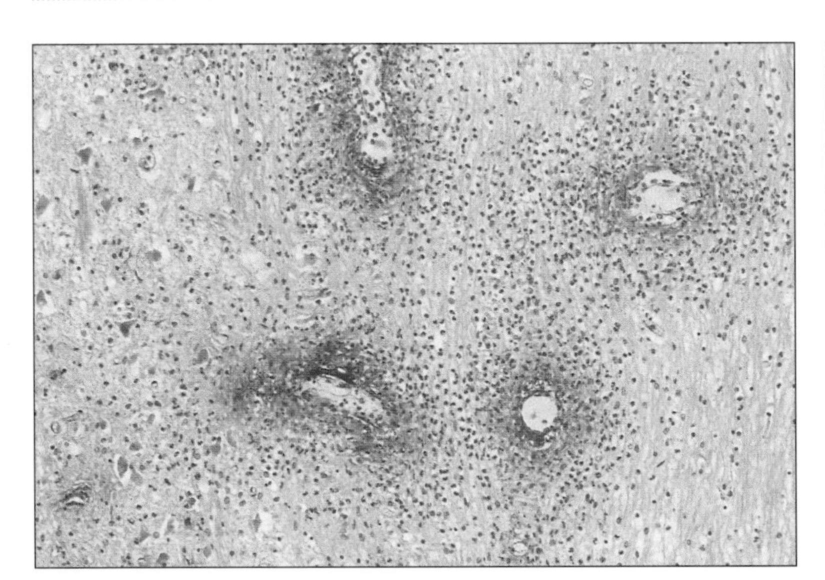

FIGURE 9-11 Acute pyogenic encephalitis. The cellular components of most microabscesses tend to be gathered together, but rarely the acute inflammatory cells may spill into the adjacent neuroparenchyma and cause a diffuse, multifocal "acute pyogenic encephalitis" (or, when in the hemispheres, a cerebritis). This photomicrograph from a septic, encephalopathic patient in whom blood culture-negative *Staphylococcus aureus* pneumonia had been proved shows dilated blood vessels of small caliber surrounded by a vasculocentric acute inflammatory infiltrate, which spreads through the parenchyma. These lesions may also represent the early phase of abscess formation in otherwise healthy patients. (Martius scarlet blue, × 38.)

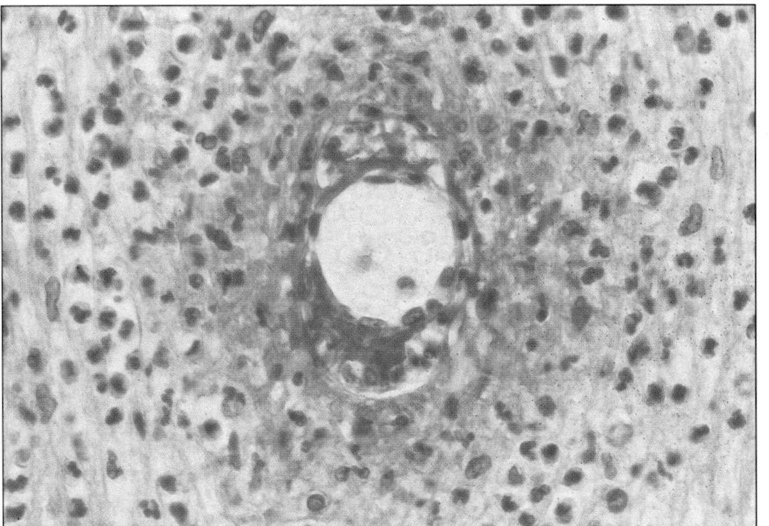

FIGURE 9-12 Acute inflammation, vascular injury. In some cases, the intensity of inflammation and nature of the organism injure the blood-brain barrier, leading to fibrin exudation (stained red) and cerebral edema, the latter causing brain swelling of variable severity. Note also in this detail from Figure 9-11 the acute perivascular inflammatory infiltrate. (A similar process in the meninges would lead to acute purulent meningitis, but an association between multiple cerebral parenchymal acute microabscesses and acute pyogenic meningitis has not yet been demonstrated.) (Martius scarlet blue, × 155.)

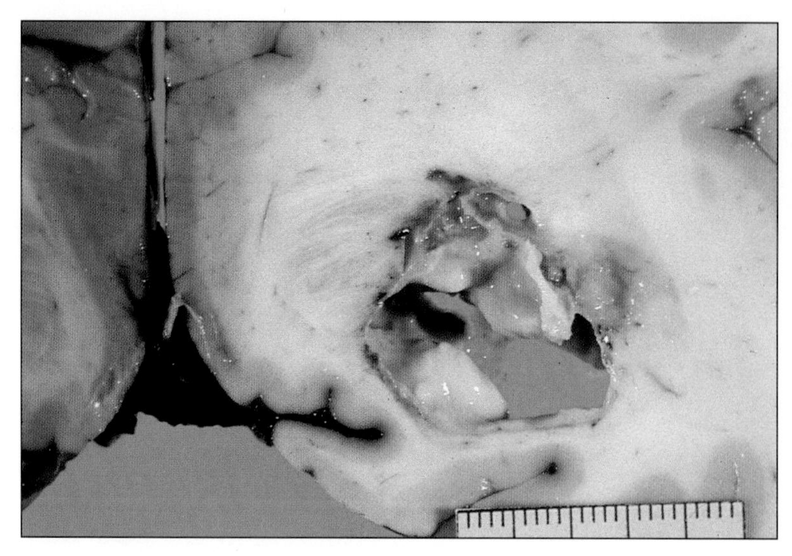

FIGURE 9-13 Acute bacterial abscess. This brain is from a patient who presented with a brief septic illness, followed by rapid neurologic deterioration. The acute bacterial abscess has ruptured into the posterior horn of the left lateral ventricle and caused pyogenic ventriculitis and choroid plexitis. A mixed flora was grown from the pus, including non–β-hemolytic streptococci and the anaerobes *Fusobacterium necrophorum* (Vincent's organism) and *Prevotella* spp., suggesting an oropharyngeal source of sepsis.

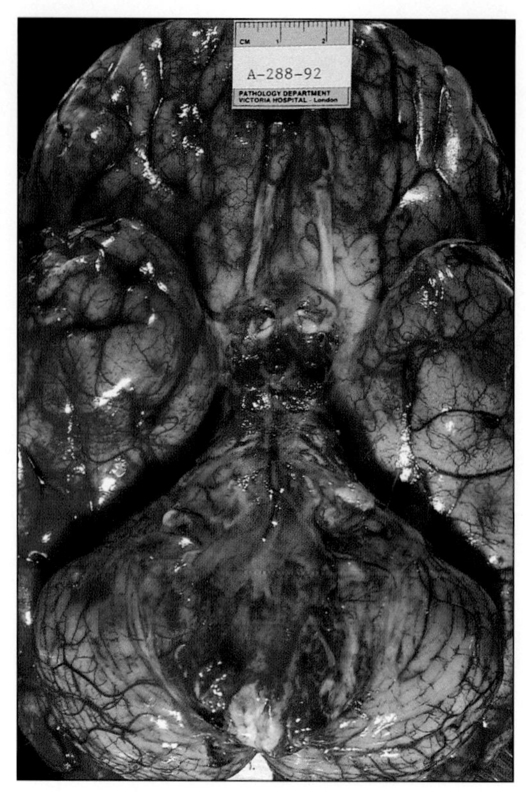

FIGURE 9-14 Acute pyogenic meningitis. Although microabscesses commonly complicate their management, septic patients are also at risk for numerous brain infections, including, as illustrated, acute bacterial meningitis. The brain shown is congested, there is diffuse opacification of the basilar meninges, and the pus is most striking around the brain stem and cerebellum. Brain swelling has caused severe cerebellar tonsillar herniation.

Other Fungal CNS Infections

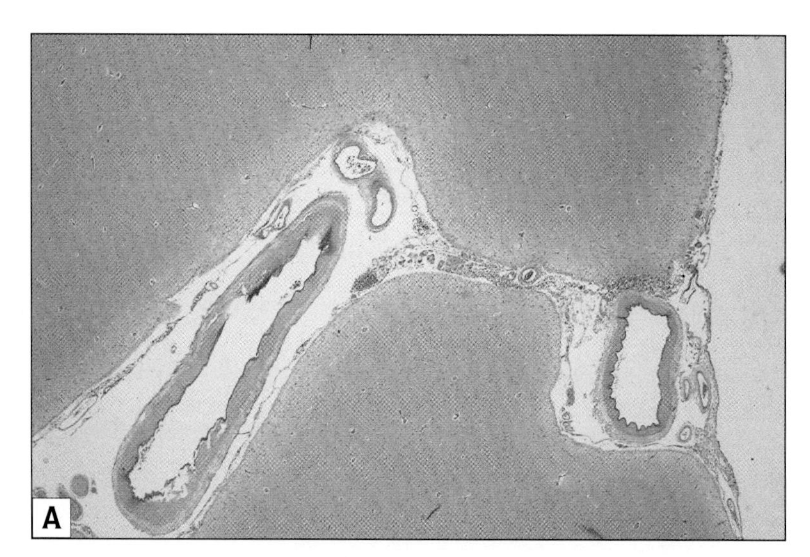

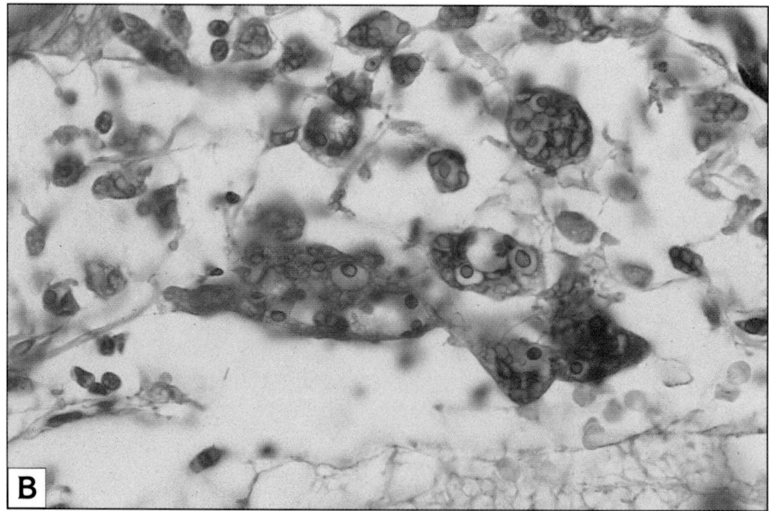

FIGURE 9-15 Chronic cryptococcal meningitis. **A** and **B**, The clinical course in septic patients may be complicated by acute pyogenic fungal meningitis (*see* Fig. 9-17) or, more commonly, chronic meningitis, as shown here. The gross appearance of chronic fungal meningitis varies from one reminiscent of acute bacterial meningitis (with a predilection for the basal meninges) to normal meninges in which microscopic examination reveals light inflammatory infiltrates in the subarachnoid space (*panel A*) and organisms (*panel B*); note in *panel B* the characteristic thick capsule of *Cryptococcus neoformans*. (*Panel A*, Hematoxylin, eosin, and solochrome, × 6. *Panel B*, Periodic acid–Schiff, × 240.)

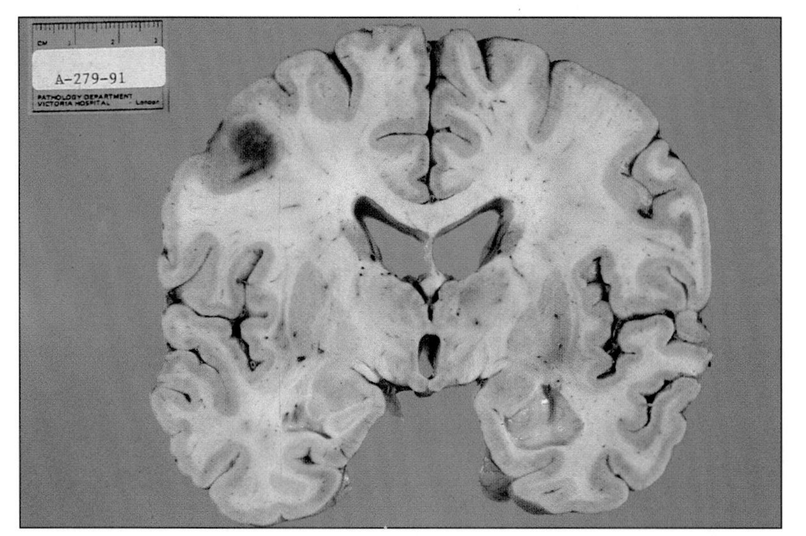

FIGURE 9-16 Aspergillus abscess. Because sepsis compromises the immune response, septic patients are prone to develop infections that are characteristically associated with conventional immunosuppression, caused, for example, by cancer chemotherapy or antirejection regimens used in organ transplantation; conversely, immunosuppressed patients have a predisposition to sepsis. This brain is from a septic patient who had received chemotherapy to treat a glioblastoma and died as a consequence of an aspergillus pneumonia. Note the hemorrhagic aspergillus-induced necrosis (aspergillus "abscess") in the left frontal region. Focal *hemorrhagic* brain necrosis is characteristic of infection by *Aspergillus* and *Phycomycetes* species; *Candida albicans* may also have a similar effect.

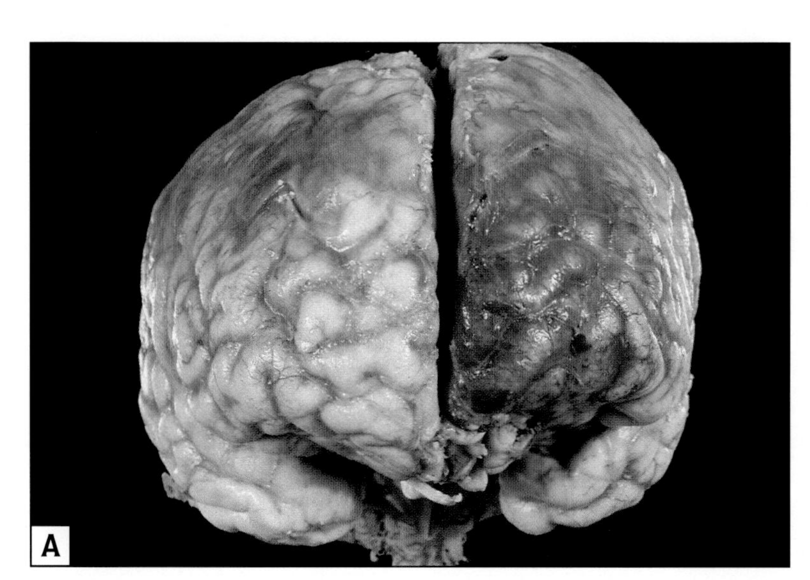

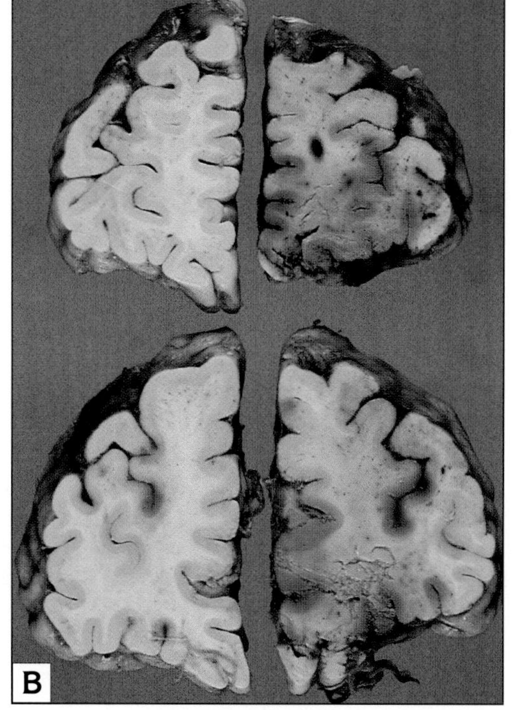

FIGURE 9-17 Acute necrotizing aspergillus meningoencephalitis. **A** and **B**, This brain is from a "failed" renal transplant recipient with aspergillus pneumonia and septicemia. Note the opacification of the meninges over the frontal poles in *panel A* (acute pyogenic meningitis) and the dusky hemorrhagic softening of left frontal lobe seen in both *panels A* and *B* (necrotizing encephalitis) owing to aspergillus vasculitis (*see* Fig. 9-19). The yellow tint indicates liver failure (part of the multiple organ failure syndrome in sepsis) and entry of bilirubin into the brain through the disrupted blood-brain barrier. Although the causes are numerous, blood-brain barrier dysfunction accounts for the common finding of cerebral edema in septic patients. In this case, an encephalopathy was thought clinically to be "metabolic" in nature, but the abnormalities shown, which were not identified before death, provide a structural explanation for sepsis-associated encephalopathy.

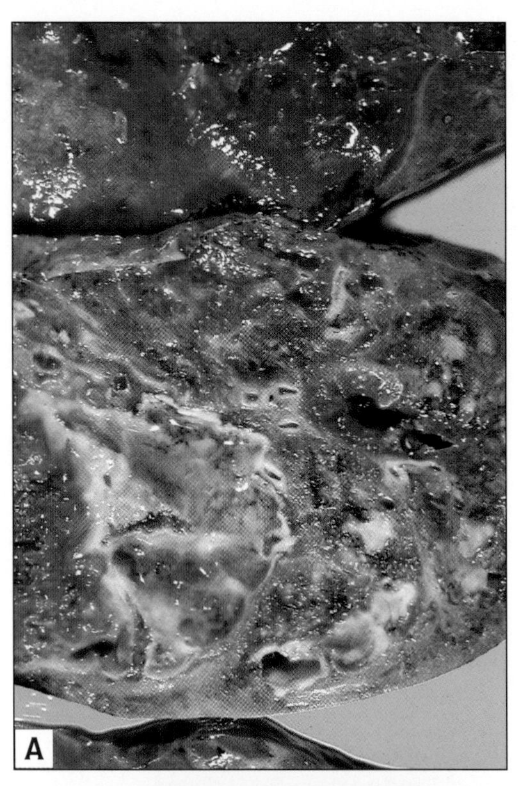

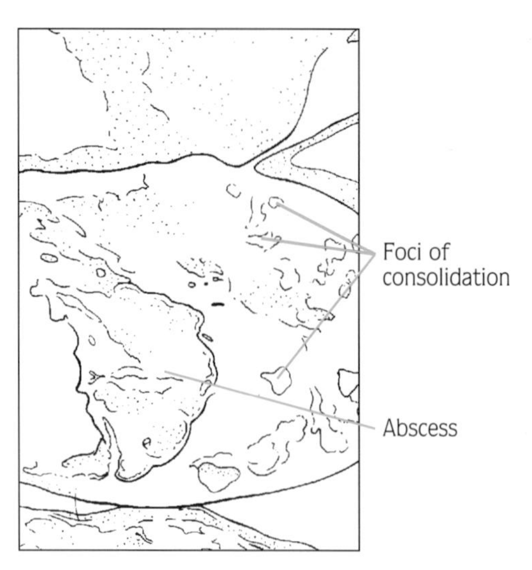

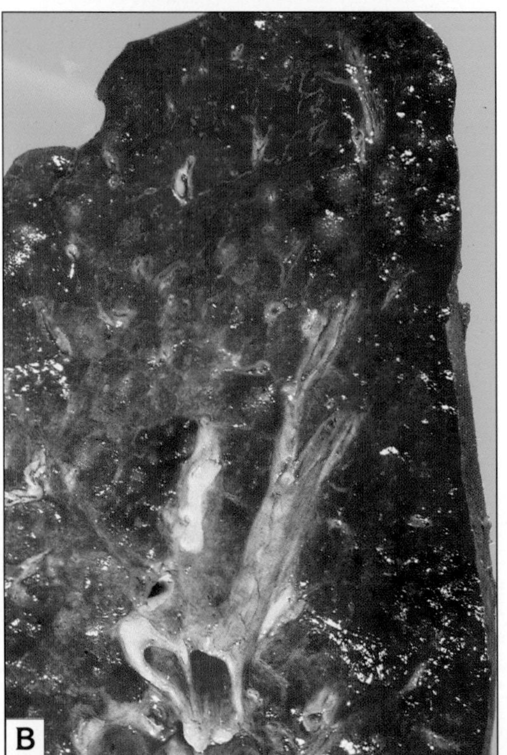

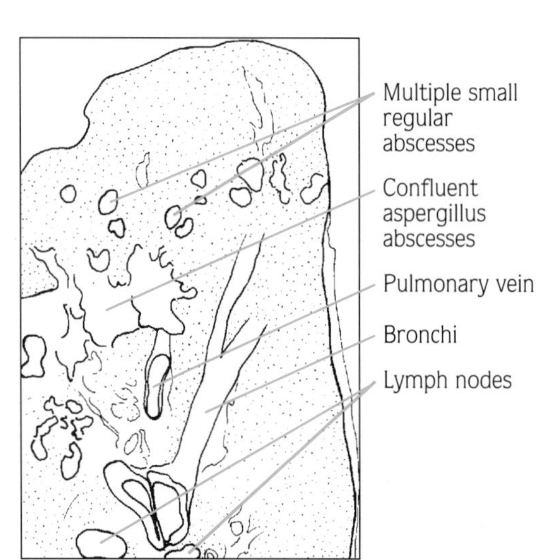

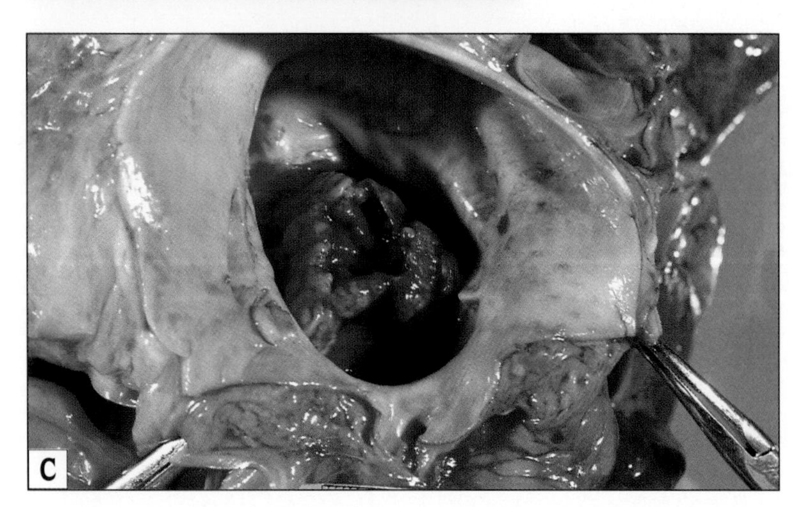

FIGURE 9-18 Sources of aspergillus sepsis. **A**, **B**, and **C**, Aspergillus and other fungal infections of the brain are customarily associated with a primary lung source, septicemia, and/or a more exotic source. **A**, A large aspergillus lung abscess is shown. **B**, Aspergillus septicemia has led to the formation of multiple small perivascular lung abscesses (some confluent). **C**, An aortic valve prosthesis bears numerous aspergillus vegetations. (*Courtesy of* Dr. D.I. Turnbull and Dr. I.D. Craig.)

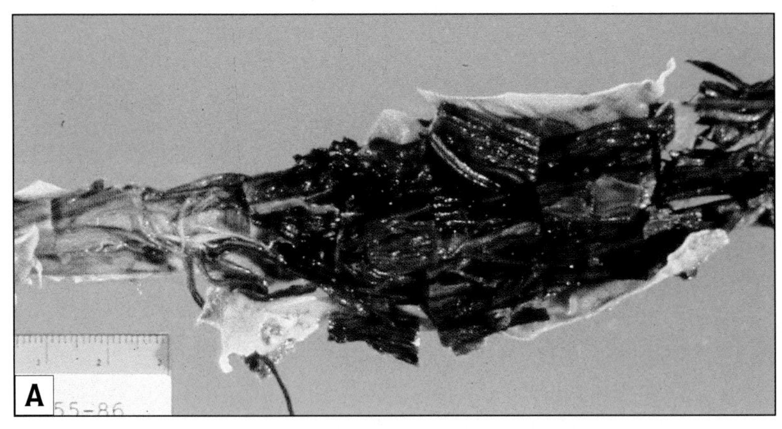

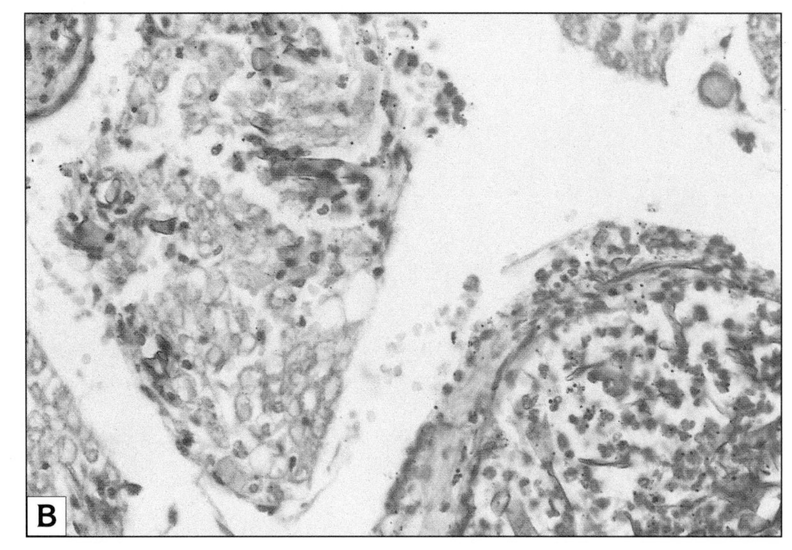

FIGURE 9-19 Mucormycotic myeloradiculitis. The septic patient is often immunosuppressed and therefore susceptible to exotic infections in unusual places. **A**, Sliced caudal spinal cord from a patient with systemic lupus erythematosus, renal failure, and sepsis. Note the hemorrhagic changes, typical of a vasculotropic fungal infection, in the lumbosacral spinal cord and cauda equina, which are rare targets for fungi. **B**, Microscopic examination of the tissue shows abundant hyphae whose morphology is diagnostic of mucormycosis. (Periodic acid–Schiff, x 38.) (*Courtesy of* Dr. J.J. Gilbert.)

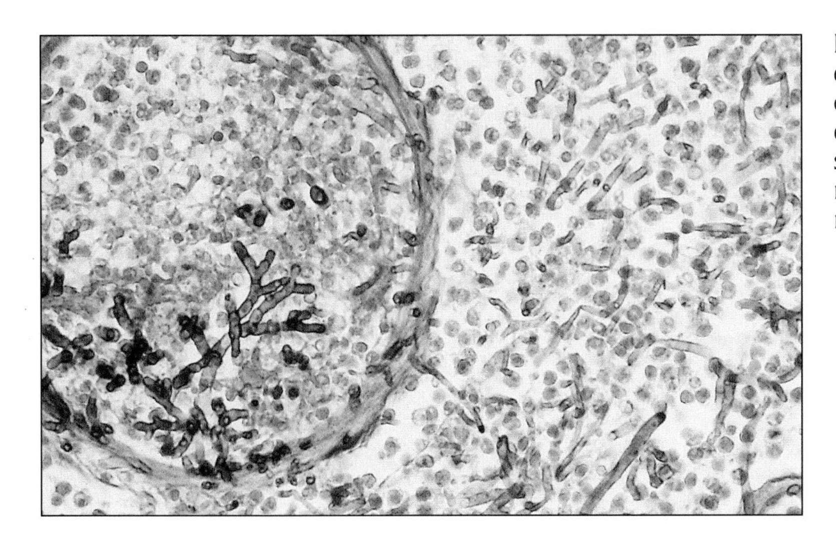

FIGURE 9-20 Aspergillus vasculitis. *Aspergillus* is a particularly destructive organism owing to its vasculotropic nature. Invasion of the venous walls, shown in this photomicrograph, leads to vascular congestion, and a fungal arteritis causes thrombotic occlusion of the vessel and infarction of the upstream neuroparenchyma. Note the brisk acute inflammatory infiltrate. (Grocott's methenamine silver, × 20.)

Indirect Complications of Sepsis

Cerebrovascular Complications of Sepsis

Cerebrovascular complications of sepsis and their underlying causes

Process	Basis
Diffuse	
Vascular encephalopathy	Cardiorespiratory arrest (ischemic encephalomyelopathy)
	Microperfusion defects owing to DIC
	Microvasculitis (associated with cerebral microabscesses)
Focal	
Watershed region infarcts	Hypotension
Cerebral infarcts	Intravascular thrombosis on atheromatous plaque
	Embolus, atheromatous or fibrin-platelet
	Infective vasculitis with secondary arterial occlusion
Venous infarct	Venous sinus thrombosis
Intracerebral hemorrhage and microhemorrhage	Altered coagulation mechanisms, iatrogenic or secondary to sepsis
	Rupture of infected vessel

FIGURE 9-21 Cerebrovascular complications of sepsis and their underlying causes. The cerebrovascular complications of sepsis may be classified as diffuse or focal. Their bases or pathophysiologic mechanisms are noted.

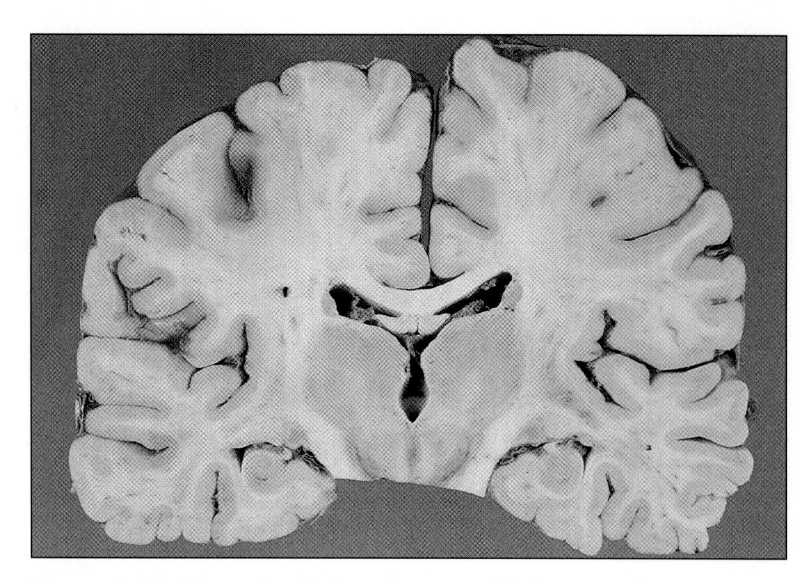

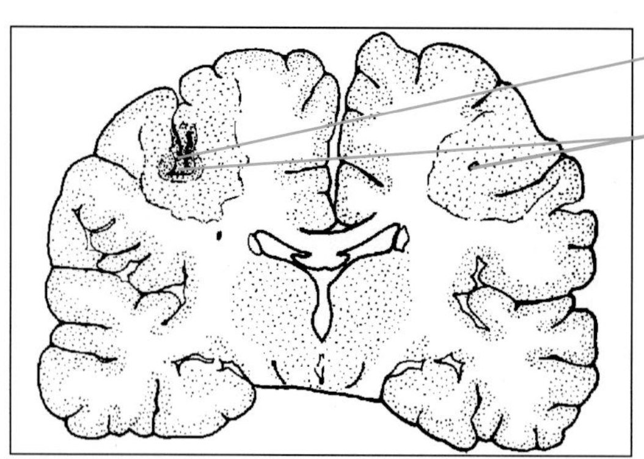

FIGURE 9-22 Watershed ischemic neuronal injury. Sepsis may be associated with a period of hypotension or circulatory arrest, which leads to ischemic brain damage, either in a "watershed" area between vascular territories or more diffusely in the form of an ischemic encephalopathy. This coronal brain slice shows faint yellow discoloration in the watershed areas between the anterior and middle cerebral arterial circulations and, on the left, a small hemorrhagic infarct. The yellow discoloration is caused by bilirubin entering the brain at sites where the blood-brain barrier has been injured by ischemia. The patient was jaundiced owing to hepatic failure, the high level of circulating bilirubin providing a useful marker for sites of blood-brain barrier incompetence.

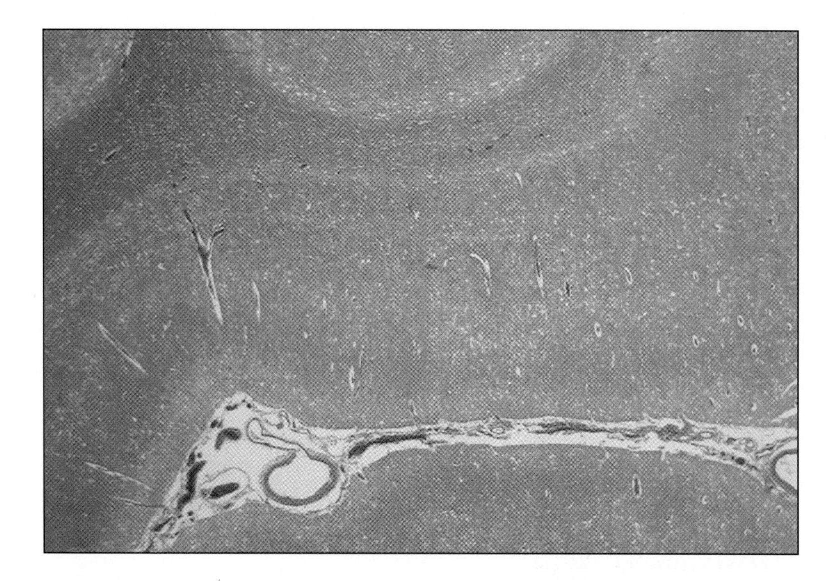

FIGURE 9-23 Ischemic encephalopathy. The widespread unevenness of staining in the cortical layer is characteristic of diffuse ischemic brain injury, which may cause an encephalopathy in some septic patients. (Hematoxylin, eosin, and solochrome, × 6.)

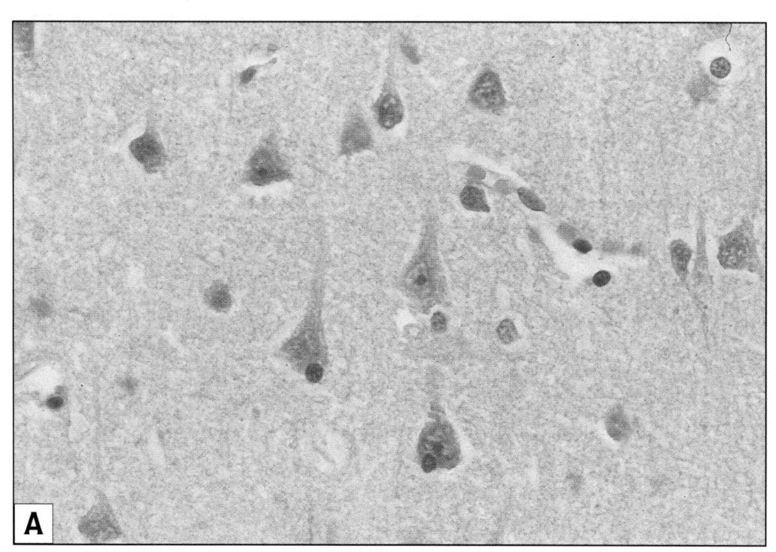

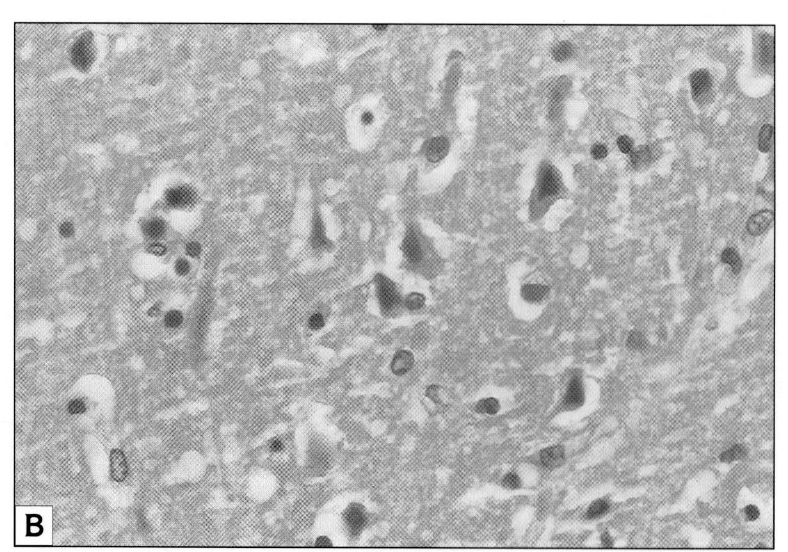

FIGURE 9-24 Ischemic neuronal necrosis. Ischemic encephalopathy is due to widespread neuronal injury (particularly to the Purkinje cells, hippocampal pyramidal cells, and neurons of the dentate gyrus) with preservation of other cellular elements in the brain (*eg*, glial cells). This pattern of injury, reflecting one aspect of the selective vulnerability of the nervous system, should not be confused with an infarct, which is, by definition, an area of ischemic pan-necrosis. **A** and **B**, In contrast to normal cerebral neurons (*panel A*), those injured by ischemia show neuronal cytoplasmic hypereosinophilia and nuclear pyknosis (*panel B*). (Hematoxylin, eosin, and solochrome, × 155.)

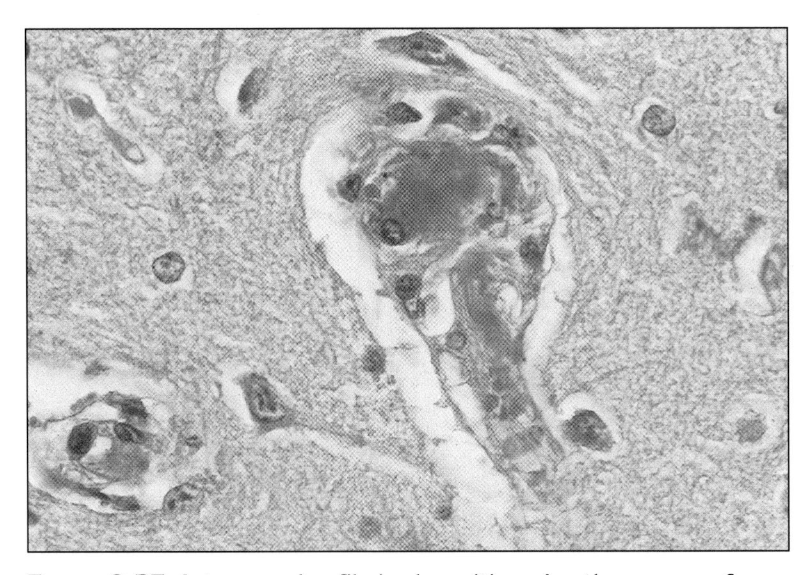

FIGURE 9-25 Intravascular fibrin deposition. Another cause of encephalopathy in septic patients is intravascular deposition of fibrin, leading to hindrance of cerebral microvascular perfusion and consequent neuronal dysfunction. The figure shows hyaline eosinophilic material in the lumen of a capillary whose endothelium is abnormally swollen. (Hematoxylin and eosin, × 155.)

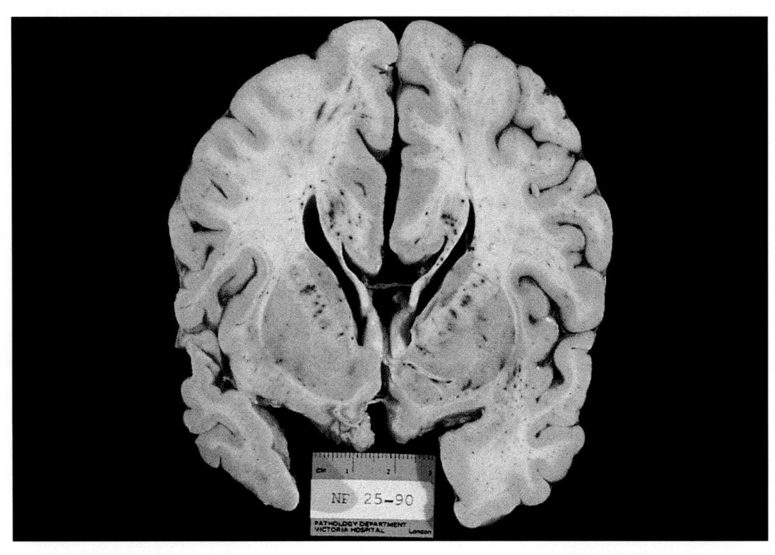

FIGURE 9-26 Acute multifocal hemorrhagic encephalopathy ("ring and ball" hemorrhages, brain purpura). In some septic patients, the hemispheric white matter and, to a lesser extent, gray matter contain numerous small and microscopic hemorrhages, many of which surround small blood vessels. A long differential is relevant for these lesions, including fat emboli, lead poisoning, blood dyscrasias, and acute hemorrhagic leukoencephalitis, but when they appear in critically ill patients in whom disseminated intravascular coagulation and related vascular damage has occurred, they may provide a structural explanation for an encephalopathy. (Agenesis of the corpus callosum is also a feature in this coronal brain slice.)

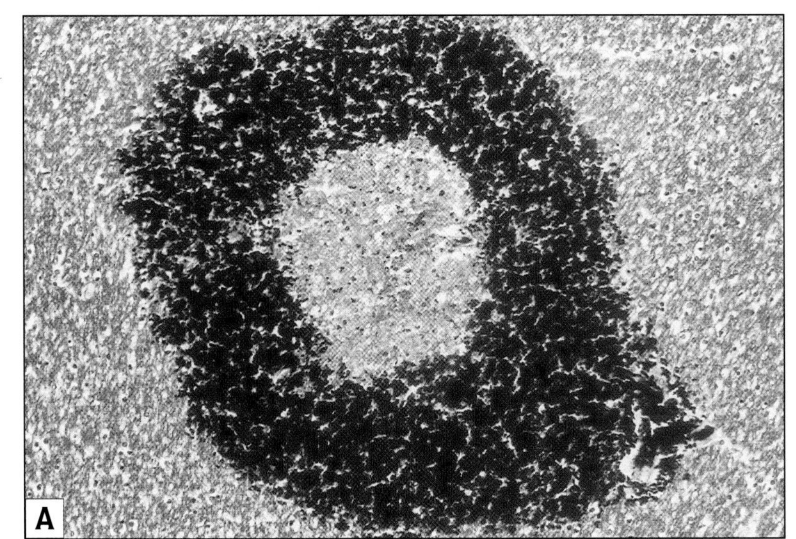

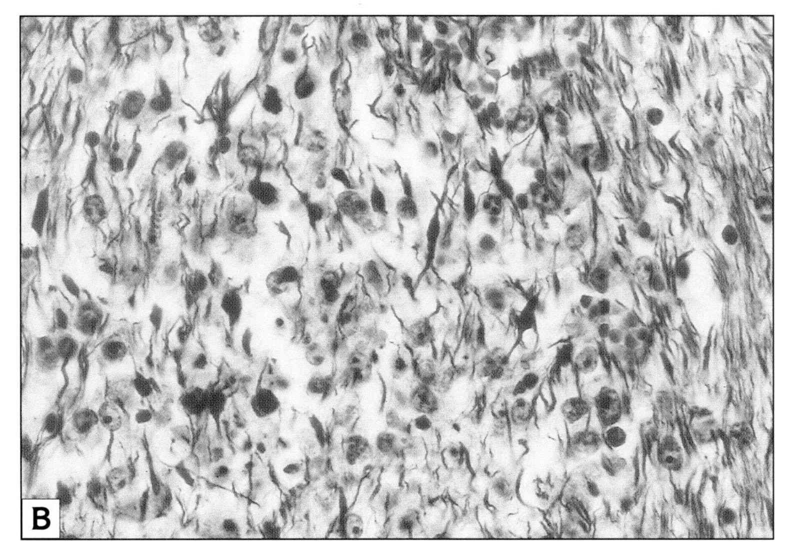

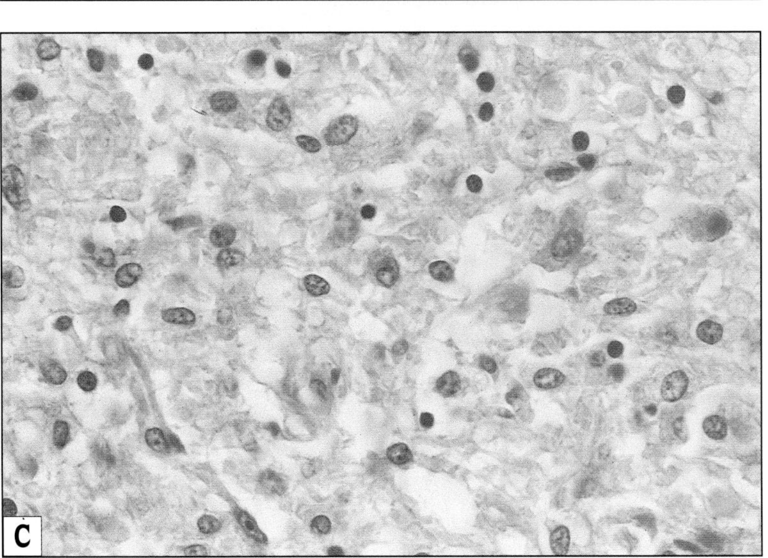

FIGURE 9-27 Histologic features of brain purpura. **A**, A typical "ring and ball" hemorrhage is characterized by a central area of necrosis (in which a capillary, occluded by fibrin or otherwise, is usually present and sometimes seen in the tissue sections) and a ring of red blood cells (*panel A*), which eventually lyse and disappear leaving multiple necrotic foci. **B** and **C**, The necrotic areas contain axonal swellings (*panel B*), degenerating myelin and axonal debris, and macrophages (*panel C*). (*Panel A*, Hematoxylin, eosin, and solochrome, × 38. *Panel B*, Bielschowsky, × 155. *Panel C*, Hematoxylin and eosin, × 155.)

Visible Metabolic Defects in Sepsis

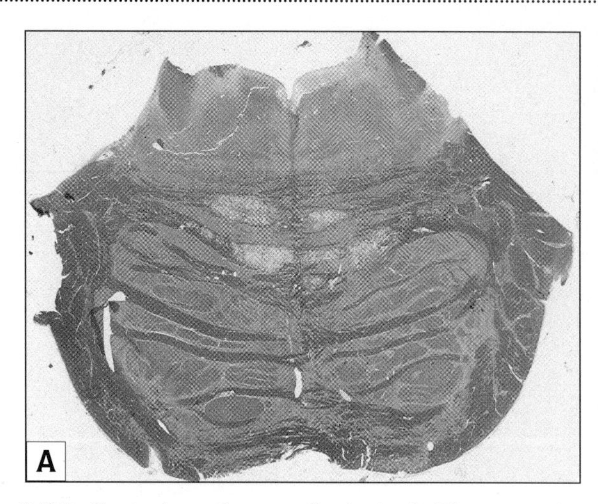

B. Serum sodium concentrations in central pontine myelinolysis

	Cases, *n*	Median	Range
[Na] on admission	30	99 mmol/L	92–115
Maximum increase in [Na]	30	21 mmol/L/d	12–38
[Na] at onset of neurologic illness	8	132 mmol/L	127–138
Time from start of [Na] correction to onset of neurologic illness	8	4.5 days	2–6

FIGURE 9-28 Central pontine myelinolysis. **A**, The pons shows centrally located, symmetrical areas of poor myelin staining in the pontocerebellar fibers, owing to vacuolation and loss of myelin with relative preservation of the other components of the neuropil. (Woelke, × 1.) **B**, Central pontine myelinolysis is normally associated with abrupt correction of severe hyponatremia. In addition to hyponatremia, serious illness such as sepsis plays a major role in the likelihood of this complication. The table shows the serum sodium concentrations ([Na]) from 30 patients with central pontine myelinolysis, 22 of whom had clinical evidence of disease and eight of whom had pathological confirmation. (Sterns RH, Riggs JE, Schochet SS: Osmotic demyelination syndrome following correction of hyponatremia. *N Engl J Med* 1986, 314:1535–1542. Brennan S, Ayus JC: Systemic disorders and cerebral demyelinating lesions. *In* Arieff AI, Griggs RC, (eds.): *Metabolic Brain Dysfunction in Systemic Disorders.* Boston: Little, Brown; 1992:247–262.)

Sepsis-Associated Encephalopathy

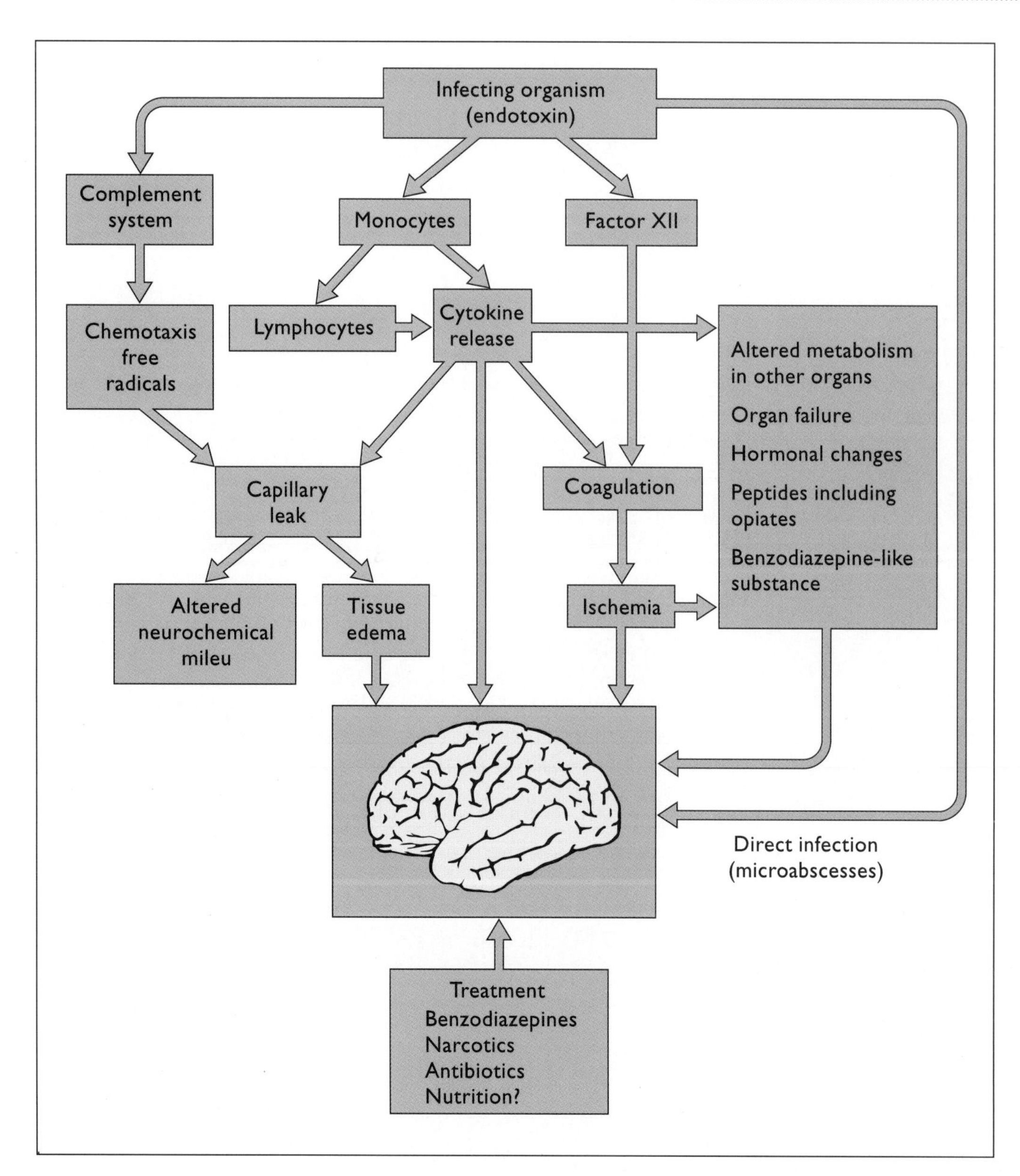

FIGURE 9-29 Mechanisms of septic encephalopathy. Many conditions can cause an encephalopathy; it is therefore crucial in septic encephalopathic patients to attempt to identify the cause of the cerebral dysfunction, bacterial meningitis and endocarditis being the most treatable. Once these disorders, the possibility of iatrogenic phenomena, and other rare causes of febrile nonseptic encephalopathy have been excluded, there remains a considerable number of septic patients in whom no structural basis or association for an encephalopathy can be proved in life or at autopsy. Possible mechanisms for this septic or sepsis-associated encephalopathy, which is a diagnosis of exclusion, are shown. The effects of sepsis on the microcirculation are central to many of the mechanisms, none of which are mutually exclusive. (*From* Bolton CF, Young GB, Zochodne DM: The neurological complications of sepsis. *Ann Neurol* 1993, 33:97; with permission.)

Causes of impaired consciousness and fever	
CNS infections	**Other intracranial events**
Meningitis (bacterial, fungal, viral, or protozoal)	Severe head injury
Encephalitis	Infarction in hypothalamus or brainstem
Brain abscess (esp. multiple)	Status epilepticus (convulsive or, rarely, nonconvulsive)
Epidural or subdural empyema	Sarcoid or tumor infiltration of hypothalamus
Systemic inflammation	**Endocrine and metabolic disturbances**
Sepsis	Thyroid storm
SIRS without infection (*eg*, following burns, trauma, or pancreatitis)	Acute adrenal insufficiency (addisonian crisis)
Pneumonia	Acute porphyria
Hepatitis	Carcinoid syndrome
Malaria	
Drug related	**Other systemic illnesses (esp. if brain involved)**
Aspirin poisoning	Systemic malignancies (carcinoma of lung, pancreas, or liver or lymphomas)
Acute porphyria (esp. with seizures)	Hematologic disorders (sickle cell crisis)
Neuroleptic malignant syndrome	Autoimmune disorders (SLE, serum sickness)
Malignant hyperthermia	**Pulmonary embolism**
Anticholinesterase toxicity	**Myocardial infarction (with failure)**
Severe withdrawal syndromes (drugs or alcohol)	**Heatstroke or heat exhaustion**
Cocaine toxicity	

FIGURE 9-30 Causes of impaired consciousness and fever. A large number of conditions may cause impaired consciousness and fever; these should be excluded before making a diagnosis of sepsis-associated encephalopathy. SIRS—systemic inflammatory response syndrome; SLE—systemic lupus erythematosus.

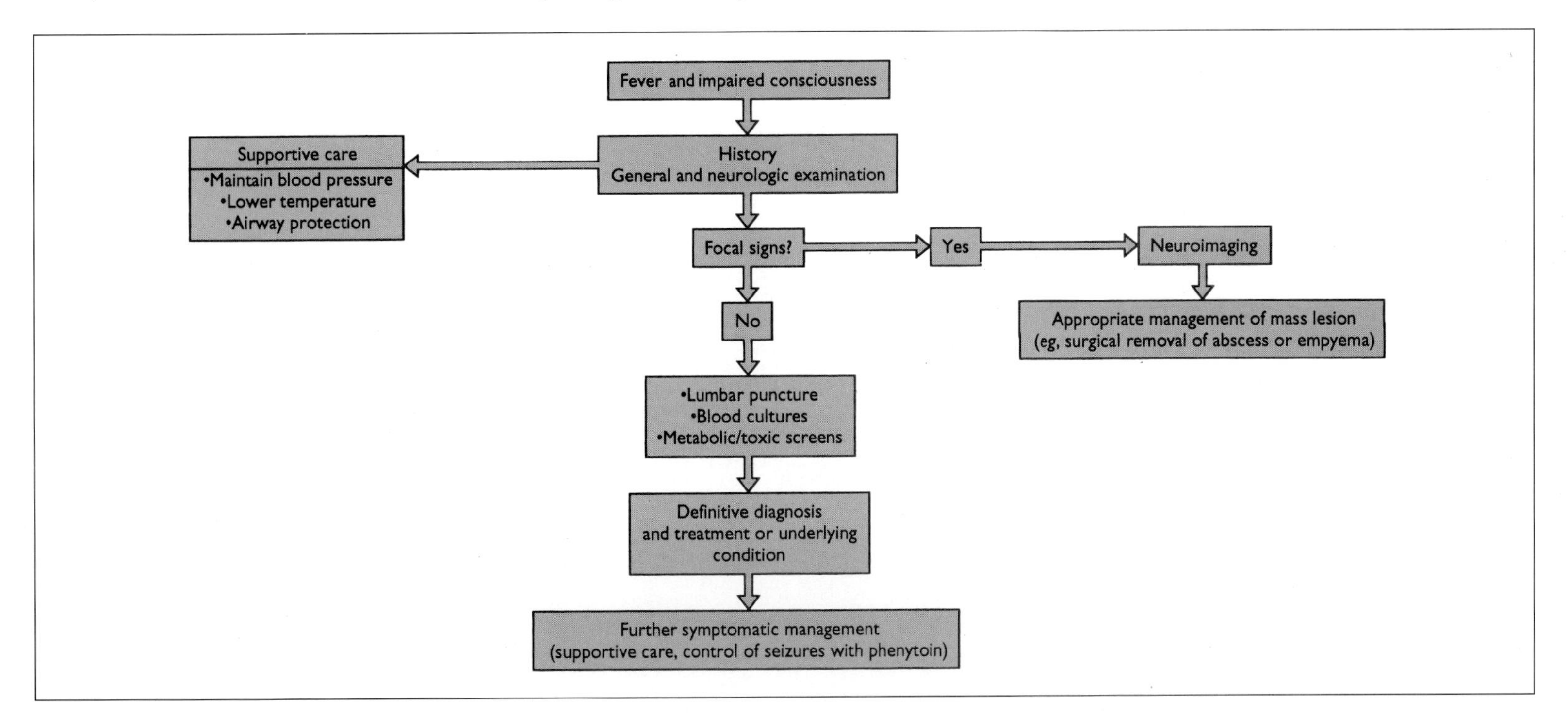

FIGURE 9-31 Diagnosis of septic encephalopathy. Although the history and physical and neurologic examinations will likely provide the diagnosis in most cases, diagnostic procedures are sometimes necessary to confirm clinical suspicions and to exclude life-threatening, treatable conditions. These tests include lumbar puncture; culture of blood, urine, sputum, and cerebrospinal fluid; toxic screen; metabolic screen for serum concentrations of electrolytes, glucose, urea, calcium, magnesium, bilirubin, ammonia, aspartate aminotransferase (AST), and phosphate; complete blood count and platelets; and blood gases. Electroencephalography (EEG) can be used to confirm altered cerebral cortical function, to exclude seizure activity, and to grade the severity of the encephalopathy. Neuroimaging (computed tomography [CT] or magnetic resonance imaging [MRI]) is indicated if there are consistent focal signs or if there is a reasonable change of an extra-axial lesion, such as a subdural hematoma, or bilateral intracerebral or extra-axial lesions. In sepsis-associated encephalopathy, the most common motor sign is *gegenhalten*, a resistance to passive movement of the limbs that is velocity dependent—*ie*, the resistance that is felt with movements at a normal rate disappears when the limb is moved slowly. Asterixis, multifocal myoclonus, seizures, and tremor are relatively infrequent. Cranial nerve functions are spared.

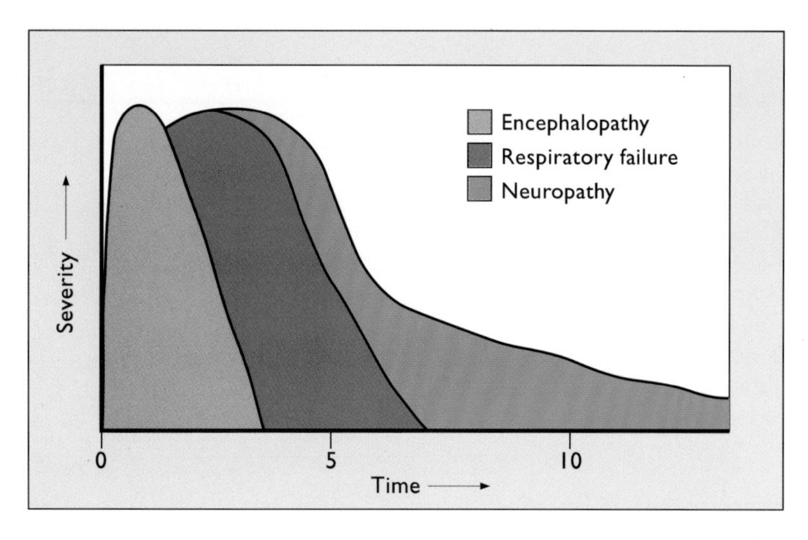

FIGURE 9-32 Clinical course of septic encephalopathy. The typical course of a severe case of septic encephalopathy is shown. The time scale on the x-axis can be in weeks or months. The encephalopathy, which occurs early in the course of a septic illness, may resolve before it is recognized that the patient is difficult to wean from the ventilator. This is usually due to a critical illness polyneuropathy (*see* Fig. 9-36), which occurs in over 70% of severely encephalopathic patients and is generally the last disorder to heal. (*From* Bolton CF, Young GB, Zochodne DM: The neurological complications of sepsis. *Ann Neurol* 1993, 33:94–100; with permission.)

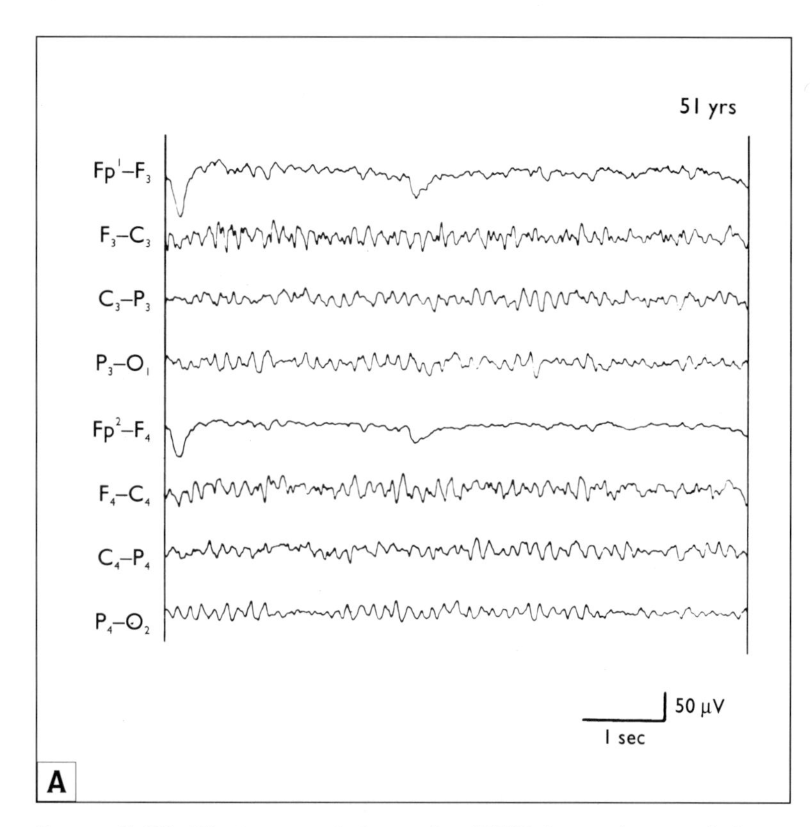

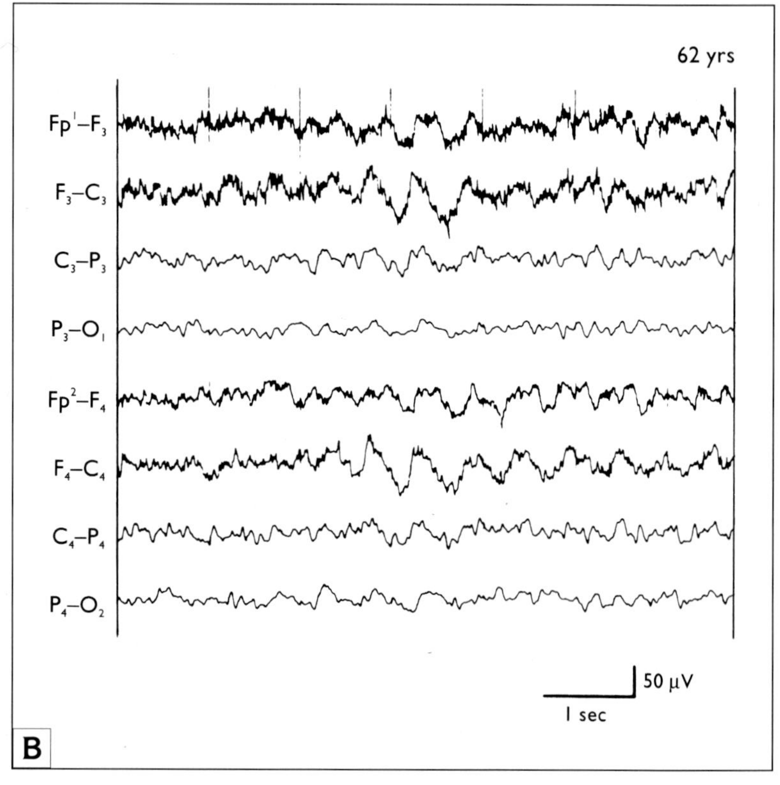

FIGURE 9-33 Electroencephalography (EEG) in septic encephalopathy. Examples of EEGs showing progressive abnormalities are illustrated. **A**, Mild cases show mild diffuse slowing. **B** and **C**, With worsening encephalopathy, generalized slow-frequency waves are intermittent (*panel B*) and then persistent throughout the record (*panel C*). (*continued*)

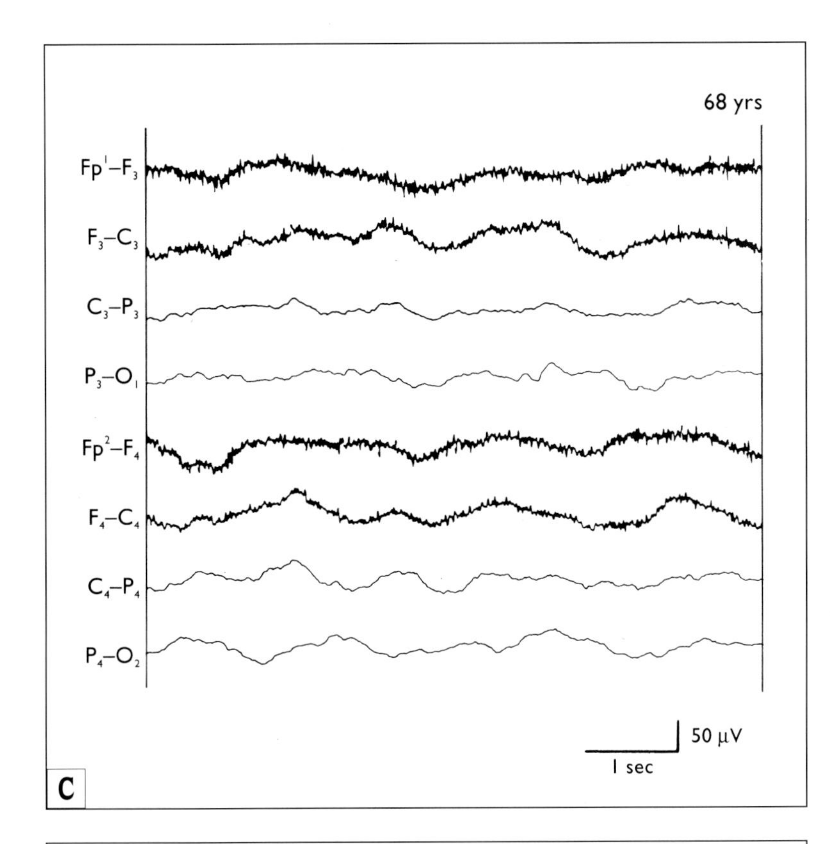

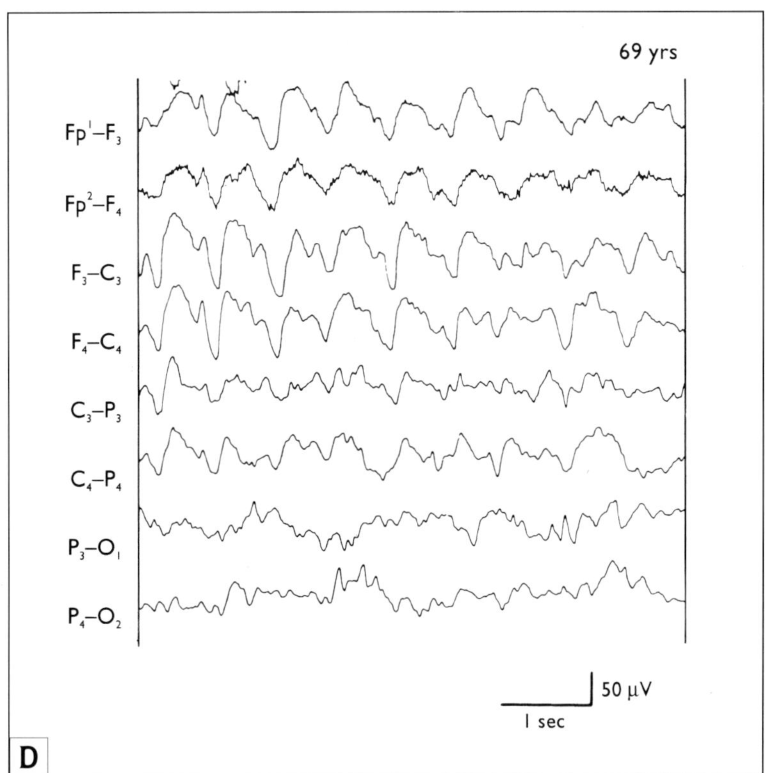

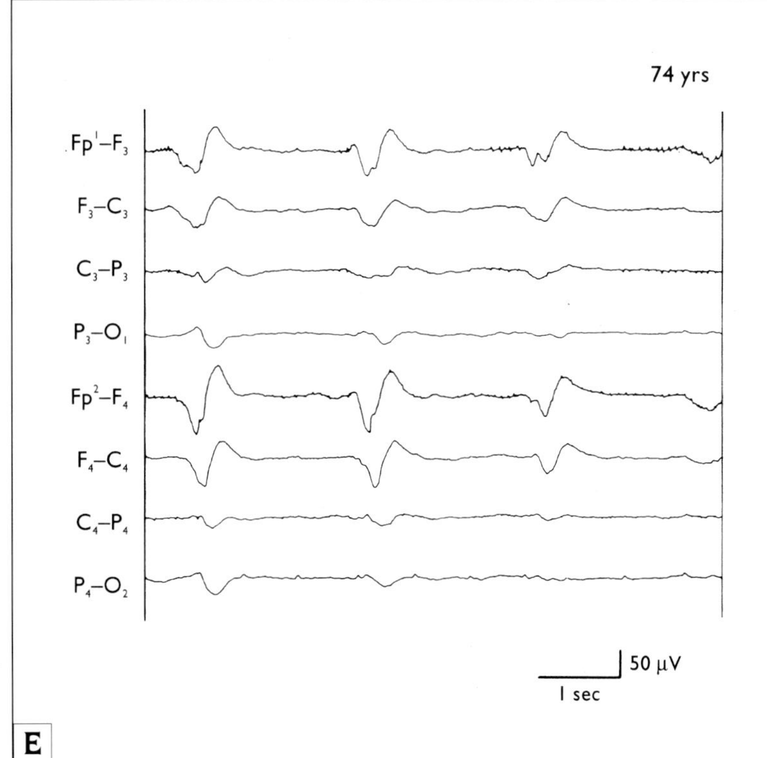

FIGURE 9-33 *(continued)* **D**, Triphasic waves are usually indicative of a severe metabolic encephalopathy. **E**, The most marked abnormality is suppression or burst-suppression, in which the voltage is generally suppressed for most of the tracing. Note, however, that these findings are not specific for sepsis-associated encephalopathy. (*From* Young GB, Bolton CF, Austin TW, *et al.*: The encephalopathy associated with septic illness. *Clin Invest Med* 1990, 13:297–304; with permission.)

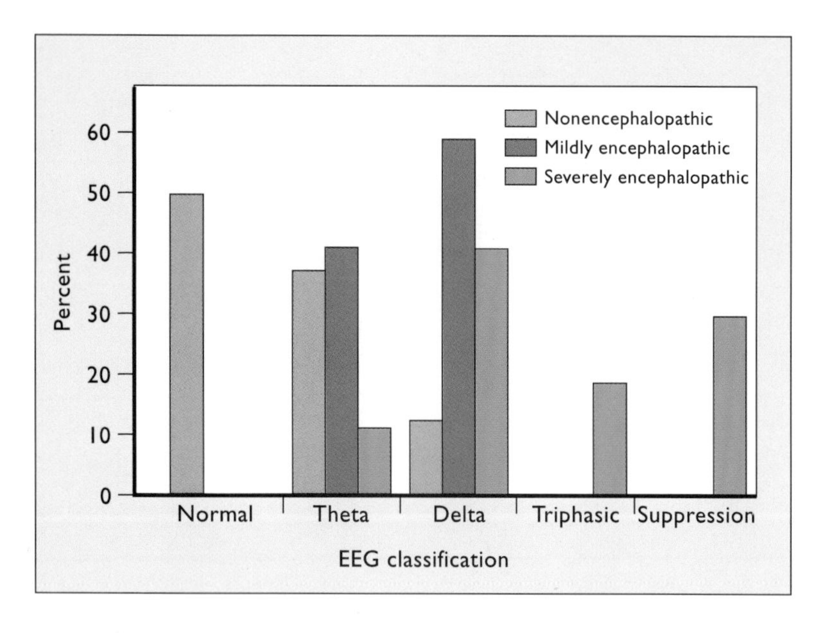

FIGURE 9-34 EEG abnormalities and severity of encephalopathy. The EEG abnormality reflects the clinical severity of the encephalopathy. In this graph, patients with severe encephalopathy associated with coma (*blue*) were the only ones with suppression or triphasic waves. Also, only 50% of the patients clinically classified as "normal" at the bedside (*yellow*) actually had normal EEGs: the EEG was more sensitive than the neurologic examination and in half the patients revealed excessive slowing, which returned to normal later. Patients with mild to moderate encephalopathy (*orange*) had EEG patterns that were intermediate in their degree of abnormality. The mortality was correlated with the severity of the encephalopathy: 0% for "nonencephalopathic" patients, 35% for the mildly-moderately encephalopathic patients, and 53% for severely encephalopathic patients. (*From* Young GB, Bolton CF, Austin TW, *et al.*: The encephalopathy associated with septic illness. *Clin Invest Med* 1990, 13:297–304; with permission. Hart RG, Foster JW, Luther MF, Kanter MC: Stroke in infective endocarditis. *Stroke* 1990, 21:695– 700. Matsushita K, Kuriyama Y, Sawada T, *et al.*: Hemorrhagic and ischemic cerebrovascular complications of active infective endocarditis of native valve. *Eur Neurol* 1993, 33:267–274.)

Abnormal blood tests in septic encephalopathy

Test	NE group	ME group	SE group	*P* Value for group differences	*P* Value for linear trend across groups
White blood count (X 10^9/L)	10.3(3.9)	16(10.5)	15.3(7.3)	<0.05	<0.05
Serum K (mmol/L)	3.7(0.6)	3.8(0.7)	4.1(0.6)	<0.05	<0.05
Serum albumin (g/L)	34(6)	27(4)	30(5)	<0.0005	<0.004
Serum urea (mmol/L)	7.14(5.57)	11.74(7.5)	18.32(9.7)	<0.0001	<0.0001
Serum creatine (μmol/L)	115(49)	128(69)	195(141)	<0.05	<0.05

FIGURE 9-35 Abnormal blood tests in septic encephalopathy. Although there is a statistically significant relationship with these laboratory values among the different severity groups, there is no evidence that the encephalopathy is secondary to the failure of other organs in most cases. It is more likely that the brain fails in parallel with other organs as part of the systemic illness. ME—mildly encephalopathic; NE—nonencephalopathic; SD—standard deviation; SE—severely encephalopathic. (Young GB, *et al.*: The electroencephalogram in sepsis-associated encephalopathy. *J Clin Neurophysiol* 1992, 9:145–152.)

SEPSIS AND THE NEUROMUSCULAR SYSTEM

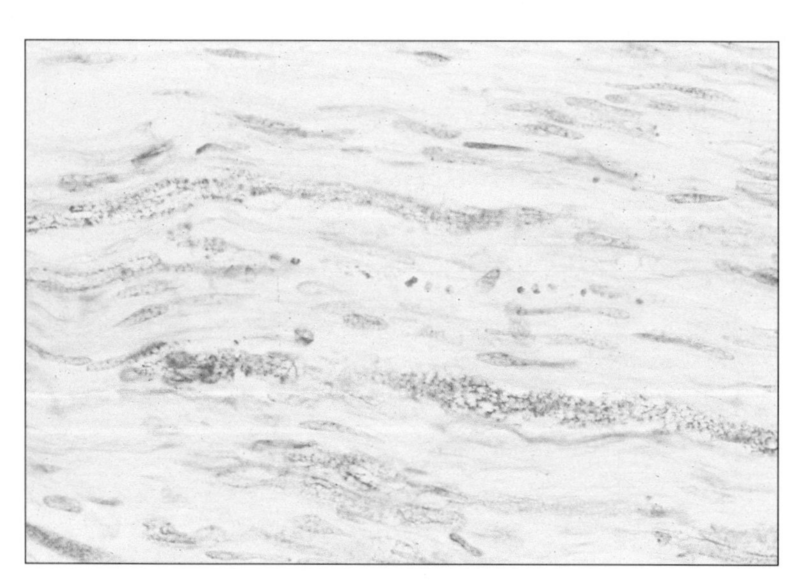

FIGURE 9-36 Critical illness polyneuropathy. A relatively common cause of weakness in critically ill septic patients, critical illness polyneuropathy is of unknown etiology. Its electrophysiologic features are of an axonal polyneuropathy, which can be difficult to distinguish from an acute necrotizing myopathy. In this photomicrograph, a line of degenerating "myelin ovoids" lies between two normal myelinated fibers and marks the course of a myelinated axon that is undergoing Wallerian degeneration. The involvement of the peripheral nervous system by this complication of sepsis is unpredictable and patchy, but degeneration of the phrenic nerve is common and may account for difficulty in weaning patients from assisted ventilation (Solochrome, × 155.) (Zochodne DW, Bolton CF, Wells GA, *et al.*: Critical illness polyneuropathy. *Brain* 1987, 110:819–842.)

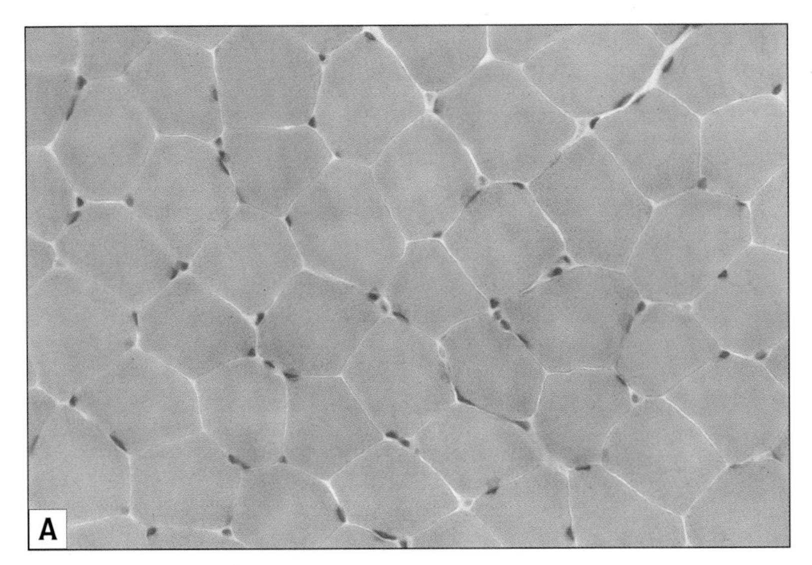

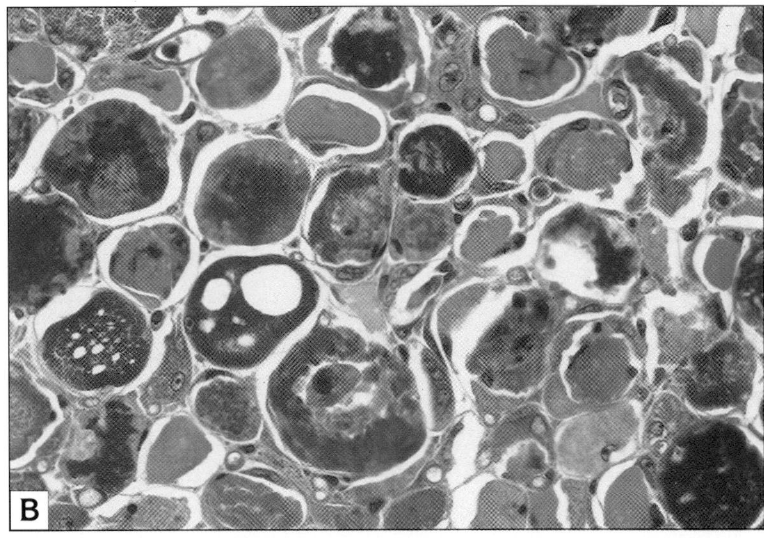

FIGURE 9-37 Acute necrotizing myopathy of intensive care. A few septic patients develop fulminant muscle necrosis, which can occur at any stage during their acute illness. The cause of the condition is unknown, but it is associated with intensive care, sepsis, corticosteroid administration, and use of nondepolarizing muscle-blocking agents. **A** and **B**, In contrast to the relatively monotonous histology of normal transversely sectioned muscle fibers (*panel A*), the sarcoplasm in acute necrotizing myopathy of intensive care shows a number of abnormalities, including multivesicular and univesicular vacuolation, hypereosinophilia (necrosis), and infiltration by macrophages (*panel B*); inflammatory changes are usually absent. (*Panel A*, Hematoxylin and eosin, × 98. *Panel B*, Hematoxylin, eosin, and saffron, × 98). (Ramsay DA, Zochodne DW, Robertson DM, *et al.*: A syndrome of acute severe muscle necrosis in intensive care unit patients. *J Neuropathol Exp Neurol* 1993, 52:387–398.)

Features of neuromuscular disorders in critically ill patients

Condition	Antecedent illness	Clinical features	Electrophysiology	Morphology	Treatment	Prognosis
Critical illness polyneuropathy	Sepsis	Absent, or signs of mainly motor neuropathy	Consistent with a primary axonal degeneration of mainly motor fibers	Primary axonal degeneration of nerve, denervation atrophy of muscle	Treat septic syndrome	Good in 40% who survive sepsis and organ failure
Neuromuscular-blocking agents and neuropathy	Sepsis	Acute quadriplegia	Neuromuscular transmission defect and/or axonal motor neuropathy	Normal or denervation atrophy on muscle biopsy	None	Good
Neuromuscular-blocking agents, steroids, and myopathy	Sepsis?	Acute quadriplegia	Neuromuscular transmission defect and/or myopathy	Thick myosin filament loss	None	Good
Panfascicular muscle fiber necrosis	Transient infection, trauma, etc.	Severe muscle weakness, increased CPK, often myoglobinuria	Positive sharp waves and fibrillation potentials on needle EMG	Panfascicular muscle fiber necrosis	None, or hemodialysis for myoglobinuria	Good
Cachectic myopathy	Severe systemic illness, prolonged recumbency	Diffuse muscle wasting	Normal	Type II fiber atrophy on muscle biopsy	Physiotherapy, improved nutrition	Good

FIGURE 9-38 Features of neuromuscular disorders in critically ill patients. The various features of the principal neuromuscular conditions encountered in septic or critically ill patients are compared. CPK—creatine phosphokinase; EMG—electromyography. (*From* Bolton CF: Neuromuscular complications of sepsis. *Intensive Care Med* 1993, 19:S58–S63; with permission.)

Neurologic Complications of Bacterial Endocarditis

Clinical Manifestations

Incidence of CNS complications in infective endocarditis

Complications	Mean % incidence (range)
Embolus	13.4 (6.7–25.9)
Meningitis	7.0 (1.1–15.1)
Encephalopathy	6.4 (0.0–8.6)
Headache	3.7 (0.0–13.9)
Hemorrhage	3.6 (0.0–13.9)
Seizure	3.5 (0.0–11.0)
Abscess	1.9 (0.0–8.6)
Mycotic aneurysm	1.5 (0.0–8.6)

Figure 9-39 Incidence of CNS complications in infective endocarditis. There is great variability in the overall incidence of CNS complications in infective endocarditis, ranging from 20% to 40% in most series. In an analysis of five series comprising 1014 patients, neurologic complications occurred in 34%, as presented in the table. Some patients had more than one complication. (*From* Tunkel AR, Kaye D: Neurologic complications of infective endocarditis. *Neurol Clin* 1993, 11:419; with permission.)

Neurologic syndromes in patients with infective endocarditis

Syndrome (main clinical presentation)	Mechanisms
Stroke (hemiplegia, aphasia)	Emboli with bland or hemorrhagic infarction Intracranial hemorrhage due to mycotic aneurysm and necrotizing arteritis Brain abscess
Meningitis (meningitis ± focal signs)	Multiple causes: microabscesses Bacterial seeding of the meninges Brain abscess
"Toxic" encephalopathy (decreased level of consciousness)	Microemboli, microabscesses, cerebritis, CNS hypertension, drug toxicity, metabolic disturbances, vasculitis, other organic CNS complications
Psychiatric abnormalities (behavioral disorders, esp. in elderly patients)	Same as "toxic" encephalopathy Reactive to conditions surrounding the diagnosis of infective endocarditis
Seizures (focal or generalized)	Any of the underlying CNS lesions Drug toxicity, metabolic imbalance, hypoxia
Brain stem (nausea, vomiting, hiccup, dyskinesia, tremor)	Emboli in the vertebrobasillar territory
Cranial nerves (visual disturbances, disorders of eye movements, palsies, sensory impairment)	Emboli, space-occupying lesions
Spinal cord and peripheral disorders (para- or tetraplegia, mononeuropathy)	Emboli, metastatic abscesses, immune injury
Severe headache (severe, often localized)	Mycotic aneurysms or other CNS lesions
Subarachnoid hemorrhage (meningismus ± decreased consciousness)	Infectious arteritis with or without detectable mycotic aneurysm

Figure 9-40 Neurologic syndromes in patients with infective endocarditis. Several complications may occur simultaneously in a single patient, or complications may occur sequentially over the course of the illness. Also, there is often considerable variability and fluctuation in the severity of the illness. (*From* Francioli P: Central nervous system complications of infective endocarditis. *In* Scheld WM, Whitley RJ, Durack DT (eds.): *Infections of the Central Nervous System*. New York: Raven Press; 1991:529; with permission.)

Organism	Cases, *n*	CNS complications, *n*	Percent (range)
Staphylococcus aureus	111	62	56 (53–65)
Staphylococci, coagulase-negative	36	10	28 (14–50)
Viridans streptococci	183	48	26 (17–41)
Streptococci group D	108	31	29 (26–30)
Streptococcus pneumoniae	16	13	81 (75–88)
Other streptococci	45	18	40 (35–57)
Other	74	29	39 (29–47)
Total	573	211	37 (33–39)

FIGURE 9-41 Microbiology of infective endocarditis in patients with CNS complications. In general, the incidence of CNS complications has been correlated with the infectious agent causing infectious endocarditis. For *Staphylococcus aureus*, the frequency of CNS involvement has ranged from 53% to 71% and was significantly higher than that for any other bacteria. Other bacteria, such as Enterobacteriaceae or anaerobes, also have been associated with a high rate of neurologic complications. For *Streptococcus pneumoniae*, which is a rare cause of infective endocarditis (causing only 1% to 3% of cases), associated meningitis is seen in 57% to 91% of cases. (*Adapted from* Francioli P: Central nervous system complications in infective endocarditis. *In* Scheld WM, Durack D, Whitley R (eds.): *Infections of the Central Nervous System*. New York: Raven Press; 1991:528; with permission.)

Pathologic Manifestations and Pathogenesis of Neurologic Complications

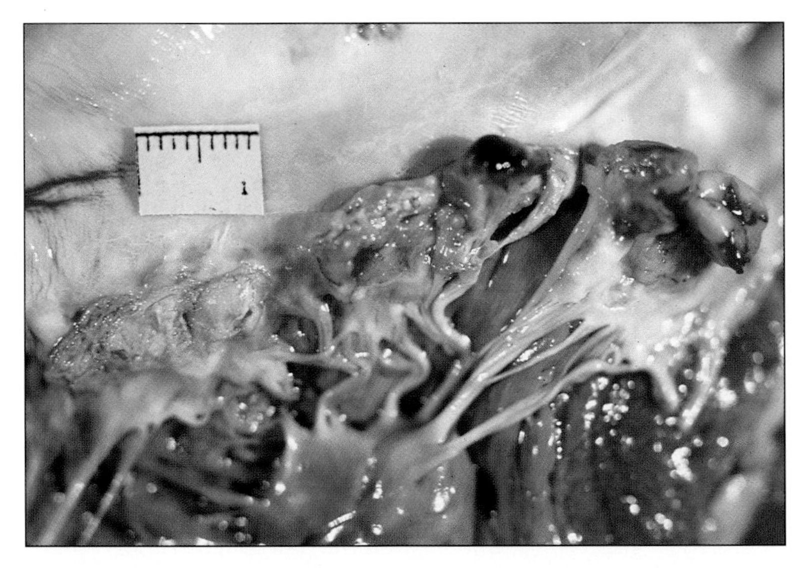

FIGURE 9-42 Bacterial endocarditis, gross appearance. Bacterial endocarditis is a special case of sepsis, owing to the protracted opportunity for direct seeding of the circulation with infected thrombi. Attached to the edges of this mitral valve are vegetations, characterized by soft, focally hemorrhagic material; the agent was a Group D *Streptococcus*. These often friable, infected thrombi are perfectly positioned to travel throughout the vascular system, and brain involvement precipitates presentation in approximately 15% of cases of native-valve bacterial endocarditis. (*Courtesy of* Dr. M.J. Shkrum.)

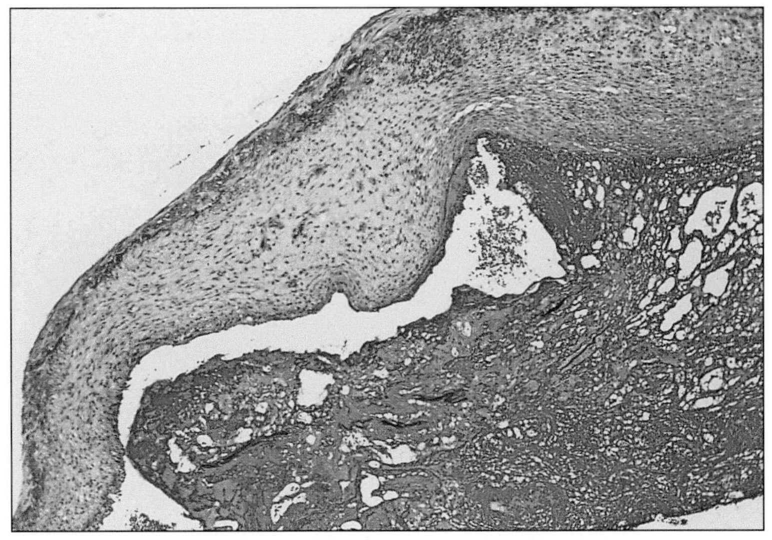

FIGURE 9-43 Bacterial endocarditis, microscopic appearance. Attached to the edge of a valve cusp (*upper part* of the photomicrograph, stained blue-green) is a thrombus (stained magenta) composed of featureless material; pieces of thrombus break off and enter the circulation, causing stroke in approximately one-fifth of all patients with native mitral and/or aortic valve endocarditis. The risk of stroke is highest in the early phase of the disease, when the valve infection is uncontrolled. Stroke, due to hemorrhage or infarction, is the characteristic neurologic complication of bacterial endocarditis, but the other complications of nonendocarditic sepsis may also occur, although less frequently. (Movats, × 15.)

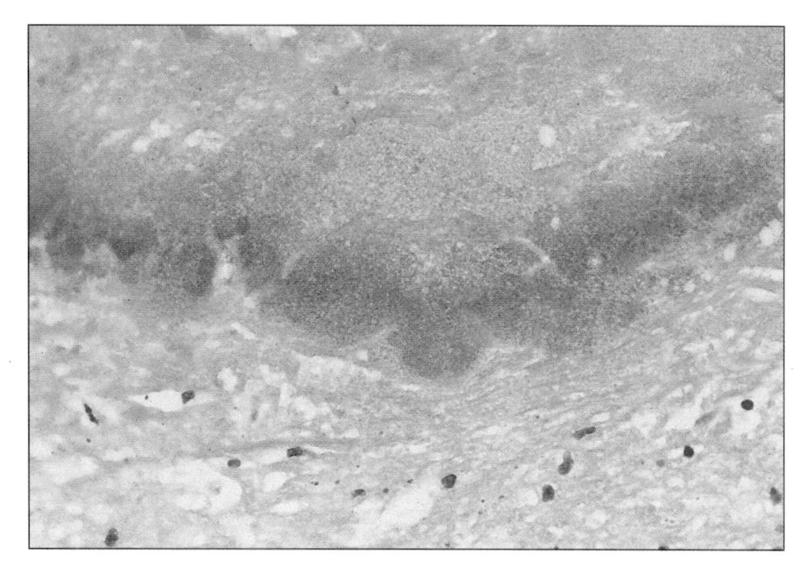

FIGURE 9-44 Bacteria in endocarditic vegetations. Elsewhere in the thrombus illustrated in Figure 9-42 are colonies of bacteria, shown here as a blue granular haze. Although *Streptococcus viridans* was once the most common cause of bacterial endocarditis, *Staphylococcus aureus* and Group D streptococci are now frequently identified. The vegetations associated with *S. aureus* tend to embolize early, and accordingly, echocardiography may fail to identify the inflamed valves in such patients; this bacterium is also apt to produce multiple brain lesions. (Hematoxylin and eosin, × 155.)

Risk factors for neurologic complications in infective endocarditis

Risk factor	Maximum risk	Comparative risk
Valve infected	76% with mitral valve	37% with other valves
Microorganism	71% with *S. aureus*	45% with other organisms
Patient age	Increased with age > 65 yrs	Relatively lower with age < 65 yrs

FIGURE 9-45 Risk factors for neurologic complications in infective endocarditis. Three risk factors—related to the specific heart valve affected (mitral), the virulent microorganism (*Staphylococcus aureus*), and patient age (> 65 years)—are associated with an increased incidence of neurologic complications.

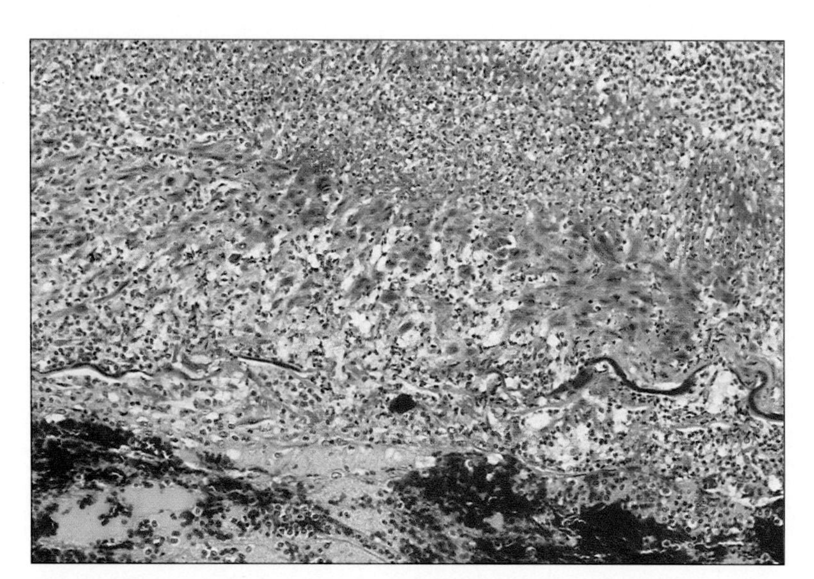

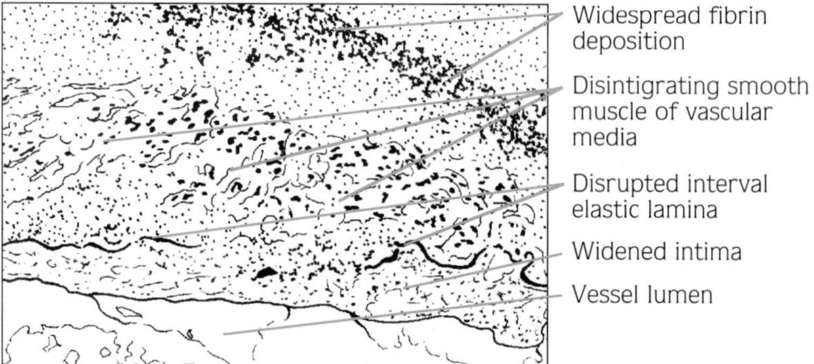

FIGURE 9-46 Mycotic arteritis. Once the infected vegetations enter the cerebrovascular circulation, they have two major effects. First, the vegetation may occlude a vessel and lead to an infarct, the size of which is related to the caliber of the occluded vessel and the competency of collateral circulation. Second, if the embolus is infected, the organisms cause acute inflammation in, and destruction of, the vessel walls. In this photomicrograph, disruption of the internal elastic lamina and disintegration of the vascular media are apparent. (Hematoxylin, phloxine, and saffron, × 38.)

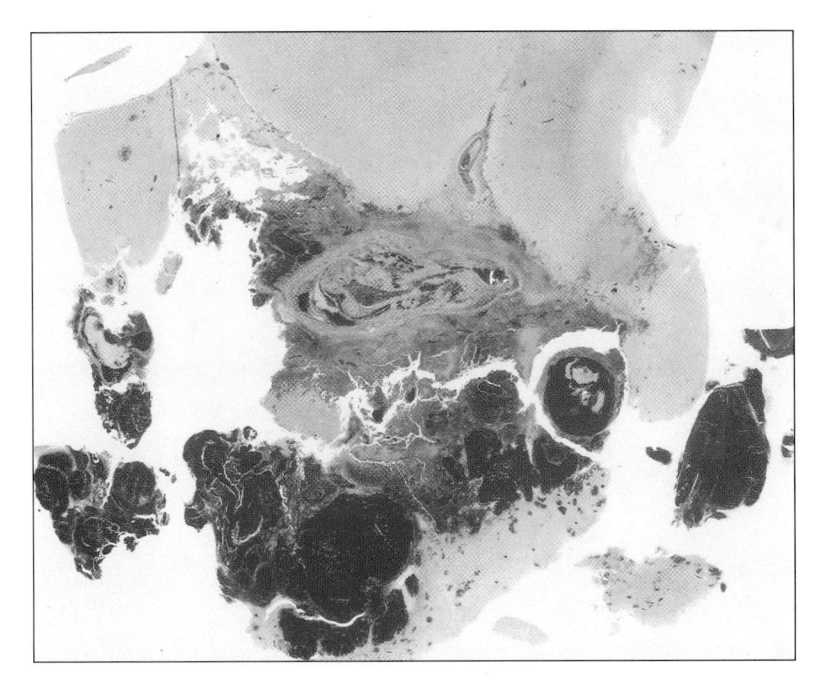

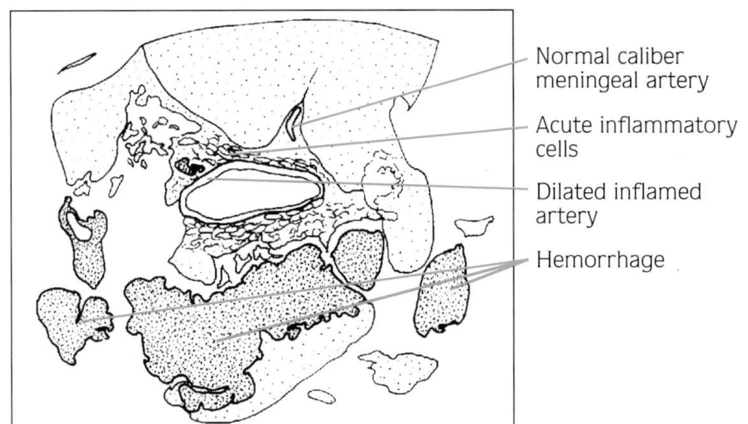

FIGURE 9-47 Septic arteritis: mechanism of arterial dilation, aneurysm formation, and rupture. The process described in Figure 9-46 weakens the blood vessel wall, which then dilates and eventually ruptures. In this figure, a greatly dilated blood vessel is surrounded by a haze of acute inflammatory cells, and a hemorrhage is obvious. (A vessel of normal caliber is identified for comparison.) Hemorrhage in most cases of *Staphylococcus aureus* endocarditis may be due to septic arteritis, whereas a closer link between streptococcal endocarditis and mycotic aneurysm rupture has been suggested. (Hematoxylin, phloxine, and saffron, × 1.) (Hart RG, Foster JW, Luther MF, Kanter MC: Stroke in infective endocarditis. *Stroke* 1990, 21:695–700).

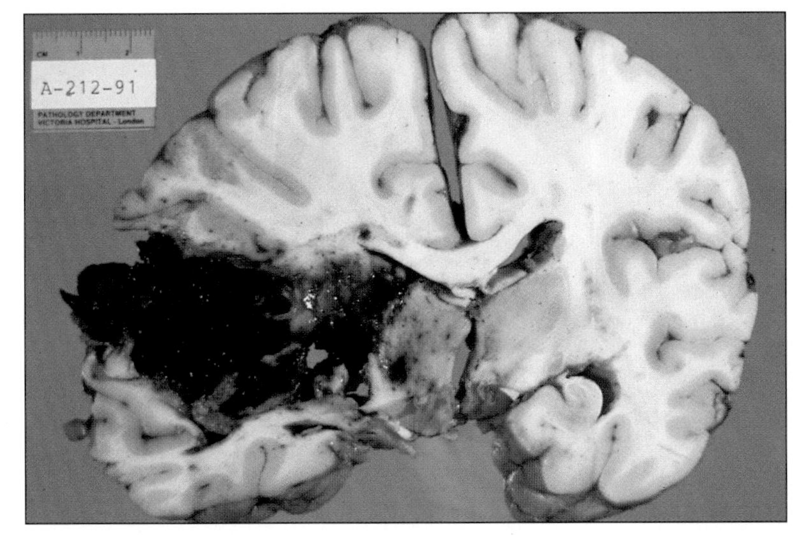

FIGURE 9-48 Endocarditic intracerebral hemorrhage. The septic arteritis illustrated in Figure 9-47 caused a fatal massive left temporal intracerebral hemorrhage. Intracerebral hemorrhage occurs in approximately 5% of patients with native-valve bacterial endocarditis, and in some cases it can be predicted by radiologic identification of "mycotic" aneurysms. Although surgical excision of these vascular abnormalities seems logical, their treatment is controversial for several reasons: they may be surgically difficult to find; they do not always rupture; rupture may occur at the site of radiologically cryptogenic septic arteritis; and prolonged antibiotic treatment alone may reduce the risk of hemorrhage. Most of the cerebrovascular complications associated with bacterial endocarditis occur early, and the risk of these complications diminishes rapidly as the infection is controlled.

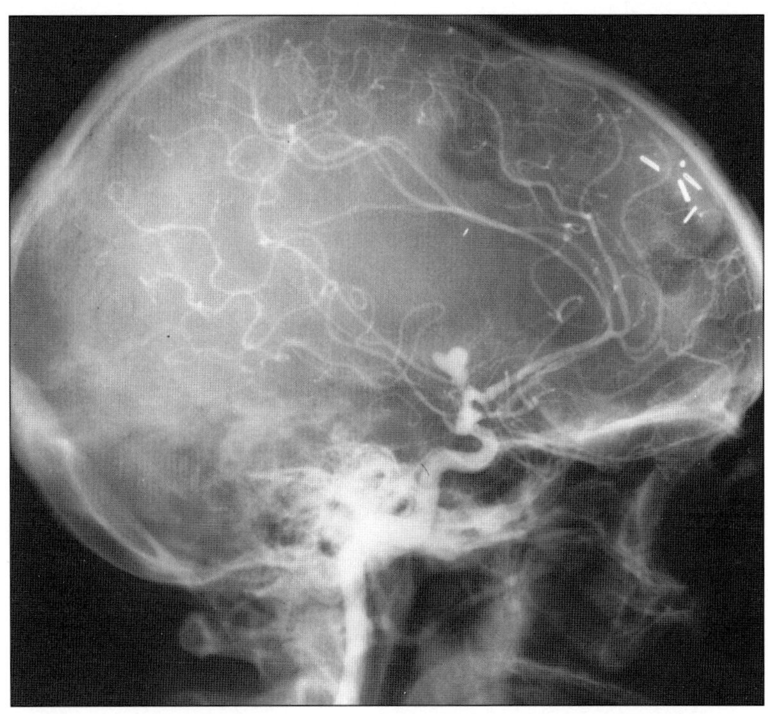

FIGURE 9-49 Angiogram showing mycotic aneurysms. Mycotic aneurysms typically involve the branch points of small, secondary arteries (the site of the clip on the angiogram). Since the clipping, a larger, multilobulated aneurysm has developed at the bifurcation of the internal carotid artery.

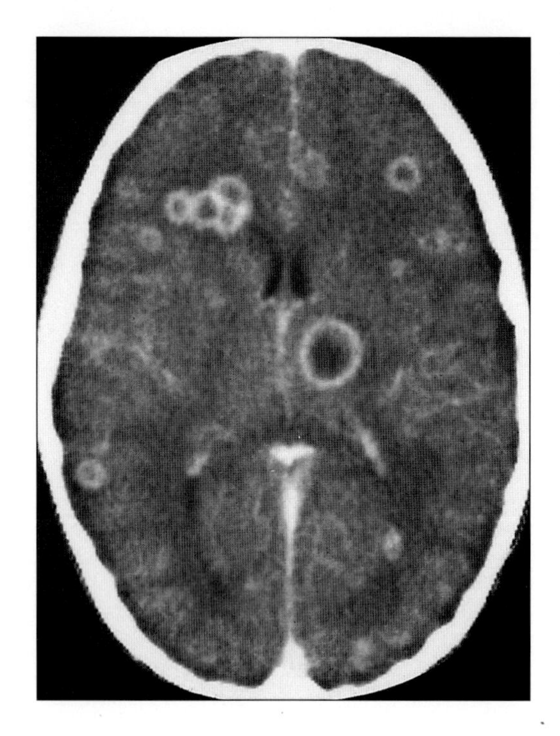

FIGURE 9-50 Multiple brain abscesses. Cranial CT scans with contrast are from a 10-year-old boy with headaches, fever, altered mental status, and frontal lobe signs. The ring-enhancing abscesses are similar to those found in bacterial endocarditis, although the cause was not found in this patient. The symptoms and radiologic signs of abscesses resolved with antibiotic therapy. (*From* Iagarashi M: Multiple brain abscesses. *N Engl J Med* 1993, 329:1083; with permission.)

Prevention and Management

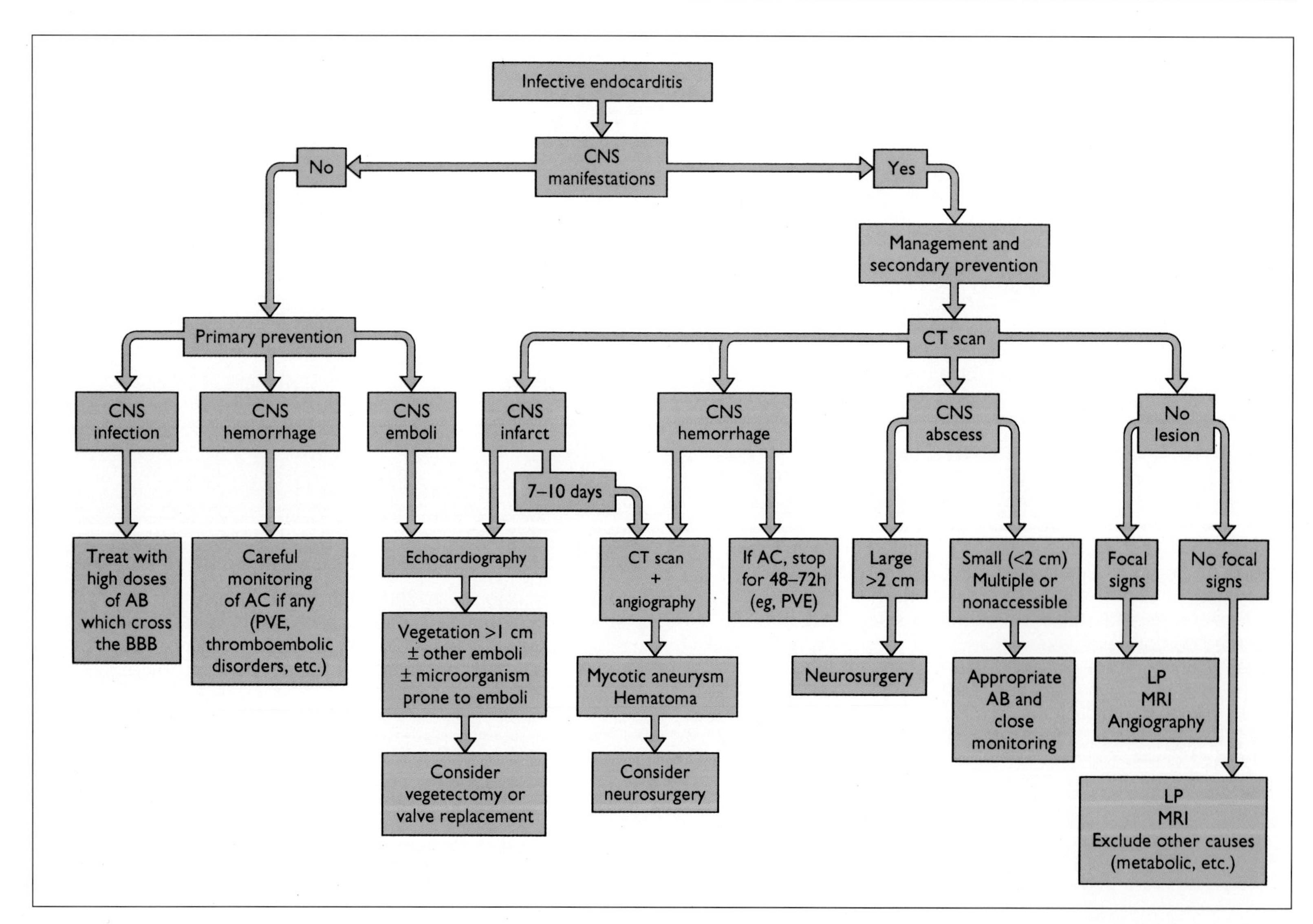

FIGURE 9-51 Prevention and management of CNS complications of infective endocarditis. AB—antibiotics; AC—anticoagulation; BBB—blood–brain barrier; LP—lumbar puncture; PVE—prosthetic valve endocarditis. (*From* Francioli P: Central nervous system complications in infective endocarditis. *In* Scheld WM, Durack D, Whitley R (eds.): *Infections of the Central Nervous System*. New York: Raven Press; 1991:536; with permission.)

Selected Bibliography

Bone RC: Sepsis syndrome: New insights into its pathogenesis and treatment. *Intensive Care World* 1992, 3:50–59.

Matsushita K, Kuriyama Y, Sawada T, *et al.*: Hemorrhagic and ischemic cerebrovascular complications of active infective endocarditis of native valve. *Eur Neurol* 1993, 33:267–274.

Ramsey DA, Zochodne DW, Robertsons DM, *et al.*: A syndrome of acute severe muscle necrosis in intensive care unit patients. *J Neuropathol Exp Neurol* 1993, 52:387–398.

Young GB, Bolton CF, Austin TW, *et al.*: The encephalopathy associated with septic illness. *Clin Invest Med* 1990, 13:297–304.

Zochodne DW, Bolton CF, Wells GA, *et al.*: Critical illness polyneuropathy: A complication of sepsis and multiple organ failure. *Brain* 1987, 110:819–842.

Chapter 10

Ocular and Orbital Infections

Thomas A. Deutsch

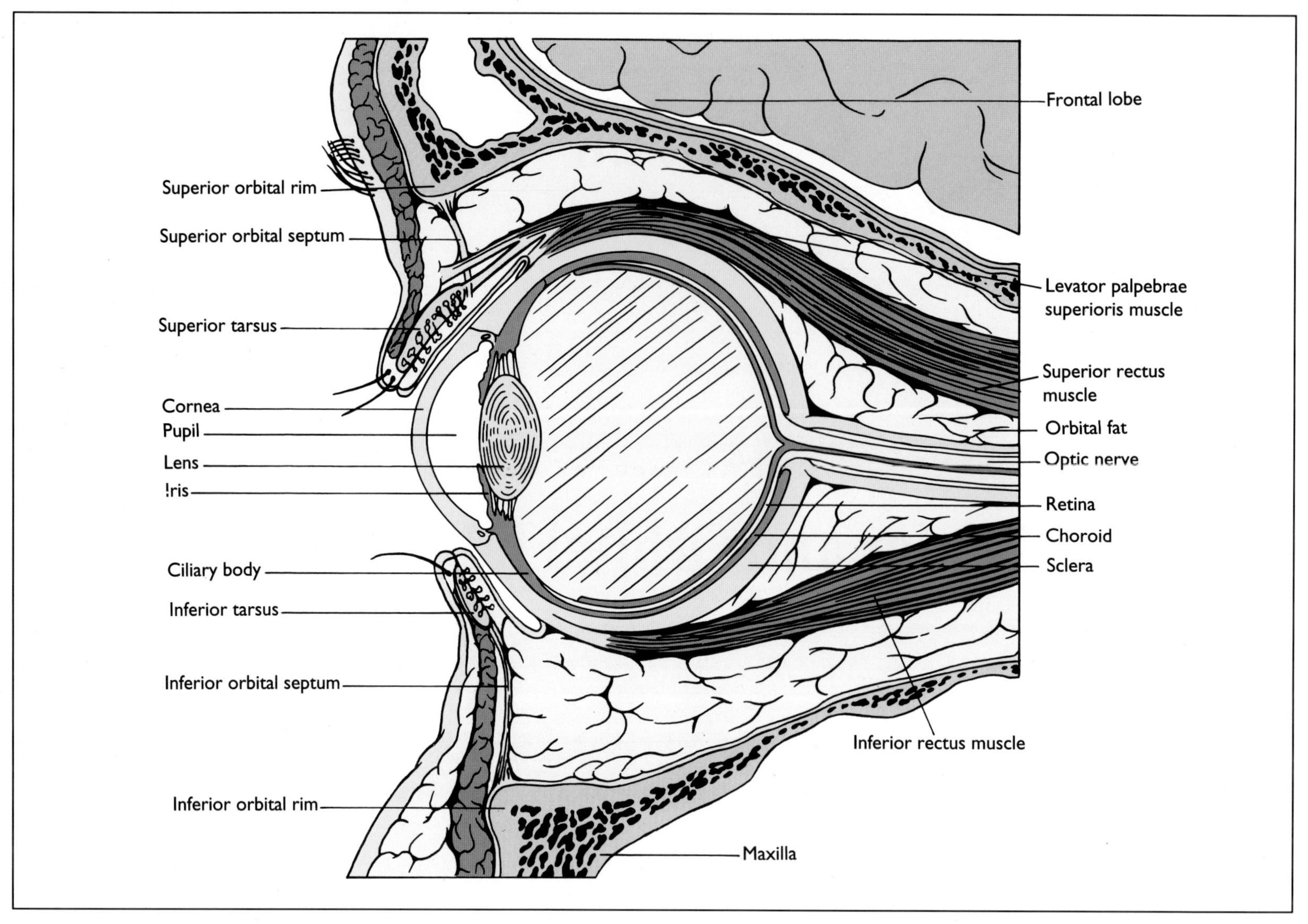

FIGURE 10-1 Sagittal section of the eye and adnexae. Note that the orbit septum separates the orbital contents from the anterior eyelids and face. (*From* Trobe JD: *The Physician's Guide to Eye Care*. San Francisco: American Academy of Ophthalmology; 1993:169; with permission.)

ORBIT AND EYELID DISORDERS

Infectious organisms in orbital cellulitis	
Bacteria	*Haemophilus influenzae* (children)
	Staphylococcus aureus
	Streptococcus pneumoniae
	Other streptococci
	Anaerobic bacteria
Fungi	Phycomycetes ((*Mucor, Rhizopus*)
	Ascomycetes (*Aspergillus*)
Parasites	Echinococcus
	Taenia solium

FIGURE 10-2 Most common infectious organisms in orbital cellulitis. Note that these are similar to the agents in acute sinus infections.

Mechanisms of infection in orbital cellulitis	
Direct inoculation	25%
Trauma, surgery	
Extension of adjacent infection	50%–75%
Acute sinus disease	
Dental abscess	
Pharyngeal infection	
Otitis media	
Hematogenous spread	< 10%
Bacterial endocarditis	
Other	

FIGURE 10-3 Mechanisms of infection in orbital cellulitis. It can be seen that the most common are direct extensions from adjacent structures, particularly the sinuses. (Westfall CT, Shore JW, Baker AS: Orbital infections. *In* Gorbach S, Bartlett J, Blacklow NR (eds): *Infectious Diseases*. Philadelphia: W.B. Saunders; 1992:1151–1155.)

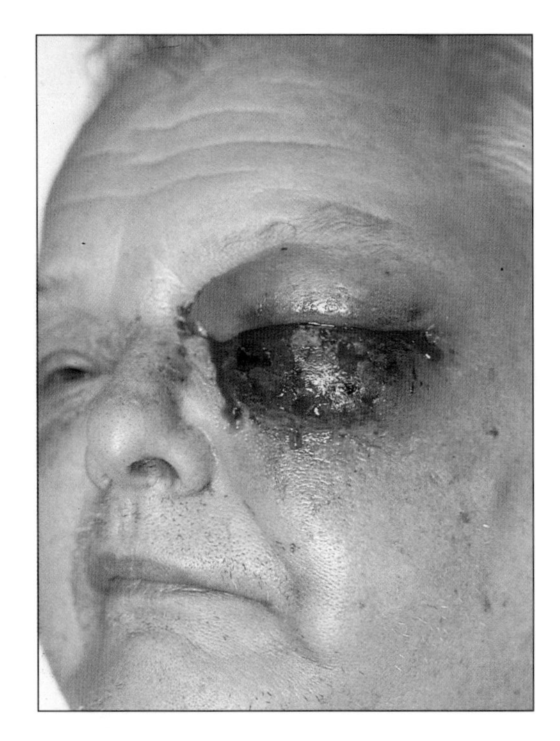

FIGURE 10-4 Preseptal cellulitis in an elderly man. This can be differentiated from orbital cellulitis by the intense preseptal inflammatory reaction, the cellulitis extending over the entire face, and extension onto the contralateral eyelids. In the presence of any recent skin injury, *Staphylococcus aureus* is a common causative organism. In the absence of any recent wound, the list of possible causative organisms is similar to that in acute sinusitis (*Haemophilus influenzae*, pneumococcus, *Streptococcus* spp., and *S. aureus*).

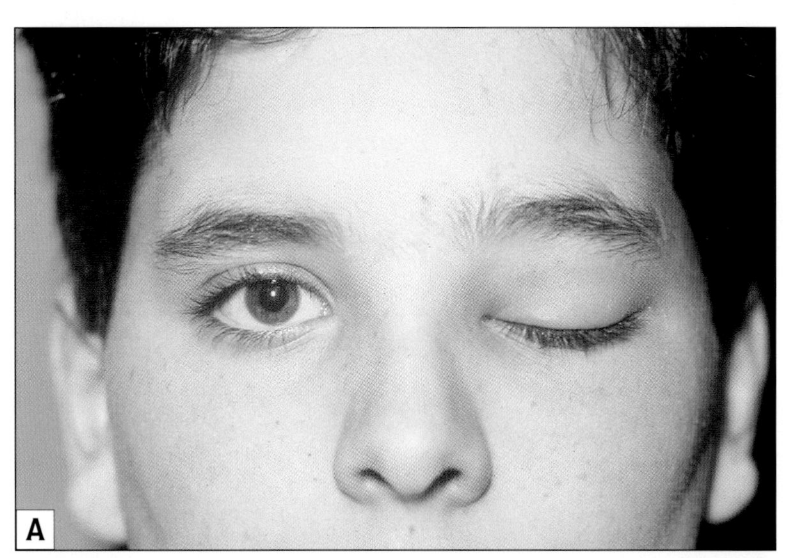

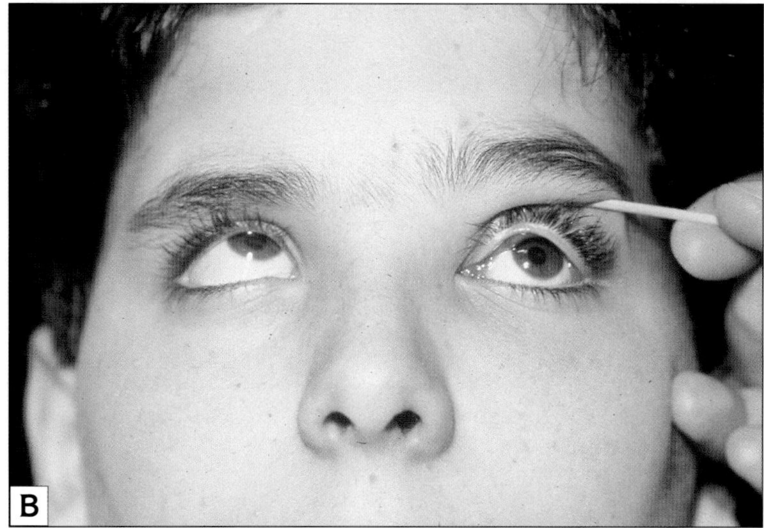

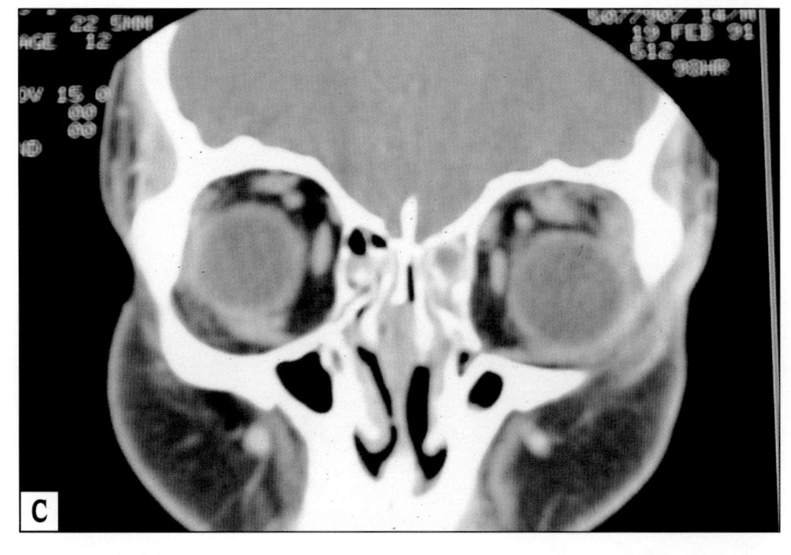

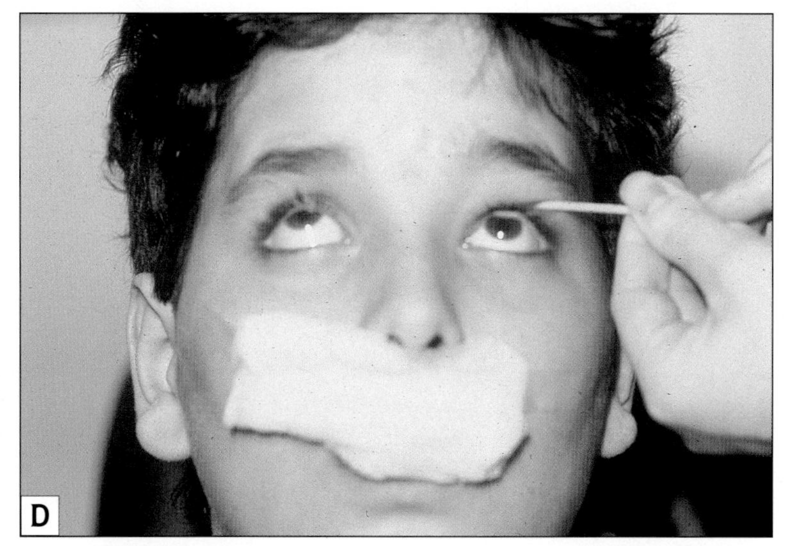

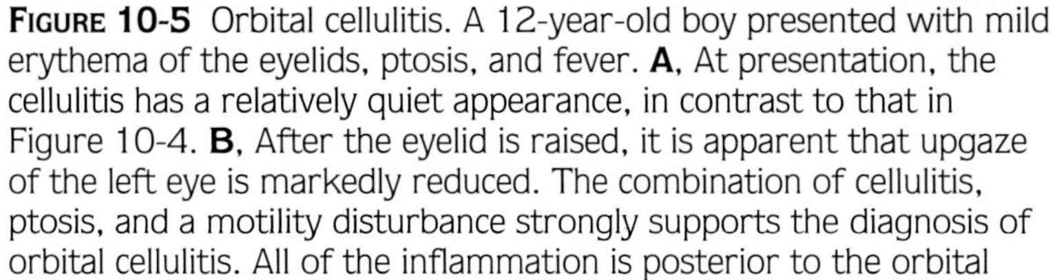

FIGURE 10-5 Orbital cellulitis. A 12-year-old boy presented with mild erythema of the eyelids, ptosis, and fever. **A**, At presentation, the cellulitis has a relatively quiet appearance, in contrast to that in Figure 10-4. **B**, After the eyelid is raised, it is apparent that upgaze of the left eye is markedly reduced. The combination of cellulitis, ptosis, and a motility disturbance strongly supports the diagnosis of orbital cellulitis. All of the inflammation is posterior to the orbital septum, which acts as a barrier, keeping much of the inflammation from the face. **C**, The computed tomography (CT) scan of the sinuses reveals extensive acute sinusitis. As with preseptal cellulitis, the microbiology of orbital cellulitis is predominantly the microbiology of acute sinusitis. **D**, Draining of the sinuses was accomplished via a Caldwell-Luc approach. On the day following surgery, the patient's ability to look up was already markedly improved. (*continued*)

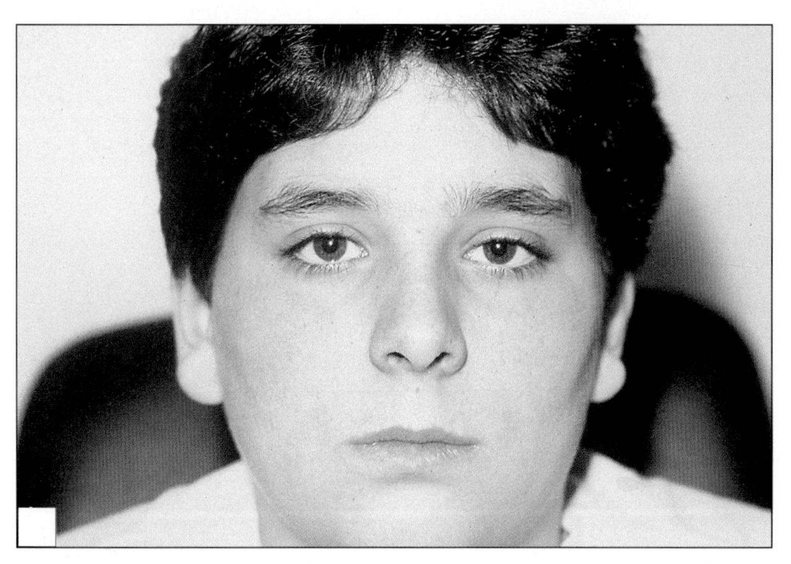

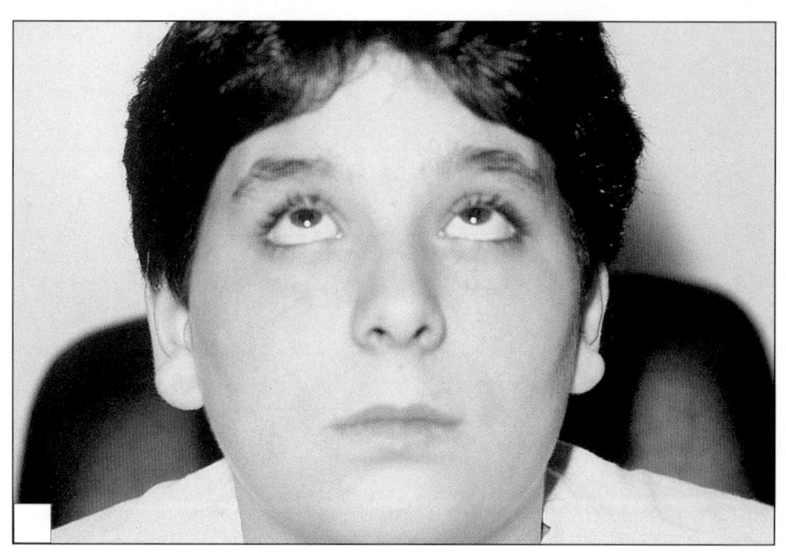

Figure 10-5 (*continued*) **E**, One month following drainage of the sinuses, the ptosis has resolved completely. Diplopia, which had been present prior to surgery when the eyelid was elevated, has completely resolved. **F**, Upgaze also had returned completely to normal.

Differentiation of preseptal versus orbital cellulitis

Preseptal	Orbital
Skin (facial) cellulitis (may be severe)	Mild to moderate skin cellulitis
Vision and pupils normal	May have decreased vision, afferent pupil defect
Normal motility	May have reduction in gaze
No proptosis	Proptosis possible

Figure 10-6 Differentiation of preseptal versus orbital cellulitis. With an increasing severity of facial skin involvement, the diagnosis of preseptal cellulitis becomes more likely. Any abnormality of vision or motility or the presence of proptosis implies orbital cellulitis.

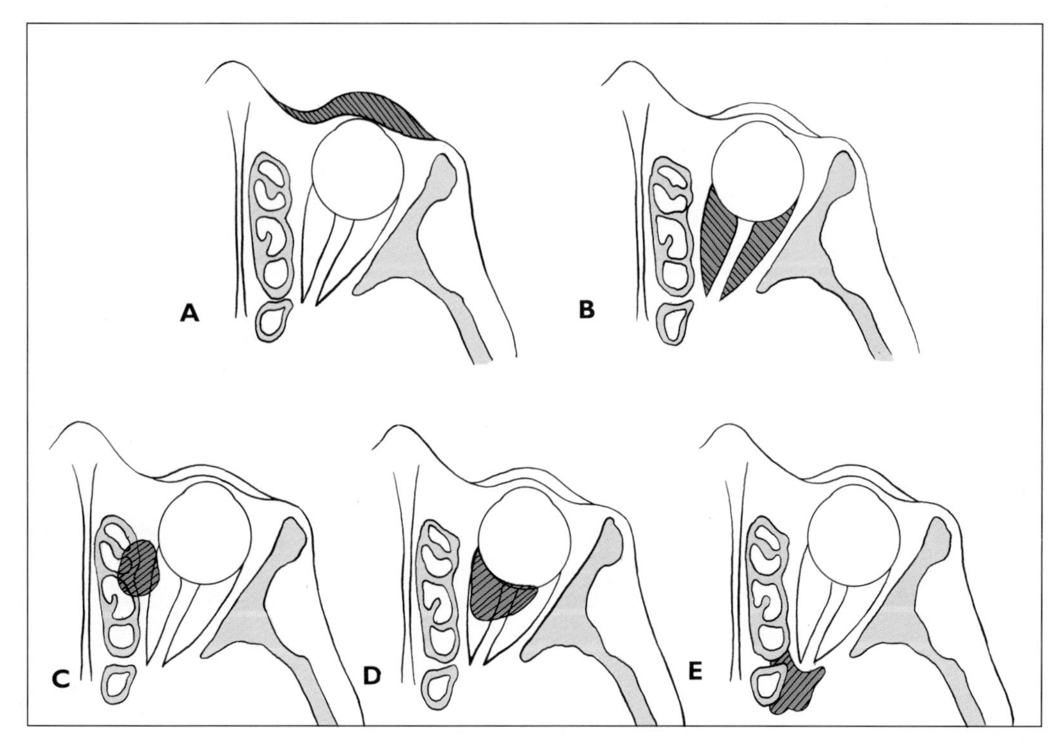

Figure 10-7 Staging of orbital cellulitis and its complications. **A**, Preseptal (periorbital) cellulitis. **B**, Orbital cellulitis. **C**, Subperiosteal abscess. **D**, Orbital abscess. **E**, Cavernous sinus thrombosis. (*Adapted from* Chandler J: Orbital cellulitis and its complications. *In* Gates G (ed.): *Current Therapy in Otolaryngology—Head and Neck Surgery*, 4th ed. Toronto: B.C. Decker; 1990:267; with permission.)

Decision making in cellulitis

Preseptal cellulitis
- Responsible adults or children with adult: oral antibiotics, outpatient care, return next day
- Children appearing systemically ill: intravenous antibiotics, inpatient care
- No CT scan

Orbital cellulitis
- All patients admitted to hospital
- Intravenous antibiotics
- CT may be delayed 24 hrs pending clinical improvement (*if* vision and pupils are normal)

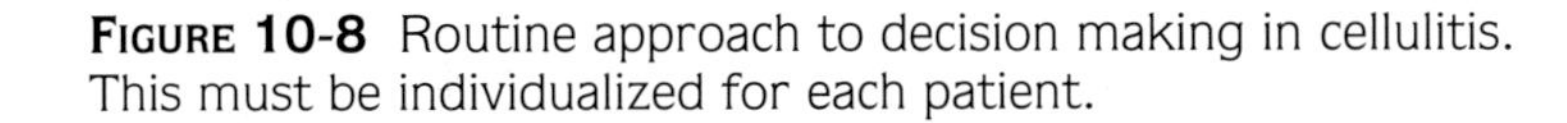

FIGURE 10-8 Routine approach to decision making in cellulitis. This must be individualized for each patient.

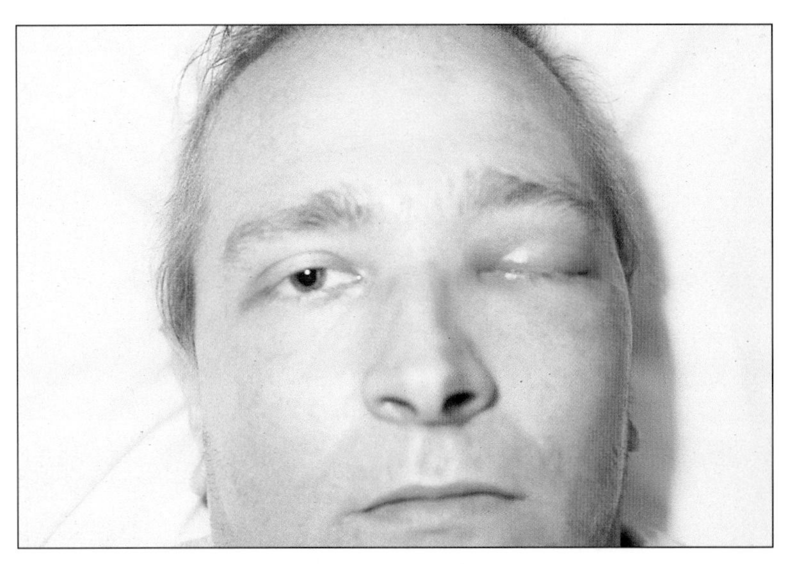

FIGURE 10-9 Leukemic infiltration of orbit. A 42-year-old man presented with acute inflammation of the left orbit and proptosis of the left eye. Although orbital cellulitis was included in the differential diagnosis, this case resulted from acute leukemic infiltration of the orbit. Orbital decompression was accomplished as an emergency procedure, and there was no growth of bacteria from the orbital contents. The patient was treated with corticosteroids and radiation, and the orbital inflammation resolved rapidly. This condition must be differentiated from infectious orbital cellulitis.

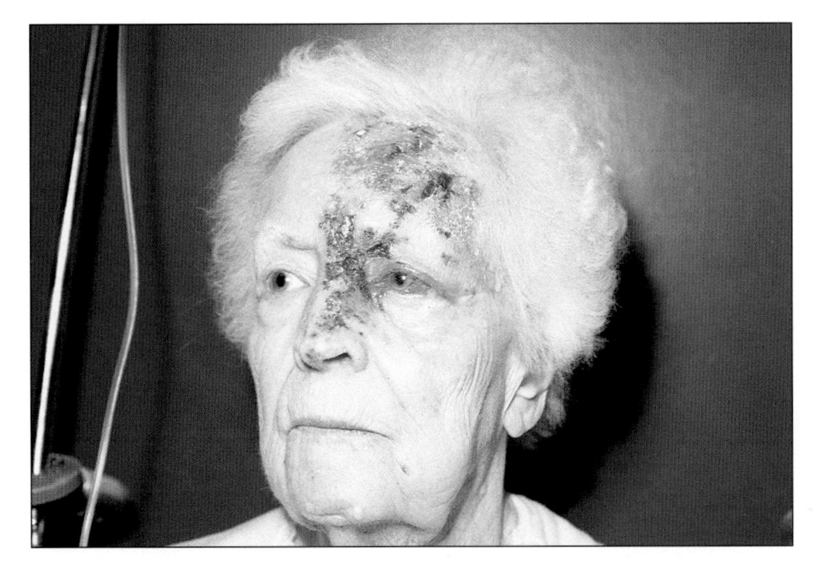

FIGURE 10-10 Acute herpes zoster ophthalmicus. An elderly woman presented with tingling and subsequent pain on the left side of her forehead. She developed vesicular lesions over the distribution of the ophthalmic branch of the trigeminal nerve. The involvement of the tip of her nose (Hutchinson's sign) suggests involvement of the nasociliary nerve, a nerve that also supplies the cornea. In this case, the cornea has become inflamed, the eye is red, and there is a danger that glaucoma will develop. Patients with acute herpes zoster ophthalmicus should be treated with acyclovir, 800 mg five times a day for 5 days, beginning within 72 hours of the onset of symptoms; this reduces the incidence of ocular involvement, but it does not alter the course of postherpetic neuralgia.

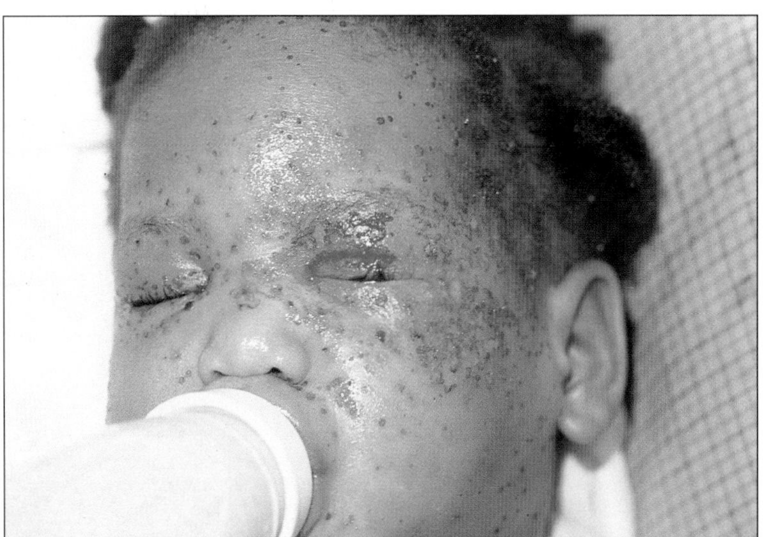

FIGURE 10-11 Primary herpes simplex virus (HSV) type-I blepharitis. Note that these vesicles extend across the bridge of the nose and onto the contralateral side. This is the primary HSV infection which nearly always precedes development of HSV keratitis by months, years, or decades. The use of acyclovir probably hastens the recovery, although primary HSV is a self-limiting condition. At the time of primary infection, many ophthalmologists recommend the use of topical antiviral drops to prevent acute HSV keratitis. However, keratitis is ordinarily a secondary condition and rarely occurs during a primary attack.

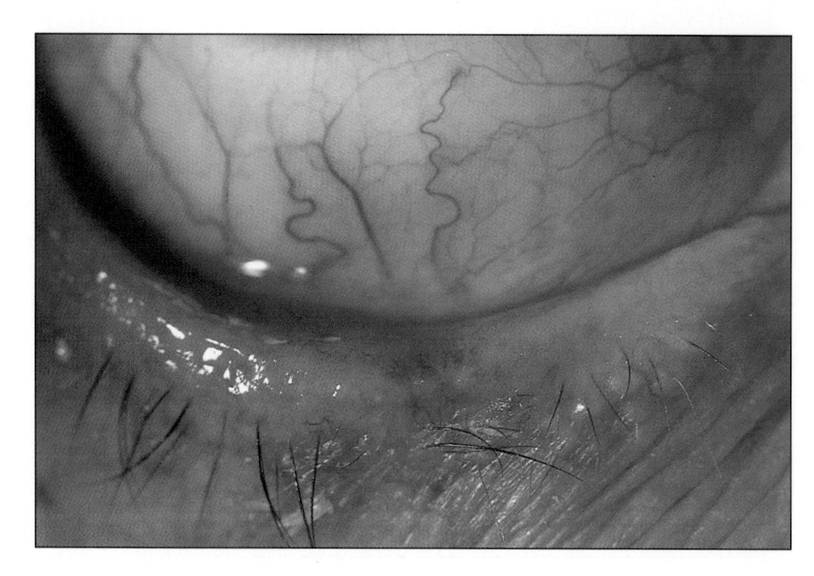

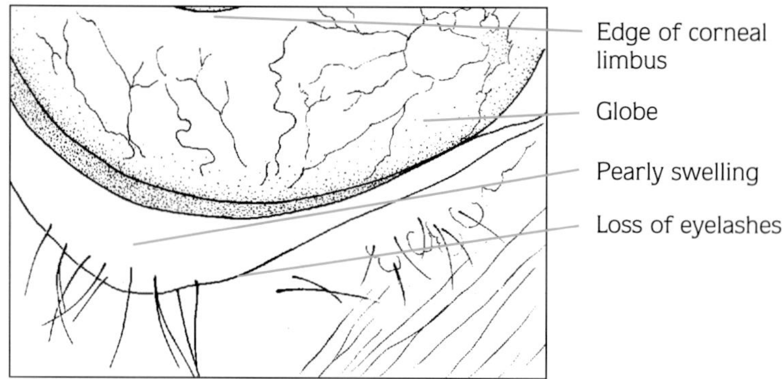

FIGURE 10-12 An inflammatory eyelid lesion must be differentiated from an infectious lesion. This is a basal cell carcinoma of the eyelid margin. Note the focal swelling next to a focal area of loss of eye lashes. The pearly appearance of the surface is typical of a basal cell carcinoma.

CONJUNCTIVAL AND CORNEAL DISORDERS

Differential diagnosis of the red eye

	Conjunctivitis	Iritis	Keratitis (corneal inflammation or foreign body)	Acute angle-closure glaucoma
Vision	Normal or intermittent blurring that clears on blinking	Slightly blurred	Slightly blurred	Marked blurring
Discharge	Usually significant, with crusting of lashes	None	None to mild	None
Pain	None or minor and superficial	Moderately severe: aching and photophobia	Sharp, severe foreign-body sensation	Very severe; frequently nausea and vomiting
Pupil size	Normal	Constricted	Normal or constricted	Fixed, dilated
Conjunctival injection	Diffuse	Circumcorneal	Circumcorneal	Diffuse, with prominent circumcorneal injection
Pupillary response to light	Normal	Minimal further constriction	Normal	Usually no reaction of mid-dilated pupil
Intraocular pressure	Normal	Normal to low	Normal	Markedly elevated to touch
Appearance of cornea	Clear	Clear or slightly hazy	Opacification present; altered light reflex; positive fluorescein staining	Hazy; altered light reflex
Anterior chamber depth	Normal	Normal	Normal	Shallow

FIGURE 10-13 Differential diagnosis of the red eye. In acute angle-closure glaucoma, it is highly desirable for an ophthalmologist to examine the patient during an acute attack to confirm the diagnosis. (*From: Managing the Red Eye*. San Francisco: American Academy of Ophthalmology; 1994:34; with permission.)

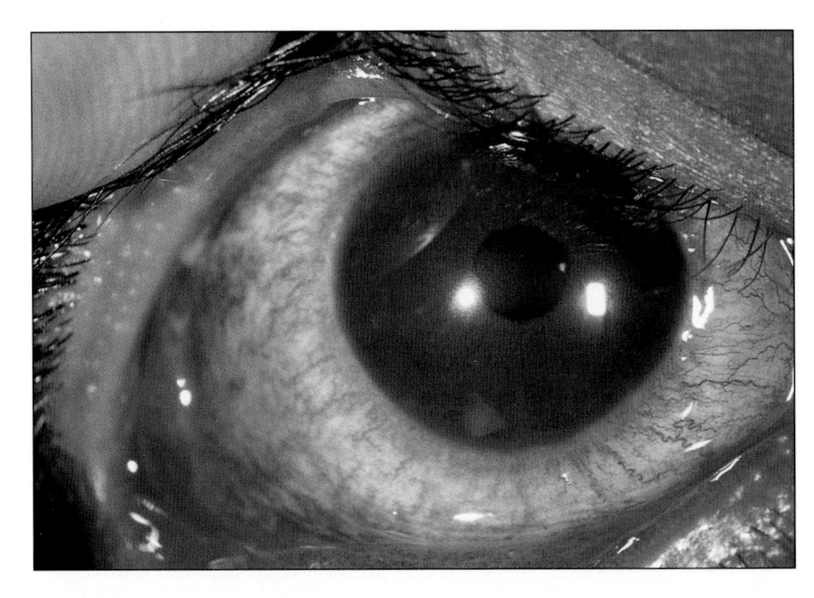

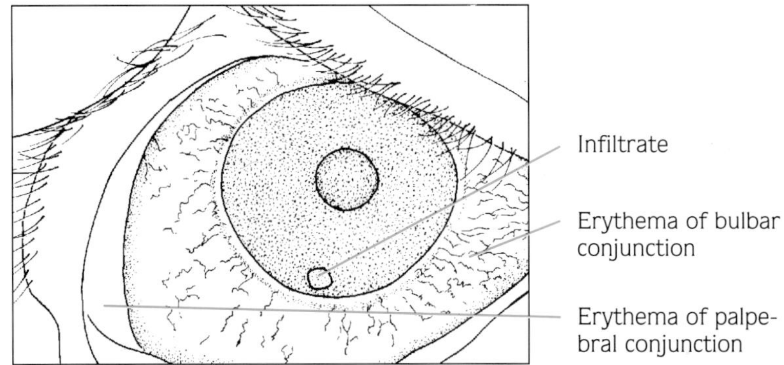

FIGURE 10-14 Hyperacute conjunctivitis. This bacterial conjunctivitis consists of diffuse erythema of the conjunctiva. Note that both the bulbar and palpebral conjunctivae are affected. A small infiltrate is seen on the surface of the inferior cornea. In hyperacute conjunctivitis, this infiltrate can proceed rapidly to perforation of the cornea, and hence prompt antibiotic treatment with ceftriaxone is necessary.

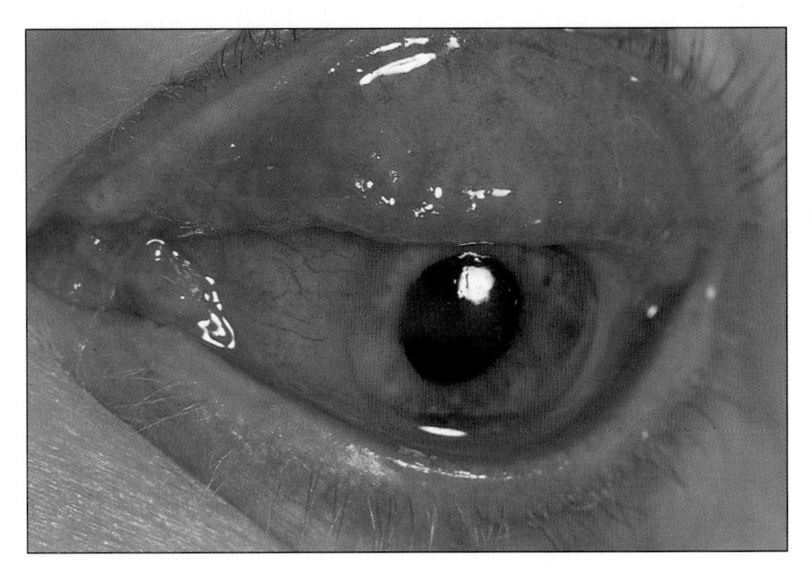

FIGURE 10-15 Intense follicular conjunctival reaction from viral conjunctivitis. This is a case of HSV conjunctivitis and highlights the danger of using topical steroids to treat viral conjunctivitis. The use of a topical steroid in this case could have resulted in HSV keratitis and permanent scarring of the cornea.

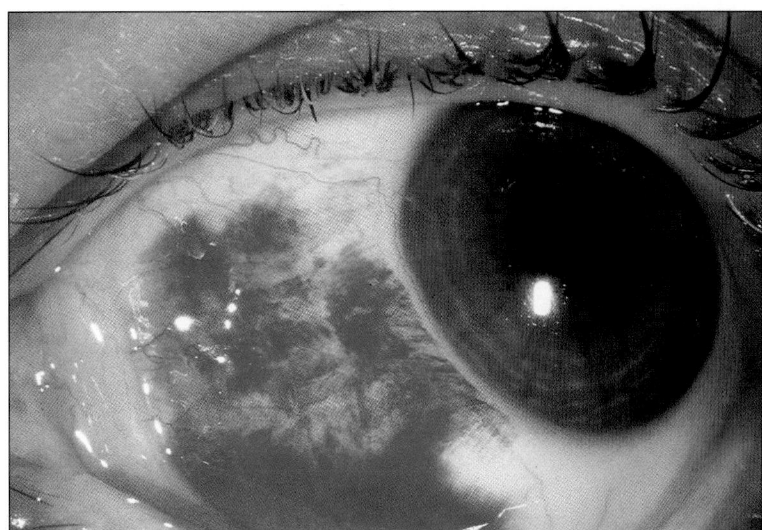

FIGURE 10-16 Subconjunctival hemorrhage. This focal area of redness contrasts with the diffuse erythema associated with conjunctivitis. This lesion is caused by a broken blood vessel, is self-limiting, and will resolve spontaneously within 10 days.

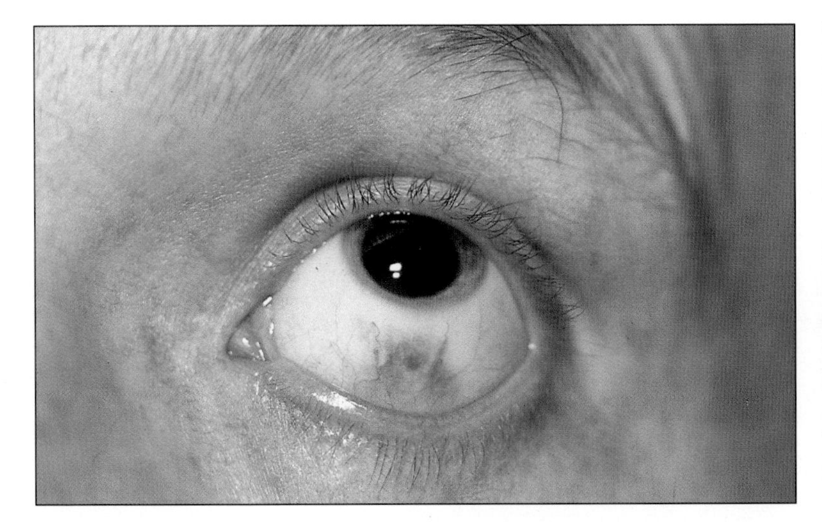

FIGURE 10-17 Kaposi's sarcoma of the conjunctiva. This red lesion is a Kaposi's sarcoma of the conjunctiva in an AIDS patient. Focal areas of erythema on the conjunctiva, when remote from the corneal limbus, are rarely infectious. In addition to subconjunctival hemorrhage and tumor, the differential diagnosis includes scleritis, an immunologic reaction of the collagen underlying the conjunctiva.

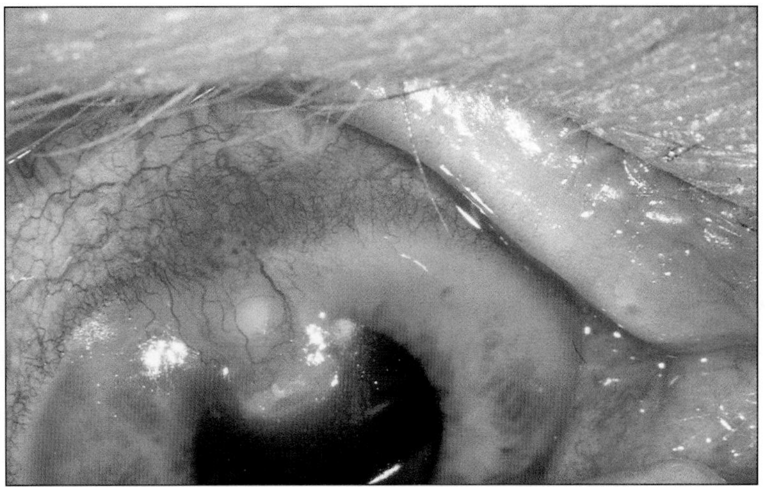

FIGURE 10-18 Focal area of erythema. This focal area of erythema is adjacent to the limbus and is associated with a raised conjunctival nodule. The "phlyctenule" is an immunologic reaction to either staphylococcal antigen or tuberculosis antigen. Although tuberculosis should be ruled out, these lesions are easily treated with topical corticosteroids.

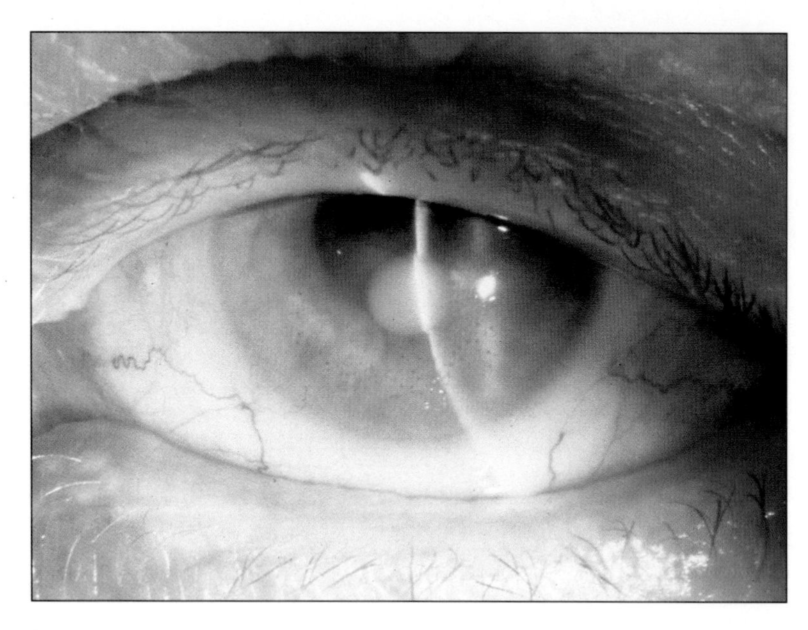

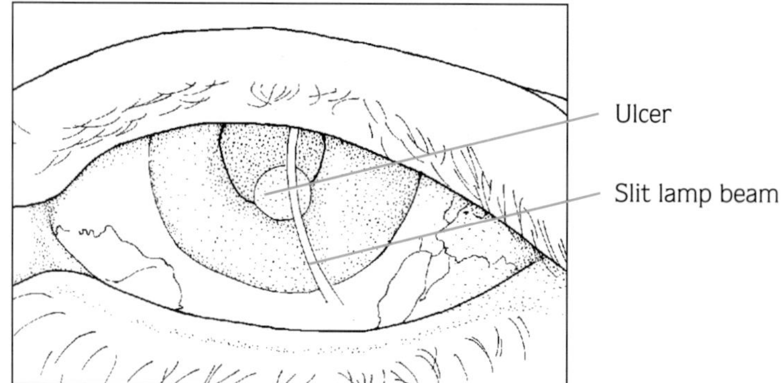

FIGURE 10-19 Bacterial corneal ulcer under a soft contact lens. The patient had been wearing extended-wear contact lenses for 2 weeks between cleanings. She developed an acute onset of irritation of this eye and was found to have a deep infiltrate of the cornea. The most common organism in this setting is *Pseudomonas* and, when present, can lead to rapid perforation of the cornea and permanent loss of vision.

UVEAL TRACT DISORDERS

Microbiology of endophthalmitis

Organism	Postoperative infections, %	Bleb-associated infections, %	Traumatic infections, %
Staphylococcus epidermidis	38	0	20
Staphylococcus aureus	21	7	0
Staphylococcus spp.	11	57	13
Bacillus spp.	0	0	27
Haemophilus influenzae	3	23	0
Other gram-negative species	13	7	20
Fungi	8	3	17
Other	6	3	3
Mixed flora	2	0	11

FIGURE 10-20 Most common organisms in endophthalmitis. Staph epidermidis also has the most favorable prognosis. (*Adapted from* Forster FK: Endophthalmitis. *In* Duane TD, Jaeger AE (eds): *Clinical Ophthalmology*, vol 4. Philadelphia: J.B. Lippincott; 1988; with permission.)

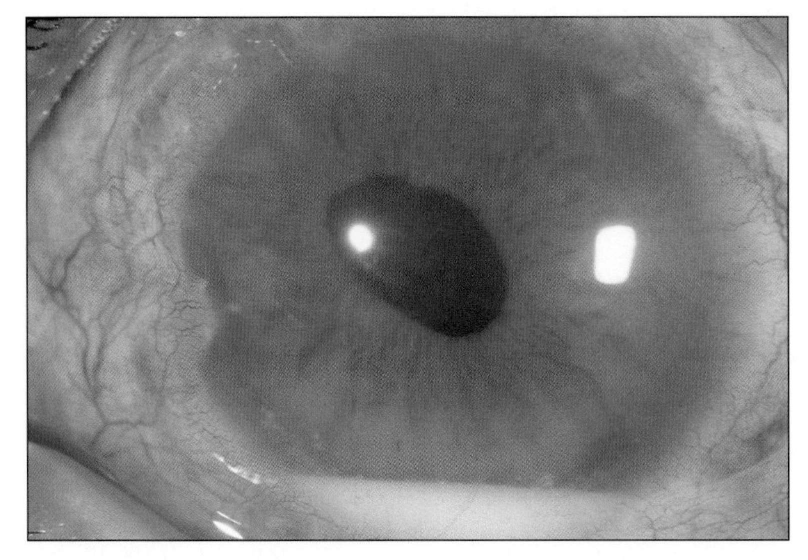

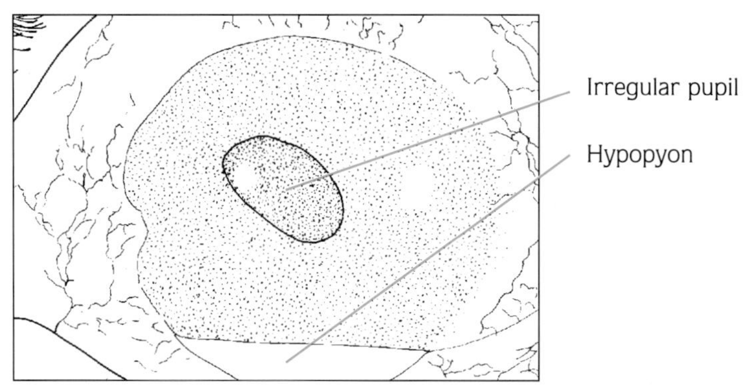

FIGURE 10-21 Endogenous endophthalmitis in an AIDS patient. This patient had an acute onset of pain and redness accompanied by decreased visual acuity. He was found to have marked inflammation, including a hypopyon (an accumulation of white blood cells in the anterior chamber). Note the layering of the hypopyon, the hazy view of the iris and pupil, and the irregularity of the pupil caused by scarring of it to the underlying lens. Systemic blood cultures can be helpful in finding the causative organism, which is most commonly treated with intravenous antibiotics. Occasionally, eyes with endogenous endophthalmitis require vitrectomy and lavage of the intraocular contents with antibiotics or antifungal agents as appropriate.

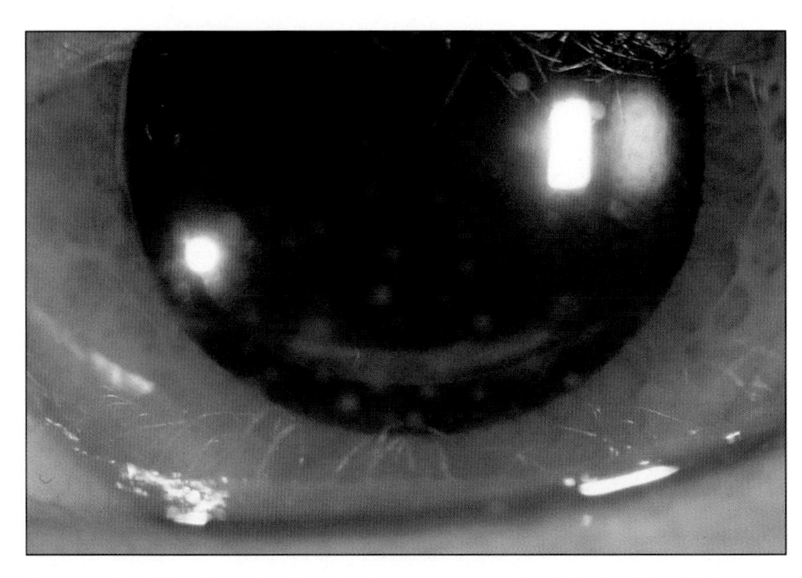

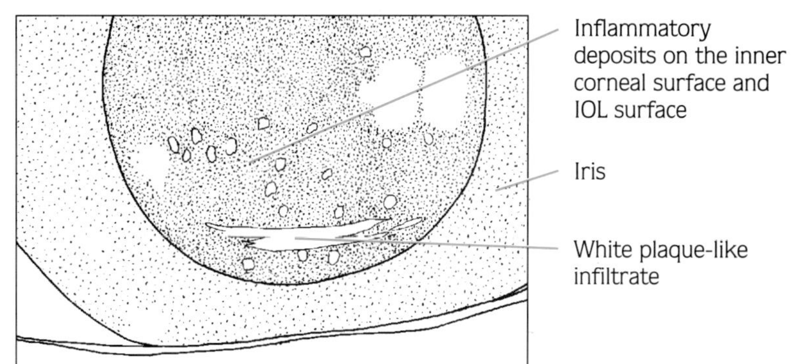

FIGURE 10-22 *Propionibacterium acnes* endophthalmitis. This patient had cataract surgery 1 year before presenting with pain and redness of the left eye. Culture of the intraocular contents revealed *P. acnes* as the causative agent of his endophthalmitis. In contrast to acute endophthalmitis seen after cataract surgery, *P. acnes* is a slow-growing and indolent organism that usually does not cause inflammation until months after the surgery. Note the inflammatory debris on the inside surface of the cornea and surface of the intraocular lens (IOL) implant. Also, note the white plaquelike material surrounding the implant. The organisms can be retrieved from this area. It appears as though *P. acnes* organisms remain walled off from the eye for some time after surgery, and when exposed, they result in a low-grade infectious and inflammatory process. Most of these eyes can be treated easily with an intraocular injection of antibiotics, usually gentamicin, clindamycin, and vancomycin.

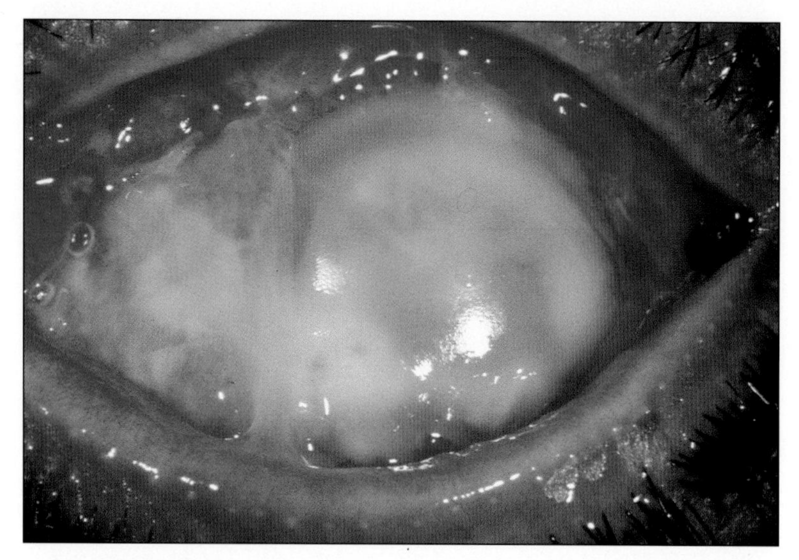

FIGURE 10-23 This patient had glaucoma surgery 5 years prior to development of acute bacterial endophthalmitis. After glaucoma surgery, there is a chronic exposure of intraocular contents to the tear film, and in some cases, endophthalmitis can develop years after the original surgery. These eyes have a poor prognosis because of the rapid development of inflammation, which damages intraocular structures such as the retina and ciliary body.

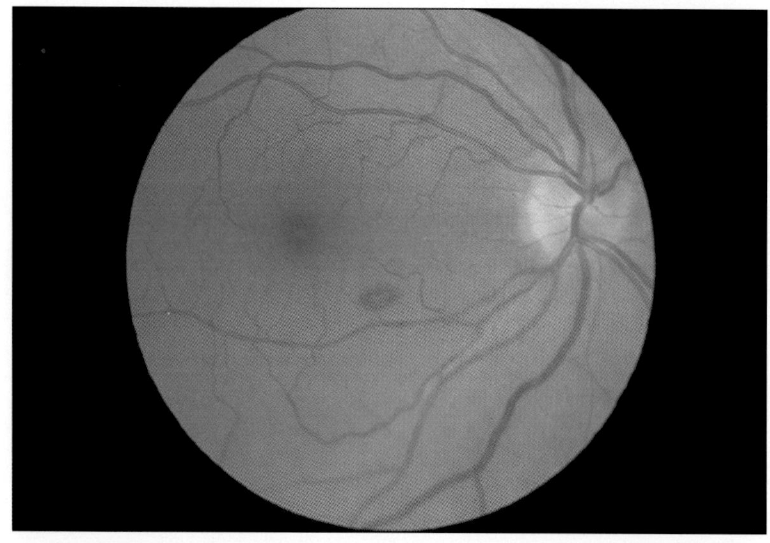

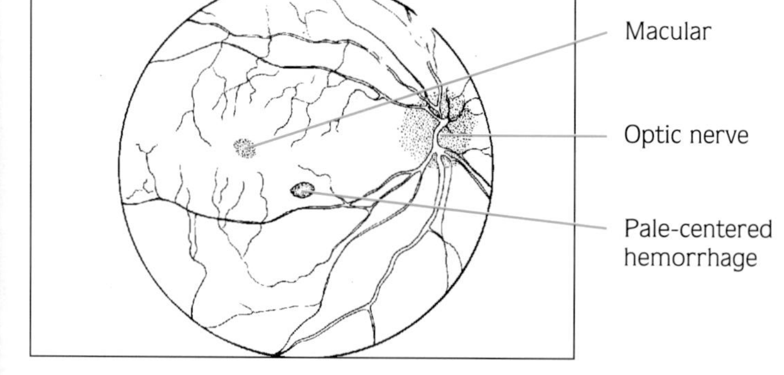

FIGURE 10-24 Roth spots. This patient has recently had a renal transplant and is now septic. The pale-centered hemorrhage between the disc and macula is known as a Roth spot. Roth spots can be seen in patients with bacterial endocarditis, sepsis, and other infectious conditions, although most are associated with hemorrhagic conditions such as acute leukemia or thrombocytopenia.

Choroid and Retinal Disorders

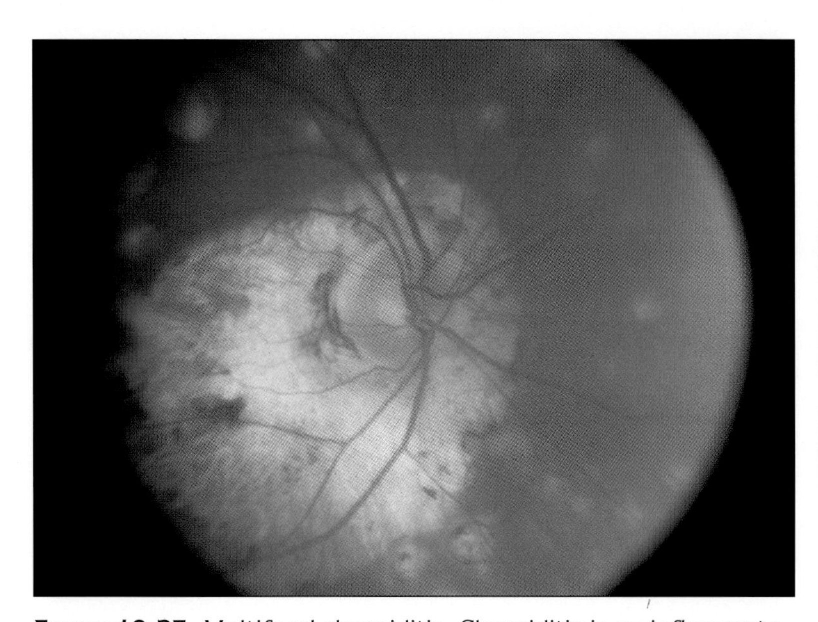

Figure 10-25 Multifocal choroiditis. Choroiditis is an inflammatory condition of the fundus associated with tuberculosis, sarcoidosis, or syphilis. The characteristic appearance is peripapillary (around the optic nerve head) atrophy with multiple, small, "punched-out," atrophic choroidal lesions and macular scarring. The most important differential diagnosis of multifocal choroiditis is ocular histoplasmosis. In ocular histoplasmosis, the retinal appearance is very similar, but there is never any inflammatory component to the ocular findings.

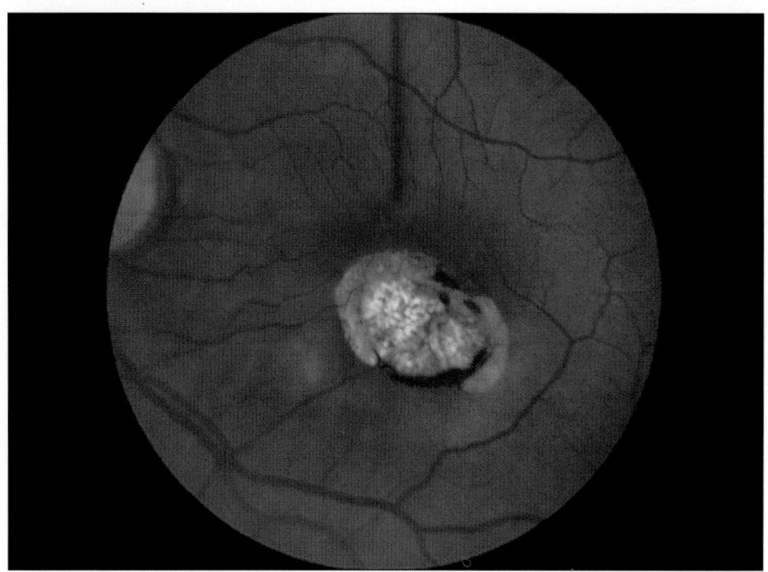

Figure 10-26 Congenital toxoplasmosis. This "punched-out" retinal and choroidal lesion is characterized by a pigmented ring around the yellow reflex from the underlying sclera. The optic nerve can barely be seen at the upper left corner of the picture and is somewhat pale because of the death of nerve fibers between this lesion and the optic nerve. The lesion was found as an incidental finding during a routine ophthalmologic examination. This eye had 20/20 vision, because the lesion did not involve the center of the fovea, shown here at the tip of the fixation pointer. It was present since birth, and if there is no reactivation of the organisms, it will remain quiet throughout the patient's life.

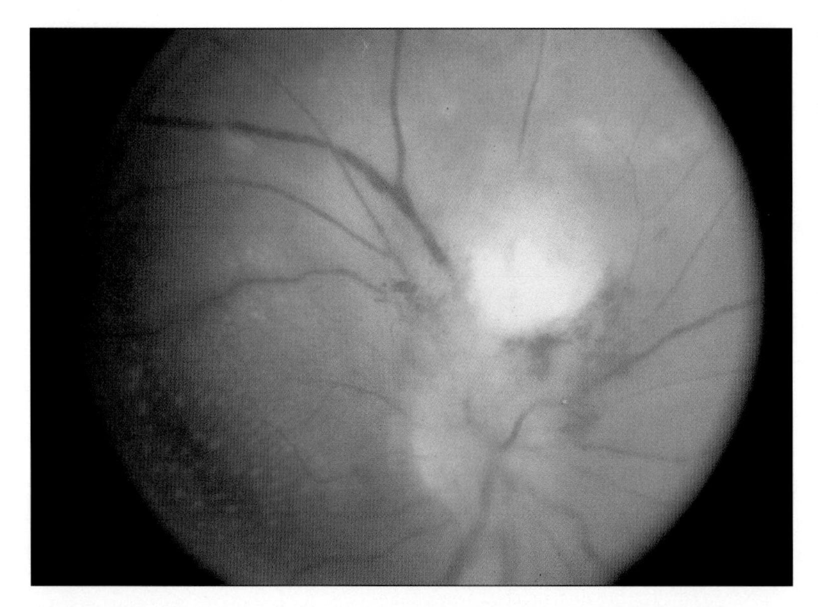

Figure 10-27 Acute acquired toxoplasmosis. A middle-aged woman developed acute toxoplasmic retinochoroiditis in the area of the optic nerve following a systemic toxoplasmosis infection. This finding is unusual in immunocompetent patients but has been seen increasingly in patients who are immunocompromised either iatrogenically or because of an underlying condition. Note the hemorrhagic and necrotic appearance of the retina, which is markedly edematous surrounding the area of infection.

Treatment of acute ocular toxoplasmosis
Trimethoprim (160 mg)–sulfamethoxazole (880 mg), orally, twice daily, for 4–6 wks
Clindamycin (300 mg), orally, four times daily, 2 wks
Prednisone (80 mg), orally, once daily, with rapid taper

Figure 10-28 Scheme for treatment of acute ocular toxoplasmosis. This scheme for treatment of acute ocular toxoplasmosis is currently recommended, but there is controversy about the best approach.

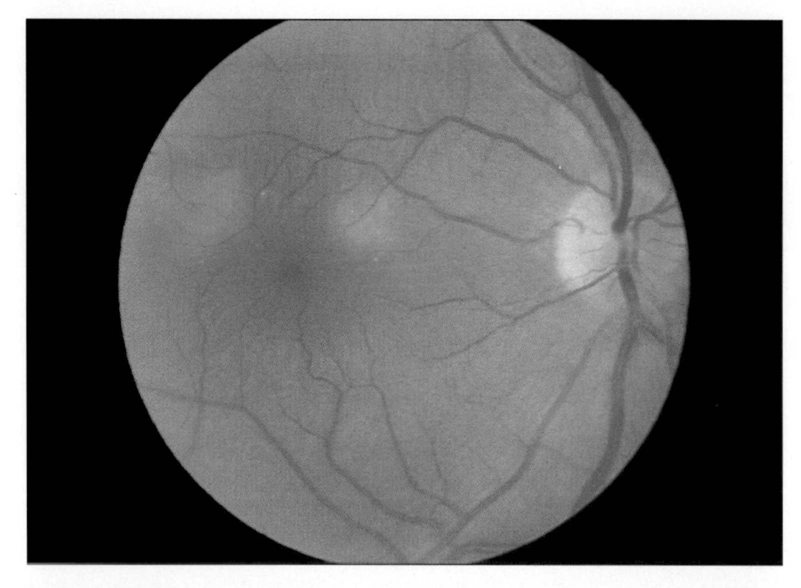

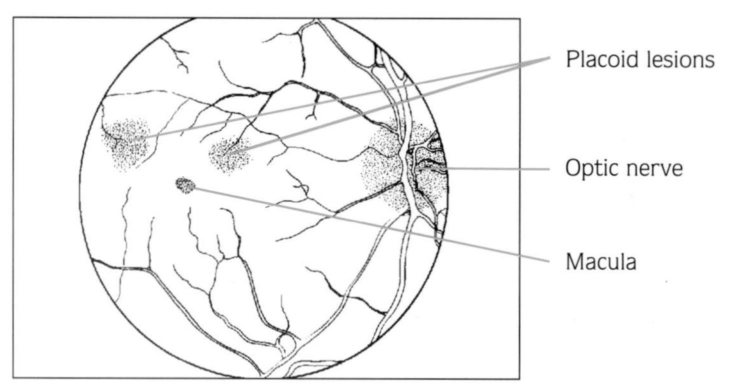

Figure 10-29 Acute posterior multifocal placoid pigment epitheliopathy. These plaque-like lesions in the posterior fundus follow a flu-like illness by about 10 days. The specific virus is not known. The visual acuity is usually slightly reduced for about 2 weeks, followed by a return to near-normal vision in most patients. It is unlikely that any medications, including corticosteroids, are of any use in this condition.

Optic Nerve Disorders

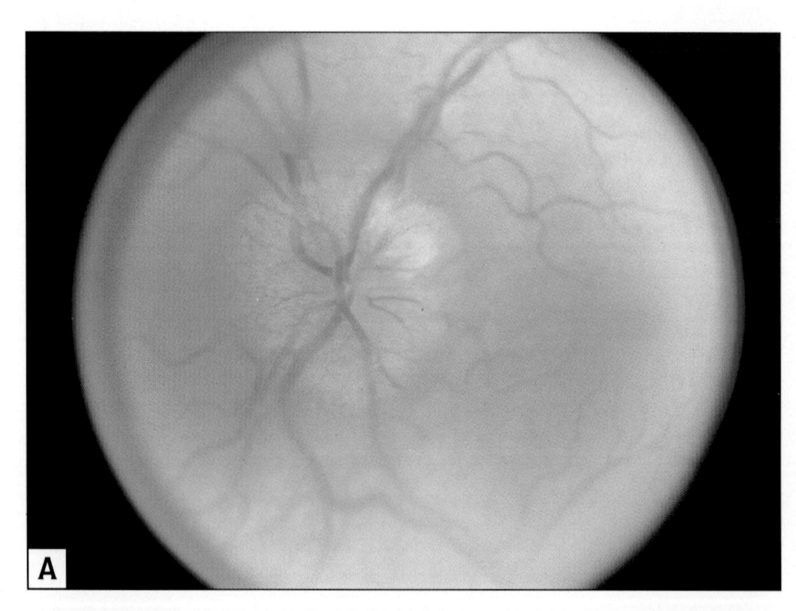

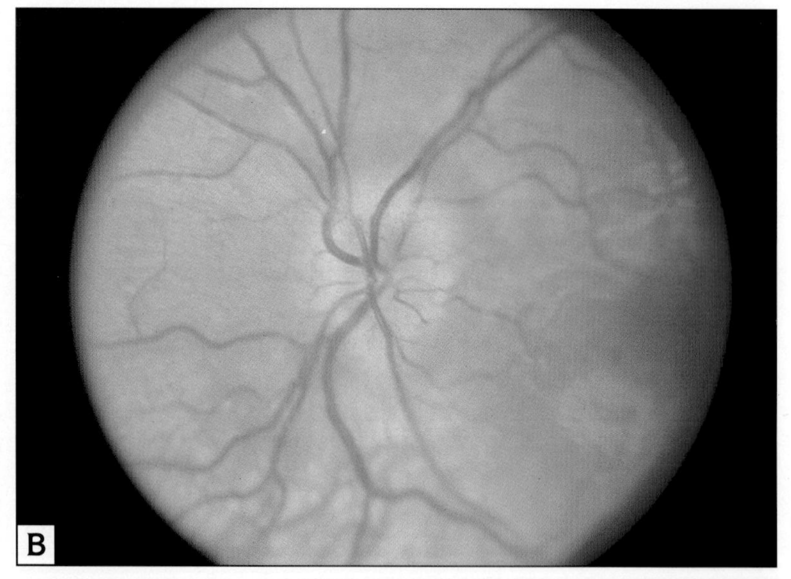

Figure 10-30 Papilledema. This patient had acute elevation of her intracranial pressure secondary to an abscess. **A**, Note that the margins of the optic nerve are blurred, there is hyperemia, and there is edema of the surrounding retina. Papilledema appears to result from pressure on the nerve axons with resultant back-up of axoplasmic flow. **B**, Three weeks following drainage of the abscess, the edema of the optic nerve has markedly abated. There remains some gliosis of surrounding tissue, but the peripapillary retina has flattened. The term *papilledema* is reserved for optic nerve swelling that is associated with elevated intracranial pressure.

AIDS-Associated Eye Disorders

HIV-related eye disease

- Kaposi's sarcoma
  - Eyelid
  - Conjunctiva
- Increased susceptibility to infection
  - Herpes zoster ophthalmicus
  - Herpes simplex keratitis
  - Conjunctivitis
  - Molluscum contagiosum
- Motility disturbances
- CNS lymphoma
- Disc edema
- AIDS retinopathy
  - Cottonwool spots
  - Hemorrhages
  - Microaneurysms
  - Vascular occlusions
- Fundus infections
  - Pneumocystis choroiditis
  - Toxoplasmosis
  - Candidiasis
  - Retinal necrosis
  - Outer retinitis
  - CMV retinitis

Figure 10-31 Ocular manifestations of HIV. This is a large, but not exhaustive list of the most common ocular manifestations of HIV infection.

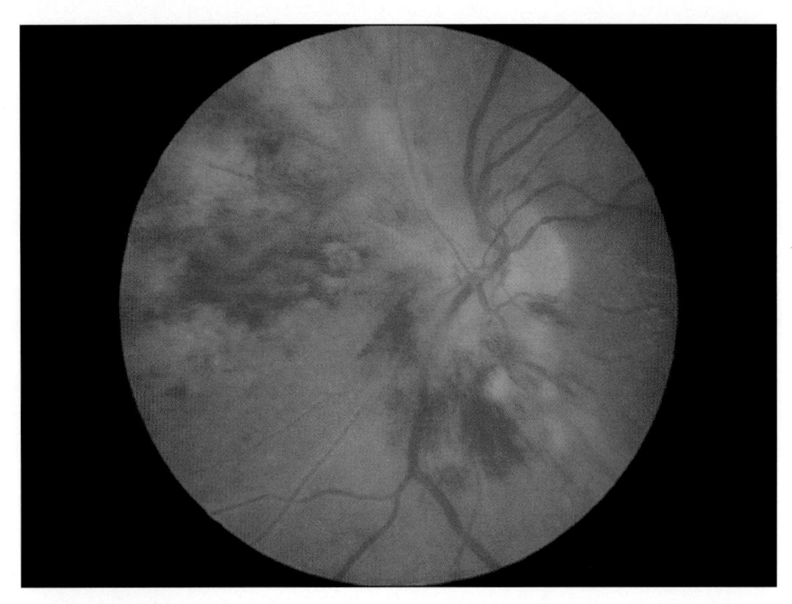

Figure 10-32 Cytomegalovirus (CMV) retinitis. This is the acute appearance of CMV retinitis affecting the posterior fundus. There is necrosis and hemorrhage of the retina and CMV optic neuritis. Following treatment with intravenous ganciclovir, the lesions lost their acute appearance and the edema subsided. However, the retinal tissue which was involved in the inflammation never recovered nor did the patient's central vision.

Treatment of cytomegalovirus retinitis

- Ganciclovir
  - Induction: 5 mg/kg twice daily for 2 wks
  - Maintenance: 5 mg/kg once daily for life
- Foscarnet
  - Induction: 180–240 mg/kg/d divided for 2 wks
  - Maintenance: 90–120 mg/kg/d for life

Figure 10-33 Treatment of cytomegalovirus retinitis. Two currently approved and efficacious approaches to the treatment of cytomegalovirus retinitis.

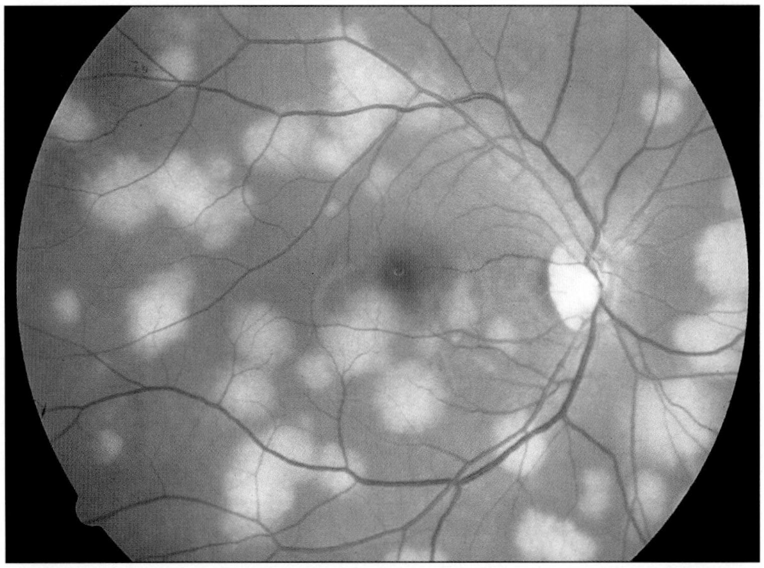

Figure 10-34 Acute pneumocystis choroiditis in AIDS. This patient had a routine ophthalmologic examination to rule out CMV retinitis. Although CMV was not present, this dramatic but asymptomatic appearance was noted. These lesions are deep to the retina in the choroid and are associated with a low-grade inflammation. They result following prophylactic inhalational pentamidine therapy to prevent pneumocystis pneumonia. These patients develop extrapulmonary pneumocystis infection, including pneumocystis choroiditis.

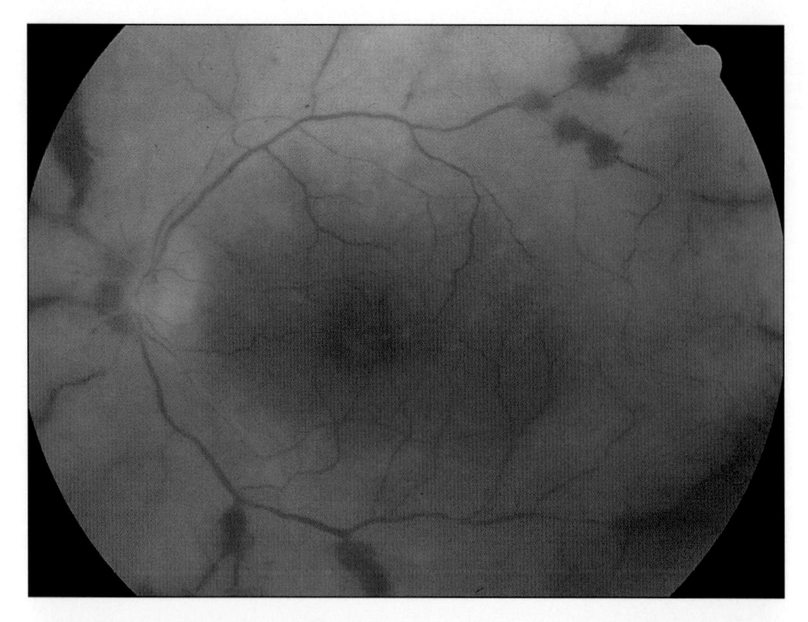

FIGURE 10-35 Inner necrotizing retinitis in AIDS. This patient had a progressive necrotizing retinal inflammation in which he lost all of the vision in both eyes over the course of 3 weeks. The retinal blood vessels are attenuated, and the retina is necrotic and only mildly hemorrhagic because of the poor blood flow. The macula itself is uninvolved, and this patient retained tunnel vision of 20/80 until the macula was completely consumed by the necrotizing process. Varicella-zoster virus is thought to be the causative organism in most cases.

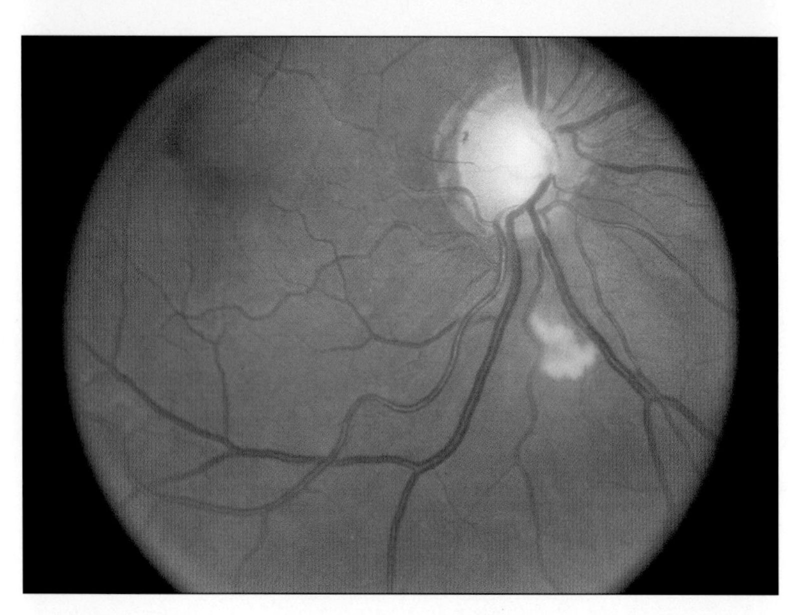

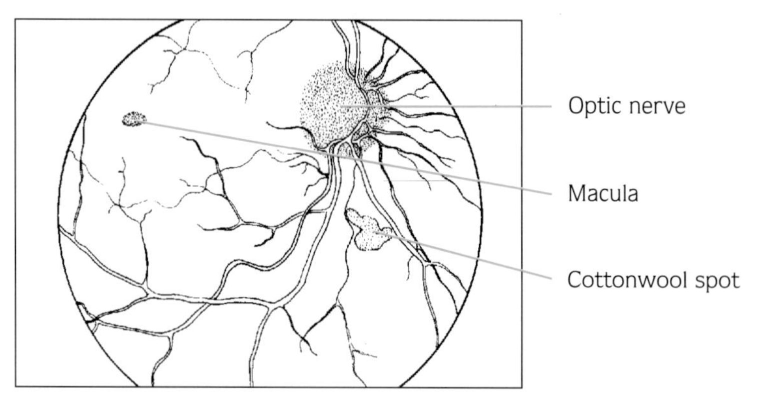

FIGURE 10-36 HIV retinopathy. The dramatic cottonwool spot seen beneath the optic nerve in this fundus is the result of ischemia to the retina. It does not appear to have any relationship to CMV retinitis, although it is often mistaken for an early CMV lesion. In addition to cottonwool spots, patients may exhibit small hemorrhages and microaneurysms, making the appearance similar to nonproliferative diabetic retinopathy. No treatment is indicated.

SELECTED BIBLIOGRAPHY

Albert DM, Jakobiec FA (eds.): *Principles and Practice of Ophthalmology.* Philadelphia: W.B. Saunders Co.; 1994:117–190.

Deutsch TA: Ophthalmic infections. *In* Brillman JC, Quenzer RW (eds.): *Infectious Disease in Emergency Medicine.* Boston: Little, Brown; 1992:887–894.

Gold DH, Weingeist TA (eds.): *The Eye in Systemic Disease.* Philadelphia: J.B. Lippincott; 1992, 8:155–276.

Chapter 11

Prion Diseases

Thomas P. Bleck
Sebastian R. Alston

Etiology and Pathogenesis

Prion diseases

Disease	Host
Scrapie	Sheep, goats
Transmissible mink encephalopathy	Mink
Chronic wasting syndrome	Mule, deer, elk
Bovine spongiform encephalopathy	Cattle
Feline spongiform encephalopathy	Cats
Kuru	Humans
Jakob-Creutzfeldt disease	Humans
Gerstmann-Sträussler syndrome	Humans
Fatal familial insomnia	Humans

Figure 11-1 Prion diseases. In 1982, Prusiner proposed the name *prion, pro*teinaceous *in*fectious particle, to describe the agent responsible for a group of chronic, progressive, neurodegenerative disorders that share similar pathologic features and are caused by an inherited and transmissible agent with unconventional biologic properties. These rare disorders affect both humans and animals.

Characteristics of prion diseases

Diseases are mostly confined to the CNS
Prolonged incubation period of months to decades
Progressive clinical course of weeks to years leading to death
All diseases exhibit reactive astrocytosis with little inflammatory response and many show neuronal vacuolation
Infectious agents (prions) show properties distinguishing them from viruses, viroids, and other infectious agents

Figure 11-2 Characteristics of prion diseases. The prion diseases are heterogeneous human and animal diseases grouped together because they share certain features. The diseases have extended incubation times that can exceed 30 years before the onset of clinical disease. The central nervous system (CNS) receives the brunt of injury, with pathologic features of neuronal loss, reactive gliosis, and neuronal vacuolation (spongiform change). (*Adapted from* Prusiner SB, Hsaio KK: Prions causing transmissible neurodegenerative diseases. *In* Schlossberg D (ed.): *Infections of the Nervous System.* New York: Springer-Verlag; 1990:153–168; with permission.)

Unusual biochemical and biophysical properties of prions

Extremely small, proteinaceous infectious particles
Resistant to chemical and physical agents that inactivate conventional viruses
Relatively sensitive to manipulations that alter, denature, or digest protein
Do not induce inflammatory or host immune responses
Lack of demonstrable nucleic acid or nonhost protein

Figure 11-3 Unusual biochemical and biophysical properties of prions. Prions are extremely small particles, filterable to an average 25- to 50-nm pore size and having a molecular weight of approximately 55,000 (minimum). They are highly resistant to inactivation by agents that disrupt nucleic acids, including heat to 80°C, nucleases, ultraviolet irradiation, ultrasonic energy, and chemical modification by nucleophiles. However, they are relatively sensitive to procedures that digest, denature, or chemically modify proteins, such as proteolytic enzymes, denaturing agents, organic solvents, chaotropic salts, and urea. These findings are interpreted to suggest that the prion is a protein or protein derivative devoid of nucleic acid. The lack of host immune response may indicate that prions are natural host-encoded proteins. Some researchers still believe that the agent could contain a small fragment of nucleic acid, but there is no direct proof of this contention.

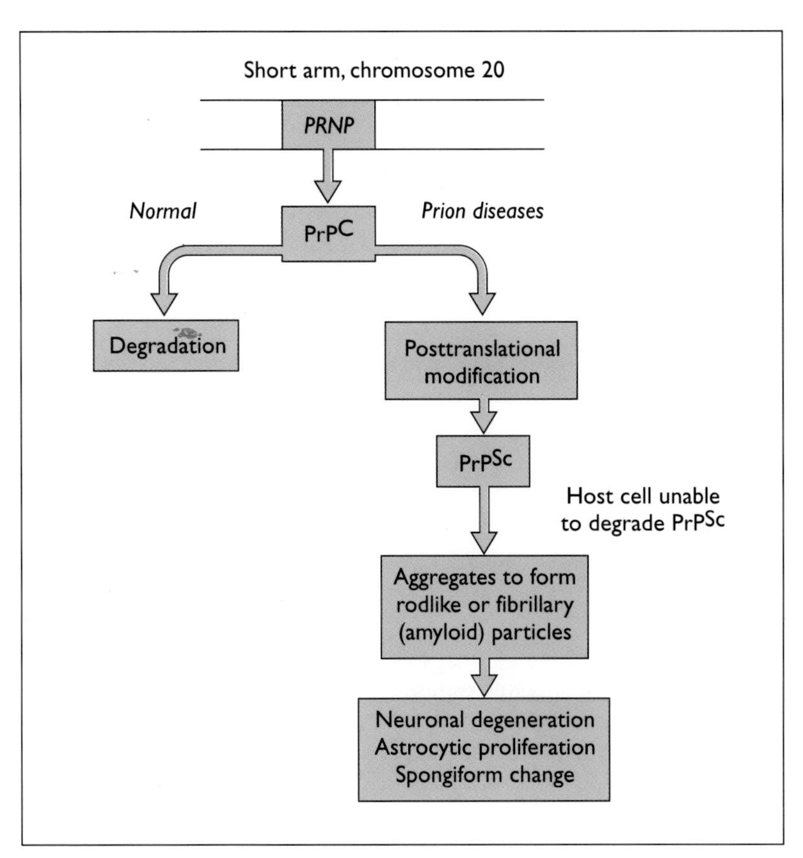

FIGURE 11-4 Pathogenesis of prion disease. Identification of the prion protein (PrP^{Sc}) in fractions of hamster brain enriched for scrapie infectivity but not in healthy controls led to localization of the gene encoding PrP on the short arm of human chromosome 20 and mouse chromosome 2. The normal cellular product of this gene is PrP^{C}, a protein of 33 to 35 kD and unknown function; this protein is expressed to similar extents in both normal (uninfected) and infected brains, and mice lacking the PrP^{C} gene have no demonstrable abnormalities. By a poorly understood process, PrP^{C} undergoes a posttranslational modification resulting in its conversion into the abnormal scrapie isoform, PrP^{Sc}, which differs from PrP^{C} in physical properties. When PrP^{C} is released from the cell surface, it is readily degraded, whereas only the amino terminal portion of PrP^{Sc} is cleared, leaving a 27- to 30-kD core, PrP 27–30, that aggregates to form scrapie-associated fibrillar structures (SAFs) or prion rods. PrP^{Sc} collects in cell vacuoles and secondary lysosomes, producing degenerative spongiform vacuolation that is characteristic of prion diseases.

Replication of prions in acquired prion disease
Protein-only hypothesis: direct action model
Protein-only hypothesis: indirect action model
Nucleoprotein hypothesis

FIGURE 11-5 Replication of prions in acquired prion disease. Prions, lacking demonstrable nucleic acids, replicate by poorly understood means. Three hypotheses for prion replication in acquired prion disorders have been outlined. Note that the hereditary forms do not appear to need any outside strains to initiate conversion.

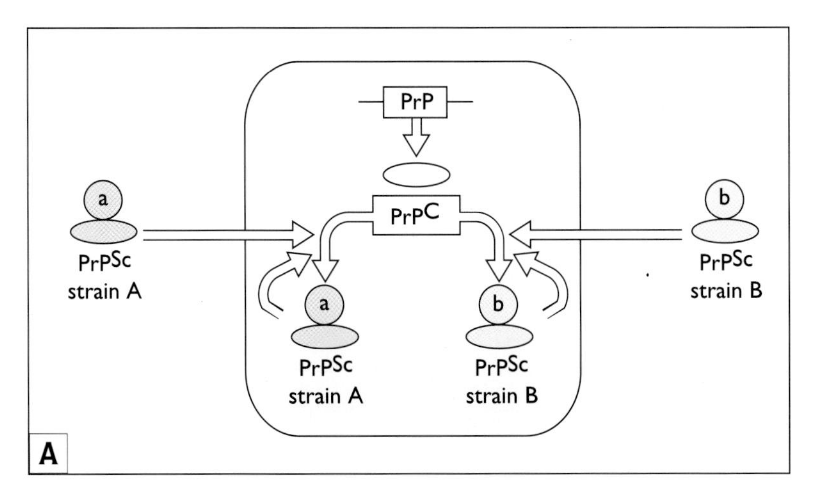

FIGURE 11-6 Protein-only hypothesis of prion replication. The protein-only hypothesis proposes that the prion, PrP^{Sc}, is a protein or protein derivative devoid of nucleic acid. Strains A and B indicate the tendency of the prion strains to "breed true" (*ie*, to remain strain-specific or species-specific). **A**, Direct action model. According to the direct action model, on infection, PrP^{Sc} converts PrP^{C} (or its precursor) into PrP^{Sc}, which in turn converts more PrP^{C}. The presence of different strains of PrP^{Sc} found in a host would be due to strain-specific modifications in PrP^{Sc} (strain A and B), which direct the conversion of PrP^{C} into PrP^{Sc} carrying the same modifications as the infecting strain. (*continued*)

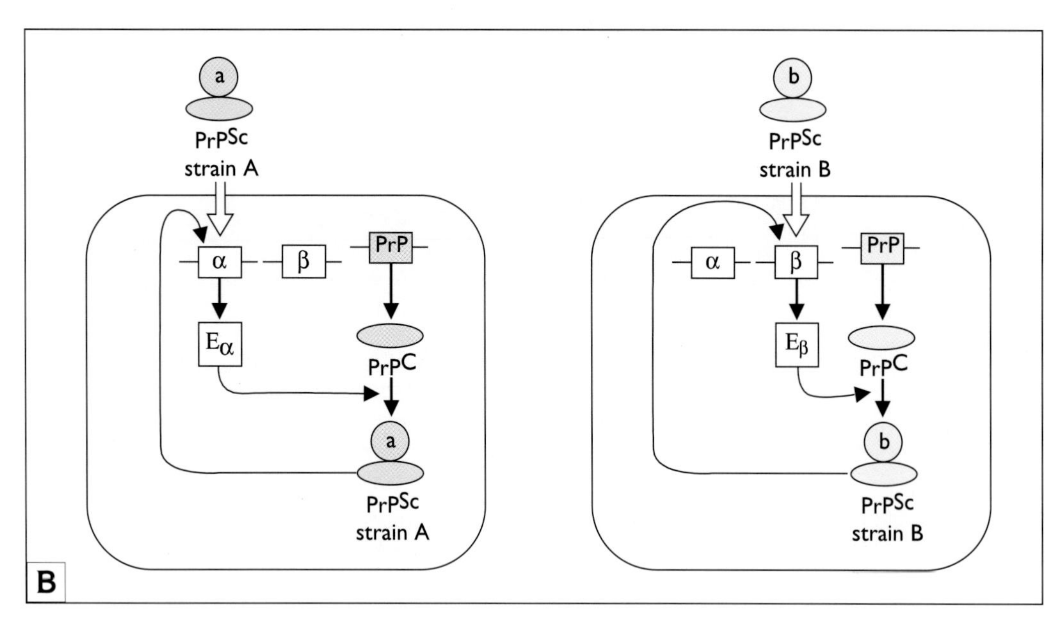

FIGURE 11-6 (*continued*) **B**, Indirect action model. In the indirect action model, PrP^{Sc} activates a cellular gene alpha, which produces a "converting enzyme" E_{α} that then converts cellular PrP^{C} into PrP^{Sc}. Propagation of different strains of PrP^{Sc} in the same host genotype would be explained by a battery of such cellular genes (alpha, beta, etc.), each encoding a different "PrP-converting enzyme." (*From* Weissman C: Sheep disease in human clothing. *Nature* 1989, 338:298–299; with permission.)

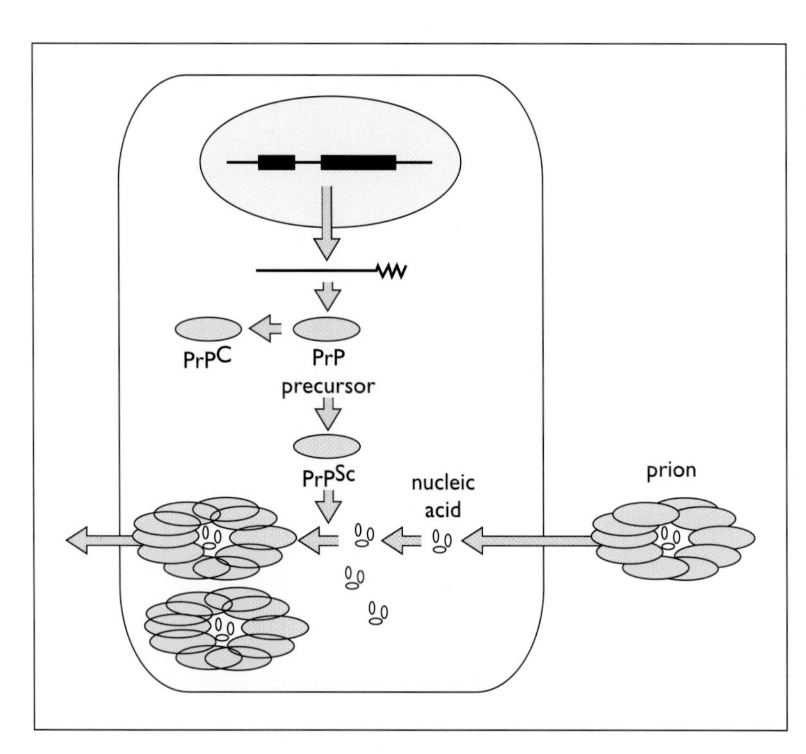

FIGURE 11-7 Nucleoprotein hypothesis of prion replication. The nucleoprotein hypothesis postulates that the prion consists of a small nucleic acid and host-encoded protein. In this model, a nucleic acid associated with host-encoded PrP^{Sc} infects the cell. After replication of the nucleic acid, infectious particles are assembled from nucleic acid and PrP. Conversion of PrP^{C} to PrP^{Sc} is caused by the association with the nucleic acid, or (as shown here) PrP^{C} or its precursor may first be converted to PrP^{Sc}. (*From* Weissman C: Sheep disease in human clothing. *Nature* 1989, 338:298–299; with permission.)

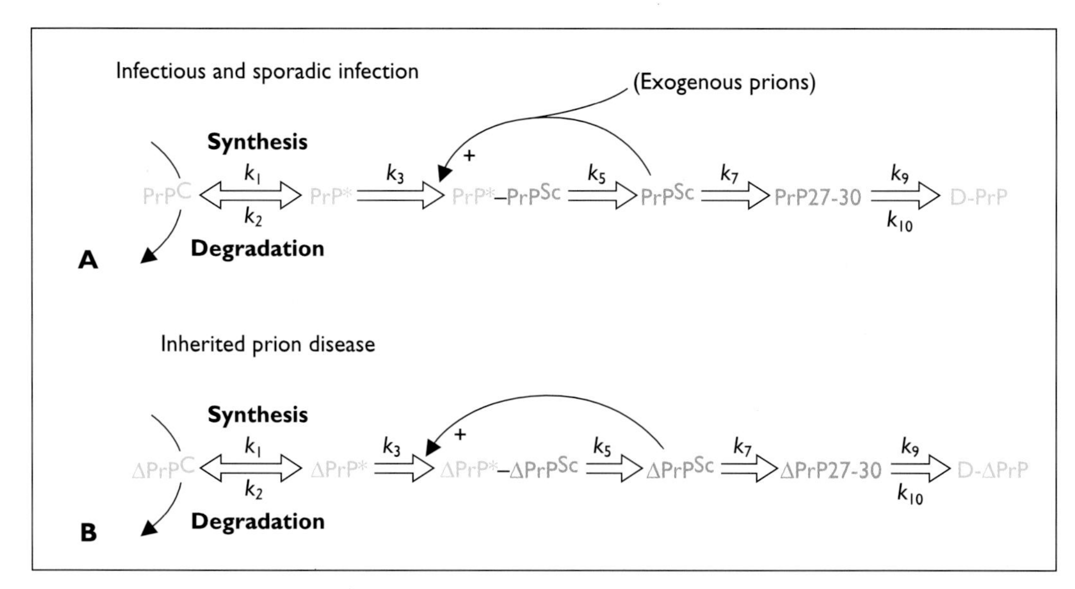

FIGURE 11-8 A conformational model for prion replication. Infectious forms of PrP are shown in *red* and noninfectious forms in *blue*. **A**, Postulated events in infectious and sporadic prion diseases. Wild-type PrP^C is synthesized and degraded as part of normal cellular metabolism. Stochastic fluctuations in the structure of PrP^C can create (K_1) a rare, partially unfolded monomer (PrP^*) that is an intermediate in the formation of PrP^{Sc}. PrP^* can revert (K_2) to PrP^C, be degraded, or form a complex (K_3) with PrP^{Sc}. Normally, the concentration of PrP^* is low and PrP^{Sc} formation is insignificant in infectious prion diseases, exogenous prions enter the cell and stimulate conversion (K_5) of PrP^* into PrP^{Sc} which is likely to be an irreversible process. In sporadic prion diseases, where there are no exogenous prions, the concentration of PrP^{Sc} may eventually reach a threshold level upon which a positive feedback loop would stimulate the formation of PrP^{Sc}. Limited proteolysis of the amino terminus of PrP^{Sc} produces (K_7) PrP 27–30, a truncated form of PrP^{Sc} that polymerizes into amyloid and has a high content of beta sheet. Denaturation (K_9) of PrP^{Sc} or PrP 27–30 into D-PrP renders these molecules protease-sensitive and abolishes scrapie infectivity; attempts to renature (k_{10}) D-PrP have been largely unsuccessful. **B**, Postulated events in inherited prion diseases. Mutant (Δ)PrP^C is synthesized and degraded as part of normal cellular metabolism. Stochastic fluctuations in the structure of ΔPrP^C is synthesized and degraded as part of normal cellular metabolism. Stochastic fluctuations in the structure of ΔPrP^C are greater than those in wild-type PrP^C; these fluctuations create (K_1) significant amounts of a partially unfolded monomer (ΔPrP^* that is an intermediate in the formation of ΔPrP^{Sc}). ΔPrP^* can revert (K_2 to ΔPrP^C), be degraded, or be converted (K_5) into ΔPrP^{Sc}. Limited proteolysis of the amino terminus of ΔPrP^{Sc} produces (K_7 ΔPrP 27–30), which in some cases may be less protease-resistant than wild-type PrP 27–30. (*From* Cohen FE, Pan K-M, Huang Z, *et al.*: Structural clues to prion replication. *Science* 1994, 264:530–531; with permission.)

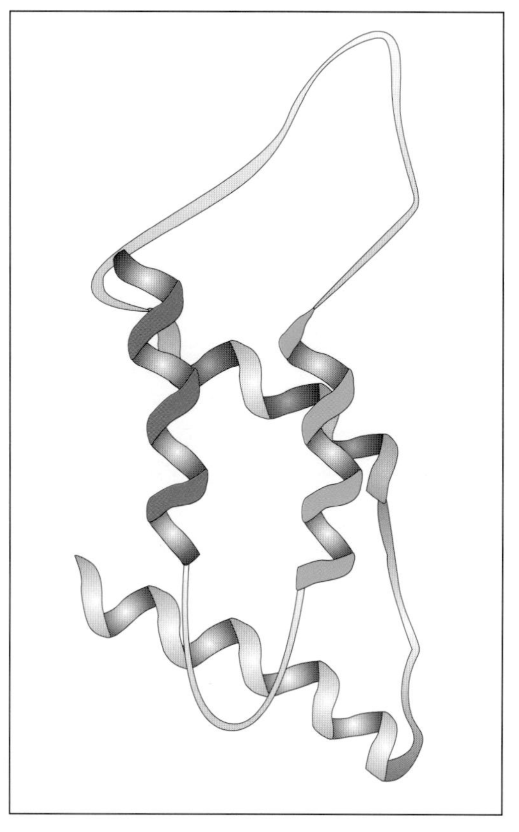

FIGURE 11-9 A plausible model for the three-dimensional structure of the cellular prion protein (PrP^c) proposed by Huang *et al.* (*Proc Natl Acad Sci USA* 1994, 91:7139–7143). The backbone of PrP^c twists into four helices. Helix one is shown in *red*, while helix two is shown in *green*. PrP^c becomes the infectious, scrapie form (PrP^{Sc}) when the backbone of helices one and two stretch out, forming so-called beta-strands (Huang Z, Prusiner SB, Cohen FE, Unpublished results. Source: Ziwe: Huang, Thomas Jefferson University; with permission.)

ANIMAL PRION DISEASES

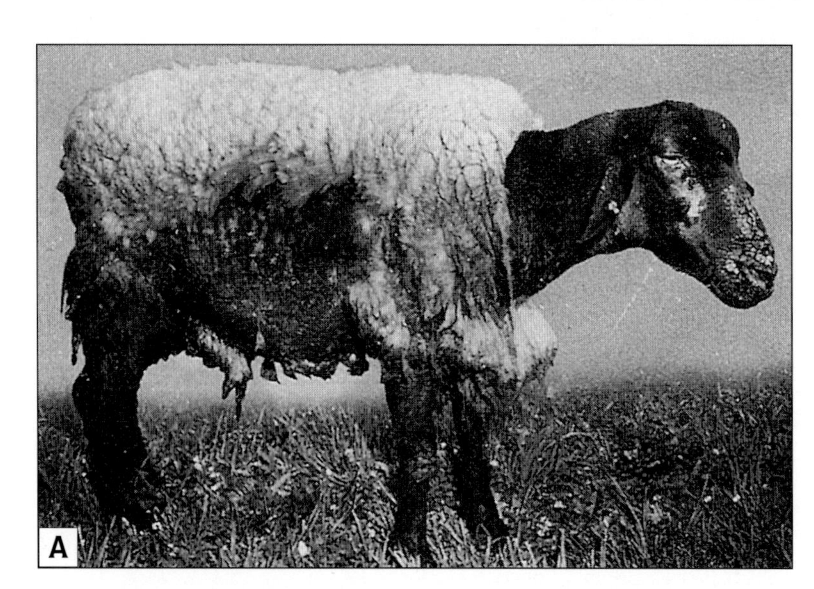

FIGURE 11-10 Scrapie. **A**, Scrapie-infected sheep. Scrapie is a naturally occurring fatal disease of sheep and goats that was first recognized over 2 centuries ago by European sheep breeders. Affected animals show progressive ataxia, tremor, wasting, and frequently severe pruritus that causes them to rub their hindquarters and flanks against fence posts, resulting in a ragged fleece. (*From* McDaniel HA: Chronic viral encephalitides of sheep. *In* Howard JL (ed.): *Current Veterinary Therapy: Food Animal Practice*. Philadelphia: W.B. Saunders; 1981:611; with permission.) **B**, Worldwide distribution of scrapie in sheep. Scrapie has widespread distribution in Europe, Asia, and America and was eradicated from Australia and New Zealand by extermination of affected flocks. (*From* Gajdusek DC: Subacute spongiform encephalopathies: Transmissible cerebral amyloidoses caused by unconventional viruses. *In* Fields BN, Knipe DM, *et al.* (eds.): *Virology*, 2nd ed. New York: Raven Press; 1990:2310; with permission.)

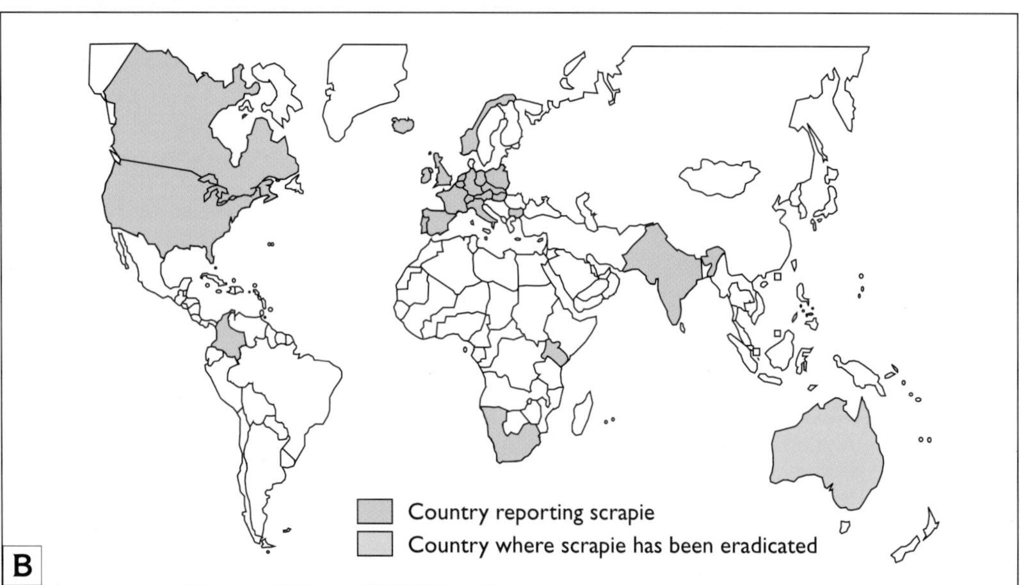

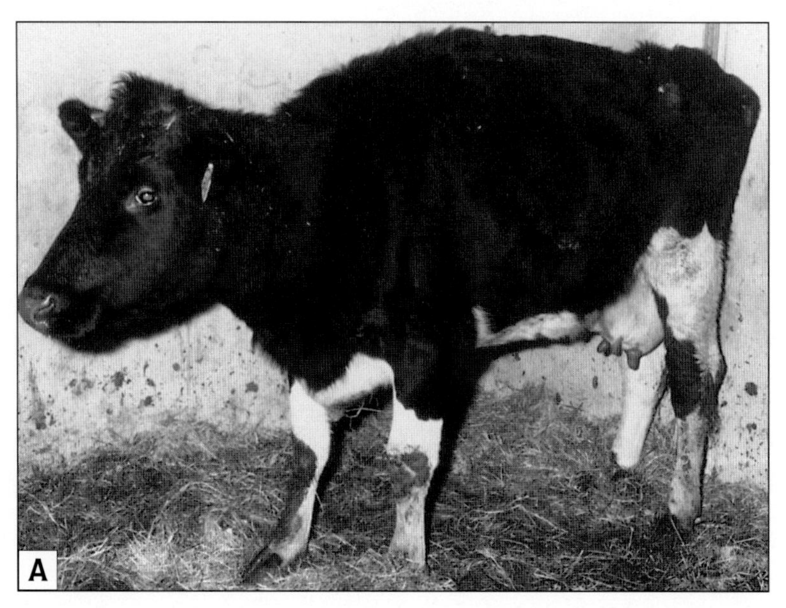

FIGURE 11-11 Bovine spongiform encephalopathy (BSE). **A**, A cow infected with BSE, or "mad cow disease," shows the typical signs of apprehension, arched back, abnormal head posture, straight abducted hind limbs, and staring eyes. (*Courtesy* of Dr. AE Wrathall, Weybridge. *From* Bradley R, Lowson RC: Bovine spongiform encephalopathy: The history, scientific, political and social issues. *In* Prusiner SB, Collinge J, Powell J, Anderton B (eds.): *Prion Diseases of Humans and Animals*. New York: Ellis Horwood (Simon & Shuster); 1992:288; with permission.) (*continued*)

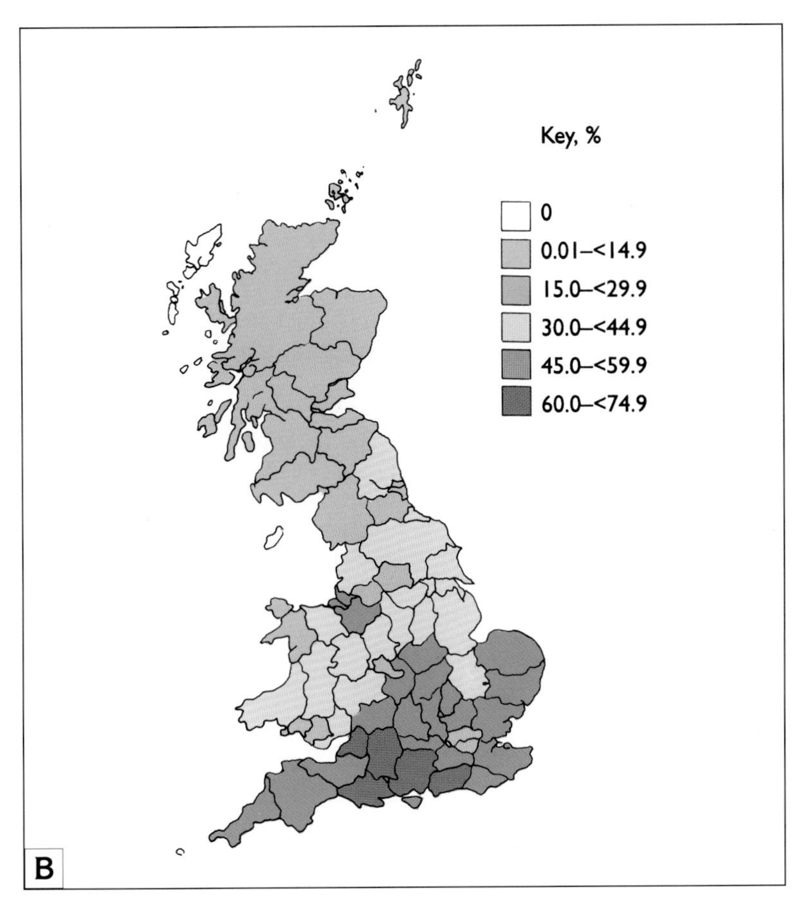

FIGURE 11-11 (*continued*) **B**, Incidence and distribution of BSE in the United Kingdom, November 1986–July 1993. In 1988, the British government banned the feeding of ruminant-derived feed, thereby preventing further scrapie and BSE infections via feed to sheep, cattle, goats, and zoo animals (exotic ungulate spongiform encephalopathy). (*From* Bradley R, Wilesmith JW: Epidemiology and control of bovine spongiform encephalopathy (BSE). *Br Med Bull* 1993, 49(4):932–959; with permission.)

HUMAN PRION DISEASES

Kuru

Clincial characteristics of kuru

Transmission	Autoinoculation/ingestion of infected brain material (ritual cannibalism)
Prevalence	Fore linguistic group of Papua New Guinea
Clinical features	Cerebellar ataxia, tremor, movement disorders (myoclonus)
	Mental impairment, emotional lability
	Frontal release signs (snout, suck, root, grasp reflexes)
Course	Fatal in 9–24 mos after onset

FIGURE 11-12 Clinical characteristics of kuru. The disease kuru ("shivering") was once endemic among the Fore linguistic group in Papua New Guinea, resulting in several hundred deaths per year among a population of 50,000 to 75,000. Since cessation in 1960 of a ritual form of cannibalism, practiced as part of a funerary rite that included ingesting the brains of deceased relatives, the incidence has declined to <10 cases/year, all occurring among older adults. Generalized tremor, which is absent at rest, is a prominent finding. Dementia occurs after motor findings have become prominent.

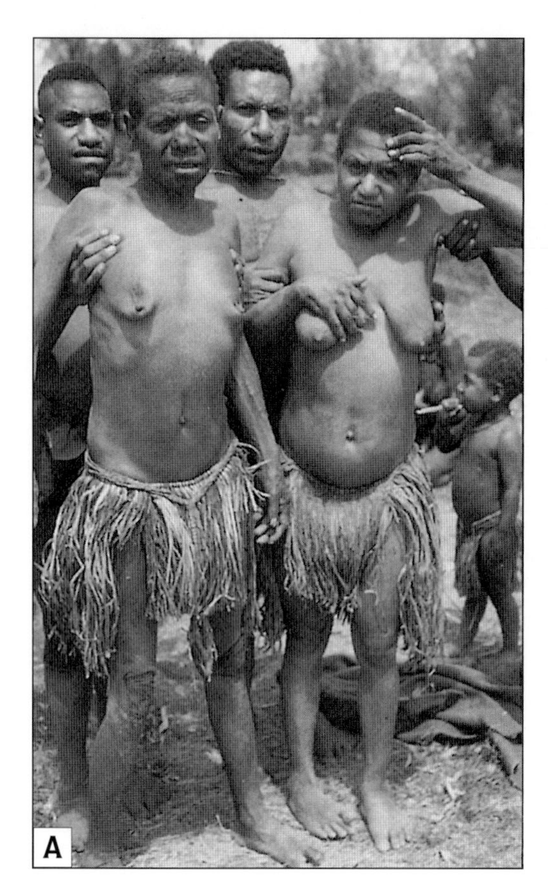

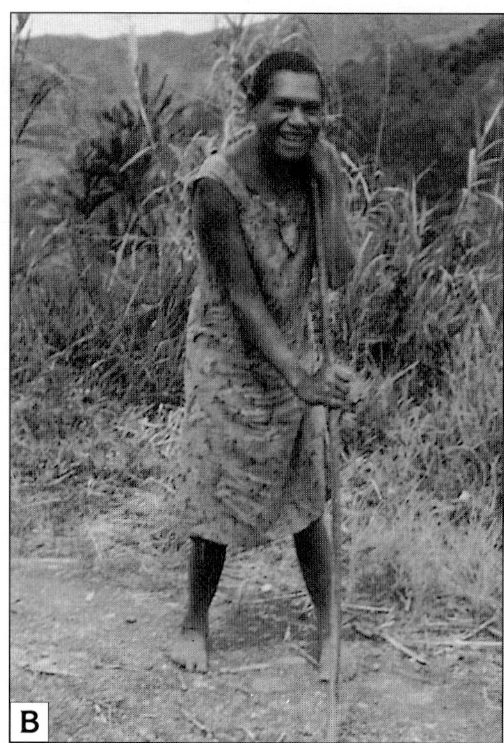

FIGURE 11-13 Ambulatory phase of kuru. **A**, Two women can no longer stand without extensive support. Symptoms and signs of kuru in this phase include instability and incoordination that progresses from the lower to upper extremities over the course of several months. (*From* Gajdusek DC: Observations on the early history of kuru investigation. *In* Prusiner SB, Hadlow WJ (eds.): *Slow Transmissible Diseases of the Nervous System*, vol 1. New York: Academic Press; 1979:7–36; with permission.) **B**, A man with moderately advanced kuru stands with a widespread stance and holds a stick for support. The patient also had moderate dementia. (*From* Hornabrook RW: Kuru and clinical neurology. *In* Prusiner SB, Hadlow WJ (eds.): *Slow Transmissible Diseases of the Nervous System*, vol 1. New York: Academic Press; 1979:37–66; with permission.)

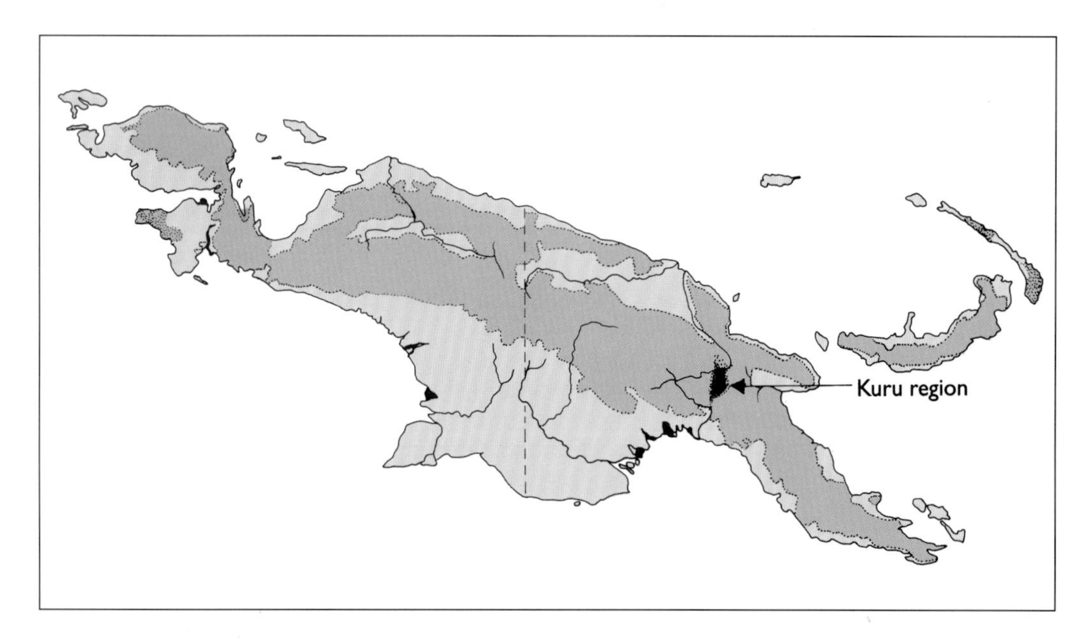

FIGURE 11-14 Geographic distribution of kuru in Papua New Guinea. Kuru is confined to the remote mountainous Eastern Highlands Province in Papua New Guinea, appearing among the native people of the Fore linguistic group. The stippled areas are over 200 m in elevation. (*From* Gajdusek DC: Subacute spongiform encephalopathies: Transmissible cerebral amyloidoses caused by unconventional viruses. *In* Fields BN, *et al.* (eds.): *Virology*, 2nd ed. New York: Raven Press; 1990; with permission.)

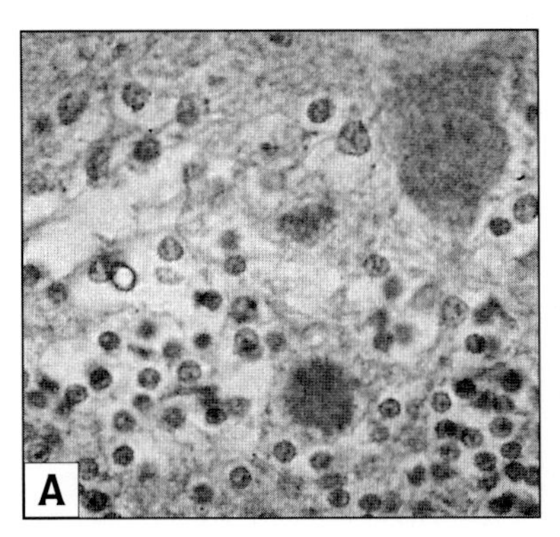

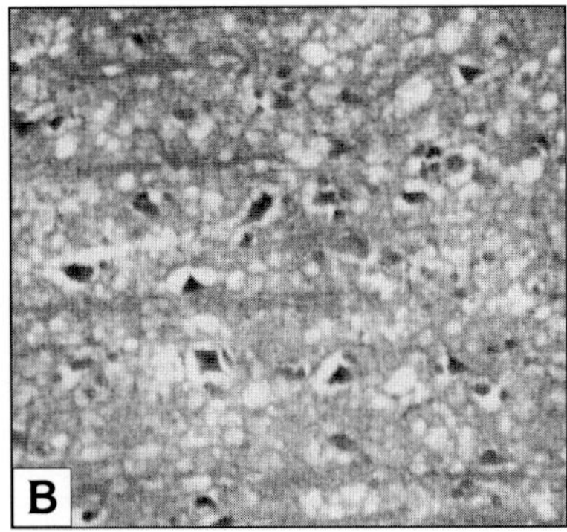

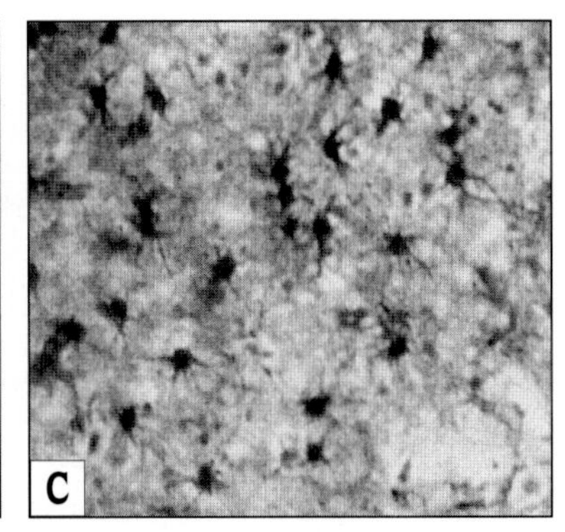

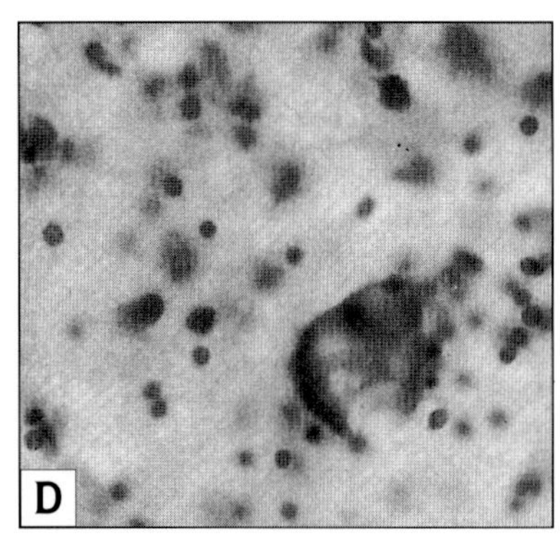

FIGURE 11-15 Neuropathologic lesions in kuru. **A**, A kuru (amyloid) plaque is seen within the granular layer of the cerebellum. Electron microscopy of these plaques reveals accumulation of amyloid-like filaments. Unlike senile plaques of Alzheimer's disease, no neuronal or glial processes surround kuru plaques. (Periodic acid-Schiff stain, × 430.) **B**, Moderate status spongiosus distributed diffusely through all layers of the cerebral cortex. (Hematoxylin-eosin stain, × 145.) **C**, Proliferation and hypertrophy of fibrous astrocytes in spongy cortices in the cerebral cortex. (Cajal stain, × 170.) **D**, Large neuron of the caudate nucleus showing multiple, coarse intracytoplasmic vacuoles. (Nissl stain, × 450.) (*From* Beck E, Daniel PM: Kuru and Creutzfeldt-Jakob disease: Neuropathological lesions and their significance. *In* Prusiner SB, Hadlow WJ (eds.): *Slow Transmissible Diseases of the Nervous System*, vol 1. New York: Academic Press; 1979:253–270; with permission.)

Jakob-Creutzfeldt Disease

Clinical characteristics of Jakob-Creutzfeldt disease

Transmission	Sporadic, familial, iatrogenic
Prevalence	Worldwide
Onset	57–62 yrs usually (range, 17–83)
Clinical features	Severe rapidly progressive dementia Myoclonus and movement disturbances Cerebellar dysfunction Visual disturbances
Course	Fatal in < 1 yr after onset
CSF findings	Typically normal
CT/MRI	Normal to generalized cortical atrophy
EEG	Periodic sharp wave complexes lasting 200–600 ms every 0.5–2.5 s (in 75%–95% of patients)

FIGURE 11-16 Clinical characteristics of Jakob-Creutzfeldt disease (JCD). JCD remains a rare disease, with a prevalence of approximately 1 case/million population worldwide, but it is the most commonly encountered of the human prion diseases. The overwhelming majority of cases (85%–95%) are sporadic. Familial transmission accounts for 5% to 15% of cases. Iatrogenic person-to-person spread is extremely rare and has followed transplantation of infected corneas or dural grafts, use of contaminated neurosurgical instruments, and use of contaminated growth hormone or pituitary gonadotropin. Dementia and myoclonus are the most prominent findings, but the clinical manifestations are highly variable, depending in part on the area of brain affected. One variant, the Heidenhain variant, has a predilection for the occipital and parietal lobes and may present with visual problems (hallucinations, hemianopia, and cortical blindness) before dementia becomes apparent.

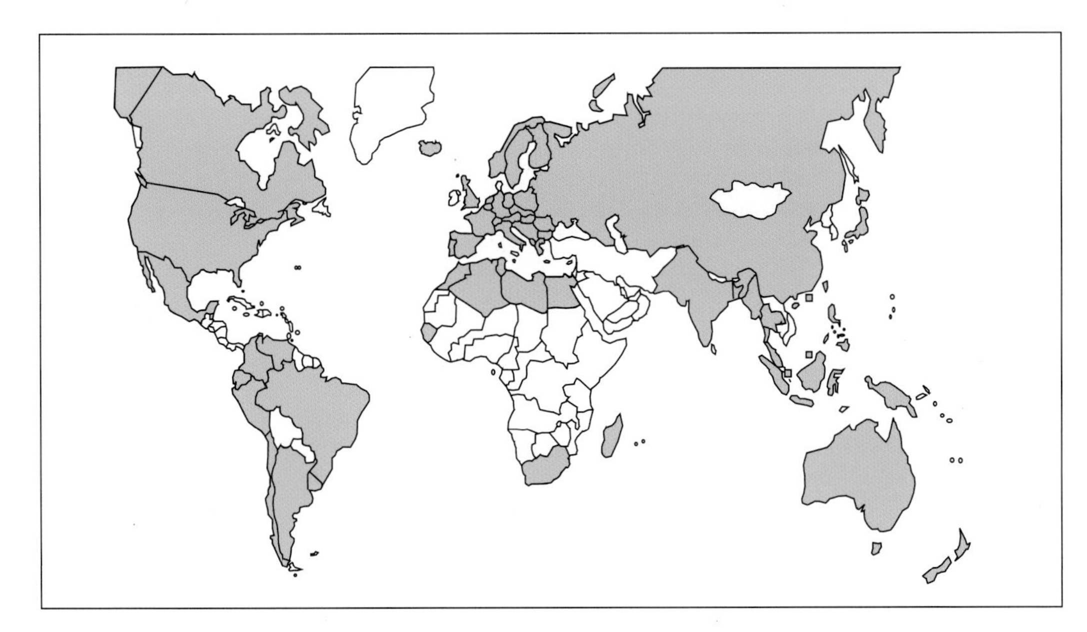

FIGURE 11-17 Geographic distribution of JCD. JCD occurs worldwide, with pockets of increased incidence among Libyan Jews living in Israel, North African immigrants to France, and parts of Slovakia. Shaded regions indicate countries reporting cases. (*From* Gajdusek DC: Subacute spongiform encephalopathies: Transmissible cerebral amyloidoses caused by unconventional viruses. *In* Fields BN, *et al.* (eds.): *Virology*, 2nd ed. New York: Raven Press; 1990: with permission.)

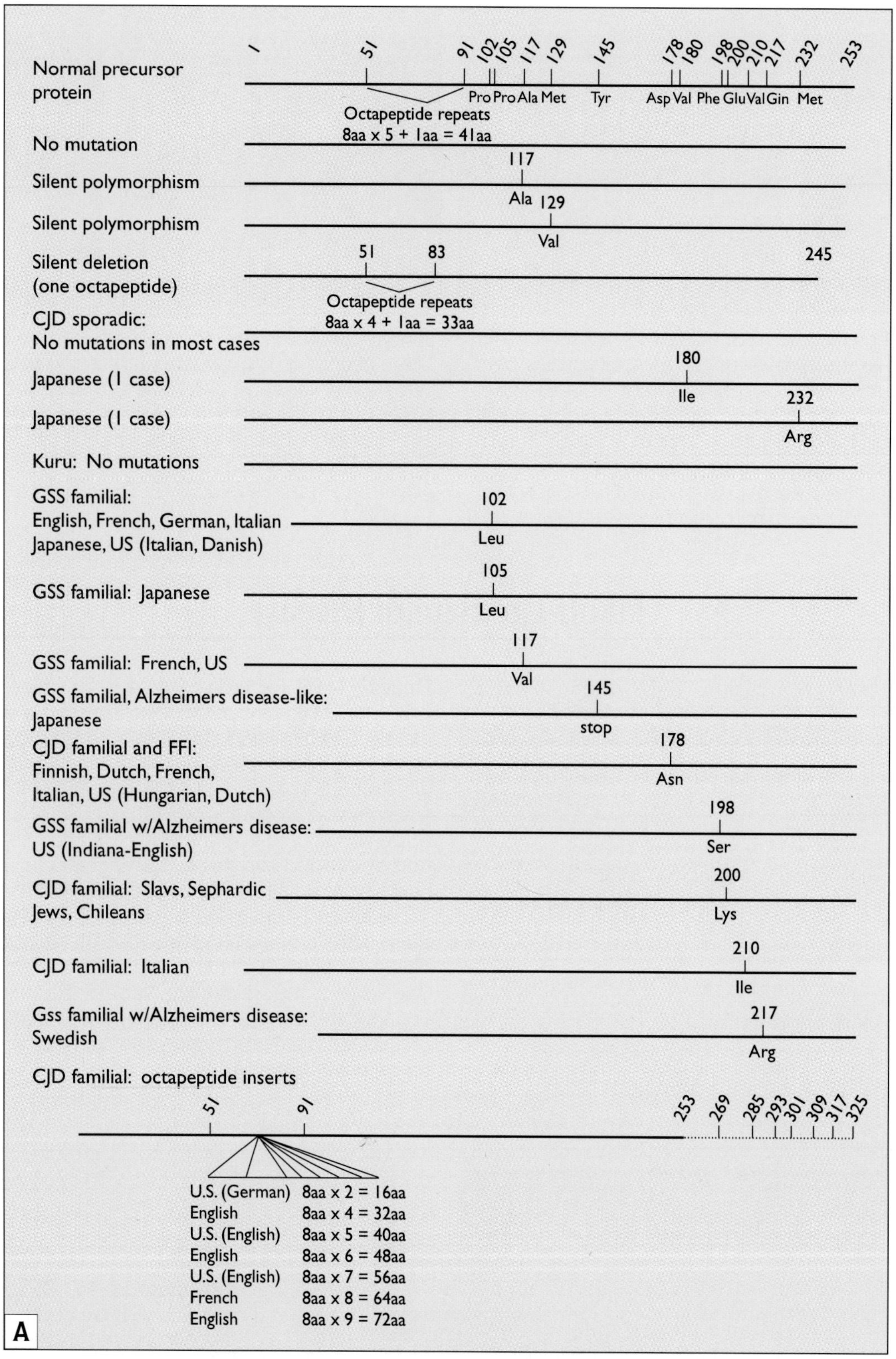

Normal precursor protein
1 51 91 102 105 117 129 145 178 180 198 200 210 217 232 253
Pro Pro Ala Met Tyr Asp Val Phe Glu Val Gln Met
Octapeptide repeats
8aa x 5 + 1aa = 41aa
No mutation
Silent polymorphism — 117 Ala
Silent polymorphism — 129 Val
Silent deletion (one octapeptide) — 51 83 245
Octapeptide repeats
8aa x 4 + 1aa = 33aa
CJD sporadic:
No mutations in most cases
Japanese (1 case) — 180 Ile
Japanese (1 case) — 232 Arg
Kuru: No mutations
GSS familial:
English, French, German, Italian
Japanese, US (Italian, Danish) — 102 Leu
GSS familial: Japanese — 105 Leu
GSS familial: French, US — 117 Val
GSS familial, Alzheimers disease-like:
Japanese — 145 stop
CJD familial and FFI:
Finnish, Dutch, French,
Italian, US (Hungarian, Dutch) — 178 Asn
GSS familial w/Alzheimers disease:
US (Indiana-English) — 198 Ser
CJD familial: Slavs, Sephardic
Jews, Chileans — 200 Lys
CJD familial: Italian — 210 Ile
Gss familial w/Alzheimers disease:
Swedish — 217 Arg
CJD familial: octapeptide inserts
51 91 253 269 285 293 301 309 317 325

U.S. (German)	8aa x 2 = 16aa
English	8aa x 4 = 32aa
U.S. (English)	8aa x 5 = 40aa
English	8aa x 6 = 48aa
U.S. (English)	8aa x 7 = 56aa
French	8aa x 8 = 64aa
English	8aa x 9 = 72aa

A

FIGURE 11-18 Genetic mutations in JCD and other infectious amyloidoses. **A**, Twenty-one different mutations in the gene specifying the host precursor molecule of JCD amyloid have been identified: 11 cause amino acid (aa) changes, 1 produces a stop codon, 1 a base change in the codon with no amino acid change, 7 are octapeptide inserts, and 1 an octapeptide deletion. Eight causing an amino acid change (102, 105, 117, 178, 200, 210, and 217) and one a stop codon (145) are found in families of diverse ethnic origins with familial JCD and its Gerstmann-Sträussler-Scheinker (GSS) and fatal familial insomnia (FFI) variants. Three are silent polymorphisms: the codon 129 substitutes valine for methionine (which is found in about 20% of the normal population), a base mutation in codon 117 causing no amino acid change, and an octapeptide deletion (in about 20% of the population). Seven additional mutations in families with JCD are insertions of octapeptide repeats into a region where there are already five copies of the same repeat. (*From* Gajdusek DC: Nucleation of amyloidogenesis in infectious and noninfectious amyloidoses of brain. *Ann NY Acad Sci* 1994, 724:173–190; with permission.) (*continued*)

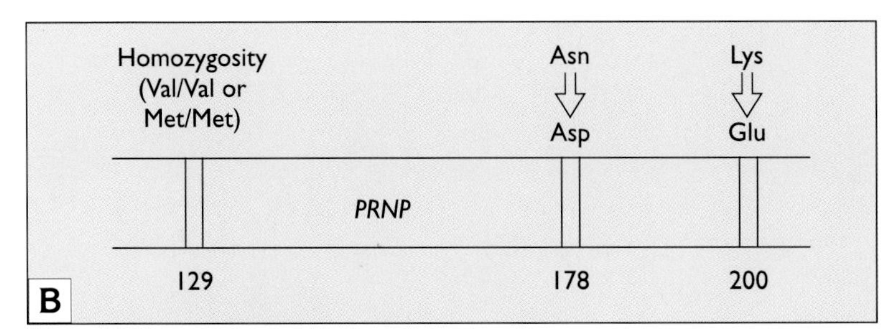

FIGURE 11-18 (*continued*) **B**, Common mutations in JCD. Familial JCD is an autosomal dominant disease. A mutation at codon 200 of the *PRNP* gene, involving a lysine-for-glutamate substitution, has been implicated. Another point mutation at codon 178, involving asparagine for aspartic acid, has been reported, as have various other insertions around codon 51. No consistent mutation has been found in patients with sporadic JCD, although a higher-than-expected rate of homozygosity has been identified at the normally polymorphic codon 129.

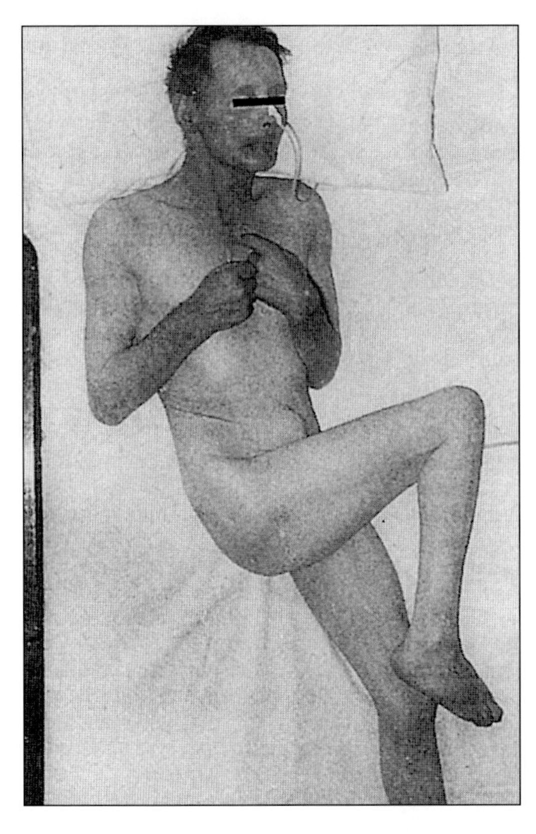

FIGURE 11-19 Patient with JCD. The patient is seen 3 months after the onset of JCD, with muteness and adopting a decorticate posture. (*From* Matthews WB: Slow viruses and the central nervous system. *In* Lambert HP (ed.): *Infections of the Central Nervous System*. Philadelphia: BC Decker; 1991:331; with permission.)

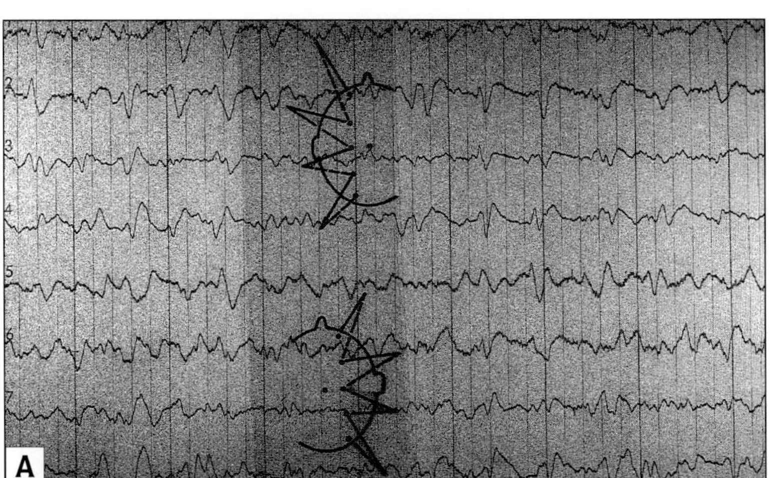

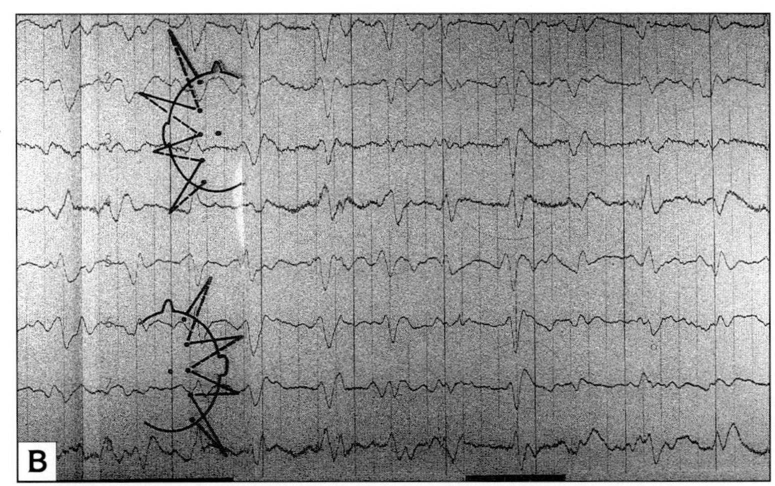

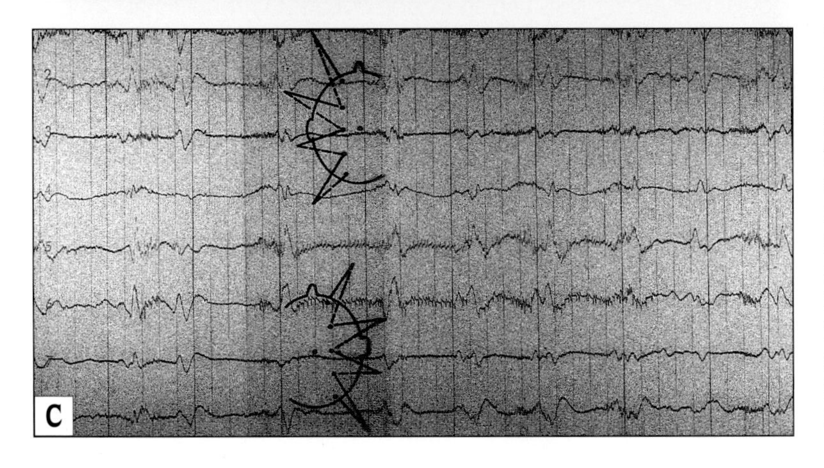

FIGURE 11-20 Characteristic electroencephalographic (EEG) changes in JCD. The EEG typically has a diffusely slow background interrupted by generalized, bilaterally synchronous, biphasic or triphasic periodic high-voltage sharp-wave complexes. These occur at intervals of 0.5 to 2.5 s and last for 200 to 600 ms. They are seen in 75% to 95% of patients. A series of three slides portray the progression of the EEG changes over 4 weeks. **A**, Periodic triphasic activity is seen on a moderately slow background. The pseudoperiodic, bisynchronous, sharply contoured triphasic activity may not be noted on presentation but typically appears within several weeks of dementia onset. It is frequently interrupted by use of intravenous benzodiazepines in the early stages of the disease. **B**, Two weeks later, the background activity is slower. **C**, At 4 weeks (2 weeks after *panel B*), the background is almost isoelectric, and the pseudoperiodic activity is less regular.

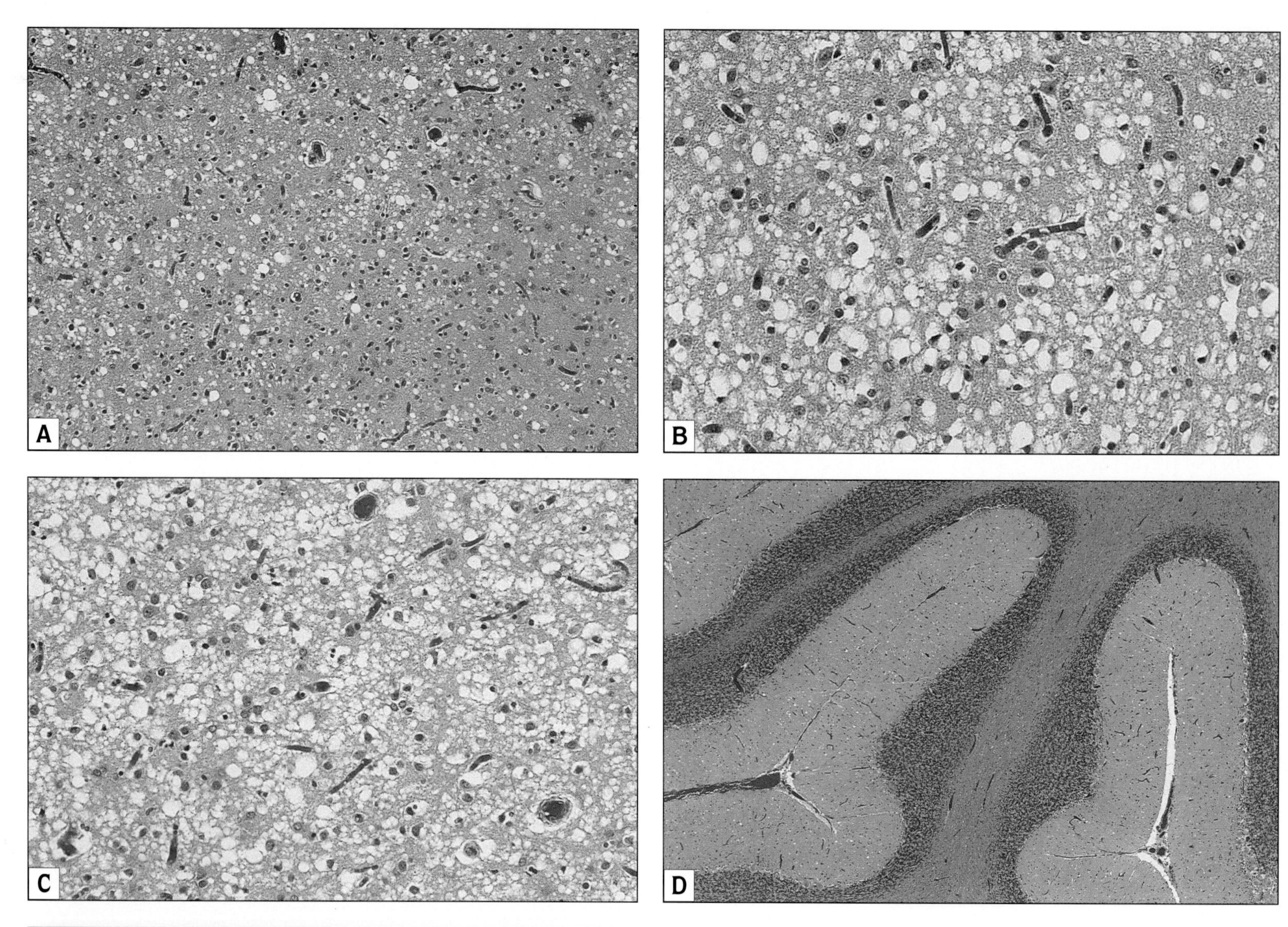

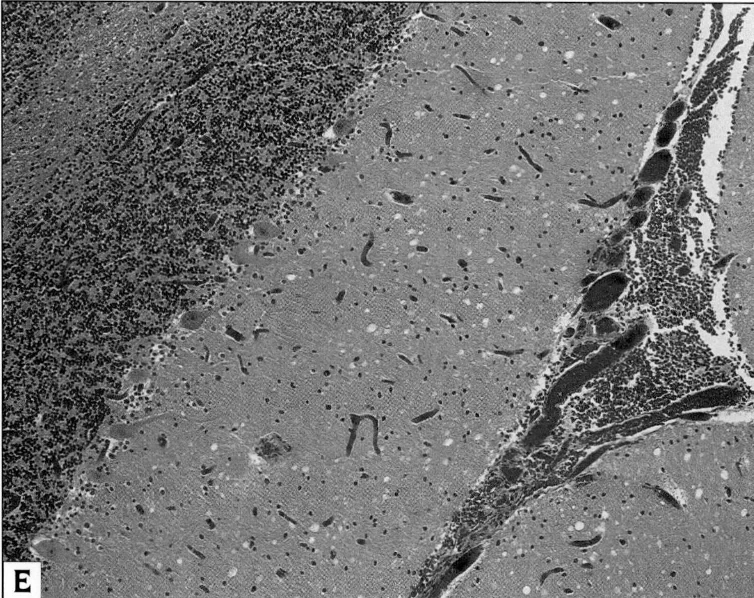

FIGURE 11-21 Spongiform encephalopathy in JCD. **A**, A low-power view of cerebral cortex shows spongiform change (vacuolization), neuronal dropout, and astrocytic proliferation. Note the absence of inflammation. Spongiform change may be seen in several other pathologic conditions and is not itself diagnostic of JCD. (Hematoxylin-eosin stain.) **B**, A higher-power view of the cerebral cortex from the same case highlights the astrocytic proliferation. This glial change occurs early and to a greater degree than would be expected as a consequence of the neuronal damage, suggesting that prion disease triggers a primary astrocytic proliferation. (Hematoxylin-eosin stain.) **C**, A high-power view shows several degenerating neurons with large, dark nuclei. (Hematoxylin-eosin stain.) **D**, A low-power view of the cerebellar cortex shows a mild degree of spongiform change. In contrast to JCD, kuru tends to affect the cerebellum more than the cerebral cortex (both pathologically and clinically). Kuru-like amyloid plaques are seldom seen in JCD (*see* Fig. 11-14) (Hematoxylin-eosin stain.) **E**, A higher-power view of the cerebellar cortex shows mild astrocytosis and spongiform change with minimal neuronal loss. However, quantitative studies show that a 20% to 30% decrease in neurons is necessary before such loss becomes visually apparent.

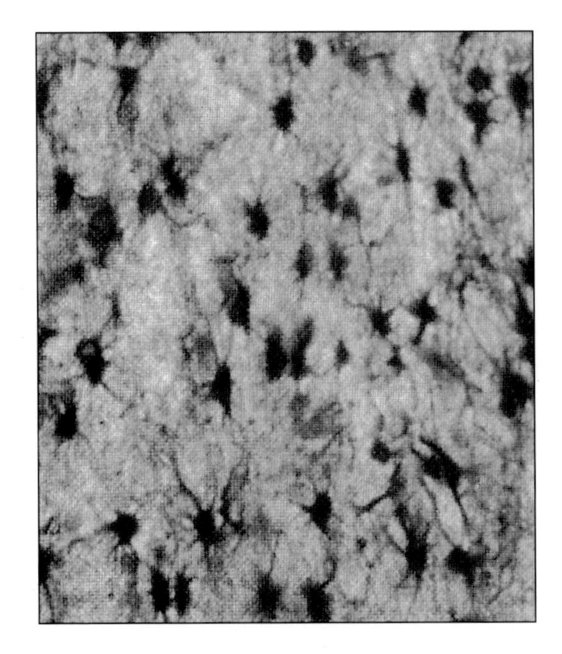

Figure 11-22 Fibrillary astrocytosis in JCD. Severe fibrillary astrocytosis of the cerebellar cortex seen under low power. (Cajal stain, × 170.) (*From* Beck E, Daniel PM: Kuru and Creutzfeldt-Jakob disease: Neuropathological lesions and their significance. *In* Prusiner SB, Hadlow WJ (eds.): *Slow Transmissible Diseases of the Nervous System*, vol 1. New York: Academic Press; 1979:253–270; with permission.)

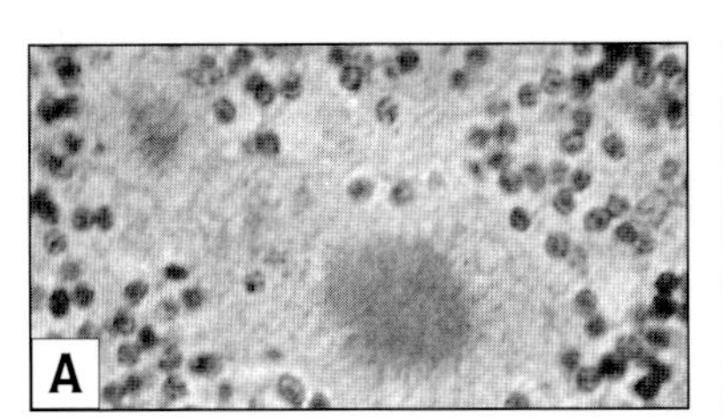

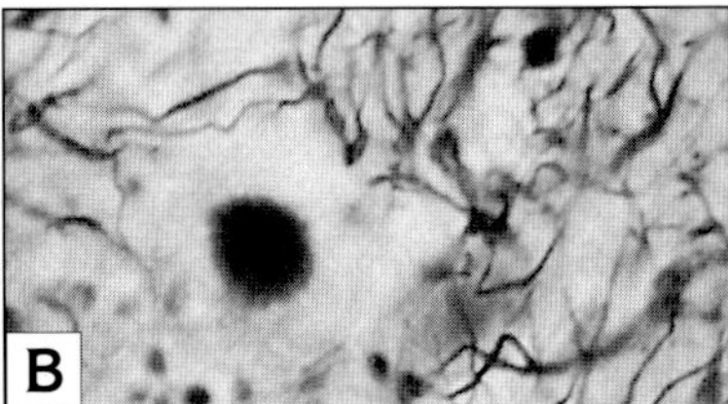

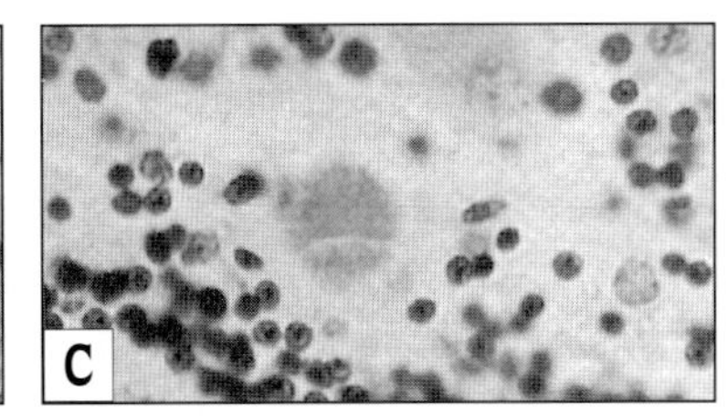

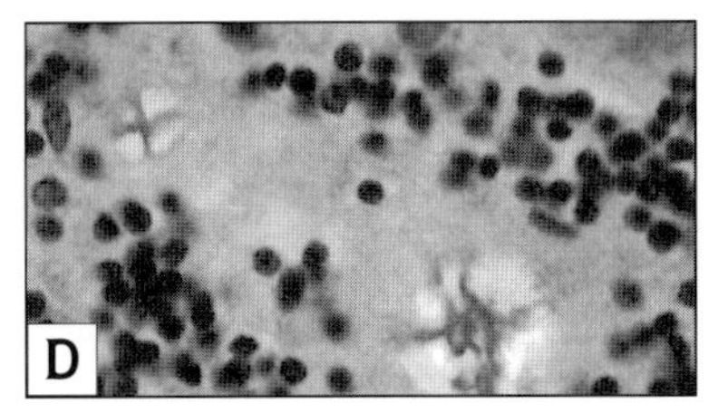

Figure 11-23 Amyloid plaques in JCD. Amyloid plaques in the cerebellum are shown as they appear in a series of different staining reactions. **A**, Periodic acid-Schiff. **B**, Palmgren silver impregnation. **C**, Congo red. **D**, Congo red stain with birefringent under polarized light. (*From* Beck E, Daniel PM: Kuru and Creutzfeldt-Jakob disease: Neuropathological lesions and their significance. *In* Prusiner SB, Hadlow WJ (eds.): *Slow Transmissible Diseases of the Nervous System*, vol 1. New York: Academic Press; 1979:253–270; with permission.)

Sterilization procedures for JCD tissues and contaminated materials

Effective (recommended) procedures
- Steam autoclaving for 1 hr at 132° C
- Steam autoclaving for 4.5 hrs at 121° C (15 psi)
- Immersion in 1 N NaOH for 1 hr at room temperature
- Immersion in 1 N NaOH for 30 min at room temperature repeated three times

Ineffective procedures
- Boiling, UV irradiation, ethylene oxide sterilization, ethanol, formalin, beta-propiolactone, detergents, quaternary ammonium compounds, Lysol, alcoholic iodine acetone, potassium permanganate

Figure 11-24 Sterilization procedures for JCD tissues and contaminated materials. Although JCD is not spontaneously contagious, cases of iatrogenic transmission are well documented but require direct inoculation, implantation, or transplantation of infected material. General precautions should be followed when caring for patients with JCD, and special precautions are needed during autopsy. UV—ultraviolet. (*From* Ravilochan K, Tyler KL: Human transmissible neurodegenerative diseases (prion diseases). *Semin Neurol* 1992, 12:178–190; with permission.)

Gerstmann-Sträussler Syndrome

Clinical characteristics of Gerstmann-Sträussler syndrome

Transmission	Hereditary (autosomal diminant)
Onset	43–48 yrs (range, 24–66 yrs)
Clinical features	Progressive spinocerebellar degeneration Unsteadiness, clumsiness, incoordination, gait disturbances (early) Ataxia, dysarthrias, tremor, nystagmus (late) Dementia (late or minor) Myoclonus absent (or minor)
Course	Fatal in approx 5 yrs

FIGURE 11-25 Clinical characteristics of Gerstmann-Sträussler syndrome (GSS). GSS is an exceedingly rare disease, with an incidence of 1 to 10 cases/100 million population/year. Most cases are familial, with an autosomal dominant pattern of inheritance and virtually complete penetrance. Approximately two dozen independent kindreds have been identified worldwide. The onset typically is in midlife, with prominent cerebellar features and absent or late dementia.

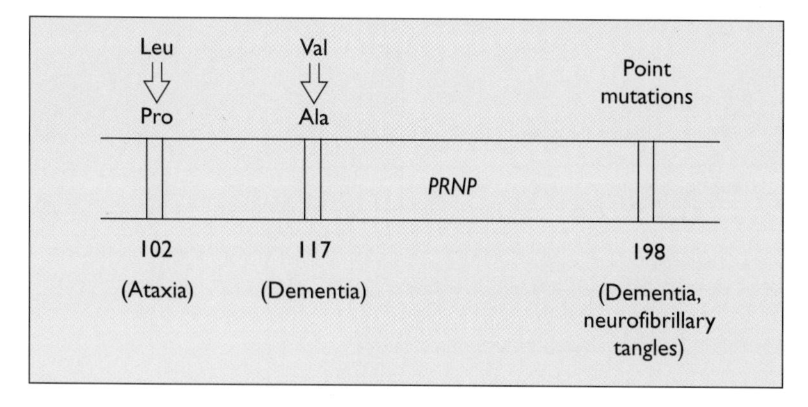

FIGURE 11-26 Genetic mutations in GSS. Several PrP gene mutations have been identified in patients with familial GSS. The most common is a leucine-for-proline substitution at codon 102. The 102 mutation appears to be associated with ataxia as a prominent clinical finding, whereas mutations at 117 have dementia as a more prominent feature and mutations at 198 have prominent dementia and neurofibrillary tangles.

Fatal Familial Insomnia

Clinical characteristics of fatal familial insomnia

Transmission	Hereditary (autosomal dominant)
Onset	Middle to late life (31–61 yrs)
Clinical features	Intractable insomnia, sympathetic hyperactivity, autonomic and endocrine disturbances, dysarthrias, motor system abnormalities Dementia not prominent Hallucinations, "enacted dreams"
Course	Fatal in approx 13 mos (range, 7–25)

FIGURE 11-27 Clinical characteristics of fatal familial insomnia (FFI). FFI is the most recently recognized of the familial prion diseases and is characterized by untreatable insomnia, autonomic dysfunction, and motor system abnormalities. Pathologically, there is selective atrophy of the anterior ventral and mediodorsal thalamic nuclei. The disease is transmitted in an autosomal dominant fashion.

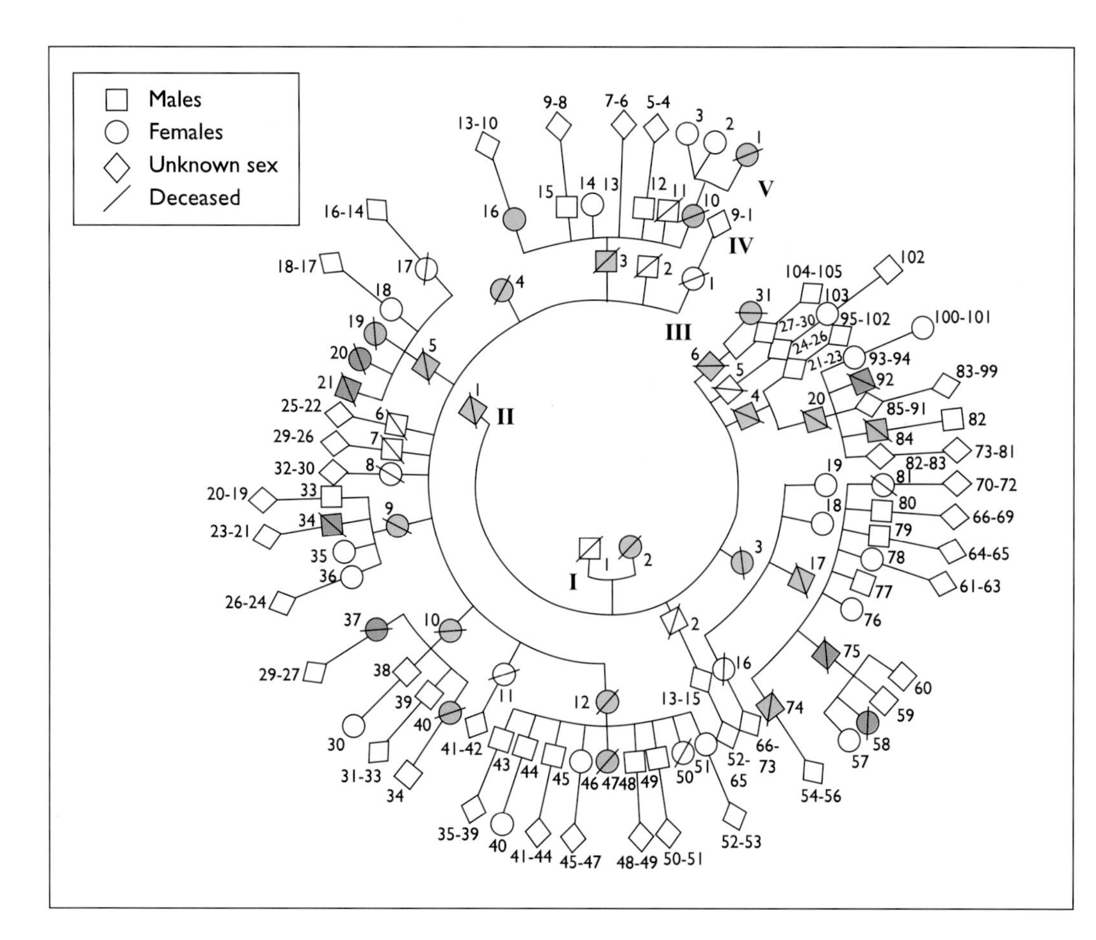

FIGURE 11-28 Pedigree of a kindred with FFI. In a family with FFI, all four affected members and 11 of 29 unaffected members who were examined had a point mutation in the PrP codon 178 involving an asparagine-for-aspartic-acid substitution and elimination of the *Tth*111 I restriction site. The *purple* symbols represent affected subjects; *blue* and *orange* symbols indicate subjects probably affected, as judged by nonmedical and medical reports, respectively. (*From* Medori R, Tritschler H-J, LeBlanc A, *et al.*: Fatal familial insomnia, a prion disease with a mutation at codon 178 of the prion protein gene. *N Engl J Med* 1992, 326:444–449; with permission.)

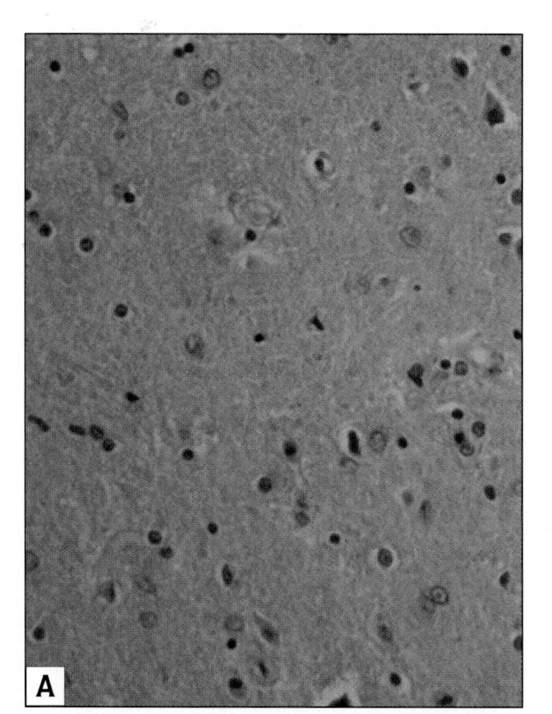

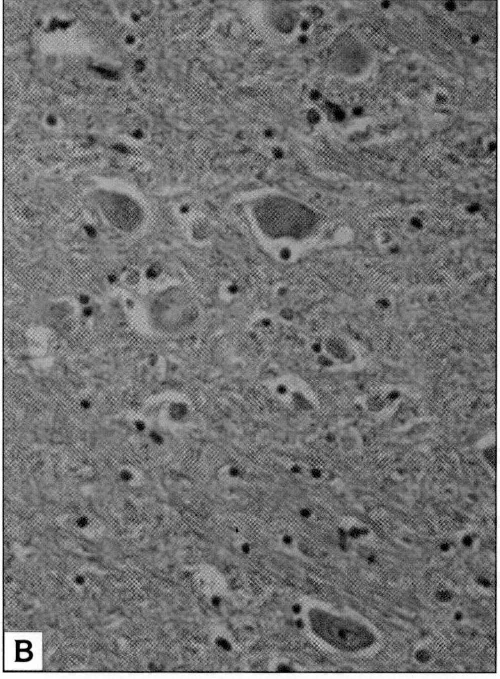

FIGURE 11-29 Neuropathologic lesions in the thalamic nuclei in FFI. **A**, Mediodorsal nucleus. **B**, Ventral lateral posterior nucleus. There is severe (>50%) neuronal loss with reactive astrogliosis in the mediodorsal nucleus, whereas the ventral lateral posterior nucleus is not affected. (Hematoxylin-eosin stain, × 220.) (*From* Manetto V, Medori R, Cartelli P, *et al.*: Fatal familial insomnia: clinical and pathologic study of five new cases. *Neurology* 1992, 42:312–319; with permission.)

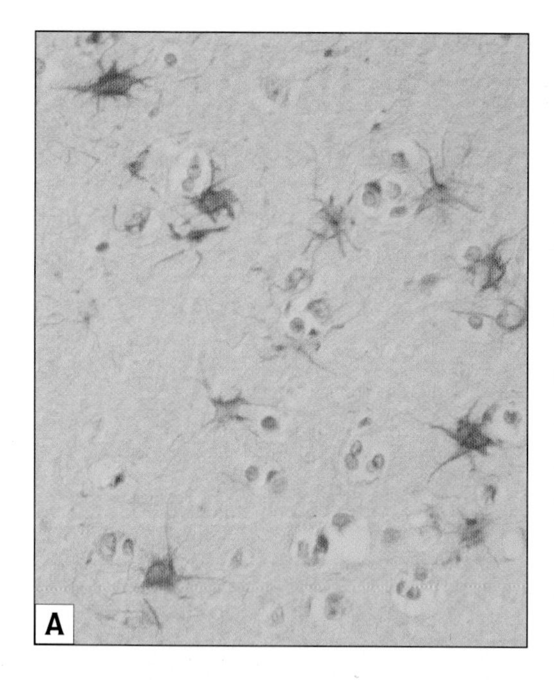

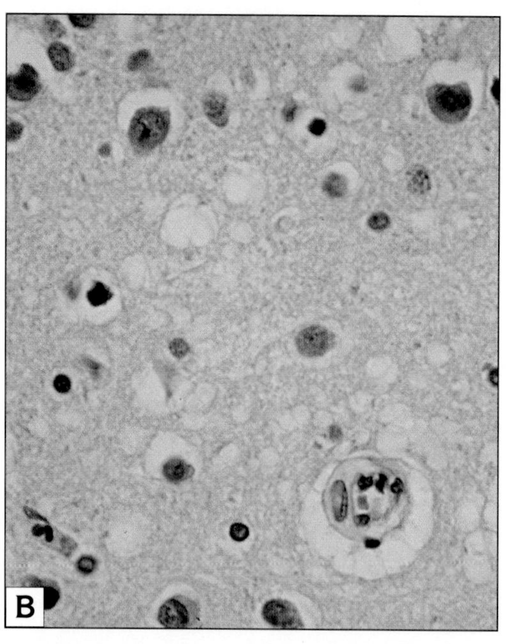

FIGURE 11-30 Neuropathologic lesions in the cerebral cortex in FFI. **A**, Astrogliosis is evident in the cerebral cortex on peroxidase-antiperoxidase immunostaining with antiserum to glial fibrillary acidic protein. (× 290.) **B**, Occipital cortex shows spongiosis. (Hematoxylin-eosin stain, × 440.) (*From* Manetto V, Medori R, Cartelli P, *et al.*: Fatal familial insomnia: clinical and pathologic study of five new cases. *Neurology* 1992, 42:312–319; with permission.)

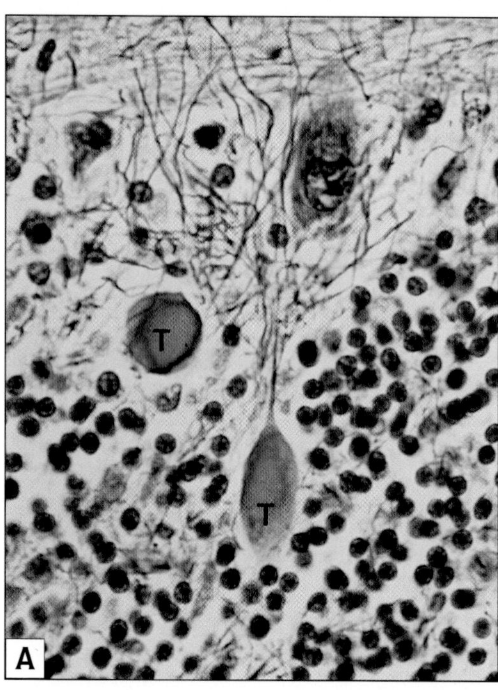

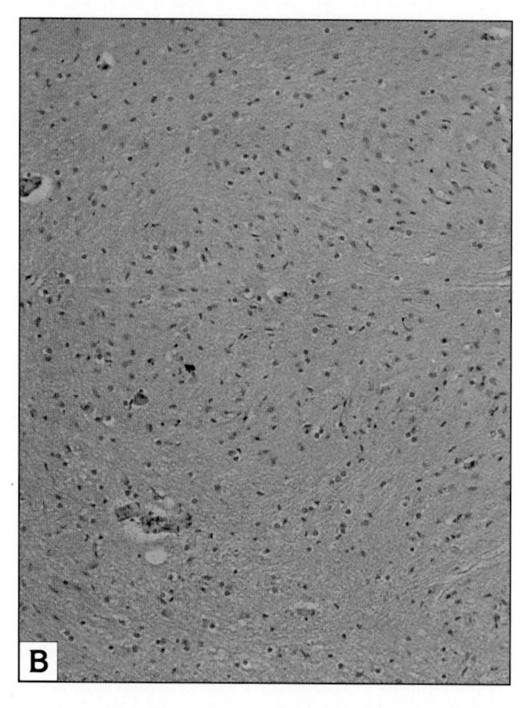

FIGURE 11-31 Neuropathologic lesions in the cerebellum and inferior olives in FFI. **A**, Torpedoes (*T*) are seen in the cerebellum. (Bodian stain, × 440.) **B**, Olivary nuclei. The cerebellum and inferior olives are variably affected in all cases examined. (Hematoxylin-eosin stain, × 110.) (*From* Manetto V, Medori R, Cartelli P, *et al.*: Fatal familial insomnia: clinical and pathologic study of five new cases. *Neurology* 1992, 42:312–319; with permission.)

SELECTED BIBLIOGRAPHY

Asher DM: Slow viral infections of the human nervous system. *In* Scheld WM, Whitley RJ, Durack DT (eds.): *Infections of the Central Nervous System*. New York: Raven Press; 1991:157.

Björnsson J, Carp RI, Löve A, Wisniewski HM (eds.): Slow infections of the central nervous system. *Ann NY Acad Sci* 1979, 274:1–495.

Prusiner SB, Hadlow WJ (eds.): *Slow Transmissible Diseases of the Nervous System*, vol 1. New York: Academic Press; 1979.

Ravilochan K, Tyler KL: Human transmissible neurodegenerative diseases (prion diseases). *Semin Neurol* 1992, 12:178–190.

Tyler KL: Prion diseases of the central nervous system (transmissible neurodegenerative diseases). *In* Mandell GL, *et al.* (eds.): *Principles and Practice of Infectious Diseases*, 4th ed. New York: Churchill Livingstone; 1995:881–885.

INDEX